EPIDEMIOLOGY AND DEMOGRAPHY IN PUBLIC HEALTH

EPIDEMIOLOGY AND DEMOGRAPHY IN PUBLIC HEALTH

EDITOR-IN-CHIEF

Japhet Killewo
Professor of Epidemiology, Muhimbili University of Health and Allied Sciences, Dar es Salaam, Tanzania

EDITORS

H. Kristian Heggenhougen
Centre for International Health, University of Bergen, Norway; Department of International Health, Boston University School of Public Health, and Department of Global Health and Social Medicine, Harvard Medical School

Stella R. Quah
Duke-NUS Graduate Medical School Singapore, Singapore

ELSEVIER

Amsterdam • Boston • Heidelberg • London • New York • Oxford
Paris • San Diego • San Francisco • Singapore • Sydney • Tokyo
Academic Press is an imprint of Elsevier

ACADEMIC
PRESS

Academic Press is an imprint of Elsevier
525 B Street, Suite 1900, San Diego, CA 92101-4495, USA
30 Corporate Drive, Suite 400, Burlington, MA 01803, USA
32 Jamestown Road, London NW1 7BY, UK
Radarweg 29, PO Box 211, 1000 AE Amsterdam, The Netherlands

British Library Cataloguing in Publication Data
A catalogue record for this book is available from the British Library

Library of Congress Catalog Number: 2010020869

ISBN: 978-0-12-382200-0

For information on all Academic Press publications
visit our website at elsevierdirect.com

CONTENTS

SECTION 2   FIELDS OF EPIDEMIOLOGY

SECTION 3   EPIDEMIOLOGY OF SPECIFIC DISEASES

SECTION 4   DEMOGRAPHY

SECTION 5   BIOSTATISTICS

SECTION 6   ETHICAL ISSUES

CONTRIBUTORS

D-M Alexe
London School of Hygiene and Tropical Medicine, London, UK

L M Anderson
US Centers for Disease Control and Prevention, Atlanta, GA, USA

N Anderson
University of Edinburgh Medical School, Edinburgh, UK

C N Antonopoulos
Athens University Medical School, Athens, Greece

I Arita
Agency for Cooperation in International Health, Kumamoto-city, Japan

R Armstrong
Cochrane HPPH Field, Victoria, Australia

A Auvinen
University of Tampere School of Public Health, Tampere, Finland

L S Bakketeig
Norwegian Institute of Public Health, Oslo, Norway

J K Bardsley
MedStar Research Institute, Hyattsville, MD, USA

J J Barendregt
School of Population Health, University of Queensland, Brisbane, Australia

P Bergsjø
Norwegian Institute of Public Health, Oslo, Norway

R Gaare Bernheim
University of Virginia, Charlottesville, VA, USA

R Boer
Erasmus MC, University Medical Center, Rotterdam, The Netherlands

J Brazier
Sheffield University, Sheffield, UK

T S Brugha
University of Leicester, Leicester, UK

H Campbell
University of Edinburgh Medical School, Edinburgh, UK

R Choi
University of Washington, Seattle, WA, USA

J G Cleland
Centre for Population Studies, London School of Hygiene and Tropical Medicine, London, UK

S S Coughlin
Centers for Disease Control and Prevention, Atlanta, GA, USA

D Czeresnia
Oswaldo Cruz Foundation (ENSP-FIOCRUZ), Brazil

E Davis
McCaughey Centre, VicHealth Centre for the Promotion of Mental Health and Community Wellbeing, School of Population Health, University of Melbourne, Carlton, VIC, Australia and School of Health and Social Development, Deakin University, Burwood, VIC, Australia

A Dobson
University of Queensland, Brisbane, QLD, Australia

J Douwes
Massey University, Wellington, New Zealand

R Engelman
Worldwatch Institute, Washington, DC, USA

R R Faden
Johns Hopkins University, Baltimore, MD, USA

C Farquhar
University of Washington, Seattle, WA, USA

L Gold
McCaughey Centre, VicHealth Centre for the Promotion of Mental Health and Community Wellbeing, School of Population Health, University of Melbourne, Carlton, VIC, Australia and School of Health and Social Development, Deakin University, Burwood, VIC, Australia

N Guttman
Tel Aviv University, Tel Aviv, Israel

J D F Habbema
Erasmus MC, University Medical Center, Rotterdam, The Netherlands

S Haddock
Population Action International, Washington, DC, USA

M Hakama
University of Tampere School of Public Health, Tampere, Finland

W R Harlan
National Institutes of Health, Rockville, MD, USA

R D Hays
University of California at Los Angeles, Los Angeles, CA, USA

H K Heggenhougen
Centre for International Health, University of Bergen, Norway; Department of International Health, Boston University School of Public Health, and Department of Global Health and Social Medicine, Harvard Medical School

T H Holtz
Centers for Disease Control and Prevention, Atlanta, GA, USA

J P A Ioannidis
Tufts University School of Medicine, Boston, MA, USA

L M Irgens
Department of Public Health and Primary Health Care, University of Bergen, Bergen, Norway and Norwegian Institute of Public Health

R Jakob
World Health Organization, Geneva, Switzerland

K Jamrozik
University of Adelaide, Adelaide, SA, Australia

S Johnson
Albany Medical College, Albany, NY, USA

N E Kass
Johns Hopkins University, Baltimore, MD, USA

J L Kelsey
University of Massachusetts Medical School, Worcester, MA, USA

A M Kimball
University of Washington, Seattle, WA, USA

M Kretzschmar
Julius Center for Health Sciences and Primary Care, University Medical Center Utrecht, Utrecht, The Netherlands

V L Lamb
North Carolina Central University, Durham, NC, USA

K C Land
Duke University, Durham, NC, USA

E Leahy
Population Action International, Washington, DC, USA

P E Leaverton
University of South Florida School of Public Health, Tampa, FL, USA

B Link
Columbia University, New York, NY, USA; New York State Psychiatric Institute, New York, USA

J H Madans
National Center for Health Statistics, Hyattsville, MD, USA

K Magruder
Medical University of South Carolina, Charleston, SC, USA

K G Manton
Duke University, Durham, NC, USA

Z Marshman
School of Clinical Dentistry, Sheffield, UK

C Mathers
World Health Organization, Geneva, Switzerland

E Mathieu
Centers for Disease Control and Prevention, Atlanta, GA, USA

J D Mayer
University of Washington, Seattle, WA, USA

H Meltzer
University of Leicester, Leicester, UK

O S Miettinen
McGill University, Montreal, QC, Canada

C Morroni
University of Cape Town, Cape Town, South Africa

L Myer
University of Cape Town, Cape Town, South Africa; Columbia University, New York, USA

D M J Naimark
University of Toronto, Toronto, Ontario, Canada

M Nakane
Agency for Cooperation in International Health, Kumamoto-city, Japan

T Nakano
National Mie Hospital, Mie, Japan

G S Norquist
University of Mississippi Medical Center, Jackson, MS, USA

S Oliver
University of London, London, UK

N Pearce
Massey University, Wellington, New Zealand

J Peto
London School of Hygiene and Tropical Medicine, London, UK and Institute of Cancer Research, Sutton, UK

E T Petridou
Athens University Medical School, Athens, Greece

M Petticrew
London School of Hygiene and Tropical Medicine,
London, UK

G A Poland
Mayo Clinic, Rochester, MN, USA

Stella R Quah
Duke-NUS Graduate Medical School, Singapore

J Ratcliffe
University of South Australia, Adelaide, Australia

O Razum
University of Bielefeld, Bielefeld, Germany

B B Reeve
National Cancer Institute, Bethesda, MD, USA

H E Resnick
MedStar Research Institute, Hyattsville, MD, USA

H Roberts
Institute of Education, University of London,
London, UK

P G Robinson
School of Clinical Dentistry, Sheffield, UK

D L Sackett
Kilgore S. Trout Research and Education Center at Irish
Lake, Markdale, ON, Canada

T T Samaras
Reventropy Associates, San Diego, CA, USA

F Samkange-Zeeb
Institute of Medical Biometry, Epidemiology and
Informatics, Mainz, Germany

A Shelly
McCaughey Centre, VicHealth Centre for the Promotion
of Mental Health and Community Wellbeing, School of
Population Health, University of Melbourne, Carlton, VIC,
Australia and School of Health and Social Development,
Deakin University, Burwood, VIC, Australia

T C Soares
Federal University in Juiz de Fora, Juiz de Fora, Brazil

Y Sodahlon
Mectizan Donation Program, Decatur, GA, USA

E Susser
Columbia University, New York, NY, USA; New York State
Psychiatric Institute, New York, USA

P V Targonski
Mayo Clinic and University of Minnesota, Rochester,
MN, USA

A Tatsioni
Tufts University School of Medicine, Boston, MA, USA

H A Taylor
Johns Hopkins University, Baltimore, MD, USA

R Taylor
University of Queensland, Brisbane, QLD, Australia

J C Thomas
University of North Carolina, Chapel Hill, NC, USA

J A Trostle
Trinity College, Hartford, CT, USA

T B Üstün
World Health Organization, Geneva, Switzerland

P A Wark
London School of Hygiene and Tropical Medicine,
London, UK

E Waters
McCaughey Centre, VicHealth Centre for the
Promotion of Mental Health and Community
Wellbeing, School of Population Health, University of
Melbourne, Carlton, VIC, Australia and School of Health
and Social Development, Deakin University, Burwood,
VIC, Australia

E Waters
University of Melbourne, Carlton, VIC, Australia

F V Wilder
The Arthritis Research Institute of America, Clearwater,
FL, USA

M E Wilson
Harvard Medical School/Harvard School of Public Health,
Boston, MA, USA

PREFACE

In a world of rapid transportation and increased movement of people across national borders, accurate knowledge of epidemiology and demography has become crucial to public health. Epidemiological and demographic issues, such as changes in the growth and health of local populations and the differences between local residents and migrant or transient populations (such as tourists, business people, immigrants, or refugees), their health status, what they do when they arrive at their destination, and their impact on local populations, are all significant public health concerns. This volume addresses the need for expert and current knowledge on those concerns and the public health dimension of epidemiology and demography by presenting a collection of 52 chapters, 50 of them from the *International Encyclopedia of Public Health* published by Elsevier in 2008 and two briefer versions of relevant articles published elsewhere. The 52 chapters are divided into six sections: overview of history, concepts, principles and methods; fields of epidemiology; epidemiology of specific diseases; demography; biostatistics; and ethical issues.

The chapters in the first section provide an overview of the history, concepts, principles, and methods of epidemiology. In his comprehensive chapter on the history of epidemiology, L.M. Irgens traces the history of the field from ancient times through the fight against the great plagues, syphilis, smallpox and other epidemics, to modern times. The concepts of health and disease and their common and scientific meanings are discussed by D. Czeresnia and T.C. Soares. The chapter by C.D. Mathers deals with the global burden of disease and disability and its impact on economic development. R. Jakob examines the development of efforts in disease classification looking into the guiding principles, accuracy, and other aspects. The discussion of efforts to classify and measure mental disorders is presented in the chapters by B. Ustun, and T.S. Brugha and H. Meltzer, respectively. In his chapter on observational epidemiology, J.L. Kelsey offers an interesting analysis of descriptive, analytical, case-control and cohort studies among other issues of study design. Health surveys that have traditionally been methodological tools in health and sociological research are becoming a regular feature in public health and J. Madans presents a wide-ranging discussion of these surveys. The chapter on clinical trials by W. Harlan provides a comprehensive discussion of the methods of testing the efficacy of medical and public health interventions. Following these methodological chapters, Arita, Nakane and Nakano's chapter on surveillance of disease offers a comprehensive discussion of systems and types of surveillance of both diseases in general and their causes.

The next three chapters in the first section of the book offer a current and precise examination of emerging and re-emerging diseases by J.D. Mayer and M. Wilson, respectively, and the factors influencing the emergence of diseases by A.M. Kimball, while the chapter by K. Jamrozik, R. Taylor, and A. Dobson analyses the risk factors for cardiovascular diseases as they are understood today. The authors discuss the impact of demographic differences like age, gender and ethnicity in addition to behavioral factors. Reflecting the impact of epidemics today, two more chapters are dedicated to their analysis: E. Mathieu and Y. Sodahlon's chapter presents the approaches to epidemic investigation; and S.R. Quah's chapter discusses the challenges faced by health authorities and communities in the management of epidemics; this chapter was originally published as Chapter 6 in the book edited by S. Quah, *Crisis Preparedness – Asian and the Global Governance of Epidemics* (APARC, Stanford University and Brookings Institution, 2007, 113–133).

The advances in disease modeling are presented in two chapters: Kretzschmar deals with infectious disease modeling while the chapter by J.D.F. Habbema, R. Boer, and J.J. Barendregt focuses on chronic disease modeling. M. Hakama and A. Auvinen's chapter on cancer screening looks critically into the suitability, validity, benefits, and harm of screening. Four additional methodological approaches in epidemiology and public health are appraised in the final four chapters of this section: the measurement and modeling of health-related quality of life by R.D. Hays and B.B. Reeve; the measurement and valuation of health for economic evaluation by J. Brazier and J. Ratcliffe; measuring the quality of life of children and adolescents by E. Davis *et al.*; and systematic review by R. Armstrong *et al.*

The second section of this volume, "Fields of Epidemiology," comprises chapters on the most important areas of the discipline. Some of the chapters focus on areas of practice and others on disciplines of epidemiology. Among the chapters on practice, D.L. Sackett and S. Kilgore's discussion of clinical epidemiology provides interesting insights into epidemiological investigations and the contributions of clinical epidemiologists to advances in health care and research in clinical settings. N. Pearce and J. Douwes's chapter on environmental and occupational epidemiology introduces readers to these active areas of epidemiology, provides examples of the types of studies conducted, and discusses critically the issues of bias and confounding. Readers unfamiliar with the impact of social factors on health and illness will find the chapter on social epidemiology by L. Myer and colleagues very informative while expert readers will benefit from the authors' clear and well-illustrated exposition of the influence of socio-economic and cultural influences on people's health. H.K. Heggenhougen analyzes the impact of social class on health and illness in his chapter on the epidemiology of inequity. This chapter first appeared in the journal *Norsk Epidemiologi—Norwegian Epidemiology* (15, 2: 127–132, 2005). The field of cultural epidemiology is carefully examined in the chapter by J. Trostle, where the author explains, among other aspects, why cultural epidemiology matters. The contrasting aspect of health and disease is presented in the chapter on genetic epidemiology by H. Campbell and N. Anderson, where they describe the key research strategies of detecting the influence of genes, gene discovery, and gene characterization. The field of dental epidemiology is discussed by P.G. Robinson and Z. Marshman; in their chapter, they highlight the measurement of oral health, risk factors, and trends. The practice of oncology is not new as a branch of medicine that deals with cancers or tumors. In their chapter on cancer epidemiology, P. Wark and J. Peto illustrate the global distribution of cancers and discuss the range of factors associated with them. Another practice field of epidemiology, psychiatric epidemiology, is the topic of the chapter by G.S. Norquist and K. Magruder, who begin with a history of the field and present the methods, assessment, types of studies, and research findings from selected studies to illustrate their arguments. The final practice chapter is on perinatal epidemiology by L.S. Bakketeig and P. Bergsjó, where, among other issues, they critically discuss the challenges of definitions as well as causes and risk factors of perinatal mortality.

Section three of this volume deals with epidemiology of specific diseases. J. Bardsley and H. Resnick's chapter on diabetes mellitus epidemiology discusses important terminology and relevant worldwide trends. The epidemiology of injuries is analyzed in the chapter by E.T. Petridou, C.N. Antonopoulos, and D.-M. Alexe; they explain the aspects of terminology, both theoretical and operational, the challenges of classification and coding systems, measures of injury burden, ethical consideration, and injury prevention. The epidemiology of tuberculosis is examined in T.H. Holtz's chapter from the perspective of the social, economic, and health burden of the disease, including the problem of drug resistance. R.R. Choi and C. Farquhar's chapter on AIDS epidemiology and surveillance presents an analysis of incidence, prevalence, and transmission modes fully illustrated with global figures and a comprehensive list of references. This section closes with the chapter on Epidemiology of Influenza by P.V. Targonski and G.A. Poland, who discuss the causes, transmission, and distribution of Influenza worldwide and the pandemics of the new influenza viruses that never circulated in humans before.

Section 4 is dedicated to the discipline of demography. Readers will find the chapters in this section useful in providing a succinct yet complete discussion of demographic topics in relation to epidemiology and public health. O.S. Miettinen's chapter, "Demography, Epidemiology and Public Health," discusses the three disciplines from the perspective of scientific research and public health practice. In their chapter on population growth, S. Haddock, E. Leahy, and R. Engelman examine the most significant population changes and trends in fertility, aging, and mortality, highlighting their impact on health. J. Cleland discusses the most significant trends in human fertility and offers an interesting classification of fertility trends in low-income countries. D.M.J. Naimark examines life expectancy measurements providing a clear explanation of the statistical approaches most commonly followed. K.G. Manton looks at the now essential concept of active life expectancy or ALE, which combines health, functional status, and longevity. Two chapters deal with the most senior cohorts: R.C. Land and V.L. Lamb present a careful and well-illustrated analysis in the chapter on the demography of aging, while T.T. Samaras focuses on the variations in longevity around the world in terms of age, gender, body height, and other factors. The case of migrant populations is examined in the final chapter in this section by O. Razum and F. Samkange-Zeeb, who identify significant health-related features such as patterns of mobility, health risks for migrants, and access to health services.

Two key chapters on the field of biostatistics are presented in Section 5. P. Leaverton and V. Wilder discuss the descriptive and analytical features of the field, its comparatively young history, and its significance for the advancement of epidemiology and public health research. A. Tatsioni and J.P.A. Ioannidis introduce readers to Meta-Analysis and its application in public health research.

As editors of this volume, we believe that it is not only relevant but also appropriate to conclude this volume with the section on ethics. Therefore, Section six begins with the chapter by H.A. Taylor, R.R. Faden, N.E. Kass, and S. Johnson on the moral obligations to communities when conducting public health research. The chapter by J.C. Thomas and R. Gaare Bernheim argues for the need for codes of ethics in public health and their functions and characteristics. The ethics of screening is examined by S.S. Coughlin from various angles including general principles, informed consent, and voluntary and mandatory screening. This section closes with the chapter on the ethics of health promotion by N. Guttman. The author argues that public health interventions that take into consideration ethical aspects are more likely to be perceived favorably by the population.

This volume is of interest to a variety of audiences, primarily epidemiologists and public health researchers and practitioners. All chapters include a list of additional references, pertinent statistical information and graphs, and are written following the guiding principle of evidence-based research.

This preface would not be complete without acknowledging those who contributed to the production of this book. We therefore acknowledge with gratitude the collaboration of all the chapter authors for accepting our invitation to include their work in this volume. We are also indebted to the Elsevier editorial team, particularly Nancy Maragioglio and Carrie Bolger, whose professionalism and cordiality made the entire enterprise a very pleasant and efficient experience. We are grateful also to the publishers of the journal *Norsk Epidemiologi—Norwegian Epidemiology* and to the Walter H. Shorenstein Asia-Pacific Research Center, Stanford University for their permission to reproduce in this volume the work of H.K. Heggenhougen and S.R. Quah, respectively.

Finally but equally important, this book would not have been possible without the support of our institutions. Our sincere gratitude goes to the Muhimbili University of Health and Allied Sciences in Tanzania for the support and encouragement provided right from the time of editing the International Encyclopedia of Public Health; the Centre for International Health, University of Bergen, Norway; the Department of International Health, Boston University School of Public Health; the Department of Global Health and Social Medicine, Harvard University Medical School; the Duke-NUS Graduate Medical School and the National University of Singapore. We therefore look forward to a wide readership of this book among health professionals and their students in these institutions and beyond.

The Editors

SECTION 1

OVERVIEW OF HISTORY, CONCEPTS, PRINCIPLES AND METHODS

History of Epidemiology

L M Irgens, Department of Public Health and Primary Health Care, University of Bergen, Bergen, Norway and Norwegian Institute of Public Health

Background

Usually, great achievements and breakthroughs in most aspects of medical care, such as procedures in diagnostics and therapy, are highly esteemed over extended periods of time, because the disease for which the procedures were introduced is still prevalent. In epidemiology, this is not necessarily the case. Here, successes, often followed by equally successful achievements in preventive medicine, may permanently eliminate the medical problem that was solved by epidemiological research, thereby relegating successes in epidemiology and preventive medicine to oblivion in the shadows of the history of medicine. Thus, the history of medicine may play a greater role in epidemiology than in most other medical disciplines.

This applies particularly to teaching. In brief, the medical student faces two essentially different didactic appraches in his or her curriculum. The first approach relates to the individual-oriented challenges represented by diagnostics and therapeutics. The second approach relates to group-oriented challenges that involve acquisition of information about health problems in the community, their causes, as well as their prevention. In medical teaching, the case history represents an invaluable didactic element, and case histories are easily available from individual-oriented clinical practice. However, successful efforts against group-oriented community challenges will inevitably transfer victory to the history of medicine with the inherent danger of being considered less relevant to current challenges or even of being forgotten; the problem is resolved and no longer represents an imminent health risk. The eradication of smallpox, which was achieved by 1977 when the last case occurred is a case in point. This leaves the history of epidemiology with an important objective related to teaching in addition to the significance of the topic *per se.*

Admittedly, the subject is vast; this article intends to identify patterns in terms of eras or paradigms as well as time trends and illustrate them by providing relevant examples rather than accounting for the complete history. Contemporary perinatal, cardiovascular, and cancer epidemiology are discussed in separate articles, as will important topics related to intrauterine programming life-course and genetic epidemiology.

Definition of Epidemiology

In *A Dictionary of Epidemiology,* epidemiology is defined as "the study of the distribution and determinants of health-related states or events in specified populations and the application of this study to control of health problems" (Last, 2001: 62).

More operationally, epidemiology can be defined as the methodology to obtain information on the distribution in the community of diseases and their determinants, e.g., according to characteristics of time, place, gender, age, and often occupation. In perinatal epidemiology, maternal age, birth order, gestational age, and birth weight are often added. The objective is to utilize this information in the search for cause(s) or the etiology of a disease or another medical outcome such as a complication, in order to prevent an adverse outcome. Thus, epidemiology may also be defined as the medical branch aiming at clarification of causes of diseases.

When does, according to this definition, the history of epidemiology actually start? When was it, for the first time, evident that the cause of a disease was of any concern? And when was the search initiated for the first time for necessary information to clarify such a cause?

Obviously, these questions are difficult to answer, but ancient sources may contribute to their elucidation. Before attempting to address the issue any further, the concept of causation and the knowledge and insights necessary to clarify the etiology of a disease should be discussed.

In brief, a factor is causal when its manipulation is followed by corresponding changes in the outcome. In a further elaboration of the issue, one often introduces the terms necessary and sufficient causes. In the first category, when the cause is necessary and sufficient, the element of randomness is nil. This is a rare situation: Measles virus in an unimmunized individual is often used as an example. In the second category, when the cause is necessary, but not sufficient, cofactors play a decisive role, e.g., in leprosy *Mycobacterium leprae* is a necessary, but not sufficient factor; poor nutrition would be needed as a cofactor. In the third category, when the cause is sufficient, but not necessary, we have multifactorial diseases, e.g., lung cancer, being caused by cigarette smoking or radon. This may be an oversimplification; in most cases cofactors would also be necessary, which brings us to the fourth category in which a factor is neither necessary nor sufficient, e.g., the large number of medical outcomes in which the etiology represents an interaction, often between genetic and environmental factors, which may be considered webs of causation.

In short, our objective is to demonstrate how the concepts of risk factors, epidemiology, and preventive medicine have evolved throughout history and to illustrate the consequences. When looking into the historical roots of epidemiology, it would be useful to contrast as a narrative thread the pattern observed in medical activities related to the individual, i.e., the patient, and activities related to the group, i.e., the community. The latter are the activities relevant to epidemiology.

Epidemiology in the Bible

Even today, it is held that knowledge of risk factors might affect the integrity, the independence, and the well-being of humans. This attitude relates to postmodernistic values in which the roles of the community in general and in particular in public health are questioned (Mackenbach, 2005). A fear of knowledge of causes of disease afflicts the basic objectives of epidemiology and needs further attention. Such thoughts are not truly novel; they may even be identified in perhaps the most important tome of Western civilization, the Bible. In Genesis, God said to Adam: "of the tree of knowledge of good and evil, thou shalt not eat for the day that thou eatest thereof, thou shalt surely die."

This statement and the subsequent eating of the fruit, after the act of the serpent, have called for a multitude of incompatible explanatory attempts (Michelsen, 1972). Nevertheless, the general interpretation of the legend implies that acquisition of knowledge *per se* is a mortal sin; this interpretation may be influential and widespread even today (**Figure 1**). Causes of unpleasant events such as disasters, catastrophes, and diseases are still often attributed to fate or God's will. On the other hand, there is also a prevalent attitude today that disease is, to a great extent, a consequence of stochastic processes with a considerable element of randomness.

Very few causal factors are sufficient (and necessary). Consequently, it is held, medical efforts should no longer focus on causes or prevention, but rather on helping the patient to cope with the situation, i.e., empower the patient. Admittedly, the role of random events definitely exists; for example, if you walk down the street and are killed by a falling roof tile, you are the victim of a process with a considerable element of randomness. Paradoxically, both a belief in fate or God's will and a belief in random events marginalize the roles of risk factors in general as well as those of epidemiology and preventive medicine in particular.

Still, there is strong evidence of the beneficial aspects of the risk factor concept and approach. If you put your baby to sleep in a face-down position, the child's risk of dying from sudden infant death syndrome increases 13-fold (Carpenter *et al.*, 2004). The child is definitely a victim of a risk factor, and the campaign advocating the supine sleeping position, the so-called back to sleep idea, has no doubt saved many infants from dying.

So far, we have only discussed the historical roots of negative attitudes to the search for causes of disease. Further examples exist in the Bible. Around 1000 BC, King David made a census of his people, admittedly not to survey their living conditions and thereby potential determinants of disease, but probably for military aims. The Lord informed David that he had sinned and punished the people with a terrible plague. The census is referred to as one of the great sins of the Old Testament (Hauge, 1973), actually without specifying why; military activities are otherwise not condemned in the Old Testament. However, the event had great impact on subsequent generations, as illustrated in a painting from the seventeenth century (**Figure 2**), and the acquisition of this type of data may have long been considered at least controversial. Thus, William the Conqueror's remarkable survey of England as of 1086, published in the Doomsday Book, was carried out against great popular resentment and was not repeated in Britain or abroad for a long time.

Ancient Roots

Where do we find the earliest roots of epidemiology? Clinical patient-oriented medicine, with thorough diagnostics and effective treatment as the paramount objective, does not include prevention among its aims; admittedly, the patient is already ill. In fact, using the term patient in our context is controversial and distracts from the aims of epidemiology and prevention; the term should

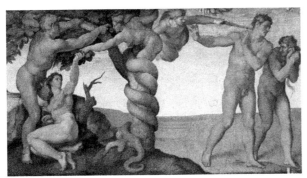

Figure 1 Temptation and Fall, Michelangelo, from the Sistine Chapel Ceiling. Source: Wikipedia.

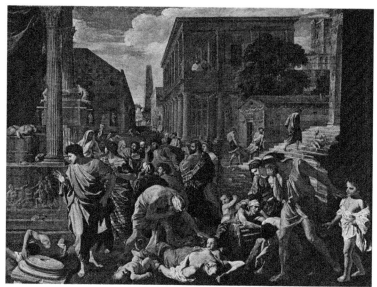

Figure 2 The Pest in Azoth; Nicolas Poussin, Louvre, Paris, France. Source: Wikipedia.

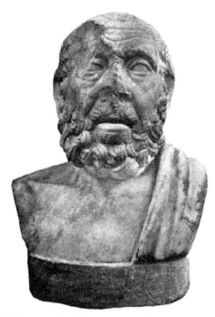

Figure 3 Hippocrates, Greek original (third century BC). Source: Wikipedia.

be replaced by population or community, terms that are much less concrete, at least to the physician. Thus, in ancient times, epidemiology and prevention were the physician's annex activities. This is amply illustrated by one of the first individual representatives of medicine; Hippocrates (460–377 BC) (**Figure 3**). He founded a school to which a series of medical texts is attributed: *Corpus Hippocraticum* (Aggebo, 1964). The authors were not only interested in clinical problems, but also in associations between health and air, water, food, dwellings, and living conditions. Recommendations to avoid diseases

were issued both to the individual and the community. In particular, the importance of good drinking water and clean processing of food was emphasized. Prudence with respect to eating and drinking, bathing, and physical exercise was most important to preserve one's health and develop a fit body.

These ideas were not restricted to individual Greek physicians. Similar concepts were found in ancient India where civil servants were appointed to be responsible for the water supply and food safety. The Babylonians and Assyrians had complex systems of water supply and sewage 3000–4000 years BC. Similar systems were established in ancient Egypt where such hygienic functions were closely attached to religion, e.g., in terms of which animals were allowed or forbidden to eat (Gotfredsen, 1964).

The strict hygiene rules detailed in the Old Testament's Books of Moses may have been influenced by Egypt; Moses lived many years in Egypt among the Jewish people. Admittedly, many of the regulations in the Books of Moses seem to reflect knowledge of risk factors and, through the wide distribution of the Bible, enormously influenced subsequent generations and their concept of risk factors and prevention up to recent time.

Still, a new concept was introduced by Hippocrates: Disease is the result of natural causes and not a consequence of infringing against God(s). These ideas, later detailed by the Hippocratic school, were further developed in subsequent generations, also in terms of practical measures. Thus, Plato (427–347 BC) suggested that civil health inspectors should be appointed for streets and roads, dwellings, and the water supply (Natvig, 1964). The ideas were applied most particularly by Roman civilization (Gotfredsen, 1964). Already by 450 BC, the Romans enforced practical regulations for food safety, water supply,

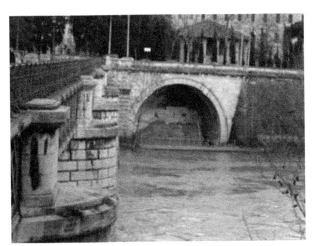

Figure 4 Outfall of Cloaca Maxima as it appears today. Source: Wikipedia.

and dead bodies. Between 300 and 100 BC, nine large aqueducts were constructed, bringing water to the city of Rome estimated at an enormous 1800 l per inhabitant per day (today's supply amounts to 300–400 l per day in most cities) (Natvig, 1964). At the same time, a complete sewage system was developed, Cloaca Maxima, which was in use until recently (**Figure 4**).

It is not certain that these elaborate hygienic systems of Antiquity were solely implemented to prevent disease. The physicians' role in their development was remarkably limited. The motivation for the systems was probably more religious in the early cultures, while the Romans were perhaps more oriented toward comfort. Furthermore, the great Roman physician, Galen (131–202 AD), seemed to be interested in nutrition and physical fitness out of clinical motivation much more than from a community health perspective (Gotfredsen, 1964).

This does not mean that physicians of Antiquity lacked interest in the causes of disease; however, their interest seemed to be more theoretical. Elaborate pathogenetic systems were established in which the four liquids – blood, yellow bile, black bile, and mucus, the four cardinal humors of the body – formed the basis of the so-called humoral pathology. Also, etiological considerations were made on causes of disease, comprising the violation of good habits with respect to food and alcohol consumption, rest and work, as well as sexual excesses. In addition, epidemic diseases were attributed to risk factors, miasmas, present in the air and exhaled from an unhealthy underground. These pathogenetic and etiological theories, first established by the Greeks and later developed by the Romans, particularly Galen, survived, even without empirical evidence, until the nineteenth century (Sigerist, 1956).

Several factors that may have been responsible for the slow progress of medicine in general and epidemiology in particular have been suggested. One is that the fall of the Roman Empire caused discontinuity in the medical sciences. The Northern peoples lacked the medical traditions developed through the centuries in Greece and Rome. Another is the new power, the Christian church, which lacked the incentive to ask questions about determinants of disease and preventive measures in the community. Even with the Biblical theses from the Books of Moses, probably aiming at prevention, the Christian spirit was dedicated to caring for the sick patient rather than protecting the community against disease. Thus, clinical functions developed in several monasteries where monks as well as nuns often organized hospital services. Furthermore, the Christian ideal, concentrating on spiritual well-being and often denying or neglecting the human body, might actually represent a threat to healthy behavior (Sigerist, 1956; Gotfredsen, 1964; Natvig, 1964).

During this period of public health deterioration, a lighthouse remained in the medieval darkness: The medical school of Salerno south of Naples in Italy, established in the ninth century (Natvig, 1964). During the twelfth and thirteenth centuries, this school developed into a center of European medicine. It became a model for subsequent schools of medicine set up within the universities to be founded in Europe. But even in Salerno, the main focus was the clinical patient. Nevertheless, a health poem written around 1100 aims at beneficial behavior in order to remain in good health, but was addressed to the individual rather than the community (Gotfredsen, 1964). Consequently, the important systems for food safety, drinking water, and sewage set up in Antiquity were neglected, and the Middle Ages were scourged by a series of epidemics that did not come to an end until the nineteenth century.

The Fight Against the Great Plagues

Epidemiology in the modern sense – clarifying the cause of a disease aiming at prevention – barely existed until 1500. Medieval public health-relevant services were probably set up for comfort rather than for disease control. If a medical interest existed in healthy behavior, it was motivated more by need for individual counseling than for public mass campaigns. Efforts aiming at establishing associations between risk factors and disease are difficult to ascertain, in part because of the notion that disease, as any other mishap, was determined by fate or God(s).

A few important exceptions to this broad statement must be mentioned. Among the epidemics pestering the medieval communities, the bubonic plague was by far the most important. Apparently, bubonic plague had existed at the time of Hippocrates and Galen and is even mentioned in Papyrus Ebers around 1500 BC. Epidemics of bubonic plague were frequent in Europe from the seventh to the thirteenth century (Gotfredsen, 1964).

The Black Death around the middle of the fourteenth century, however, surpassed any previous epidemic in terms of mortality and case fatality. Of a population in Europe of 100 million, more than 25 million died (Gotfredsen, 1964). Even if the plague was considered to be a punishment from God, fear of contagion was widespread, and the idea existed that isolation might be beneficial. In some cases, attempts were made to isolate a city, but with no convincing effect; the city might already have been infected or isolation was impossible to obtain since the germ was spread also by birds. Still, during subsequent plague epidemics in the fourteenth century, rational and effective measures were taken. For example, in 1374, the city council of Ragusa (Dubrovnik), Croatia, ordered all suspect vessels to be kept in isolation for 30 days. In 1383, a similar regulation was introduced in Marseille, now amounting to 40 days of isolation. Thereby the concept of quarantine (from the French: *quarante* = 40) was introduced, which came to influence the fight against infectious diseases far into the twentieth century.

Isolation was also effective against another killer of the Middle Ages, more silent and less dramatic, but still highly influential in people's minds: leprosy. Leprosy has been known in Europe since the fifth century when the first leprosy hospitals were built in France. Knowledge of the infectiousness of the disease was established, and isolation of the infected patients was attempted, for example by regulations in Lyon (583) and in northern Italy (644) (Gotfredsen, 1964). In the wake of the crusades, the incidence of leprosy increased considerably, and leprosy hospitals were set up in most cities, almost always outside the city walls. Usually, leprosy patients were forced to live in these institutions with very limited rights to move outside. On the continent and in Britain, leprosy was more or less eradicated by the end of the sixteenth century, presumably because of strict rules aiming at isolation of infectious cases. A new wave of leprosy culminated in Norway around 1850, and an important factor in the subsequent eradication of the disease by 1920 was isolation, as documented by the National Leprosy Registry of Norway (see the section titled 'Registry-based epidemiology) (Irgens, 1973).

The Search for the Cause of Syphilis

The Renaissance introduced new ideas that brought medicine far beyond what was achieved in Antiquity. Girolamo Fracastoro (1483–1553) of Padua, Italy (**Figure 5**), has been considered the great epidemiologist of the Renaissance. In 1546, he published a booklet on infectious

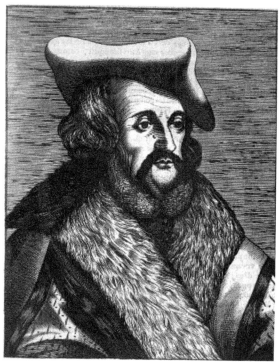

Figure 5   G. Fracastoro; Il Torbido. Source: Wikipedia.

diseases, including smallpox, measles, leprosy, tuberculosis, rabies, plague, typhus, and syphilis. Fracastoro suggested the existence of germs that could be disseminated from person to person, through clothes and through the air (Gotfredsen, 1964).

No doubt syphilis was at this time a novelty, the reason why the new ideas were developed and caught attention. Even if it has been claimed that syphilis existed in Europe before 1500, it is generally agreed that Columbus brought the disease back from his discovery of America in 1492. Fracastoro suggested that most patients got the disease from being infected through sexual intercourse, even if he had seen small children who were infected by their wet-nurse. The spread of the disease from 1495, when besieging soldiers outside Naples were infected, was most remarkable and corresponded to where the troops went after the campaign. Already the same year, the disease became well known in France, Switzerland, and Germany and in 1496 in the Netherlands and Greece. During the following years, syphilis was introduced in most European countries, to a great extent following soldiers, who went where battles might be fought.

Interestingly, the disease was named after the country in which it supposedly originated: In Italy it was called the Spanish disease, in France the Italian disease, in Britain the French disease, in the Nordic countries the German disease, etc. Fracastoro coined the term syphilis when in 1530 he published the poem *Syphilis or the French illness*, in which the hero Syphilis is a shepherd who convinces the people of the benefits of betraying the God of the Sun. Consequently, the God punishes the people with a terrible epidemic disease, named after the perpetrator. The poem may be considered an elegant example of the importance in research of convincing people of the validity of one's findings, a function one might denote scientific rhetoric. The poem was used to call attention to urgent scientific results.

Venereal diseases such as syphilis set the stage for a remarkable event in the history of medicine, which truly illustrates the search for etiology as well as the concept of experimentation. John Hunter (1728–93) (**Figure 6**), a Scottish surgeon, considered the most influential in scientific surgery in his century, was intrigued by the question of whether syphilis and gonorrhea were the same disease with a variety of symptoms dependent on a series of cofactors. Hunter presented this hypothesis in *A Treatise on the Venereal Disease* in 1786, in which he provided evidence supporting this assertion derived from an experiment conducted on himself. He inoculated his own penis with pus taken from a gonorrhea patient and eventually developed typical syphilis. Apparently, his patient had a mixed infection with both gonorrhea and syphilis.

The publication and the findings of this experiment caused heated debate on whether experiments like this were ethically acceptable. Further experiments in Edinburgh published in 1793 concluded that inoculation from a chancre (i.e., syphilis) produces a chancre and inoculation from gonorrhea produces gonorrhea (Gotfredsen, 1964).

Smallpox: Pitfalls and Victory

Smallpox (variola) remained one of the scourges of ancient time. It had been observed that a person very rarely was affected by smallpox twice. This had led to the so-called variolation by which pus from a case was inoculated into the skin of another person, a practice developed in the Orient, spreading to Europe in the eighteenth century. Lady Mary Wortley Montagu (**Figure 7**), the wife of the British ambassador to Turkey, was instrumental in the introduction of the variolation to Europe; another example of rhetoric related to research, even if the research part in this case was rather remote. In 1717, Lady Montagu wrote a letter to smallpox-infested Britain, saying that no one died of smallpox in Turkey, and she had her son inoculated accordingly. Back in London, she started a campaign to introduce variolation in Britain (Gotfredsen, 1964; Natvig, 1964). Voices raised against the practice, in part since the method actually contributed to the spread of the disease (inoculated persons might cause disease in noninoculated persons), in part since some of the inoculated persons died from smallpox. Thus, toward the end of the century, variolation had shown no breakthrough.

Nevertheless, it may have paved the way for the vaccination against smallpox that was introduced by Edward Jenner (1749–1823) (Henderson, 1980). Jenner (**Figure 8**) was a student of John Hunter and worked as a general practitioner in Berkeley, England. A smallpox-like disease in cattle was prevalent in his region, and he observed that, to a large extent, children who were variolated had no clinical symptoms after the variolation. People thought

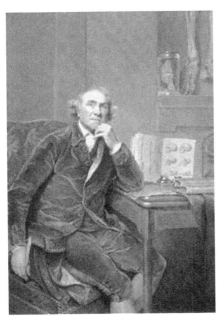

Figure 6   J. Hunter; J. Reynolds, Royal College of Physicians, London, UK. Source: Wikipedia.

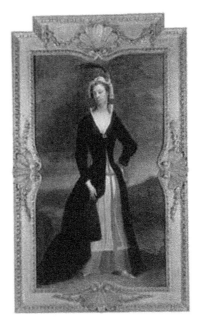

Figure 7   Lady Mary Worley Montagu, 1716 by Charles Jervis. Source: Wikipedia.

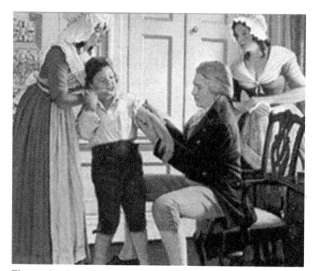

Figure 8   Jenner vaccinating a boy. Source: Wikipedia.

this was because previous exposure to cattle-pox disease was protective. In 1796, Jenner conducted an experiment in which he vaccinated a boy with pus from a milkmaid's hand. Later, Jenner put the boy into bed with smallpox-infected children and also variolated him. The boy did not get smallpox and had no symptoms after variation. Jenner interpreted this as a protective effect of the inoculation and tried to publish his findings, but the article was rejected for lack of firm evidence. Two years later, Jenner published his treatise *An Inquiry into the Causes and Effects of the Variolae Vaccinae* in which he accounted for another seven children vaccinated and a further 16 individuals with previous cattle-pox disease, all with no symptoms after variation by Jenner (Gotfredsen, 1964). His conclusion was that the inoculation with cattle-pox pus, i.e., vaccination, provided the same protection as variation, and that the new method, contrary to variation, did not involve any risk of infecting other people. Furthermore, the method was seemingly harmless to the persons vaccinated (Henderson, 1980).

As compared to the syphilis experiments, this elegant trial was ethically far less controversial even if the question was raised as to whether such an inoculation with an animal disease might cause an unknown number of new diseases in humans, a pertinent question at that time and even today in other contexts. Still, in a very short time, Jenner's conclusions received broad support. The concerns appeared far less important than feared, and in 1802, an institution for vaccination was established in Britain, in 1808 organized as The National Vaccine Establishment. An international vaccination movement was established, promoting this protective measure on a large scale and as a mass campaign. Already in 1810, vaccination was made compulsory by legislation in Denmark and Norway (Gotfredsen, 1964). In addition, the introduction of vaccination indicates the importance

in science of convincing people of the validity of one's findings, virtually a prerequisite of success in epidemiology and public health.

The Epidemiological Avenue

Before further exploring the history of epidemiology, an overview of the analytic methods aiming at establishing an association between a factor and a medical outcome should be made (Rothman and Greenland, 1998). The basic principle in epidemiology is that individuals exposed to a risk factor should have a higher occurrence of a disease than nonexposed individuals. Such an association between a risk factor and a disease can be established by different methods, which have been referred to as the epidemiological avenue.

First comes the case study, which does not at all take the nonexposed into consideration and for that reason is not included in the avenue by many epidemiologists. Today, the results of a case study will never be published, but still a case study will often be the first observation that sheds light on a problem on which a hypothesis is formulated. A case study will be particularly relevant if exposure and outcome are rare or new. In such a situation, the outcome may be considered not to occur in the unexposed. A case study will be followed by a subsequent study along the epidemiological avenue, often a case–control study. The history of epidemiology offers many examples of interesting case studies, often reported by clinicians who have observed a particular risk factor in a rare disease. Thus, the British surgeon Percival Pott (1714–88) found that almost all of his patients with the very rare scrotal cancer were or had been chimney sweeps (Gotfredsen, 1964). He concluded that chimney sweeps were exposed to some etiological agent in their work, in which they often had to scrub the chimneys by passing their own bodies through the narrow flues. More recently, the association between phocomelia, a very rare birth defect, and the drug thalidomide, was ascertained by clinicians who observed that in these cases, all mothers had taken thalidomide during the first trimester (Warkany, 1971).

Next on the avenue is the ecological design that characterizes a group of individuals with respect to exposure rather than the individual *per se*. Typically, the group may represent a nation and the exposure may, for example, be average consumption of salt, while mortality due to stroke may represent the outcome. If a number of countries are included, it becomes apparent that countries with a low intake of salt have a low stroke mortality and vice versa, suggesting a cause–effect association. Misinterpretation of such observations is the background for the term ecological fallacy. Still, a missing association at a group level is a serious argument against an association observed at an individual level being interpreted as causal.

Further down the avenue are the survey, the case–control study, and the cohort study, which are all based on data characterizing the individual rather than the group. In a survey, all individuals of a population are characterized at the same time with respect to exposure and outcome, while in a cohort study all individuals are initially characterized with respect to exposure and are followed up subsequently with respect to outcome. In the more parsimonious but still powerful case–control study, cases are selected among sick individuals and controls among healthy individuals who are then studied with respect to previous exposure.

Finally, there is the experiment, in epidemiology often called a randomized controlled trial, in which a more or less homogeneous population is randomized into groups exposed to various protective agents and compared to a nonexposed group, which may be given a placebo. The roots of this method are found in a rudimentary form in the Old Testament where King David ordered some of his servants to eat of the king's food, a procedure reiterated throughout history and even today when the host tastes his wine before serving his guests.

Evidence-Based Epidemiology

Methods and concepts developed for epidemiological aims may be relevant in a clinical setting as well, and particularly concepts related to experiments. During the first half of the nineteenth century, one finds the first roots of evidence-based medicine. Pierre Charles Alexandre Louis (1787–1872) at the Charité hospital in Paris called attention to the need for more exact knowledge in therapy. He questioned the benefits of venesection in different diseases and particularly pneumonia. In 1835, he published his treatise *Recherches sur les effects de la saignee.* Venesection was the standard treatment in pneumonia, and for ethical reasons he was unable to undertake an experiment in which a group of patients was not given this treatment. However, he categorized his pneumonia patients according to the time when they had their venesection. Among those treated during the first 4 days, 40% died versus 25% among those treated later (Gotfredsen, 1964). Even if these data may be subject to selection bias, the more serious cases having an initial treatment, the results raised skepticism against venesection as treatment of pneumonia.

Louis was also interested in the causes of disease and conducted studies for example on tuberculosis, in which he obtained data questioning the role of heredity in this disease and the benefits of a mild climate. In his conclusion he used terms such as "the exact amount of hereditary influence" that may lead our thoughts to the concept of attributable risk, and one of his students, W. A. Guy (1810–85), conceptualized what we now refer to as the odds ratio (Lilienfeld and Lilienfeld, 1980).

Louis's work also paved the way for the development of medical statistics in general, which was strongly boosted by Jules Gavarret (1809–90), who in *Principes généraux de statistique médicale* in 1840 concluded that medical theories should not be based on opinion, but rather on evidence that could be measured (Gotfredsen, 1964).

The contributions by Louis and Gavarret may be considered consequences of a public health movement that developed in France during the first half of the nineteenth century. Even if the roots of epidemiology, as we have seen, are traceable back to Hippocrates, the growth of modern epidemiological concepts and methods took place in the postrevolutionary Parisian school of medicine. The French Revolution may have eliminated many medical beliefs and broadened the recruitment to the medical profession, which was called upon when Napoleon Bonaparte (1769–1821) reorganized France. However, the era of the French public health movement came to an end toward the middle of the nineteenth century, possibly due to the lack of public health data; France did not develop a vital statistics system (Hilts, 1980; Lilienfeld and Lilienfeld, 1980).

In England, epidemiology flourished because of the presence of such a system, which to a large extent was attributable to William Farr (1807–83) (**Figure 9**), a physician who has been considered the father of medical statistics (Eyler, 1980). As chief statistician of England's General Register Office, which he commanded over a period of 40 years, Farr became a man of influence and also a prominent member of what may be called a statistical movement of the 1830s, itself a product of the broader reform movement (Hilts, 1980). The members of the

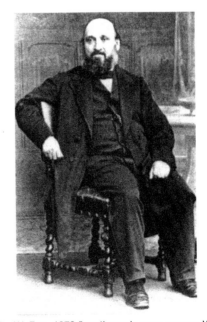

Figure 9 W. Farr, 1870 (location unknown; source: Wikipedia).

statistical movement saw in the use of social facts a valuable weapon for the reform cause. They considered statistics a social rather than a mathematical science. It has been said that few members of this movement mastered more mathematics than rudimentary arithmetic.

The hospital as the arena of observation and evidence-based medicine was explicitly highlighted by Benjamin Phillips (1805–61), who in 1837, after years of experience as a doctor at Marylebone Infirmary, read a paper before the Royal Medical and Clinical Society referred to in the *Journal of the Statistics Society of London*, 1838. The editor claimed that the article had "... great interest, because so few attempts have been made in this country to apply the statistical method of enquiry to the science of surgery. The object of the enquiry was to discover whether the opinion commonly entertained with respect to the mortality succeeding amputation is correct...." And Phillips wrote:

> In the outset, I am bound to express my regret, that the riches of our great hospitals are rendered so little available for enquiries like the present, that these noble institutions, which should be storehouses of exact observation, made on a large scale, and from which accurate ideas should be disseminated throughout the land, are almost completely without the means of fulfilling this very important object. (Phillips, 1838: 103–105)

These critical statements were representative of the statistical movement. Most general in nature, the ambitions were amply illustrated by the achievements of Ignaz Philipp Semelweiss (1818–65) (**Figure 10**), with an influence far beyond clinical epidemiology. During the first half of the nineteenth century, puerperal fever caused serious epidemics at the large European maternity hospitals in which large proportions of all women giving birth died. The general opinion was that the

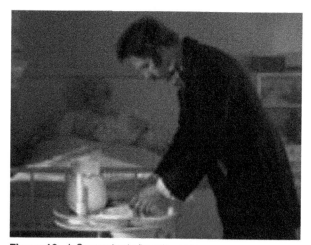

Figure 10   I. Semmelweis (location unknown; source: www.dasErste.de).

contagion was miasmatic, related to atmospheric or telluric conditions. Consequently, the institutions were often moved to other locations, but with no beneficial effect (Gotfredsen, 1964).

In 1847, Semmelweis, a Hungarian gynecologist working in Vienna, made an observation that led him to the etiology of puerperal fever (Loudon, 2000; Lund, 2006). A pathologist at the hospital died from septicemia after being injured during an autopsy, with symptoms and findings identical to those observed in puerperal fever. Thus, Semmelweis hypothesized that puerperal fever was caused by doctors and medical students involved both in autopsies and obstetrics, bringing a germ from one activity to the other. He found that the rate of lethal puerperal fever was 114 per 1000 births at the ward attended by medical students versus 27 per 1000 at the ward attended by students of midwifery, who did not participate in autopsies. After a campaign, instructing everyone attending a birth to wash their hands in chloride of lime, the rate declined to 13 per 1000 in both departments. Semmelweis's findings experienced the consequences of a lack of a convincing presentation. Rather the opposite happened: In a discrediting confusing presentation, he made a number of enemies by accusing colleagues of indolence and negligence. Still, he had conducted an elegant experiment with convincing results, shedding light on the etiology of an important disease long before the dawn of the bacteriological era.

Cholera, Right or Wrong

To many epidemiologists, John Snow's fight against cholera represents the foundation of modern epidemiology (Sigerist, 1956; Natvig, 1964). Cholera is assumed to have been endemic in India in historic time, but was unknown in Europe until the nineteenth century when Europe was hit by a series of pandemics. The first started around 1830, causing an estimated 1.5 million deaths (Gotfredsen, 1964). To the population in Europe, this first wave of cholera demonstrated that the disease represented a most serious threat to the community. However, knowledge of the etiology of the disease was scarce. Obviously, cholera was an epidemic disease, but whether it spread from person to person or was a result of miasma diffusing up from a contaminated ground, the ancient etiological concept, was uncertain. An apparent failure of quarantine to constitute an effective measure against the spread of the disease suggested the latter etiological mechanism.

Thus, when the second pandemic hit, lasting from 1846 to 1861, no effective preventive measure existed. Europe remained unprepared, and the challenge to epidemiology and public health was enormous. In 1848, John Snow (1813–58) (**Figure 11**) was working as a general

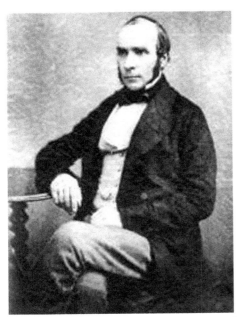

Figure 11   J. Snow (location unknown; source: wikipedia).

practitioner in London when an epidemic of cholera occurred among his patients. In a publication of 1849, Snow presented his observations of the distribution of the disease according to time, place, age, gender, and occupation. He concluded that the agent causing cholera entered the human body by eating or drinking, that the agent was present in the stools of the patients and that the disease was propagated by sewage containing the agent that contaminated the drinking water. To the extent that this publication received any attention, its conclusions were rejected.

However, during the summer of 1854, a new epidemic hit London, and now Snow achieved important practical results when he managed to close down the public well in Broad Street. Snow had observed that a frequent finding among his patients was the use of water from this pump and that people in the same area who did not get cholera, did not take water from the well. Here, Snow more or less laid down the principles of the case–control study. However, even if the pump handle of this well was removed and the local epidemic came to an end, the health authorities and the local medical establishment were not convinced; Snow's hypothesis, that an infectious agent in the drinking water represented the etiological mechanism, was not easy to accept.

Snow was not defeated, nor was the cholera. New local epidemics occurred. Encouraged by reform-minded people such as William Farr, Snow wanted to test his drinking water hypothesis. The water supply system in London at that time offered the possibility to conduct a most elegant study. Two waterworks, Lambeth & Co. and Southwark & Vauxhall, provided drinking water to large areas of London, and both companies were within the same districts. The former took water from farther up the river than the latter, which consequently had a much poorer quality and even a high sodium content. Snow hypothesized that the occurrence of cholera in the population receiving poor-quality drinking water would be much higher, and he was right: Mortality due to cholera was 14 times higher.

Here, Snow had conducted an elegant cohort study in which the population was grouped according to exposure. Due to the situation with two waterworks delivering water in the same districts, one might assume that the only relevant difference between the two groups would be the source of water supply, thus eliminating possible confounding factors. In a critical perspective, this might not necessarily be true; the best drinking water might have been more expensive, introducing a socioeconomic confounder, but the socioeconomic gradient in cholera was allegedly low. Perhaps more important in those days was that the poorer drinking water was presumably delivered to the lower floors, which would be compatible with the alternative hypothesis of miasmas from the ground water. Still, Snow concluded that drinking water was the source, and he added that one must not believe that simply unclean water was sufficient; only when the specific etiological agent finds its way into the water is the disease disseminated. Snow died in 1858 without having been recognized as the scientist who had clarified the etiology of cholera, but his work had great impact on the subsequent development of the London water supply and in the rest of the world.

On the continent, epidemiological research on cholera followed another path. Max von Pettenkofer (1818–1901) (**Figure 12**) was in many ways Snow's extreme opposite, being a member of the German medical establishment. As professor of hygiene, his assistance was requested by the authorities in organizing the fight against cholera when Munich was hit by an epidemic in 1854. His conclusions, even if they were later proved to be wrong, were recognized by his contemporaries and gave him widespread respect. Nevertheless, Pettenkofer was a meticulous observer and collected epidemiologically relevant data in much the same way as Snow. He found that houses in which many cases occurred and particularly the initial cases, were located at a lower altitude than houses without cholera cases. After some time, the disease also spread to other houses. Furthermore, uncleanliness was an important factor, but this factor was also present in non-cholera houses. Consequently, Pettenkofer inferred that cholera was caused by contaminated ground water in which the agent was derived from human stools and subsequently transferred to a gas fuming into the dwellings above; in principle not far from the miasma theory of Antiquity. Pettenkofer even claimed that houses built on rock would never be affected.

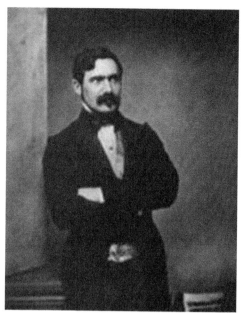

Figure 12   M. von Pettenkofer (location unknown; source: www.wikipedia).

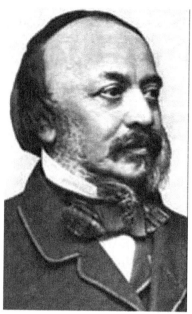

Figure 13   E. Chadwick (location unknown; source: www.wikipedia).

Finally, in 1892, Pettenkofer's fallacy was dramatically demonstrated in his remarkable experiment on himself (Gotfredsen, 1964). After Robert Koch (1843–1910) had discovered the cholera bacillus in 1883, many years after Snow's and Pettenkofer's initial research, Pettenkofer felt that his ground water theory was losing support. Thus, when an epidemic hit Hamburg in that year, Pettenkofer obtained a culture of the bacillus and on 7 October drank 1 ml of it. He did not get ill, only a slight diarrhea a few days afterward. On 17 October, his assistant did the same experiment on himself and he got typical rice-water-like stools. They both had bacilli in their stools for several weeks. Even now, Pettenkofer was not convinced. He was not impressed by his own symptoms and still held that the ground water theory was correct. His opponents attributed his lack of symptoms to the epidemic of 1854, when Pettenkofer also had contracted the disease and presumably received lasting immunity.

Nevertheless, Pettenkofer's efforts to establish adequate sewage systems and to drain the surroundings were instrumental in the fight not only against cholera, but also typhoid and dysentery. His research led to impressive achievements in public health and sanitation, not only in Germany, but throughout Europe and the rest of the world. Pettenkofer's work again demonstrates both the importance, but also the potential perils of rhetoric in the dissemination of scientific results and how rhetoric may compensate for lacking validity of the conclusions. Snow was right and for a long time forgotten, while Pettenkofer was wrong and for a long time celebrated.

Furthermore, the work of both these scientists represents what has later derogatorily been referred to as black box epidemiology: Observing effects and trying to attribute them to causal factors without being able to account for the intermediate mechanisms. In short, Snow's work demonstrates the usefulness of black box epidemiology; an effective fight against cholera was possible without having seen the bacillus. On the other hand, Pettenkofer's inferences from much the same observations illustrate the potential pitfalls involved. Knowledge of details relating to the pathway between the factor and the outcome is evidence that an association is causal. Nevertheless, the principle of not publishing anything until all intermediate mechanisms are clarified in every detail is hardly sustainable.

The Public Health Perspective

Cholera was spectacular. The disease was new and involved serious consequences, not only medically, but also in the community at large in terms of loss of productivity: Cholera was a major and evident challenge to the nation. Far less attention was paid to diseases and epidemics in general and the lack of hygiene.

In Britain, Edwin Chadwick (1800–90) (**Figure 13**) in 1838 started a crusade in which he highlighted these problems and their inherent consequences to the community (Natvig, 1964). As the secretary to a poor-law commission, he gave an influential report on the miserable housing conditions in London's East End. Consequently, Chadwick was asked by the Parliament to conduct a similar survey throughout the country, which was published as *Report on the Sanitary Conditions of the Labouring Population of Great Britain in 1842.*

Statistics on outcomes such as morbidity and mortality as well as risk factors, e.g., housing conditions, unemployment, and poverty in general, produced compelling evidence explaining the high morbidity and mortality rates. This statistical evidence also paved the way for adopting special health legislation, the first of its kind, and for establishing the first board of health, in London in 1848. Chadwick, together with William Farr, were the chief architects of the British Health Administration built up during these years.

In the United States, similar pioneering work was conducted by Lemual Shattuck (1793–1859), who was appointed chairman in a commission reporting on the hygienic conditions in Massachusetts and giving recommendations for future improvements. Shattuck also provided statistical data on the most important causes of death and their distribution according to season, place, age, sex, and occupation. The commission stated that the mean age at death might be considerably increased, that annually, thousands of lost lives could have been saved and that ten thousands of cases of disease could have been prevented, that these preventable burdens cost enormous amounts of money, that prevention would have been much better than cure and, most importantly, that means were available to prevent these burdens (Natvig, 1964). Contrary to Chadwick, Shattuck did not succeed with his campaign in his lifetime, but the next generations have seen the importance of his work.

Registry-Based Epidemiology

Until the middle of the nineteenth century, the data necessary to clarify etiological issues had been scarce. Initially, the nature of the data needed was not clear; even the school of Hippocrates, which considered disease to be the result of natural causes, did not start systematic data collection on a large scale. In the Middle Ages, the challenges related to epidemics were overwhelming, precluding any efforts to collect data. The substantial progress in the fight against smallpox was based on a low number of experiments, and the elucidation of the epidemiology of cholera comprised relatively small-scale *ad hoc* studies. The large hospitals that saw the studies of puerperal fever and pneumonia were, in their clinical records, managers of enormous amounts of data, as pointed out by interested doctors who realized their assets, although it was kept in a form that prohibited use in research. As pointed out by Florence Nightingale, the data did exist but were inaccessible.

Thus, in 1856 a new paradigm was introduced when the first national registry for any disease was established: the National Leprosy Registry of Norway. Prophetically, its initiator, Ove Guldberg Höegh (1814–62) (**Figure 14**), stated that it was by means of this registry that the

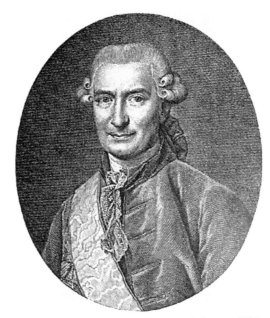

Figure 14 Ove Guldberg Höegh (1814–62). Source: Wikipedia.

etiology of leprosy would be clarified. At that time, the prevailing opinion among the medical establishment was that the disease was hereditary; it seemed to run in families. Another group claimed that leprosy was caused by harsh living conditions in general, while quite a few considered leprosy to be a contagious or infections disease spreading from one person to another. Thus, there was an urge for clarification of the etiology of the disease.

Still, other motivations may have been more important for the establishment of the registry. A need was expressed from a humanitarian point of view to provide care for patients. Consequently, one had to know the patients and their whereabouts. Furthermore, there was a need for health surveillance to obtain reliable information on the occurrence of the disease, whether it was increasing or propagating to parts of the country in which it had not been observed previously (Irgens, 1973).

Already in one of his first annual reports, Höegh presented evidence from the Leprosy Registry of an association between isolation of cases in terms of admission to leprosy hospitals and the subsequent occurrence of the disease. On this basis, he inferred that leprosy was an infectious disease. In 1874, when Gerhard Henrik Armauer Hansen (1841–1912) (**Figure 15**) published his detection of the leprosy bacillus, he first accounted for an elaborate epidemiological analysis along the same lines as Höegh's in which he confirmed the association between isolation and subsequent fall in incidence. Next, he described the bacillus which, he claimed, represented the etiological agent in leprosy.

Altogether, 8231 patients were recorded with primary registration data and with follow-up data, e.g., on hospital

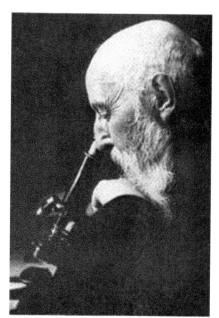

Figure 15 Gerhard Armauer Hansen. Source: Wikipedia.

admissions, until death. In the 1970s, the Leprosy Registry was computerized and utilized in epidemiological studies of the disease (Irgens, 1980), showing that the mean age at onset increased steadily during the period when leprosy was decreasing (**Figure 16**), an observation useful in leprosy control in countries where a national registry does not exist. A similar pattern is to be expected whenever the incidence of a disease with a long and varying incubation period decreases over an extended period of time.

Later, new challenges such as tuberculosis and cancer paved the way for the establishment of similar registries in many other countries. The final step on this registry path was the establishment of medical birth registries comprising the total population, irrespective of any disease or medical problem. The first, the Medical Birth Registry of Norway, has kept records from 1967. The medical birth registries were set up in the wake of the thalidomide tragedy in the late 1950s to prevent similar catastrophes in the future. In other countries, permanent case–control studies were set up with similar aims, cooperating in the International Clearinghouse for Birth Defects Surveillance and Research and EUROCAT (European Surveillance of Congenital Anomalies).

These medical registries, with long time series of observations, provide unique analytical opportunities, particularly in the field of cohort analysis. In 1875, Wilhelm Lexis (1837–1914), in Strasbourg, Alsace (France), set up the theoretical statistical framework for following individuals from birth onward. The question often being addressed was whether an effect seemingly attributed to age is truly the result of age or rather the effect of year of birth, i.e., a birth cohort effect. For example,

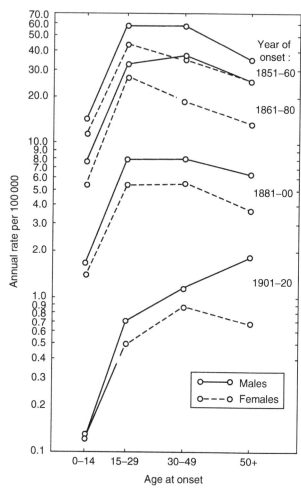

Figure 16 Age- and sex-specific incidence rates of leprosy by year of onset in Norway 1851–1920. Reproduced from Irgens LM (1980) Leprosy in Norway. An epidemiological study based on a national patient registry. *Leprosy Review* 51 (supplement 1): 1–130. With permission from Leprosy Review.

in conventional cross-sectional analyses, performed in the 1950s, the mortality of lung cancer peaked around 65 years of age, an observation leading to speculations that most individuals who are susceptible to lung cancer would have had their onset of the disease at this age and older individuals would be resistant. However, when analyzed according to year of birth, the mortality increased continuously by age in all birth cohorts (**Figure 17**). Still, due to the increasing prevalence of smoking, the incidence increased from one cohort to the next, causing the artifactual age peaks that represented a cohort phenomenon (Dorn and Cutler, 1959).

In infectious diseases with long incubation periods such as tuberculosis and leprosy, a similar cohort phenomenon has been observed. In both diseases, it appeared in cross-sectional analyses that during decreasing rates, the mean age at onset increased by year of onset. The inference was drawn that when the occurrence is low, the time necessary to be infected and to develop

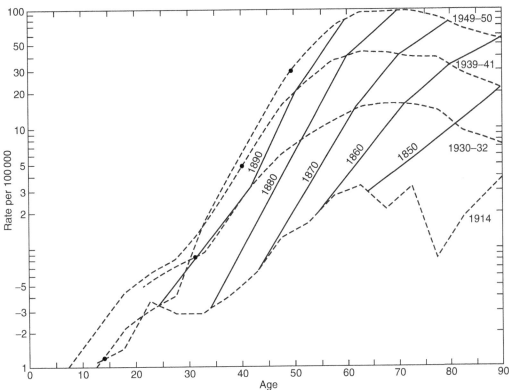

Figure 17   Age-specific mortality rate from lung cancer by year of death (broken lines) and year of birth (solid lines). Source: Dorn HF and Cutler SJ, (1959) Morbidity from cancer in the United States. *Public Health Monographs No. 56*. Washington, DC: US Govt Printing Office.

the disease would be longer than when the occurrence is high. This may in some cases be true, but does not account for the increasing age at onset. In analyses by year of birth, it has appeared that from one birth cohort to the next, the age of the peak occurrence did not increase. Consequently, the pattern observed in the cross-sectional analyses represented a cohort phenomenon (**Figures 16, 18** and **19**).

The detection of such cohort phenomena requires long series of observations, which in practice are available only in registries. The enormous amounts of data in the registries, covering large numbers of individuals over extended periods of time, combined with the analytical power offered by the computer-based information technologies, have caused epidemiologists to talk about megaepidemiology, and registry-based epidemiology will no doubt play an important role in future epidemiological research.

Causality in the Era of Microbiology

Armauer Hansen's detection of *M. leprae* in 1873 was a pioneering achievement, not only in leprosy but in infectious diseases in general. As we have already seen, the concept that some diseases are contagious, spreading from one individual to the next, had existed since Antiquity

or before. However, not until 1863, when Casimir Davaine (1812–82) saw the anthrax bacillus and demonstrated that the disease could be reproduced in animals after inoculation of blood from infected animals, were the general etiological principles of infectious diseases clarified. Anthrax is an acute disease that was generally considered infectious. Leprosy is a chronic illness, and in the middle of the nineteenth century, the confusion was great as to its etiology. Even if a microorganism had been observed in a disease, it was not necessarily the cause of the disease, but possibly a consequence or even a random observation. Jacob Henle (1809–85) had enlarged on these problems already in 1840, and prerequisites necessary to establish a microorganism as the cause of a disease were later known as Koch's postulates (Gotfredsen, 1964). These prerequisites are:

- The microorganism should be found in every case of the disease.
- Experimental reproduction of the disease should be achieved by inoculation of the microorganism taken from an individual suffering from the disease.
- The microorganism should not be found in cases of other diseases.

Paradoxically, Armauer Hansen was not able to meet any of these prerequisites, but still *M. leprae* eventually was accepted as the cause of leprosy; already in 1877 a

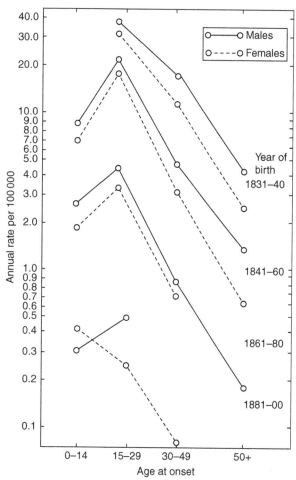

Figure 18 Age and sex-specific incidence rates of leprosy by year of birth in Norway 1851–1920. Reproduced from Irgens LM (1980) Leprosy in Norway. An epidemiological study based on a national patient registry. *Leprosy Review* 51 (supplement 1): 1–130. With permission from Leprosy Review.

bill aiming at preventing the spread of leprosy by isolating the infectious patients was enacted (Irgens, 1973).

In their considerations as to the etiological role played by microorganisms, Henle and Koch touched on general problems related to the association between a potential factor and a medical outcome; whether the association is causal or not. In 1965, A. Bradford Hill (1897–1991) published a comprehensive list of prerequisites of a causal association known as Hill's criteria:

- The association is consistently replicated in different settings and by different methods.
- The strength of the association in terms of relative risk is sufficient.
- The factor causes only one specific effect.
- A dose–response relationship is observed between the factor and the outcome.
- The factor always precedes the outcome.
- The association is biologically plausible.

- The association coheres with existing theory and knowledge.
- The occurrence of the medical outcome can be reduced by manipulating the factor, e.g., in an experiment.

The importance of these criteria differs and the criterion of specificity, stating that a factor causes only one specific effect is not valid: Cigarette smoking causes a variety of adverse outcomes. Nor is specificity in the opposite direction valid: Lung cancer may be caused by a variety of factors. The discussion of such criteria and their shortcomings has continued since the middle of the nineteenth century, and taking the complexity of causal inference into consideration, the progress in microbiological research until the turn of the nineteenth century was amazing.

On the other hand, the conditions necessary to undertake this research had existed for almost two centuries, and one may ask why this progress did not occur earlier. The concept of infectious agents, e.g., in the air or spreading from person to person, had been accepted since Antiquity, and around 1675, Anthony van Leeuwenhoek (1632–1723) constructed the microscope. In 1683, he even described various types of microorganisms, apparently cocci and rods, which he referred to as small animals. Still, the implications of his observations were not recognized. Again lack of scientific rhetoric to convince himself and others of the significance of his findings seems to have been the case. Furthermore, it has been speculated that the spirit of the eighteenth century, attempting to organize assumed knowledge into systems, in medicine originating with Galen and Hippocrates, detrimental to new empirical evidence-based knowledge, was a major obstacle to further progress (Sigerist, 1956).

Two hundred years later, the time was ripe. In 1882, 9 years after Armauer Hansen's discovery of *M. leprae*, Koch detected *Mycobacterium tuberculosis*, cultivated it, and produced disease after inoculation in research animals, as he had done for anthrax in 1876, and did for cholera in 1883. Over the next 30 years, Koch's discoveries were followed by similar achievements by which a large number of microorganisms were discovered.

During the same period, the concept of vaccination, introduced a century earlier, was further advanced by Louis Pasteur (1822–95) (**Figure 20**). Pasteur was also involved in anthrax research, and in 1881 he inoculated anthrax in cattle both protected and unprotected by a vaccine; none of the vaccinated cattle became infected versus all of the nonvaccinated animals, of which a large fraction died (Gotfredsen, 1964). Thus the concept of vaccination was introduced into the fight against diseases other than smallpox, but the term relating to where the vaccine originated (*vacca* = cow) was retained.

Pasteur's efforts to achieve protection against infectious diseases by inoculation of antigens producing antibodies against infectious agents were further expanded

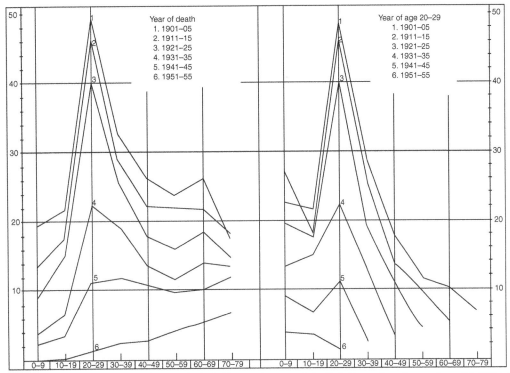

Figure 19   Age-specific mortality rates of tuberculosis in Norway by year of death (left panel) and year of age 20–29 (right panel). Source: Central Bureau of Statistics Norway (1961) *Trend of Mortality and Causes of Death in Norway 1856–1955*. Oslo, Norway: Central Bureau of Statistics Norway.

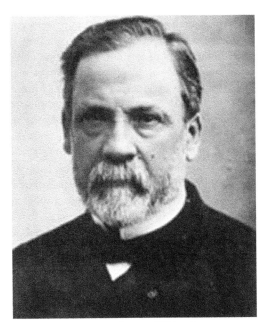

Figure 20   Louis Pasteur. Source: Wikipedia.

by himself and several successors. Interestingly, Pasteur's achievements obtaining top publicity was not the vaccinations to protect the community, but a vaccine produced for clinical purposes, i.e., his vaccine against rabies. Pasteur had succeeded in attenuating the infectious agent in this disease, later identified as a virus, which was inoculated in individuals who had been bitten by rabid dogs. The popular press at the time abounded with reports on how 19 bear hunters, bit by a rabid wolf, were sent on the Trans-Siberian Express to Paris to be inoculated by Pasteur. The inoculation should be made as soon as possible after the bite, but although the journey took 15 days, only three persons (15.8%) died (Gotfredsen, 1964); untreated, the case fatality rate ranges from 60 to 90%, and after onset, the disease is almost always fatal.

During the last half of the twentieth century, the importance of infection in the causation of disease seemed to diminish. In part, this may have resulted from reduced pathogenicity of some previously important infectious agents, e.g., streptococci, which used to cause rheumatic fever as well as kidney and cardiac complications. But decreasing attention and interest can hardly be disregarded. Thus, *Helicobacter pylori* as a causative agent in ulcers of the stomach was detected as late as 1990. Around the turn of the twentieth century, infectious diseases again hit the tabloid headlines due to increased pathogenicity and resistance against antibiotics.

Vitamins and the Web of Causation

In many ways, the history of the study of avitaminoses parallels the history of infectious diseases. Both topics attracted great attention around the turn of the nineteenth century, and both survived a period of negligence to resurrect on top of the list of important medical issues among lay persons as well as the learned. Furthermore, in the history of epidemiology, both infectious diseases and avitaminoses occurred epidemically, and since their etiologies are essentially different, this caused considerable confusion. Thus, beriberi (avitaminosis B_1), pellagra (avitaminosis B_2), and scurvy (avitaminosis C), important diseases in the Middle Ages as well as more recently, were all at some time considered to be infectious or attributed to miasma. Also, the etiological avitaminosis research to some extent recalled black box epidemiology: The most important aim was to find measures to prevent the diseases more or less irrespective of the pathogenetic mechanisms involved.

Beriberi (meaning I cannot, i.e., work), is a polyneuritic disease that was particularly prevalent in East Asia. In 1886, Christjaan Eijkman (1858–1930) set up a bacteriological laboratory in Jakarta to find the cause of the disease (Gotfredsen, 1964). After several years of experiments on chickens, he concluded that the etiology of the disease was lack of a factor that was found in cured but not in uncured rice. To find out whether this also applied in humans, an experiment was conducted in 1906 in a mental hospital in Kuala Lumpur, Malaysia, where two different wards were given cured and uncured rice, respectively (Fletcher, 1907). The occurrence of beriberi was much lower in patients given cured rice produced in a process by which this factor was preserved. To test the alternative hypothesis, that the difference in occurrence of beriberi was caused by the dwelling, i.e., miasma, all patients in the first ward were moved to the second ward and vice versa, but still retained their diet; and the difference in occurrence persisted. When the diet was changed from uncured to cured rice, the occurrence changed accordingly.

This experiment illustrates inherent ethical dilemmas in epidemiology and public health work and would hardly be permitted today. However, its potential benefits to large numbers of people were a question of life and death. Later, in 1926, the active substance was identified and called vitamin B_1, or thiamin.

Pellagra (*pelle agra* = rough skin) was described as a nosological entity in the eighteenth century and was considered infectious until Joseph Goldberger (1874–1929) and coworkers clarified its etiology. Pellagra was manifested by skin, nervous system, and mental symptoms. The disease occurred most frequently among the economically deprived and particularly in areas where the diet was high in maize (corn) intake. The disease was common in many areas in Europe, Egypt, Central America, and the southern states of the United States. The largest outbreak occurred in the United States from 1905 through 1915. Goldberger considered the cause of pellagra to be lack of a factor found in yeast, milk,

and fresh meat. In 1937, the factor was isolated and called vitamin B_2, or niacin.

Scurvy (Latin *scorbutus*, possibly derived from a Norse name referring to edema) was the first major disease found to be associated with a nutrient when a Scottish naval doctor, James Lind (1716–94), in 1753 published *A Treatise of the Scurvy* (Gotfredsen, 1964). He recommended lemon or lime juice as both a preventive and curative measure that had proved effective aboard Dutch vessels. From 1795, a daily dose was compulsory in the Royal Navy and from 1844 in the merchant navy, after which scurvy disappeared. However, being a curse during the Crusades, the disease had been recognized much earlier. In wartime, the disease caused high mortality in armies, navies, and besieged cities. But most importantly, scurvy was the disease of the sailing ships of the great exploratory expeditions. The disease was of some importance as recently as World War II. Great progress in the understanding of its etiology was made by Axel Holst (1860–1931) and Theodor Frølich (1870–1947) who, based on a series of experiments, concluded in 1907 that scurvy was an avitaminosis (Natvig, 1964; Norum and Grav, 2002). The active agent, vitamin C, or ascorbic acid, was isolated around 1930.

The clarification of the etiology of rachitis illustrates the importance of interacting risk factors in the web of causation. The disease had been described as a nosological entity around 1650 and later attributed to both genetic and infectious factors. However, its prevention by cod liver oil represented the only firm etiological evidence. In the 1920s, a component derived from cod liver oil was identified and referred to as vitamin D. At the same time, an antirachitic effect of ultraviolet light was demonstrated. Only in the early 1930s, the antirachitic factor, calciferol, was isolated and the role played by ultraviolet radiation was established. Previously as in the developing world today, rachitis was and is a disease caused by vitamin D deficiency. Today in the developed world, with adequate nutrition, rachitis can still be observed, but here the disease represents a genetic metabolic disorder. A similar shift is observed in tuberculosis: In the past as in the developing world today, the whole population being infected, tuberculosis was, and still is, related to genetic susceptibility, or other cofactors such as protein deficiency. Today, in the developed world, tuberculosis is dependent on risk of infection. These examples shed light on the concept of sufficient and necessary etiological factors and illustrate how the etiological web of a disease can vary according to time and place.

Vitamins and their relevance to disease in humans were more or less forgotten after the etiology of the avitaminosis had been clarified and the preventive measures taken. However, the observation in the early 1990s case–control studies that use of folic acid very early during pregnancy significantly reduced the occurrence of congenital neural tube defects, contributed to a change of attitude. Later, it appeared that the occurrence of birth defects in general also might be reduced. Subsequent research has focused on folic acid and the relationship with homocysteine, a risk factor in cardiovascular disease. An inverse association between folic acid intake and serum homocysteine has suggested a protective affect of folic acid. Also, a protective effect in cancer has been suggested, but this is still far from clarified.

Sudden Infant Death Syndrome and Evidence-Based Recommendations

Sudden infant death syndrome (SIDS) brings us back to the beginning, to the Bible, in which an account is given of an infant smothered to death during the night by its mother. More recent sources also give information about this condition in which a seemingly completely well infant suddenly dies. In the middle of the nineteenth century, the sociologist, Eilert Sundt (1817–75) conducted an epidemiological study in which he accounted for the occurrence of SIDS in Norway.

Growing interest attached to the condition when, in the 1970s, the occurrence seemed to be increasing in many countries. However, based on mortality statistics, this trend was questioned, particularly by pathologists who claimed that the new trend was caused by increasing interest and awareness, whereby cases previously diagnosed as pneumonia, for example, now were diagnosed as SIDS by a process of transfer of diagnosis. Early epidemiological studies had established that SIDS occurred after the first week of life and throughout the first year, with a highly conspicuous peak around 3 months. When time trend studies of the total mortality in a window around 3 months of life showed the same secular trend as the alleged SIDS trend, a transfer of diagnosis was ruled out and there was a general agreement that an epidemic of SIDS was under way.

This epidemic occurred in most countries where reliable mortality statistics were available. In some countries, all infant deaths that had occurred during an extended period of time were revised on the basis of the death certificate, and it appeared that the increase in the SIDS risk had been even steeper than previously thought. Thus, in Norway, the SIDS rate increased threefold from 1 per 1000 in 1969 to 3 in 1989. Consequently, national research councils in many countries earmarked funds for SIDS research and comprehensive efforts were made to resolve the so-called SIDS enigma. Also, influential national parent organizations were set up and international associations were established for research. The increasing SIDS rates even caused general public awareness and concern.

In initial case–control studies and registry-based cohort studies, risk factors for SIDS were identified, such as low maternal age and high parity. Furthermore, social gradients existed with strong effects of marital status and maternal education. However, none of these risk factors could explain the secular increase. Even if genetic factors did not account for the increase, great concern attached to the risk of recurrence among siblings. In early case–control studies, more than tenfold relative recurrence risks had been reported, but in registry-based cohort studies, the relative risk was found to be around 5, a relief for mothers who had experienced a SIDS loss. The difference was most likely attributable to selection bias in the case–control studies; in a non-population-based case–control study, a mother with two losses would be more likely to participate than a mother with only one loss.

Eventually, infant care practices were the focus in large comprehensive case–control studies. In the late 1980s, the first evidence, observed in Germany, was published, indicating that the face-down, prone sleeping position was harmful, with a relative risk versus the supine position of around 5. Later, this finding was confirmed by studies in Australia, New Zealand, Scandinavia, Britain, and on the European continent, with far higher relative risks. The side sleeping position was also found to be harmful, as was maternal cigarette smoking, co-sleeping, non-breastfeeding, and overheating. The use of a pacifier was found to be protective.

The distribution of the information that prone (face-down) sleeping was a serious risk factor had a dramatic effect. In Norway, this information was spread by the mass media in January 1990. The SIDS rate in Norway dropped from 2.0 per 1000 in 1988 to 1.1 in 1990. In a retrospective study, it appeared that the prone (face-down) sleeping position after having continuously increased from 7.4% in 1970, was reduced from 49.1% in 1989 to 26.8% in 1990 (Irgens *et al.*, 1995) (**Figure 21**). The example again illustrates how important it is to provide scientifically convincing evidence, pivotal to bring results of epidemiological research into practice.

The SIDS experience raises important questions with respect to the reliability of recommendations given to the public based on epidemiological studies. The prone sleeping position had been recommended by pediatricians since the 1960s to avoid scoliosis as well as cranial malformations. Even though a case–control study in Britain early on in the period had observed an increased relative risk, no action was taken; again an example of the necessity to convince scientifically.

Future Directions

Even if epidemiology and particularly observational studies from time to time have been criticized and accused of giving misleading conclusions, the search for knowledge on the determinants of disease, in order to take effective preventive measures will no doubt prevail, providing an important future role for epidemiology. New challenges are life-course epidemiology, addressing major causes

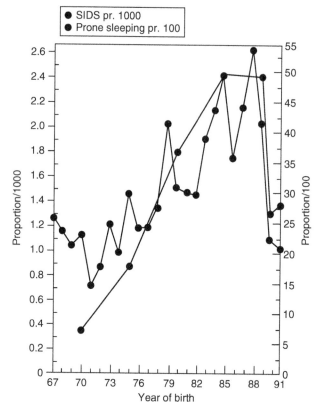

Figure 21 Occurrence (%) of prone sleeping at three months of age and SIDS rate (per 1000) by year of birth, Norway (1967–1991). Reproduced from Irgens LM, Markestad T, Baste V, Schreuder P, Skjærven R, and yen N (1995) Sleeping position and SIDS in Norway 1967–71. *Archives of Diseases in Childhood* 72: 478–482, with Permission.

of adult diseases and deaths, as well as the study of interactions between environmental and genetic factors. Further progress will require the population to understand the necessity for providing data, often based on the suffering of the individual, to benefit the community and future generations, an ethical principle underlying all epidemiological research and of utmost importance to providing data necessary to the search for causes in medicine.

See also: Demography, Epidemiology and Public Health; Observational Epidemiology; Surveillance of Disease.

Citations

Aggebo A (1964) *Hvorfor Altid den Hippocrates?* Aarhus, Denmark Universitetsforlaget i Aarhus.

Carpenter RG, Irgens LM, Blair P, et al. (2004) Sudden unexplained infant death in 20 regions in Europe: Case–control study. *Lancet* 363: 185–191.

Dorn HF and Cutler SJ (1959) Morbidity from cancer in the United States. *Public Health Monographs No. 56.* Washington, DC: US Govt Printing Office.

Eyler JM (1980) The conceptual origins of William Farr's epidemiology: Numerical methods and social thought in the 1830s. In: Lilienfeld AM

(ed.) *Times, Places and Persons,* pp. 1–21. Baltimore, MD: Johns Hopkins University Press.

Fletcher W (1907) Rice and beri-beri: Preliminary report of an experiment conducted at the kuala Lumpur Lunatic Asglum. *Lancet* 1: 1776–1779.

Gotfredsen E (1964) *Medicinens Historie.* Copenhagen, Denmark: Nyt nordisk forlag Arnold Busck.

Hauge D (1973) Fortolkning til Samuelsbøkene (In Bibelverket). Oslo.

Henderson DA (1980) The History of smallpox eradication. In: Lilienfeld AM (ed.) *Times, Places and Persons,* pp. 99–114. Baltimore, MD: Johns Hopkins University Press.

Hilts VL (1980) Epidemiology and the statistical movement. In: Lilienfeld AM (ed.) *Times, Places and Persons,* pp. 43–55. Baltimore, MD: Johns Hopkins University Press.

Irgens LM (1973) Epidemiology of leprosy in Norway. An interplay of research and public health work. *International Journal of Leprosy* 41: 189–198.

Irgens LM (1980) Leprosy in Norway. An epidemiological study based on a national patient registry. *Leprosy Review* 51 (supplement 1): 1–130.

Irgens LM, Markestad T, Baste V, Schreuder P, Skjærven R, and Øyen N (1995) Sleeping position and SIDS in Norway 1967–71. *Archives of Diseases in Childhood* 72: 478–482.

Last JM (2001) *A Dictionary of Epidemiology.* Oxford, UK: Oxford University Press.

Lilienfeld DE and Lilienfeld AM (1980) The French influence on the development of epidemiology. In: Lilienfeld AM (ed.) *Times, Places and Persons,* pp. 28–38. Baltimore, MD: Johns Hopkins University Press.

Loudon I (2000) *The Tragedy of Childbed Fever.* Oxford, UK: Oxford University Press.

Lund PJ (2006) Semmelweis – en varsler. *Tidsskrift for den Norske Lœgorening* 126: 1776–1779.

Mackenbach J (2005) Kos, Dresden, Utopia . . . A journey through idealism past and present in public health. *European Journal of Epidemiology* 20: 817–826.

Michelsen LM (1972) Fortolkning til 1. Mosebok (In Bibelverket). Oslo Bibelverket.

Natvig H (1964) *Lœrebok i Hygiene.* Oslo: Liv og helses forlag.

Norum KR and Grav HJ (2002) Axel Holst og Theodor Frølich. Pionerer i bekjempelsen av skjørbuk. *Tidskrift for Den Norske Lœgeforening* 122: 1686–1687.

Phillips B (1838) Mortality of Amputation. *Journal of the Statistical Society of London* 1: 103–105.

Rothman K and Greenland S (1998) *Modern Epidemiology.* Philadelphia, PA: Lippincott, Raven Publishers.

Sigerist HE (1956) *Landmarks in the History of Hygiene.* London: Oxford University Press.

Statistics Norway (1961) Dødeligheten og dens årsaker i Norge 1856–1955. Trend of motality and causes of death in Norway 1856–1955. *Statistisk Sentrallgyriǎ,* Oslo No. 10, 132.

Warkany J (1971) *Congenital Malformations.* Chicago, IL: Year Book Medical Publishers Inc.

Relevant Websites

http://search.eb.com/eb/article-9040540 – Encyclopedia Britannica Online.

http://www.jstor.org/ – Journal Storage, the Scholarly Journal Archive.

http://www.lshtm.ac.uk/library/archives/farr.html – London School of Hygiene and Tropical Medicine, Behind the Frieze – William Farr (1807–83).

http://www.spartacus.schoolnet.co.uk/PHchadwick.htm – The National Archives, Edwin Chadwick.

http://www.civeng.ucl.ac.uk/edwin.htm – UCL Civil and Environmental Engineering, Sir Edwin Chadwick, KCB.

http://www.gesundheit.de/wissen/persoenlichkeiten-medizin/ignaz-philipp-semmelweis-kindbettfieber/printer.html – Wer war Ignaz Philipp Semmelweis?.

http://en.wikipedia.org/wiki/Cloaca_Maxima – Wikipedia, Cloaca Maxima.

Concepts of Health and Disease

D Czeresnia, Oswaldo Cruz Foundation (ENSP-FIOCRUZ), Brazil
T C Soares, Federal University in Juiz de Fora, Juiz de Fora, Brazil

Health, Illness, and Disease

Ask a person what it means to be healthy. If you repeat the question several times, you are certain to get different answers. It is impossible to provide a precise, generic definition, because there are various ways of experiencing health. The concept of health is a qualification of existence, and there are different ways of existing with quality of life. Health is not amenable to scientific definition; it is first and foremost a philosophical question and relates to each person's life, as stated by French philosopher Georges Canguilhem (1990).

Another point of view was proposed by Boorse (1977), who stated that the medical concept of health can be described by two elements: Biological function and statistical normalcy. According to Boorse, the concept of health as absence of disease provides a value-free scientific definition.

Health has become a vast scientific field. Public health itself can be defined as an area of knowledge and practice focused on the health of populations. However, circumscribing health as a scientific issue and one involving the application of science-based technologies, led to a problem in the shaping of health practices. The relation between health care and other ways of expressing reality, such as art, philosophy, and politics has been overlooked (Czeresnia, 1999).

The definition of health by the World Health Organization (WHO) as "a state of complete physical, mental, and social well-being, and not merely the absence of disease or infirmity" has been criticized in its philosophical manifestation on the grounds that it expresses hope for a reality free of obstacles, an ideal situation unrelated to the life of any human being.

Health cannot be conceived statically, which may explain why it is almost always approached in reference to illness. Health and disease occur in a dynamic process. Ask anyone if they have ever been ill, and it is highly unlikely that you will get a negative answer. There is no such thing as perfect health, and disturbances are part of life. What is healthy in a given condition may not be in another; movement is a basic condition for adjusting to new situations. The capacity to bring about change and preserve one's integrity under varying circumstances is a fundamental resource for health. Health is a way of approaching existence with the ability to create new forms of life, to find alternatives in order to deal with the inherent difficulties of living.

In a meaning linked to biology, health is defined by Canguilhem as "a margin of tolerance for the inconsistencies of the environment" (Canguilhem, 1975). Dubos presents a similar definition when he states, based on Claude Bernard, that health is "the ability of the organism to resist the impact of the outside world and maintain constant within narrow limits the physicochemical characteristics of its internal environment" (Dubos, 1996: 119).

Health as the ability to withstand the difficulties of the environment is a concept that is also applied to psychology and psychiatry. The concept of resilience has been introduced recently to operationally approach individuals' resources to face, react to, preserve themselves, and recover from adverse situations (Rutter, 1987).

All these definitions highlight the inseparability between individuals and their environment. Health thus relates to living conditions, which for human beings are a set of physical, social, economic, cultural, and ecological circumstances. This observation led to health being defined as the responsibility of the state and a citizen's right, an approach to health which is at the very basis of the institutional organization of modern public health (Rosen, 1993), reaffirmed in the discourse of health promotion in the contemporary world.

Meanwhile, health as the result of a unique process of preservation of integrity in relation to the environment, highlights the meaning of health as a personal value and responsibility. Even so, health as a personal criterion is also mediated by societal values. The way a society conceives health interferes in, or even constitutes, individual options. There is no way to disassociate the value individuals create, when relating to their bodies in health or in disease, from the way society conceives health and disease and operates them in practice.

Nevertheless, we need to distinguish between the feeling of being healthy or ill and the scientific concept of disease. Here, we should highlight that health can only be defined scientifically as the absence of disease, as proposed by Boorse. Thus, the difference between illness and having a diagnosed disease should have an equivalent for the concept of health. That is, there should be a way of differentiating between feeling healthy and not having a disease. However, we only have terms to designate this distinction in relation to disease, namely illness, for the subjective experience, and disease, for the scientific concept.

For illness, what is expressed is suffering. Meanwhile, disease means living with a diagnosis mediated through a set of interventions by the health system. One meaning does not correspond exactly to the other. For example, there are circumstances in which a person does not feel ill, but has been diagnosed with a lesion that may not have produced clinical symptoms, characterizing the presence of a potential disease. On the other hand, the expression of suffering may not be translated as the diagnosis of a disease.

There is a controversial relationship between the way a health system is structured as a field of social intervention and individuals' need for health. The first is a peculiarity of a given concept of disease that imposes itself and creates technologies and demands. The latter involves individuals' need from the point of view of the primary intuition that each human being experiences as a unique person. Discrepancies often arise between the way medicine intervenes and the way individuals feel their own bodies.

Scientific medical knowledge is not always capable of dealing adequately with the subjective dimension of human suffering that comes from living with illness and the proximity of death. Works like *The Magic Mountain* by Thomas Mann and *The Death of Ivan Illich* by Tolstoy have shown how literature is complementary to medicine in this sense.

When people turn to a health professional or service, they are seeking relief for their pain, and not only a treatment plan based on tests and medication. Medicine needs to be humanized, as observed by those who contend that treatment technique should include a dialogical relationship: The convergence between the technique *per se*, communication, and affect, since treating and healing are more than simply medicating.

Tables 1 and **2** systematize the concepts approached in this subitem. **Table 1** presents the distinction between health as a scientific concept and as a philosophical issue. **Table 2** provides the differences in meaning between the terms illness and disease.

Table 1   Health

Scientific concept	Philosophical question
Absence of disease	Value
Statistical normalcy	Normativeness
Biological function	Capacity to withstand environmental adversities

Table 2   Illness × disease

Illness	Disease
Subjective experience	Objective scientific concept
Suffering	Disease diagnosis
Primary intuition	Medical intervention
Need	Demand

Influence of Medical Science

Throughout history, concepts of disease have been produced in the context of disputes between philosophical perspectives. Until the nineteenth century, the predominant idea was that of disease as an imbalance or disharmony between individuals and their environment. With the emergence of modern medicine, disease was conceptualized as clinical signs and symptoms arising from injury originating from specific causal agents.

Medical science successively located diseases in organs, tissues, cells, genes, and enzymes. Diagnostic and therapeutic techniques were transformed with the progressive introduction of methods involving clinical analysis, imaging, discovery of new etiological mechanisms, and interventional technologies. Since the initial discoveries by bacteriology, the tendency to prioritize the investigation of lesions and their causes has been the defining trait in the monumental development of biomedicine in the twentieth century.

It is a challenge to establish the connection between the biological, psychological, and social dimensions of disease. Many medical, social, and behavioral studies use the concept of stress to make this link. However, stress is not a highly explanatory concept, and there is no clear and accepted definition of a state of stress or how it leads to alterations in the organism's internal functions (Hinkle, 1987).

Without a doubt, a more adequate explanation is still needed for the relations between general living conditions, the psyche, and disease. The concept of somatic disease tended to circumscribe medical care mainly to specific, individualized interventions, with progressive specialization and incorporation of technology. Patients and their environment were in a sense carved out according to guidelines for medical intervention in this narrow sense and were thus relegated to a secondary plane. However, there was still a conflict between this trend and those who contended that the health/disease process required a broader approach, and that the health sector should be linked to other areas of knowledge and intervention.

Disease Prevention

The preventive medicine movement emerged in the first half of the twentieth century. The work of Leavell and Clark (1965) in this context was important for the organizational structure of health systems worldwide and therefore merits our dwelling on their concept of prevention.

Prevention is defined as "anticipatory action based upon knowledge of the natural history to make the onset of further progress of the disease unlikely" (Leavell and Clark, 1965: 20). Natural history, in turn, is defined as

> all the interrelations of the agent, host, and environment affecting the complete process and its development, from the first forces which create the disease stimulus in the environment or elsewhere (pre-pathogenesis), through the resulting response of man, to the changes which take place leading to defect, disability, recovery, or death (pathogenesis)   (Leavell and Clark, 1965: 18)

Prevention permeates all phases of intervention by the health system and appears at three levels – primary, secondary, and tertiary – from the process prior to onset of the disease until rehabilitation, including diagnostic and therapeutic measures. The origin of the disease is seen as a continuous chain of causes and effects and not merely the result of specific causes. The multicausal model proposed by Leavell and Clark is based on the relations between agent, host, and the environment.

Although still heavily focused on the disease dimension and health services organization, the preventive medicine approach proposes health promotion as one level of primary prevention, defined as measures devoted to health in general, not oriented specifically to a single disease or disorder.

Epidemiology and Risk

The intense changes in the demographic and epidemiological profile of populations, especially in developed countries, has raised the need to adjust the idea of multicausality to the study of chronic, noncommunicable diseases. Epidemiology had already been structured as a scientific discipline since the early twentieth century, but after World War II, it gained a new configuration with the development and refinement of techniques and study designs for the analysis of causal factors for diseases (Susser, 1985).

Epidemiological risk estimates are now the principal source for organizing scientific activity to determine disease etiology and evaluate medical procedures. Epidemiological studies build concepts and orient risk-control practices. Increasingly, statistical techniques have been developed for the evaluation of the causal nature of associations and interaction among causes and to guarantee the quality of findings by avoiding errors such as bias, chance, and confounding.

Epidemiological studies contribute to legitimizing changes in the ways of conceiving diseases and acting to prevent, control, and treat them. These changes can be illustrated by gastric ulcer, the example used by Thagard (1998). A person with stomach pain who consulted a physician in the 1950s would have been advised to take it easy and drink milk. In the 1970s and 1980s, ulcer was considered a disease resulting from increased gastric acidity, and treatment was thus based on antacids. Beginning in the 1990s, it became an infection with *Helicobacter pylori* and medication shifted to a combination of antibiotics.

Another important dimension of risk studies is the construction of a rationale for attributing positive or negative meanings to exposures, habits, or behaviors related to eating, exercise, sex, smoking, and various toxic agents. The concept of risk in the contemporary world is a central element for individual and collective decision making, and various authors have developed critical research on its implications (Lupton, 1999).

What meanings are generated socially by establishing that given habits and behaviors risk harming health? The border between health and disease becomes tenuous: in addition to persons with established diseases, there are now individuals with merely a diagnosis of potential disease, thus raising an ethical dimension. For instance, with very few exceptions, disorders classified as genetic actually involve multiple factors. Genetic tests only indicate a statistical risk that may not even materialize, and thus end up inappropriately medicalizing the individual's life (Melzer and Zimmern, 2002).

Health Promotion

The exponential technological progress of biomedicine has led to an equivalent increase in the costs of financing medical procedures. This has helped revive the idea that health is a good that needs to be guaranteed before disease appears.

In an official report in 1974, the Canadian government proposed the concept of health field, consisting of four components: Human biology, the environment, lifestyle, and organization of health care. The document, known as the Lalonde Report (1981), expresses the need to reorient health expenditures. According to the report, most costs come from the health-care component, yet most causes of disease and death are located in the other three.

The reinvigorated discourse advocating the importance of investment in the promotion of better living and work conditions (to impact the structure that underlies health problems) has oriented the search for intersector strategies (Terris, 1990). The sector responsible for organizing health care should be linked to broader social policies. Meanwhile, health promotion programs emphasize the dimension of individual responsibility, that is, proposing to capacitate individuals and social groups to deal with and struggle for their health. Health promotion discourse covers from personal uniqueness to the broader dimension of state policies.

Concepts and approaches such as vulnerability have been incorporated more recently in the search to innovate knowledge and instrumentalize practices aimed at interconnecting the multiple dimensions of health problems.

Table 3   Approaches to health and disease

Causal model	Components	Emphasis	Protection	Actors
Ecological triad	Agent, Host, Environment	Health services organization	Disease prevention	Health professionals
Health field	Human biology, Environment, Lifestyle, Organization of health care	Intersectorality, Empowerment	Health promotion	Individuals, Social movements, Governments
Risk	Statistical association between exposure and disease	Risk management	Disease prevention	Individuals, Health professionals and managers
Vulnerability	Individual, social and health-program aspects	Empowerment	Health promotion	Individuals, Social movements

The concept of vulnerability originated in the international human rights movement, to deal with the citizens' rights of disempowered individuals or groups. The concept was introduced into public health to investigate conditions favoring the occurrence of HIV infection and AIDS. It takes into consideration and seeks to comprehensively integrate dimensions related to individual, social, and health-program aspects.

It is important to emphasize that health promotion strategies are operationalized through the disease prevention and risk control approaches described in the sections above. This can lead to prevention and promotion practices not being distinguished. The difference between them depends on a clear understanding of the limits of scientific concepts to deal with the uniqueness of experiencing health and disease by persons and social groups (Czeresnia, 1999).

Table 3 systematizes the approaches to health and disease presented in this article.

Citations

Boorse C (1977) Health as a theoretical concept. *Philosophy of Science* 44(4): 542–573.
Canguilhem G (1975) *Le normal et le pathologique*, 3ème edn. Paris, France: PUF (Coll. Galien).
Canguilhem G (1990) *La Santé: Concept vulgaire et question philosophique*. Paris, France: Sables.

Czeresnia D (1999) The concept of health and the difference between promotion and prevention. *Cadernos de Saúde Pública* 15(4): 701–710.
Dubos R (1987) *The Mirage of Health. Utopias, Progress and Biological Change*, 2nd edn. New Brunswick, NJ: Rutgers University Press.
Hinkle L (1987) Stress and disease: the concept after 50 years. *Social Science and Medicine* 25(6): 561–566.
Lalonde M (1981) *A New Perspective on the Health of Canadians*. Ottawa, Canada: Ministry of Supply and Services, Canada.
Leavell HR and Clark EG (1965) *Preventive Medicine for the Doctor in His Community*. New York: McGraw-Hill.
Lupton D (1999) *Risk: Key Ideas*. London: Routledge.
Mann J and Tarantola DJM (eds.) (1996) *AIDS in the World II*. New York: Oxford University Press.
Melzer D and Zimmern R (2002) Genetics and Medicalisation. *British Medical Journal* 324: 863–864.
Rosen G (1993) *A History of Public Health*, expanded edn. Baltimore, MD: Johns Hopkins University Press.
Rutter M (1987) Psychosocial resilience and protective mechanisms. *American Journal of Orthopsychiatry* 57(3): 316–331.
Susser M (1985) Epidemiology in the United States after World War II: The Evolution of Technique. *Epidemiologic Reviews* 7: 147–177.
Terris M (1990) Public Health Policy for the 1990s. *Annual Review of Public Health* 11: 39–51.
Thagard P (1998) Explaining disease: Correlations, causes and mechanisms. *Minds and Machines* 8: 61–78.

Further Reading

Kleinman A, Eisenberg L, and Good B (1978) Culture, illness, and care: Clinical lessons from anthropological and cross-cultural research. *Annals of Internal Medicine* 88(2): 251–258.
Susser M (1973) *Causal Thinking in the Health Sciences*. New York: Oxford University Press.

Global Burden of Disease

C Mathers, World Health Organization, Geneva, Switzerland

Introduction

A common approach for describing and quantifying the health of populations is to aggregate individual-level data to generate estimates of quantities such as the proportion of the population (or of a particular age-sex group) suffering from a particular health problem or dying from a specific cause in a defined time period. When we are interested in assessing all important causes of loss of health, the numbers of statistics that must be compared rapidly become large, and we also face difficulties in comparing indicators relating to different health states, mortality risks, or disease events.

Such statistics also suffer from several other limitations that reduce their practical value for policy makers: first, they are partial and fragmented. Basic information on causes of death is not available for all important causes in many countries, and mortality statistics fail to capture the impact of nonfatal conditions, such as mental disorders, musculoskeletal disorders, or blindness or deafness. Second, analyses of incidence, prevalence, or mortality for single causes often result in under- or overestimates when not constrained to fit within demographically plausible limits or to be internally consistent.

Governments and international agencies are faced with setting priorities for health research and investment in health systems and health interventions in a context of increasing health-care costs, increasing availability of effective interventions, and numerous and diverse priorities and interest groups. One of the key inputs to such decision making should be detailed and comprehensive assessments of the causes of loss of health in populations, that incorporates both causes of death, as well as the main causes of nonfatal illness and their long-term sequelae. Broad evaluation of the effectiveness of health systems and major health programs and policies also requires assessments of the causes of loss of health that are comparable not only across populations, but also over time.

The World Bank's 1993 World Development Report, Investing in Health, recommended cost-effective intervention packages for countries at different levels of development. Underpinning these analyses was the first Global Burden of Disease (GBD) study, carried out by Chris Murray at Harvard University and Alan Lopez at the World Health Organization (WHO), in collaboration with a global network of over 100 scientists. As well as generating a comprehensive and consistent set of estimates of mortality and morbidity by age, sex, and region for the world, the GBD study introduced a new metric – the disability-adjusted life year (DALY) – to simultaneously quantify the burden of disease from premature mortality and the nonfatal consequences of over 100 diseases and injuries (Murray and Lopez, 1996a).

Global Burden of Disease Studies

The initial GBD study was commissioned by the World Bank to provide a comprehensive assessment of disease burden in 1990 from more than 100 diseases and injuries, and from ten selected risk factors (Murray and Lopez, 1996a, 1996b; World Bank, 1993). Earlier attempts by Lopez and others to quantify global cause-of-death patterns had been largely restricted to broad cause-of-death groups and did not address nonfatal health outcomes.

The results of the original GBD study were surprising to many health policy makers, more familiar with the pattern of causes represented in mortality statistics. Neuropsychiatric disorders and injuries were major causes of lost years of healthy life as measured by DALYs, and were greatly undervalued when measured by mortality alone. More broadly, noncommunicable diseases, including neuropsychiatric disorders, were estimated to have caused 41% of the global burden of disease in 1990, only slightly less than communicable, maternal, perinatal, and nutritional conditions combined (44%), with 15% due to injuries. The GBD study stimulated a number of similar studies at national and subnational level, and also contributed to the setting of global health research priorities (World Health Organization, 1996).

Between 1998 and 2004, WHO undertook a new assessment of the global burden of disease for the years 1999 to 2002, under the leadership of Chris Murray, with annual assessments published in annex tables to the World Health reports. These were based on an extensive analysis of mortality data for all regions of the world together with systematic reviews of epidemiological studies and population health surveys, as well as incorporating a range of methodological improvements. Additionally, a major and expanded research program, the Comparative Risk Assessment (CRA) project, was undertaken to quantify the global and regional attributable mortality and burden for 26 major risk factors.

The WHO GBD analysis for the year 2001 was used as the framework for cost effectiveness and priority setting analyses carried out for the Disease Control Priorities Project, a joint project of the World Bank, WHO, and the National Institutes of Health, funded by the Gates Foundation. The GBD results were documented in detail, with information on data sources and methods as well as uncertainty and sensitivity analyses, in a book published as part of the Disease Control Priorities Project (Lopez et al., 2006).

The basic units of analysis for the first GBD study were the eight World Bank regions defined for the 1993 World Development Report. The heterogeneity of these large regions limited their value for comparative epidemiological assessments. For the recent GBD assessments by WHO, a more refined approach was followed. Mortality estimates by disease and injury cause, age, and sex were first developed for each of the 192 WHO member states using different methods for countries with different sources of information on mortality. Epidemiological estimates for incidence, prevalence, and years lost due to disability (YLD) were first developed for 17 groupings of countries, and then imputed to country populations using available country-level information and methods to ensure consistency with the country-specific mortality estimates. The resulting country-level estimates were made available by WHO at a summarized level, and also facilitated the production of regional estimates for any desired regional groupings of countries.

Analytic Methods

The DALY – Construction and Concepts

The DALY extends the concept of potential years of life lost due to premature death (PYLL) to include equivalent years of 'healthy' life lost from living in states of poor health or disability. One lost DALY can be thought of as one lost year of 'healthy' life (either through death or illness/disability), and total DALYs (the burden of disease) as a measurement of the gap between the current health of a population and an ideal situation in which everyone in the population lives into old age in full health.

DALYs for a specific disease or injury cause are calculated as the sum of the years of life lost due to premature mortality (YLL) from that cause and the YLD for incident cases of the disease or injury. The YLL are calculated from the number of deaths, d_x, at each age x multiplied by a global standard life expectancy, L_x, which is a function of age x:

$$YLL_x = \sum_x d_x \times L_x$$

The GBD 1990 study chose not to use an arbitrary age cutoff such as 70 years in the calculation of YLL, but rather specified the loss function L_x in terms of the life expectancies at various ages in standard life tables with life expectancy at birth fixed at 82.5 years for females and 80.0 years for males (**Figure 1**). The loss function was specified to be the same for all deaths of a given age and sex, in all regions of the world, irrespective of other characteristics such as socioeconomic status or relevant current local life expectancies.

Because YLL measure the incident stream of lost years of life due to deaths, an incidence perspective is also taken for the calculation of YLD. The YLD for a particular cause in a particular time period are calculated by multiplying the number of incident cases i_x, at each age x in that period, by the average duration of the disease for each age of incidence, l_x, and a weight factor dw_x, that reflects the severity of the disease on a scale from 0 (full health) to 1 (dead):

$$YLD_x = \sum_x i_x \times l_x \times dw_x$$

YLD are generally calculated either for the average incident case of the disease, or for one or more disabling sequelae of the disease. For example, YLD for diabetes are calculated by adding the YLD for uncomplicated cases and the YLD for sequelae such as diabetic neuropathy, retinopathy, and amputation.

Murray and Lopez chose to apply a 3% time discount rate to the years of life lost in the future to estimate the net present value of years of life lost in calculating DALYs. Based on a number of studies that suggest the existence of a broad social preference to value a year lived by a young adult more highly than a year lived by a young child or an older person, Murray also incorporated nonuniform age weights. When discounting and age weighting are both applied, a death in infancy corresponds to 33 DALYs, while deaths at ages 5 to 20 equate to around 36 DALYs (**Figure 2**). Discounting and age weighting essentially

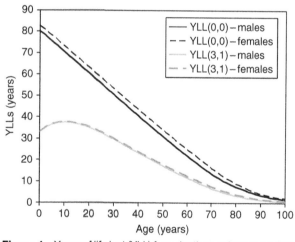

Figure 1 Years of life lost (YLL) for a death at various ages. The upper curves show the undiscounted, nonage-weighted YLL used in the calculation of DALYs based on the life expectancy at each age in standard life tables (Coale and Demeny West Model Level 26) with life expectancy at birth fixed at 82.5 years for females and 80.0 years for males. The lower curves show the effects of age-weighting and discounting on the YLL lost per death at various ages for males and females. YLL(r,K) denotes YLL calculated with discount rate r (%) and standard age-weighting (K = 1) or uniform age-weighting (K = 0). Reproduced from Mathers CD, Salomon JA, Ezzati M, Begg S, and Lopez AD (2006) Sensitivity and uncertainty analyses for burden of disease and risk factor estimates. In: Lopez AD, et al. (eds.) Global Burden of Disease and Risk Factors, pp. 399–426. New York: Oxford University Press.

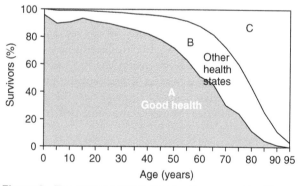

Figure 2 The relationship between health gaps and health expectancies in a stationary population. The health gap is area C + f(B) where f(B) is a function of B in the range 0 to area B representing the lost equivalent years of full health lived in states B. The health expectancy is the area A + g(B), where G(B) = B − f(B) represents the equivalent years of full health lived in states B. DALYs are the best known example of a health gap indicator; examples of health expectancies include disability-free life expectancy (DFLE) and health-adjusted life expectancy (HALE). Reproduced from Murray CJL, Salomon JA, Mathers CD, and Lopez AD (2002) Summary measures of population health: Concepts, ethics, measurement and applications. Geneva: WHO.

modify the loss function L_x in the calculation of YLL and the average duration, l_x, in the calculation of YLD. A more complete account of the DALY, calculation formulae, and the philosophy underlying parameter choices, is given by Murray and Lopez (1996a).

The 'valuation' of time lived in nonfatal health states formalizes and quantifies social preferences for different states of health as disability weights (dw_x). Depending on how these weights are derived, they are variously referred to as disability weights, quality-adjusted life year (QALY) weights, health state valuations, or health state preferences. Because the DALY is measuring loss of health (unlike the QALY that measures equivalent healthy years lived), the disability weights for DALYs are inverted, running from 0 (ideal health) to 1 (state comparable to death).

The original GBD study used two forms of the person trade-off method to value health states and asked participants in weighting exercises to make a composite judgment about the severity distribution of the condition and the preference for time spent in each severity level. This was largely necessitated by the lack of population information on the severity distribution of most conditions at the global and regional levels.

A Dutch disability weight study attempted to address this problem by defining the distribution of health states associated with each sequela using the EuroQol health profile to describe the health states (Stouthard et al., 1997). Using similar methodology to the original GBD study with three panels of public health physicians and one lay panel, this study concluded that it makes little difference whether the valuation panels comprise medical experts or lay people, as long as accurate functional health state profiles are provided.

Relationship to Other Summary Measures of Population Health (SMPH)

The DALY is one example of a time-based summary measure of population health that combines mortality and morbidity into a single indicator (Murray et al., 2002). Two classes of SMPH have been developed: health expectancies (e.g., disability-free life expectancy, active life expectancy, healthy life expectancy) and health gaps (e.g., disability-adjusted life years, healthy life years, etc.). Health expectancies extend the concept of life expectancy to refer to expectations of various states of health, or of the overall expectation of years of equivalent full health, not just of life per se (see **Figure 2**).

Health gaps are a complementary class of indicators that measure lost years of full health against some normative ideal (see **Figure 2**). Measures of potential YLL have been used for many years to measure the mortality burden of various causes of death. The DALY is one of several examples of a health gap indicator which extends the

notion of mortality gaps to include time lived in states with other than excellent health.

A health gap measure was chosen for the GBD studies because it allows the use of categorical attribution to attribute the fatal and nonfatal burden of diseases and injuries to an exhaustive and mutually exclusive set of disease and injury categories. The lost years of health (or DALYs) on one hand are additive across such a set of disease or injury categories. However, health expectancy measures, on the other, do not naturally lend themselves to disaggregation by categorically defined causes. Instead, counterfactual methods, such as 'disease elimination,' are required to quantify the contribution of disease causes to overall health expectancy measure, as well as for dealing with risk factors. Health gap measures also generally require counterfactual analysis to attribute the burden of disease to health determinants and risk factors.

Dealing with Incomplete and Partial Data

The GBD study developed methods and approaches to make estimates for causes of burden for which there were limited data and considerable uncertainty, to ensure that causes with limited information were not implicitly considered to have zero burden and hence ignored by health policy makers (Murray et al., 2003). The basic philosophy guiding the GBD approach is that there is likely to be useful information content in many sources of health data, provided they are carefully screened for plausibility and completeness, and that internally consistent estimates of the global descriptive epidemiology of major conditions are possible with appropriate tools, investigator commitment, and expert opinion.

This philosophy has remained central to the WHO updates of the GBD, which incorporated a range of new data sources both for mortality (YLL) and YLD calculations (Lopez et al., 2006). Despite this, there remains very considerable uncertainty in cause-specific mortality estimates for Africa and many other developing countries, and also for YLD for many diseases in both developed and developing countries (Mathers et al., 2006). To address criticisms about lack of transparency in the GBD enterprise, substantial effort was also put into documenting cause-specific analyses and the overall analytical approach (Mathers et al., 2006).

Estimation of Mortality Levels and Causes of Death

For the most recent GBD estimates at WHO, life tables specifying mortality rates by age and sex for 192 WHO member states were developed for 2002 from available death registration data (112 member states), sample registration systems (India, China), and data on child and adult mortality from censuses and surveys such as the

Demographic and Health Surveys (DHS) and UNICEF's Multiple Indicator Cluster Surveys (MICS).

Death registration data containing useable information on cause-of-death distributions were available for 107 countries, the majority of these in the high-income group, Latin America and the Caribbean, and Europe and Central Asia. Population-based epidemiological studies, disease registers, and notifications systems (in excess of 2700 data sets) also contributed to the estimation of mortality due to 21 specific communicable causes of death, including HIV/AIDS, malaria, tuberculosis, childhood immunizable diseases, schistosomiasis, trypanosomiasis, and Chagas' disease. Almost one-third of these data sets related to sub-Saharan Africa.

To address information gaps relating to other causes of death for populations without useable death registration data, models for estimating broad cause-of-death patterns based on GDP and overall mortality levels were used. The approach to cause-of-death modeling used for the GBD 1990 study was substantially revised and enhanced for the 2000–02 study to estimate deaths by broad cause group in regions with limited information on mortality (Salomon and Murray, 2002).

Data and Methods for Estimation of YLD

Estimating YLD requires systematic assessments of the available evidence on incidence, prevalence, duration, and severity of a wide range of conditions, often based on inconsistent, fragmented, and partial data available from different studies. Data sources included disease registers, epidemiological studies, health surveys, and health facility data (where relevant).

Two key tools in dealing with limited or missing data were to carefully screen sources of health data for plausibility and completeness, drawing on expert opinion and on cross-population comparisons, and to explicitly ensure the internal consistency of estimates of incidence, prevalence, case fatality, and mortality for each specific disease cause. A software tool called DisMod was developed for the GBD study to help model the incidence and duration parameters needed for YLD calculations from available data, to incorporate expert knowledge, and to check the consistency of different epidemiological estimates and ensure that the estimates used were internally consistent. **Figure 3** shows the underlying model used by DisMod (Barendregt *et al.*, 2003).

Around 8700 data sets were used to quantify the YLD estimates for GBD 2000–02, of which more than 7000 related to Group I causes. One-quarter of the datasets relate to populations in sub-Saharan Africa, and around one-fifth to populations in high-income countries. Together with the more than 1370 additional data sets used for the estimation of YLL, the 2000–02 GBD study incorporated information from over 10 000 data sets relating to population

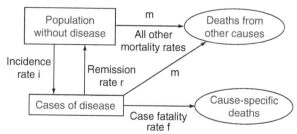

Figure 3 The basic disease model underlying DisMod. For a given population with specified all cause mortality rates, the three transition rates for incidence (i), remission (r) and cause-specific mortality (f) completely determine the prevalence of cases of the disease, and the average duration of cases. As well as calculating solutions when the 3 hazard rates (for incidence, remission, and mortality) are provided as inputs, DisMod allows other combinations of inputs such as prevalence, remission, and case fatality. In these cases, DisMod uses a goal-seeking algorithm to fit hazards such that the model reproduces the available input variables. DisMod may thus be used either to estimate parameters needed for YLD calculations (incidence and average duration) from other available epidemiological information, or to check the internal consistency of the various parameter estimates from available studies. Reproduced from Mathers CD, Lopez AD, and Murray CJL (2006) The burden of disease and mortality by condition: Data, methods and results for 2001. In: Lopez AD, et al. (eds.) *Global Burden of Disease and Risk Factors*, pp. 45–240. New York: Oxford University Press. Copyrights International Bank for Reconstruction and Development, The World Bank.

health and mortality. This almost certainly represents the largest synthesis of global information on population health ever carried out.

Latest Results

This section gives a brief overview of results for the year 2002 grouped in World Bank regions, with high-income countries grouped together separately. Diseases and injuries are classified in the GBD using a tree structure based on the International Classification of Diseases. The highest level of aggregation consists of three broad cause groups: Group I (communicable, maternal, perinatal, and nutritional conditions), Group II (noncommunicable diseases), and Group III (injuries). Group I causes are those conditions that typically decline at a faster pace than all-cause mortality during the epidemiological transition, and occur largely in poor populations. **Figure 4** compares the distribution of deaths and DALYs across the three groups in 2002 for high-income countries and low- and middle-income countries.

Global and Regional Mortality in 2002

Slightly over 57 million people died in 2002, 10.4 million (or nearly 20%) of whom were children younger than 5 years of age. Of these child deaths, 99% occurred in

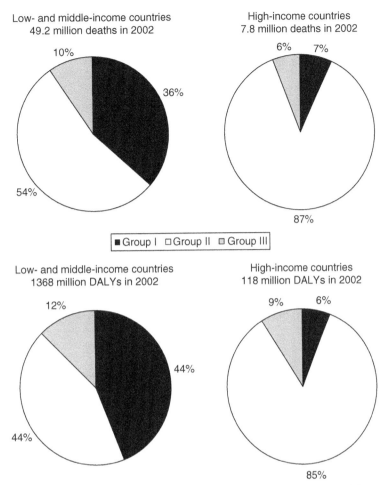

Figure 4 Distribution of deaths and DALYs by broad cause group, for low- to middle-income countries and high-income countries, 2002. Group I conditions include communicable diseases, and maternal, perinatal, and nutritional conditions, Group II conditions include noncommunicable diseases, and Group III includes unintentional and intentional injuries. Source: World Health Organization.

low- and middle-income countries. Worldwide, one death in every three is from a Group I cause. This proportion remains almost unchanged from 1990, with one major difference. Whereas HIV/AIDS accounted for only 2% of Group I deaths in 1990, it accounted for 16% in 2002.

The risk of a child dying before age 5 ranged from 17% in sub-Saharan Africa to 0.7% in high-income countries in 2002. Low- and middle-income countries accounted for 99% of global deaths among children under the age of 5 years and 85% of these were in the low-income countries. Just five preventable conditions – pneumonia, diarrheal diseases, malaria, measles, and perinatal causes are responsible for 70% of all child deaths (**Figure 5**).

In developing countries, Group II causes (noncommunicable diseases) were responsible for more than 50% of deaths in adults aged 15–59 in all regions except South Asia and sub-Saharan Africa, where Group I causes including HIV/AIDS remained responsible for one-third and two-thirds of deaths, respectively (**Figure 6**). In other words, the epidemiologic transition is already well established in most developing countries.

Table 1 summarizes estimated numbers of deaths and DALYs in 2002 for diseases and injuries causing more than 1% of global deaths or DALYs. Ischemic heart disease (IHD) and cerebrovascular disease (stroke) were the leading causes of death in both high-income countries and low- and middle-income countries in 2002, together responsible for more than 20% of all deaths worldwide (**Table 2**). Four of the top ten causes of death in the world are related to smoking (ischemic heart disease, stroke, chronic obstructive pulmonary disease, and lung cancer). In low- and middle-income countries, five of the leading ten causes of death remain infectious diseases, including lower respiratory infections, HIV/AIDS, diarrheal diseases, tuberculosis, and malaria.

Leading Causes of Disability

The overall burden of nonfatal disabling conditions is dominated by a relatively short list of causes. In all regions, neuropsychiatric conditions are the most important causes of disability, accounting for over 37% of YLDs

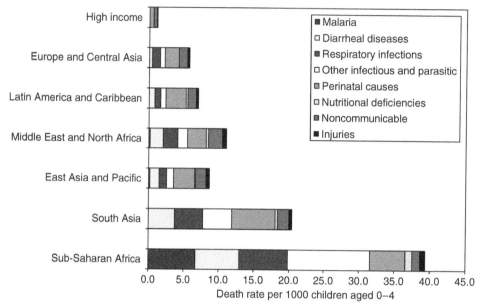

Figure 5 Death rates by disease group and region for children aged 0–4 years, 2002. For all the World Bank geographical regions, high-income countries have been excluded and are shown as a single group at the top of the graph. Source: World Health Organization.

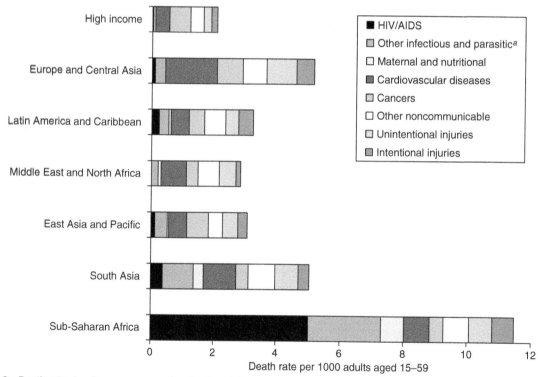

Figure 6 Death rates by disease group and region for adults aged 15–59 years, 2002. For all the World Bank geographical regions, high-income countries have been excluded and are shown as a single group at the top of the graph. [a]The category 'Other infectious and parasitic diseases' includes acute respiratory infections such as influenza and pneumonia. Source: World Health Organization.

among adults aged 15 years and over. While depression is the leading cause of disability for both males and females, the burden of depression is 50% higher for females than males, and females also have higher burden from anxiety disorders, migraine, and senile dementias. In contrast, the male burden for alcohol and drug use disorders is nearly six times higher than that for females, and accounts for one-quarter of the male neuropsychiatric burden.

Table 1 Estimated deaths and burden of disease by cause – low- and middle-income, high-income countries, and world, 2002 [a]

All causes	Low- and middle-income		High-income[b]		World	
	Deaths	DALYs	Deaths	DALYs	Deaths	DALYs
Total number (thousands)	49 164	1 368 156	7847	118 093	57 011	1 486 249
Rate per 1000 population	9.3	259.0	8.4	126.7	9.2	239.2
Age-standardized rate per 1000[c]	11.4	261.5	4.9	111.5	10.0	239.6
Selected cause groups:	Number (thousands)					
I. Communicable, maternal, perinatal, and nutritional conditions						
Group I Total	17 840 (36.3)	601 885 (44.0)	539 (6.9)	7162 (6.1)	18 378 (32.2)	609 047 (41.0)
Perinatal conditions	2428 (4.9)	96 798 (7.1)	30 (0.4)	1438 (1.2)	2459 (4.3)	98 236 (6.6)
Lower respiratory infections	3603 (7.3)	92 186 (6.7)	336 (4.3)	1303 (1.1)	3939 (6.9)	93 489 (6.3)
HIV/AIDS	2833 (5.8)	81 771 (6.0)	20 (0.3)	609 (0.5)	2853 (5.0)	82 380 (5.5)
Diarrheal diseases	1863 (3.8)	64 445 (4.7)	6 (0.1)	315 (0.3)	1868 (3.3)	64 759 (4.4)
Malaria	911 (1.9)	34 758 (2.5)	0 (0.0)	2 (0.0)	911 (1.6)	34 760 (2.3)
Tuberculosis	1550 (3.2)	34 454 (2.5)	15 (0.2)	149 (0.1)	1565 (2.7)	34 602 (2.3)
Maternal conditions	509 (1.0)	32 957 (2.4)	1 (0.0)	479 (0.4)	510 (0.9)	33 436 (2.2)
Measles	607 (1.2)	20 953 (1.5)	0 (0.0)	3 (0.0)	607 (1.1)	20 955 (1.4)
Protein-energy malnutrition	251 (0.5)	16 740 (1.2)	9 (0.1)	98 (0.1)	260 (0.5)	16 838 (1.1)
II. Noncommunicable diseases						
Group II Total	26 630 (54.2)	596 788 (43.6)	6843 (87.2)	100 291 (84.9)	33 473 (58.7)	697 079 (46.9)
Unipolar depressive disorders	11 (0.0)	56 474 (4.1)	3 (0.0)	10 588 (9.0)	13 (0.0)	11 (0.0)
Ischemic heart disease	5856 (11.9)	51 646 (3.8)	1340 (17.1)	7502 (6.4)	7195 (12.6)	5856 (11.9)
Cerebrovascular disease	4736 (9.6)	43 748 (3.2)	766 (9.8)	5708 (4.8)	5502 (9.7)	4736 (9.6)
Chronic obstructive pulmonary disease	2442 (5.0)	24 176 (1.8)	304 (3.9)	3873 (3.3)	2746 (4.8)	2442 (5.0)
Hearing loss, adult onset	0 (0.0)	21 978 (1.6)	0 (0.0)	3974 (3.4)	0 (0.0)	0 (0.0)
Cataracts	0 (0.0)	24 780 (1.8)	0 (0.0)	376 (0.3)	0 (0.0)	0 (0.0)
Alcohol-use disorders	67 (0.1)	14 767 (1.1)	23 (0.3)	5471 (4.6)	90 (0.2)	67 (0.1)
Diabetes mellitus	775 (1.6)	13 044 (1.0)	208 (2.7)	3121 (2.6)	983 (1.7)	775 (1.6)
Schizophrenia	21 (0.0)	14 631 (1.1)	2 (0.0)	1458 (1.2)	23 (0.0)	21 (0.0)
Asthma	212 (0.4)	13 333 (1.0)	28 (0.4)	1908 (1.6)	240 (0.4)	212 (0.4)
Osteoarthritis	2 (0.0)	12 163 (0.9)	3 (0.0)	2648 (2.2)	5 (0.0)	2 (0.0)
Congenital heart anomalies	249 (0.5)	14 508 (1.1)	12 (0.2)	802 (0.7)	262 (0.5)	249 (0.5)
Vision disorders, age-related	0 (0.0)	12 975 (0.9)	0 (0.0)	1127 (1.0)	0 (0.0)	0 (0.0)
Bipolar disorder	0 (0.0)	12 437 (0.9)	0 (0.0)	1467 (1.2)	1 (0.0)	0 (0.0)
Cirrhosis of the liver	668 (1.4)	12 233 (0.9)	117 (1.5)	1685 (1.4)	785 (1.4)	668 (1.4)
Trachea, bronchus, lung cancers	786 (1.6)	7751 (0.6)	456 (5.8)	3497 (3.0)	1242 (2.2)	786 (1.6)
Nephritis and nephrosis	561 (1.1)	7802 (0.6)	115 (1.5)	585 (0.5)	676 (1.2)	561 (1.1)
Stomach cancer	707 (1.4)	7061 (0.5)	142 (1.8)	1028 (0.9)	850 (1.5)	707 (1.4)
Hypertensive heart disease	783 (1.6)	6995 (0.5)	126 (1.6)	693 (0.6)	908 (1.6)	783 (1.6)
Liver cancer	514 (1.0)	6275 (0.5)	104 (1.3)	813 (0.7)	617 (1.1)	514 (1.0)
Colon and rectum cancer	365 (0.7)	3759 (0.3)	256 (3.3)	2051 (1.7)	621 (1.1)	365 (0.7)
III. Injuries						
Group III Total	4694 (9.5)	169 483 (12.4)	465 (5.9)	10 640 (9.0)	5159 (9.0)	180 123 (12.1)
Road traffic accidents	1071 (2.2)	35 158 (2.6)	118 (1.5)	3085 (2.6)	1189 (2.1)	38 244 (2.6)
Violence	536 (1.1)	20 373 (1.5)	22 (0.3)	780 (0.7)	558 (1.0)	21 153 (1.4)
Self-inflicted injuries	750 (1.5)	18 149 (1.3)	123 (1.6)	2327 (2.0)	873 (1.5)	20 475 (1.4)
Falls	320 (0.7)	14 876 (1.1)	71 (0.9)	1240 (1.1)	391 (0.7)	16 116 (1.1)

Note: Numbers in pararentheses indicate % of column total.

Source: World Health Organization.

[a]Within each major group, disease and injury causes resulting in greater than 1% of total deaths or DALYs are shown, ranked within each group by global DALYs.

[b]High-income countries are those countries with gross national income per capita of $9206 or more in 2001, according to the World Bank's 2003 World Development Report. This group includes the countries of Western Europe, North America, Australia, New Zealand, Japan, the Republic of Korea, Singapore, and four of the Gulf States.

[c]Age-standardized using the WHO World Standard Population.

Table 2   Fifteen leading causes of death, world, 2002

		Total deaths (millions)	% of total deaths
	All causes	57.01	100.0
1	Ischemic heart disease	7.20	12.6
2	Cerebrovascular disease	5.50	9.7
3	Lower respiratory infections	3.94	6.9
4	HIV/AIDS	2.85	5.0
5	Chronic obstructive pulmonary disease	2.75	4.8
6	Perinatal conditions[a]	2.46	4.3
7	Diarrheal diseases	1.87	3.3
8	Tuberculosis	1.56	2.7
9	Trachea, bronchus, lung cancers	1.24	2.2
10	Road traffic accidents	1.19	2.1
11	Diabetes mellitus[b]	0.98	1.7
12	Malaria	0.91	1.6
13	Hypertensive heart disease	0.91	1.6
14	Suicide	0.87	1.5
15	Stomach cancer	0.85	1.5

Source: World Health Organization.

[a]Includes 'causes arising in the perinatal period' as defined in the International Classification of Diseases, and does not include all causes of deaths occurring in the perinatal period.

[b]Does not include renal failure deaths attributable to diabetic nephropathy or cardiovascular disease deaths attributable to diabetes mellitus as a risk factor. Taking these attributable deaths into account, a total of approximately 3 million deaths are attributable to diabetes mellitus.

Vision disorders, hearing loss, and musculoskeletal disorders are also important causes of YLD, in both developed and developing countries (**Figure 7**).

The Burden of Diseases and Injuries

HIV/AIDS is now the third-leading cause of burden of disease globally, and the leading cause in sub-Saharan Africa, followed by malaria. Five other Group I causes also appear in the top ten causes for low- and middle-income countries (**Table 3**). Group I conditions accounted for 73% of the burden of disease in sub-Saharan Africa, and 47% of the burden in South Asia (**Figure 8**). In other low- and middle-income regions, Group I conditions account for a little under one-quarter of the disease burden. Total disease burden in Europe and Central Asian countries increased by nearly 40% over the period since 1990 and was higher in 2002 than for other developing regions of the world apart from South Asia and sub-Saharan Africa.

The epidemiological transition in low- and middle-income countries has resulted in a 20% reduction since 1990 in the per capita disease burden due to Group I causes (communicable, maternal, perinatal, and nutritional conditions). Without the HIV/AIDS epidemic and the associated lack of decline in tuberculosis burden, this reduction would have been substantially greater, closer to 30% over the period.

The burden of noncommunicable diseases accounted for nearly half of the global burden of disease in 2002, a 10% increase from estimated levels in 1990. Indeed, almost 50% of the adult disease burden in low- and middle-income countries of the world is now attributable to noncommunicable disease. The burden of disease in Europe and Central Asia was dominated by ischemic heart disease and stroke, which together accounted for more than one-quarter of total disease burden. In contrast, in Latin America and Caribbean countries, these diseases accounted for 8% of disease burden. However, there were very high levels of diabetes and endocrine disorders in this region, compared to others.

Road traffic accidents are among the top 10 causes of DALYs for both high-income and low- and middle-income countries. Violence is also the fourth leading cause of burden in Latin America and Caribbean countries. In these countries, as well as the Europe and Central Asian region, and the Middle East and North Africa, more than 30% of the entire disease and injury burden among male adults aged 15–44 is attributable to injuries, including road traffic accidents, violence, and self-inflicted injuries. Additionally, injury deaths are noticeably higher for women in some parts of Asia and the Middle East and North Africa, in part due to high levels of suicide and violence.

Applications of Burden of Disease Analysis

The GBD studies have provided a base or starting point for a number of analytic exercises to provide inputs to international and national health policy and priority setting. Apart from the application to health research priority

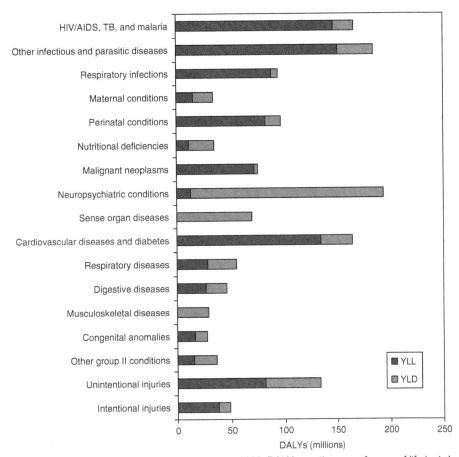

Figure 7 Global YLD, YLL, and DALYs for major disease groups, 2002. DALYs are the sum of years of life lost due to premature mortality (YLL) and years lived with disability (YLD). Source: World Health Organization.

Table 3 The ten leading causes of burden of disease, DALYs by broad income group, 2002

	Low- and middle-income countries				*High-income countries*		
	Cause	*DALYs (million)*	*% of total DALYs*		Cause	*DALYs (millions)*	*% of total DALYs*
1	Perinatal conditions	96.8	7.1	1	Unipolar depressive disorders	10.6	9.0
2	Lower respiratory infections	92.2	6.7	2	Ischemic heart disease	7.5	6.4
3	HIV/AIDS	81.8	6.0	3	Cerebrovascular disease	5.7	4.8
4	Diarrheal diseases	64.4	4.7	4	Alcohol use disorders	5.5	4.6
5	Unipolar depressive disorders	56.5	4.1	5	Alzheimer and other dementias	4.1	3.5
6	Ischemic heart disease	51.6	3.8	6	Hearing loss, adult onset	4.0	3.4
7	Cerebrovascular disease	43.7	3.2	7	Chronic obstructive pulmonary disease	3.9	3.3
8	Road traffic accidents	35.2	2.6	8	Trachea, bronchus, lung cancers	3.5	3.0
9	Malaria	34.8	2.5	9	Diabetes mellitus	3.1	2.6
10	Tuberculosis	34.5	2.5	10	Road traffic accidents	3.1	2.6

setting mentioned earlier, the GBD has also provided a population base for the calculation of the potential health gains through cost-effective interventions, and for the analysis of priorities for health interventions and investments in low- and middle-income countries (Jamison

et al., 2006; Tan-Torres Edejer *et al.*, 2003). Perhaps the major methodological advance has been in the quantification of the attributable burden for 26 global risk factors.

During the years 2000–03, WHO reported on the average levels of population health for its 192 member countries

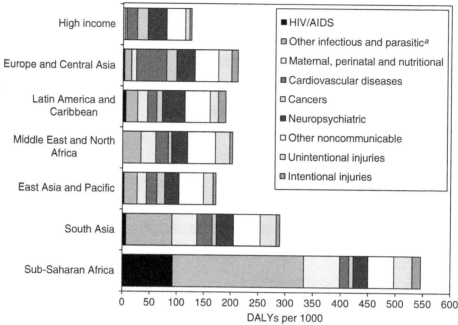

Figure 8 DALYs per 1000 population, by region and cause group, all ages, 2002. For all the World Bank geographical regions, high-income countries have been excluded and are shown as a single group at the top of the graph.[a]The category 'Other infectious and parasitic diseases' includes acute respiratory infections such as influenza and pneumonia. Source: World Health Organization.

using a health expectancy measure, healthy life expectancy (HALE). The HALE calculations were based substantially on imputed national-level data from the GBD study as difficulties in comparing self-reported health data across populations severely limited the information input from population-representative surveys (Mathers *et al.,* 2004). HALE was also used as one of the key outcome measures in WHO analysis of the overall performance, or efficiency, of national health systems (Murray and Evans, 2003).

Projections

The original GBD study included projections of mortality and burden of disease by cause, age, and sex for the eight GBD regions for the years 2000, 2010, and 2020. These projections have been widely used and quoted, and due to ongoing demand, WHO prepared updated projections to the year 2030 using similar but updated methods (Mathers and Loncar, 2006).

According to these projections, overall (age-standardized) mortality rates worldwide are expected to decline by 0.6–1.0% per year over the next 30 years, but at two to three times this rate for most major communicable diseases, the exception being HIV/AIDS. Indeed, by 2030, global HIV/AIDS mortality is expected to double from the 2005 annual toll of just under 3 million deaths. **Table 4** shows the projected ten leading causes of death globally in 2030. Total tobacco-attributable deaths will rise from 5.4 million in 2005 to 8.3 million in 2030, 11% of all deaths globally. The three leading causes of burden of

disease in 2030 are projected to be HIV/AIDS, unipolar depressive disorders, and ischemic heart disease.

National Burden of Disease Studies

The methods and findings of the original GBD study stimulated quite a number of national disease burden studies of varying scope and methodological rigor during the 1990s. The earliest comprehensive studies were for Mexico and Mauritius, followed by studies in the late 1990s in the Netherlands and Australia. In the last few years, comprehensive national burden of disease studies have also been carried out in countries such as Brazil, Malaysia, Turkey, South Africa, Zimbabwe, Thailand, and the United States, and studies are under way in Canada and several other countries. (A reasonably up-to-date list of references and links may be found on the WHO website; see section titled 'Relevant websites' later in this article.)

Criticisms and Controversies

The burden of disease methodology and the DALY have been controversial in the international and national health policy arenas, in the health economics and epidemiological research communities, and among disability interest groups (Fox-Rushby, 2002). Criticisms of the GBD approach fall into three main groups: (1) those concerned with the extrapolation of population health estimates in which data are limited, uncertain, or missing; (2) those concerned

Table 4   Projected leading causes of death, by income group, 2030

Both sexes			*Both sexes*		
Rank	*Disease or injury*	*% total deaths*	*Rank*	*Disease or injury*	*% total deaths*
World			Middle-income countries		
1	Ischemic heart disease	13.4	1	Cerebrovascular disease	14.4
2	Cerebrovascular disease	10.6	2	Ischemic heart disease	12.7
3	HIV/AIDS	8.9	3	COPD	12.0
4	COPD	7.8	4	HIV/AIDS	6.2
5	Lower respiratory infections	3.5	5	Trachea, bronchus, lung cancers	4.3
6	Trachea, bronchus, lung cancers	3.1	6	Diabetes mellitus [b]	3.7
7	Diabetes mellitus [b]	3.0	7	Stomach cancer	3.4
8	Road traffic accidents	2.9	8	Hypertensive heart disease	2.7
9	Perinatal conditions [a]	2.2	9	Road traffic accidents	2.5
10	Stomach cancer	1.9	10	Liver cancer	2.2
High-income countries			Low-income countries		
1	Ischemic heart disease	15.8	1	Ischemic heart disease	13.4
2	Cerebrovascular disease	9.0	2	HIV/AIDS	13.2
3	Trachea, bronchus, lung cancers	5.1	3	Cerebrovascular disease	8.2
4	Diabetes mellitus [b]	4.8	4	COPD	5.5
5	COPD	4.1	5	Lower respiratory infections	5.1
6	Lower respiratory infections	3.6	6	Perinatal conditions [a]	3.9
7	Alzheimer and other dementias	3.6	7	Road traffic accidents	3.7
8	Colon and rectum cancers	3.3	8	Diarrheal diseases	2.3
9	Stomach cancer	1.9	9	Diabetes mellitus [b]	2.1
10	Prostate cancer	1.8	10	Malaria	1.8

Reproduced from Mathers CD and Loncar D (2006) Projections of global mortality and burden of disease from 2002 to 2030. *Public Library of Science Medicine* 3(11): e442.

[a] Includes 'causes arising in the perinatal period' as defined in the International Classification of Diseases, and does not include all causes of deaths occurring in the perinatal period.

[b] Does not include renal failure deaths attributable to diabetic nephropathy or cardiovascular disease deaths attributable to diabetes mellitus as a risk factor.

about a number of issues in how the DALY summarizes fatal and nonfatal health outcomes; and (3) some well-known health economists who have argued that burden of disease analysis is irrelevant or potentially misleading for setting health priorities.

The GBD analyses have been criticized for making estimates of mortality and burden of disease for regions with limited, incomplete, and uncertain data, and have even been characterized by some critics as having at best only tenuous links to empirical evidence (Cooper *et al.*, 1998). Murray and colleagues have argued that health planning based on uncertain assessments of the available evidence – which attempt to synthesize it while ensuring consistency and adjustment for known biases – will almost always be more informed than planning based on ideology; there will be practically no cases in which we are totally ignorant about an issue to the point where there is no alternative to ideology (Murray *et al.*, 2003). The GBD analytic approach has been strongly influenced by demographic and economic traditions of making the best possible estimates of quantities of interest for populations from the available data, using a range of techniques depending on the type and quality of evidence.

The second group of criticisms has largely focused on the disability weights, social value choices such as age

weights, and on concepts of health incorporated in the DALY (Anand and Hanson, 1997; Williams, 1999). The DALYs have received a great deal of criticism from disability advocates and some health analysts, who have seen the inclusion of disability in the DALY as implying that people with disability are less valued than people in full health. Some of this criticism relates to claims that cost-effectiveness analysis imposes an implicit utilitarianism on policy choices, but a more fundamental criticism is that the conceptualization of disability found in the DALY confounds the ideas of 'health' and 'disability,' whereas in fact people with disabilities may be no less healthy than anyone else.

In response to these critics, the conceptual basis for the measurement of health and the valuation of health states in the DALY has been further developed and clarified (Salomon *et al.*, 2003). As used in the DALY, the term disability is essentially a synonym for health states of less than full health. The DALY is actually attempting to quantify loss of health, and the disability weights should thus reflect social preferences for health states, not broader valuations of 'quality of life,' 'well-being,' or 'utility.' Thus disability weights should reflect judgments about the 'healthfulness' of defined states, not any judgments of quality of life or the worth of persons. A high disability weight for a health state then implies that people place a high social value on preventing such health states or on provision of treatment interventions that replace them by states closer to full health.

The valuation methods used in the original GBD have also been criticized on the grounds that the groups used to elicit weights were not representative of the general global population, and that the person trade-off method used in the GBD is unethical, in that it involves hypothetical scenarios trading off saving the lives of people in full health versus saving the lives of people with specified health conditions (Arnesen and Nord, 1999). Subsequent GBD work on eliciting health state valuations has moved away from reliance on the person trade-off method, and has also made use of large representative population surveys, although a full revision of the weights used in the GBD has not yet been carried out.

Finally, some economists have expressed concern that burden of disease analysis might result in priority setting solely on the basis of the magnitude of disease burden and that burden of disease studies are irrelevant for priority setting (Mooney *et al.*, 1997). Although this view has little credibility among policy makers, who are generally very interested to understand the patterns of causes of loss of health in populations, and the changes in these over time, it is a misrepresentation of the purpose of burden of disease analysis. Both the original GBD study, and the later round of GBD work at WHO, have been accompanied by substantial efforts in cost-effectiveness analysis and an explicit recognition that health priority setting requires not only information on the size and causes of health problems, but also on the cost-effectiveness of interventions and on other information relating to equity and social values (Jamison *et al.*, 2006; Tan-Torres Edejer *et al.*, 2003; World Bank, 1993).

Future Priorities and Developments

While methodological and data developments over the past decade have improved the empirical base for disease burden assessment, there are still very substantial data gaps and uncertainties, particularly for causes of death and levels of adult mortality in Africa and parts of Asia. Improving the population-level information on causes of death, and on the incidence, prevalence, and health states associated with major disease and injury causes, remains a major priority for national and international health and statistical agencies.

The Bill and Melinda Gates Foundation has provided funding for a new GBD 2005 study, to be carried out over 3 years, commencing in 2007. The study will be led by the new Institute for Health Metrics and Evaluation at the University of Washington, headed by Chris Murray, with key collaborating institutions including Harvard University, the World Health Organization, Johns Hopkins University, and the University of Queensland. The GBD 2005 study will include a comprehensive revision of disability weights, and assess trends from 1990 to 2005, and will be completed in 2010.

As international programs and policies to improve health worldwide become more widespread, so too will the need for more comprehensive, credible, and critical assessments to periodically monitor population health and the success, or not, of these policies and programs. Repeated one-off assessments of global burden of disease do not provide comparability over time due to improvements in data and methods. There is a need to move beyond these, toward truly consistent and comparable monitoring of the world population's health over time.

See also: Measurement and Modeling of Health-Related Quality of Life; Methods of Measuring and Valuing Health.

Citations

Anand S and Hanson K (1997) Disability-adjusted life years: A critical review. *Journal of Health Economics* 16(6): 685–702.

Arnesen T and Nord E (1999) The value of DALY life: Problems with ethics and validity of disability adjusted life years. *British Medical Journal* 319(7222): 1423–1425.

Barendregt J, van Oortmarssen GJ, Vos T, and Murray CJL (2003) A generic model for the assessment of disease epidemiology: The computational basis of DisMod II. *Population Health Metrics* 1: 4.

Cooper RS, Osotimehin B, Kaufman JS, and Forrester T (1998) Disease burden in sub-Saharan Africa: What should we conclude in the absence of data? *The Lancet* 351(9097): 208–210.

Fox-Rushby JA (2002) *Disability Adjusted Life Years (DALYS) for decision-making? An overview of the literature.* London: Office of Health Economics.

Jamison DT, Breman JG, Measham AR, *et al.* (2006) *Disease Control Priorities in Developing Countries,* 2nd edn. Oxford, UK: Oxford University Press.

Lopez AD, Mathers CD, Ezzati M, Murray CJL, and Jamison DT (2006) *Global Burden of Disease and Risk Factors.* New York: Oxford University Press.

Mathers CD, Iburg K, Salomon J, *et al.* (2004) Global patterns of healthy life expectancy in the year 2002. *BioMed Central Public Health* 4(1): 66.

Mathers CD and Loncar D (2006) Projections of global mortality and burden of disease from 2002 to 2030. *Public Library of Science Medicine* 3(11): e442.

Mathers CD, Lopez AD, and Murray CJL (2006) The burden of disease and mortality by condition: Data, methods and results for 2001. In: Lopez AD, *et al.* (eds.) *Global Burden of Disease and Risk Factors,* pp. 45–240. New York: Oxford University Press.

Mathers CD, Salomon JA, Ezzati M, Begg S, and Lopez AD (2006) Sensitivity and uncertainty analyses for burden of disease and risk factor estimates. In: Lopez AD, *et al.* (eds.) *Global Burden of Disease and Risk Factors,* pp. 399–426. New York: Oxford University Press.

Mooney G, Irwig L, and Leeder S (1997) Priority setting in Healthcare Unburdening from the burden of disease. *Australian and New Zealand Journal of Public Health* 21: 680–681.

Murray CJL and Evans DA (2003) *Health Systems Performance Assessment: Debates, Methods and Empiricism.* Geneva, Switzerland: World Health Organization.

Murray CJL and Lopez AD (1996a) *The Global Burden of Disease: A Comprehensive Assessment of Mortality and Disability from Diseases, Injuries and Risk Factors in 1990 and Projected to 2020.* Cambridge, MA: Harvard University Press.

Murray CJL and Lopez AD (1996b) *Global Health Statistics*. Cambridge, MA: Harvard University Press.

Murray CJL, Salomon JA, Mathers CD, and Lopez AD (2002) *Summary Measures of Population Health: Concepts, Ethics, Measurement and Applications*. Geneva, Switzerland: WHO.

Murray CJL, Mathers CD, and Salomon JA (2003) Towards evidence-based public health. In: Murray CJL and Evans D (eds.) *Health Systems Performance Assessment: Debates, Methods and Empiricism*, pp. 715–726. Geneva, Switzerland: World Health Organization.

Salomon J, Mathers CD, Chatterji S, Sadana R, Ustun TB, and Murray CJL (2003) Quantifying individual levels of health: Definitions, concepts and measurement issues. In: Murray CJL and Evans D (eds.) *Health Systems Performance Assessment: Debates, Methods and Empiricism*, pp. 301–318. Geneva, Switzerland: World Health Organization.

Salomon JA and Murray CJL (2002) The epidemiologic transition revisited: Compositional models for causes of death by age and sex. *Population and Development Review* 28(2): 205–228.

Stouthard M, Essink-Bot M, Bonsel G, Barendregt J, and Kramers P (1997) *Disability Weights for Diseases in the Netherlands*. Rotterdam, the Netherlands: Department of Public Health, Erasmus University.

Tan-Torres Edejer T, Baltussen R, Adam T, *et al.* (2003) *WHO Guide to Cost-effectiveness Analysis*. Geneva, Switzerland: WHO.

Williams A (1999) Calculating the global burden of disease: time for a strategic reapprisal. *Health Economics* 8: 1–8.

World Bank (1993) *World Development Report 1993. Investing in Health*. New York: Oxford University Press for the World Bank.

World Health Organization (1996) Investing in health research and development. *Report of the Ad Hoc Committee on Health Research Relating to Future Intervention Options*. Geneva, Switzerland: WHO.

Further Reading

Murray CJL (2007) Towards good practice for health statistics: Lessons from the Millennium Development Goal health indicators. *The Lancet* 369: 862–873.

Relevant Websites

http://www.hsph.harvard.edu/Organizations/bdu – Burden of Disease Unit, Center for Population and Development Studies at the Harvard School of Public Health.

http://www.dcp2.org/pubs/GBD – Disease Control Priorities Project, Global Burden of Disease and Risk Factors.

http://www.globalhealth.harvard.edu – Harvard Initiative for Global Health.

http://www.who.int/evidence/bod – World Health Organization, Burden of Disease Statistics.

Disease Classification

R Jakob, World Health Organization, Geneva, Switzerland

Classifications are essential for science, as they define the universe of entities that are studied and highlight the relevant aspects of these entities. Internationally endorsed classifications facilitate the storage, retrieval, analysis, and interpretation of data and their comparison within populations over time and between populations at the same point in time, as well as the compilation of internationally consistent data. Populations may be nations, states and territories, regions, minority groups, or other specified groups.

In many areas of the world, a large proportion of the population has no access to health care provided by medically qualified personnel. In these areas, health care is often provided by lay or paramedical personnel and is based on traditional methods or elementary medical training. These same personnel also must produce the health information needed to indicate the existence of a health problem or to facilitate the management of health-care systems.

Use

The purpose of classifying diseases is manifold. In epidemiology and prevention, a classification of diseases is used to alert the health authorities to the emergence of a health problem (for example, an increase in cases of an infectious disease indicating the possible start of an epidemic).

Management of health depends on information about disease frequency for planning, operations, or evaluation. Knowledge is needed regarding diseases that cause high mortality and morbidity to allocate health-care workers, medications, devices, and facilities needed for treatment and prevention.

Available funds for providing health-care services and improving health are always limited. Statistics that are compiled with the aid of a classification of diseases allow spending the money in the most useful way for the population health. Prevention and health programs can be improved, for example, by analyzing differences between two regions in terms of maternal deaths.

There are many different diseases. In order to understand the disease pattern of a population, one needs to have a unique classification system so that the results can be displayed and reported in a systematic way. Agreeing on how to classify (group) diseases at a regional, national, and international level enables comparing results and merging such information into larger-scale statistics (Jakob *et al.*, 2007; WHO, International Classifications, 2007).

Principles of Classification

Statistical classification is a procedure in which individual items are placed into groups based on quantitative information on one or more characteristics inherent in the items (referred to as traits, variables, characters, dimensions, etc.) (Bailey, 1994).

Any classification groups information according to the detail relevant to a specific scope. Compromises have to be made in the specificity of categories of a classification in which several scopes have to be served.

Classification of diseases has to follow common classification principles (Bailey, 1994; Pavillon, 1998; Wikipedia, 2007):

- A classification of diseases must have a category for every disease. Some single diseases are represented by an individual category. Other categories may group together several diseases that have a relevant aspect in common.
- There must be no overlap between the categories. This means that no disease can be placed in two different categories at the same time.
- There must be at least one disease for every category; no category may be empty.

The categories of a classification of diseases may be designed to serve public health, epidemiology, and treatment and allow comparison of frequencies of diseases from the community level up to the whole world. A classification can best be implemented in systems for routine information collection, if it can be used in several settings, such as primary care, secondary care, for legal purposes, or policy making.

Public health could be described as the efforts organized by society to protect, promote, and restore the people's health. A classification of diseases that serves public health would be shaped to identify diseases in a way that allows formulation, monitoring, and improvement of public health interventions, such as CHOICE (CHOosing Interventions that are Cost-Effective). This project is a WHO initiative developed in 1998 with the objective of providing policy makers with the evidence for deciding on the interventions and programs that maximize health for the available resources. To achieve this, WHO-CHOICE reports the costs and effects of a wide range of health interventions in the 14 epidemiological subregions (world divisions based on geographical location and epidemiological profiles). The results of these cost-effectiveness analyses are assembled in regional databases, which policy makers can adapt to their specific country setting (WHO, 2007).

The Dimensions of Disease

There are several ways of defining an individual disease entity. There exists an international definition for 'health' – "a state of complete physical, mental, and social well-being and not merely the absence of disease, or infirmity" (WHO) – but none for 'disease.' In clinical medicine such a definition may relate to a phenotype (a set of symptoms, signs, complaints, and findings), which is recognizable clinically and which has a unique management approach. However, in public health the notion of a phenotype may be broader. Public health interventions may be aimed at the treatment of individuals or at a prevention program for a population and therefore any relevant costs should be taken into account. Aspects of cost-effectiveness have to be included (Giere, 2007; Jakob *et al.*, 2007; Ustun *et al.*, 2007).

The real world of diseases is multidimensional. A disease is defined through a set of dimensions:

- Symptomatology – manifestations: Known pattern of signs, symptoms, and related findings.
- Anatomy: The organ or organ system primarily affected by the disease, as 'ear' by 'otitis.'
- Histology: The changes in the tissues, such as 'adenocarcinoma' for a specific cancer that starts in a glandular tissue.
- Etiology: An underlying explanatory mechanism, as in infection by a virus.
- Course and outcome: A distinct pattern of development over time, as 'persisting over years' and having sequelae, as paralysis of a leg.
- Age of onset: Some diseases are different when they occur in children instead of in adults.
- Severity/extent: A heart disease can become manifest under physical exercise or at the slightest effort, or malignant neoplasm may be *in situ* or spread throughout the body.
- Treatment response: A known pattern of response to specific interventions.
- Linkage to intrinsic (genetic) factors: Genotypes, phenotypes, and endophenotypes.
- Gender: Some diseases affect only one gender.
- Linkage to interacting environmental factors.

Other personal factors, as pregnancy, young age, old age may be additional elements in the definition of a specific disease. Diseases may present differently and be treated differently whether occurring in a child, an adult, or a pregnant woman.

Multiple classification systems of diseases have been created. They are used in particular contexts. **Figure 1** illustrates the diversity in the example of a disease, adrenoleukodystrophy, for which several such classifications exist (Orphanet, 2007). For pragmatic use in public health, the emphasis of a classification would be its suitability for monitoring health programs and policy making.

Classifications and Terminologies

A classification involves clustering information according to logical rules. The way of grouping is driven by a

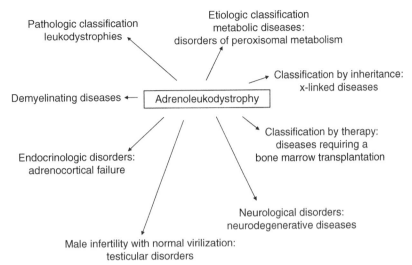

Figure 1 Several classifications for one disease. (With kind support of Dr. Ana Rath and Dr. Ségolene Aymé, Orphanet.)

specific purpose. Terminology contains information bits at higher granularity; for example, body parts, findings, or other elements that constitute a disease. With the aid of terminologies, information can be recorded at a higher level of detail. In a terminology, a disease can be defined, for example establishing linkages between its elements, such as anatomy or findings. Specific aggregation rules will even allow grouping relevant elements of a terminology (e.g., diseases) for specific purposes, thus creating a classification. Terminologies are able to retain the information without emphasizing any aspect of the recorded information. In contrast, classification allows identification of 'relevant parts' of the content, for example for public health. International agreement about these relevant parts makes sure that the aggregated information is internationally comparable. It does not matter whether an aggregation logic is incorporated in a terminology or displayed separately as a classification. The result will be the same: comparability. And international agreement processes are necessary in both cases – and should be the same as soon as the same question has to be answered by the aggregation/classification. Terminologies and classifications should be considered complementary.

Losing Detail – Gaining Overview

The detail retained and highlighted by a classification of disease will depend on what one wants to identify. ICD-10 categorizes external causes of disease or injury in Chapter 20, including 'accidents.' Specific aspects of an accident may be highlighted by grouping such an accident in one or another way:

The case: A car driver is killed when his car crashes into a tree as a result of driving with excessive speed. A classification of accidents may allow retaining different aspects of this case: the classification may categorize this specific case to 'car crash,' 'traffic accident,' 'excessive speed,' driver killed,' or killer-trees (or any combination of the above). The detail that one finally wants to retain will depend on the scope of the classification one is using. For example, retaining the type of the crashed vehicle ('car') would allow compiling statistics that potentially identify dangerous vehicles.

Groups in a classification are created in the way that each event can be assigned to one – and only one – category. Assigning them to two overlapping categories would cause double counts. It has already been noted that in a disease classification, every possible disease should be included in a group. Rare diseases might be grouped in a category named 'other specified diseases of . . .', imprecise disease descriptions may go into broad categories of the type 'unspecified diseases of . . .'.

In the field of diseases it may be challenging to decide upon the relevant detail to be retained. For example, a genetic defect may cause diabetes mellitus. The diabetes may lead to arteriosclerosis but also to kidney disease. Nevertheless, other diseases, as shown in **Figure 2**, can cause arteriosclerosis and kidney disease. It has to be decided which aspect is retained in the category of a classification. Recent approaches to classification of diseases allow adding information from several of the dimensions mentioned above to a disease category. In such a way, different views (serializations) of disease categories can be created, such as an anatomical or an etiological one. In addition, relationships between diseases and the different elements of the linked dimensions can be expressed, thus culminating in an ontology (National Center for Biomedical Ontology, 2007; National Library of Medicine, 2007; Wikipedia, 2007).

The information collected with a classification may be aggregated at a higher level for statistical presentation, thus eliminating varying levels of detail of the several

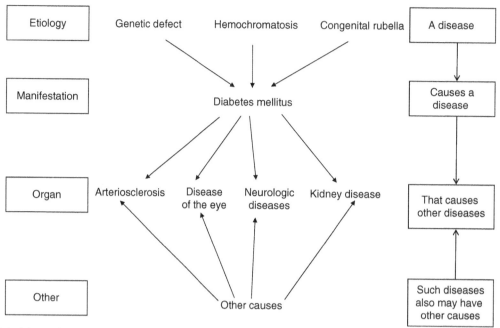

Figure 2   Principles and challenges in classification of diseases.

sources of data. Such aggregations are listed as special tabulation lists in the ICD. Different ones are used, for example, in the World Health Report, in international statistics on hospital activity, and Organization for Economic Cooperation and Development (OECD) reports (WHO, International Classifications, 2007). These lists should never be used for reporting – too much detail of information would get lost from the very beginning. Data comparison between data collections that use different aggregation logic may be challenging or merely impossible.

Granularity of the Categories

The size of categories of a classification of diseases and the facets of the original information that are vitally important to mortality and morbidity have to be defined. Doctors and health-care workers need detailed information to provide better patient care and prevent disease. Less detail is needed for resource allocation, reimbursement (case-mix systems) or broad prevention programs (screening and therapy), which may be of interest at the level, for example, of a government.

Reification – Unknown Etiology

Classification of diseases with unknown etiology differs from classification of other diseases. A set of challenges has to be faced. The scientific understanding of diseases for which nothing or little of etiology is known is usually in the early stages; there are rarely objective medical tests or

replicated risk genes. Such diseases are identified by symptom clustering, such as in mental disorders. (Most other diseases are defined by etiology and other known mechanisms; see 'Dimensions of disease'). The reliability of making such a diagnosis has to be balanced with its validity, for example, in clinical context. Reification of poorly validated entities impairs scientific progress and treatment development, and may have financial and political implications. However, standardization in this field allows for comparability in research and treatment approach. In mental health, the Diagnostic and Statistical Manual of Mental Disorders (DSM) (American Psychiatric Association, 2000) and ICD Chapter 5, 'Mental and Behavioural Disorders' (WHO, 1994), define diseases through symptom clustering, and thus allow compilation of statistics, comparative studies, and treatment guidelines.

Diagnostic Accuracy

The quality of information depends on diagnostic accuracy. The availability of diagnostic procedures is relevant to the certainty of a diagnosis. For example, in some settings, breast cancer may be diagnosed through palpation of a lump in a breast and a history of cachexia. In other settings, it is feasible to have a microscopic examination of the tissue and determination of genetic pattern.

Diagnostic accuracy relates also to the accuracy of a postmortem examination before the cause of death is reported. In some countries, postmortem may be carried out by nonmedical staff or may be limited as a result of legislation or cultural background.

The access to preexisting information about an ill or dead person (e.g., patient record) influences diagnostic accuracy. Interviewing friends or relatives who have been in contact with a person before he or she died may contribute to assessing the cause of death. Such techniques are called 'verbal autopsy' or 'lay reporting.' The method is used when no routine postmortem is available or the deceased was not attended by medical personnel during his or her illness (Shibuya et al., 2007). In classification of diseases it has to be decided whether the degree of diagnostic accuracy should be a dimension that is relevant to the aggregation logic.

Reporting

In public health, information on disease is frequently gathered in routine processes such as vital registration. The quality and standardization of reporting influences the outcome of the information collection. A classification of diseases has to acknowledge this fact in providing suitable categories, and has indeed been taken into account since the formulation of the first drafts of the ICD over 120 years ago. Furthermore, agreement has been achieved on standards for selection of the most relevant cause of death and a standard form for reporting the cause of death (WHO, 2007).

Political and Financial Aspects

In a classification of diseases, each disease is included as a specific code. Such a code may be used by physicians to specify a diagnosis, by insurance companies to provide payment, and by advocacy groups to promote treatment and prevention and to assure that new diseases are officially recognized. Health-care industries, such as pharmaceutical companies, develop products based on the characterization of diseases displayed in ICD.

Classification of Diseases and Health Information Systems

Mortality, prevalence, measure evaluation, reimbursement, pharmacovigilance, cancer control, rehabilitation, medical documentation, and resource allocation are a small sample of domains that inform a health system. Classification of diseases is just one element of this information framework.

A set of international classifications is designed to cover all domains of health. This is the WHO Family of International Classifications.

International Classification of Diseases (ICD)

The aim of the ICD is to categorize diseases, health-related conditions, and external causes of disease and injury in order to be able to compile useful statistics in mortality and morbidity. Its categories are also useful for decision support systems, reimbursement systems, and as a common denominator to be used in language-independent documentation of medical information.

The history of the systematic statistical classification of diseases dates back to the nineteenth century. Groundwork was done by early medical statisticians, such as William Farr (1807–1883) and Jacques Bertillon (1851–1922). The French government convened the first International Conference for the revision of the Bertillon or *International Classification of Causes of Death* in August 1900. The next conference was held in 1909, and the French government called succeeding conferences in 1920, 1929 and 1938. With its 6th revision in 1948, WHO became the custodian of the ICD. The ICD-6 extended the scope of the classification to nonfatal diseases, and WHO has continued to be responsible for periodic revisions of the classification. With a need to create comparability at the international level in public health as well as in clinical research, more and more clinical concepts have been introduced. The current revision, the ICD-10, consists of three volumes, and for correct coding all three volumes are necessary. Volume I contains the tabular list, as well as some definitions and the WHO nomenclature regulations. Volume II is the manual with extensive description of the classification and methods for use in mortality and morbidity, including short lists. Volume III is the alphabetical index. It contains separate indices for diseases, external causes, and drugs/substances.

Since its publication in 1992, an updating mechanism allows yearly updates and major revisions every 3 years. However, the structure and the content of ICD-10 are mainly based on scientific knowledge at the time of its creation, as well as on previous editions, and deserve thorough revision. The revision process toward ICD-11 started in 2006 for publication by 2015 (Ustun et al., 2007; World Health Organization, International Classifications, 2007).

ICD-10 can be looked up online in English and French at WHO (World Health Organization, International Classifications, 2007), and accessed in other languages through the relevant national institutions (WHO Collaborating Centres for the Family of International Classifications, 2007). Overall, ICD-10 is available in 42 languages.

Some countries have created clinical modifications for morbidity applications, principally as extensions of the international classification. Special adaptations have been created by medical scientific societies for clinical and research use in the relevant specialties (see 'Modifications and adaptations').

Implementation

ICD-10 has been implemented in the majority of WHO Member States as the standard for coding diseases in mortality and/or morbidity (statistics, reimbursement, resource allocation, administration, treatment, and research), and ICD is in the process of being implemented in many other Member States. For example, the ICD is used in systematic full mortality registration in more than 117 countries, as displayed in **Figure** 3. However, implementation is not easily defined, because it gives no indication of the level of use of ICD-10 within the whole health sector. For example, a government might decide to implement ICD-10 for coding mortality; however, this represents only a fraction of the use of ICD-10 within a health system, and use in morbidity may relate only to pilot projects or specific diseases. If a country has fully implemented ICD-10 at a national level, this would mean that it has mandated the use of ICD-10 for coding mortality and morbidity across the whole health sector, as in the UK, South Africa, and many other countries. This means that all health-care providers (or the appropriate allied personnel) will be required to code every death and every patient discharge, thus using ICD-10 for death registration, claims, and reimbursement purposes. In these cases, if the health-care providers do not use ICD-10 codes on their claims, their claims will be rejected.

Modifications and Adaptations

Although some countries found ICD sufficient for clinical reporting, many others felt that it did not provide adequate detail for clinical and administrative uses. Also, neither ICD-9 nor ICD-10 provided codes for classification of operative or diagnostic procedures. As a result, clinical modifications of ICD were developed, often along with procedure classifications.

In the United States the U.S. Department of Health and Human Services developed an adaptation of ICD-9, the ICD-9-CM (Clinical Modification) for use in health statistics and health sector reimbursement. The ICD-9-CM categories are more precise than those needed for mortality coding and for international reporting. The diagnosis component of ICD-9-CM is consistent with ICD-9 codes. A procedure classification for in-patient discharges, ICD-9-CM, Volume 3, also was developed. Based on the ICD-9-CM, the United States developed a patient classification system for reimbursement in the health sector, known as diagnosis-related groups. The ICD-9-CM has evolved over the past 30 years continuously, with annual updates. It is deeply integrated in reporting, retrieval, insurance, and reimbursement throughout the whole health sector. Several countries have adopted the U.S. reimbursement system and thus the ICD-9-CM

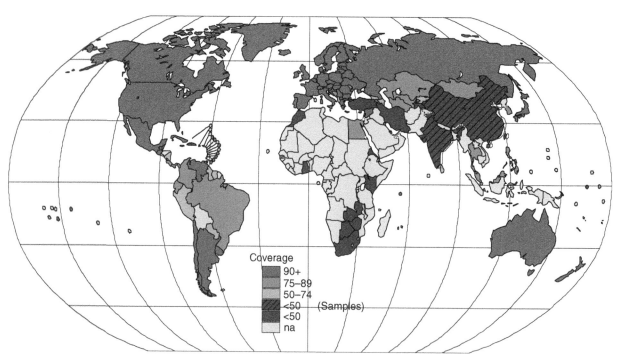

Figure 3 Registration of causes of death mortality (since 1995) with cause of death available to WHO.

in the context of their national health reimbursement systems, including Spain, Italy, Austria, Taiwan, Philippines, Costa Rica, and Guam (2007). Since 1997, an ICD-10-CM has been under development. It takes into account the evolution in medical knowledge and experience with ICD-9-CM, and provides more clinical detail; its adoption would solve the comparability issues between mortality and morbidity data, as ICD-10 has been used in the United States for mortality reporting since 1999. ICD-9-CM, Volumes 1 and 2, and ICD-10-CM (Clinical Modification) have been developed and are maintained by the U.S. National Center for Health Statistics (see Relevant Websites).

Australia adopted ICD-9-CM in 1994. In the following years, the ICD-9-CM was developed to meet the needs of the Australian health reimbursement system. In 1998, Australia developed its own patient classification system and changed to its own modification of ICD-10, the ICD-10-AM (Australian Modification). A classification of procedures was published at the same time (ACHI: Australian Classification of Health Interventions). In the past years, this complementary set of classifications was exported for use in reimbursement systems to several countries, such as Solomon Islands, Samoa, Fiji, Ireland, Romania, Slovenia, and Germany. The ICD-10-AM is maintained by the Australian National Centre for Classifications in Health (NCCH) (see Relevant Websites).

In 2003–04, Germany created the ICD-10-GM (German Modification) based on the ICD-10 AM for national in-patient reimbursement purposes. In contrast to the Australian approach, the system is designed to cover all specialties. The ICD-10-GM is maintained by the German Institute for Medical Documentation and Information (DIMDI, Deutsches Institut für Medizinische Dokumentation und Information) (see Relevant Websites).

In Canada, the Canadian Institute for Health Information (CIHI) (see Relevant Websites) developed and published an enhanced version of ICD-10 for morbidity classification in 2001, the ICD-10-CA, and a companion classification for coding procedures, CCI (Canadian Classification of Interventions). The ICD-10-CA replaces ICD-9 and ICD-9-CM in Canada for morbidity coding.

Clinical modifications for reimbursement or resource allocation also have been developed by other countries, such as France, maintained by the ATIH, and Thailand.

Adaptations of ICD for dentistry and stomatology, dermatology, mental health, neurology (NA), oncology (ICD-O), pediatrics, orthopedics and rheumatology, and other disciplines accommodate the need for more detail in these specialties (WHO, International Classifications, 2007).

See also: Concepts of Health and Disease; Demography, Epidemiology and Public Health; Surveillance of Disease.

Citations

American Psychiatric Association (2000) *Diagnostic and Statistical Manual of Mental Disorders*, rev. 4th edn. Washington, DC: APA.

Bailey KD (1994) Typologies and taxonomies: An introduction to classification techniques. In: *Sage University Papers Series on Quantitative Applications in the Social Sciences*, pp. 7–102. Thousand Oaks, CA: Sage.

Giere W (2007) Classification in Medicine [Klassifikation in der Medizin]. In: *Bundesgesundheitsblatt* Vol. 50. Berlin/Heidelberg: Springer.

Jakob R, Ustun B, *et al.* (2007) The WHO Family of international classifications. *Bundesgesundheitsblatt* Vol. 50. Berlin/Heidelberg: Springer.

National Center for Biomedical Ontology (2007) http://www.bioontology.org (accessed January 2008).

National Library of Medicine (2007) *Mesh, NLM classification.* http://www.nlm.nih.gov (accessed January 2008).

Orphanet (2007) *Rare Diseases, Different Classifications.* http://www.orpha.net (accessed January 2008).

Pavillon G (ed.) (1998) *Challenges of the International Health Related Classifications.* [Enjeux des classifications internationals en sante] Paris, France: Edition Inserm.

Shibuya K, *et al.* (2007) Setting international standards for verbal autopsy. *Bulletin of the World Health Organization* 85(8): 569–648.

Ustun B, Jakob R, *et al.* (2007) ICD; *Revision Process: Towards ICD-11.* extranet.who.int/icdrevision/help/docs/ICDRevision.pdf (accessed November 2007).

Wikipedia (2007) Classifications. http://www.wikipedia.org (accessed January 2008).

World Health Organization (1994) *International Statistical Classification of Diseases and Related Health Problems.* (10th edn.). Geneva, Switzerland: WHO.

World Health Organization (2007) *Choosing Interventions that Are Cost-Effective.* http://www.who.int/choice/ (accessed January 2008).

World Health Organization, Collaborating Centres for the Family of International Classifications (2007) http://www.who.int/classifications/network/collaborating (accessed January 2008).

World Health Organization, International Classifications (2007) *ICD and Other Classifications of the WHO Family of International Classifications.* http://www.who.int/classifications (accessed January 2008).

Relevant Websites

http://www.who.int/classifications – WHO Classifications.

http://www3.fhs.usyd.edu.au/ncchwww/site/ – Australian National Centre for Classifications in Health, NCCH.

http://secure.cihi.ca/cihiweb/splash.html – Canadian Institute for Health Information (CIHI).

http://www.dimdi.de/static/en/index.html – German Institute for Medical Documentation and Information, DIMDI.

http://www.cdc.gov/nchs/icd9.htm – U.S. National Center for Health Statistics, NCHS.

Classification of Mental Disorders

T B Üstün, World Health Organization, Geneva, Switzerland

Introduction

The diagnosis and classification of mental disorders has been a controversial issue throughout history. Multiple philosophical and theoretical approaches have been put forward to understand the nature of mental disorders in their various forms and types. Only in the last half of the twentieth century have systematic efforts toward an operational classification enabled scientific studies regarding the description, possible causes, and treatment responses to mental disorders. A common way of defining, describing, naming, and classifying mental disorders was made possible by the International Classification of Diseases (ICD) Mental Disorders (World Health Organization, 1992, 1993) developed by the World Health Organization and also the Diagnostic and Statistical Manual (DSM) of Mental Disorders (American Psychiatric Association, 1994). General acceptance of the ICD and DSM rests on the merits of their descriptive and operational approach toward diagnosis (Stengel, 1959). Operational criteria are logical descriptive statements about the clinical features of the disorders, which can be observed or measured if possible, and as a whole identify similar groups of disorders. These classifications have greatly facilitated practice, teaching, and research by distinguishing the mental illnesses from each other. The absence of etiological information linked to brain physiology, however, has limited the understanding of mental illness.

Classification of mental disorders creates great interest because it offers a synthesis of our current knowledge of mental disorders. A classification represents a way of seeing the whole spectrum of mental disorders and hence provides a general overview. As an accepted standard of theory and knowledge, a classification reflects both the nature of mental disorders and our approach to knowing them. The classification of mental disorders may thus yield some knowledge about the essence of the underlying mechanisms of mental disorders and it may offer some clues toward an understanding of how the brain works. At the same time, the organization of the classification may reflect the conceptual path of how we know and group various mental disorders. Having all this knowledge organized in a classification presents a challenge in terms of consistency and coherence. It also helps us to identify the limits of our knowledge and leads to further research on unresolved issues.

Uses of Mental Health Classifications

Classification of mental disorders has traditionally started from practical efforts to seek similarities and differences among patient groups. Today its greatest use is for administrative and reimbursement purposes. In addition, researchers use mental disorder classifications to identify homogeneous groups of patient populations so as to explore their characteristics and possible determinants of mental illness such as the cause, treatment response, and outcome. Use of mental disorder classifications has also gained importance as a guide in teaching and clinical practice. Earlier practice of psychiatry and behavioral medicine was mainly based on clinical judgment and speculative theories about etiology; the introduction of operational diagnostics has demystified aspects of various practices: Identification of a clinical feature should be defined, observed, and if possible measured in a similar way independent of the assessor. One of the greatest achievements of mental disorder classifications so far has been understanding that mental illnesses could be explained as brain dysfunctions. For example, schizophrenia, which was seen as a myth or a societal label, was defined as an integration of mental functions originating in the brain: Errors in thought processing, for example, result in this mental disorder.

Epistemological State of Mental Health Classifications

The current classifications of mental disorders have largely been built on observation of so-called pathological human behaviors or deviant mental states. They identify patterns of signs or symptoms that are observable and relatively stable over time, across different cultural settings, that can be informed by new knowledge of the way the mind and brain work. Such a classification is a reflection of (a) natural observable phenomena; (b) cultural ways of understanding these; and (c) the social context in which these experiences occur. Since one of the major purposes of a diagnostic classification is to help clinicians communicate with each other by identifying patterns linked to disability, interventions, and outcomes, these classifications have often evolved based on the sorting techniques that clinicians use. All psychiatric classifications are therefore human tools intended for use within a social system. Therefore in thinking about the classification of mental

Table 1 Timeline of landmark events in psychiatric classification in the twentieth century

Late nineteenth century	Human-rights-based treatment of mentally ill (Pinel, Tuke, Rush and others)
1895	Freud asserts mental disorders are caused by the unconscious mechanisms and uses the psychoanalytic method for assessment and therapy
1910	Watson and Skinner founded behaviorism, which advocates the use of experimental procedures to study observable behavior in relation to the environment
1917	Precursor of DSM: the American Medico-Psychological Association and the United States Bureau of the Census produced the statistical manual including 59 mental illnesses to classify mental inpatients
1922	Krapelin stressed the likely physiological causes of mental disorders and their study through well-defined tests and measurements
1930	ECT was introduced as a reliable method to treat depression
1948	ICD-6 and DSM-I (1952) listing 106 mental illnesses
1955	Major psychotropic drugs introduced to alleviate symptoms of mental illness
1959	Stengel: quest for operational criteria
1960	Deinstitutionalization of mental patients started in Italy, United States, UK
1967	Lin et al.: WHO Programme on Diagnosis of Mental Disorders
1968	ICD-8 and DSM-II
1970	Robins and Guze criteria for validity of mental disorders, including clinical description (symptom clusters); laboratory studies; treatment response; family studies and long-term follow-up
1980	DSM-III: fulfilling Stengel's operational criteria quest and paralleling ICD-9 from 1975
1994	ICD-10 and DSM-IV: following a 5-year global collaborative effort

disorders, multiple factors need to be taken into account, simply because our understanding of genetics, physiology, individual development, behavioral patterns, interpersonal relations, family structures, social changes, and cultural factors all affect how we think about a classification. The twentieth century was marked by several distinct phases in the way mental phenomena and disorders have come to be understood (see **Table 1**). The determinism of psychoanalysis and early behaviorism has been superseded by the logical empiricism of biological psychiatry that is searching for the underpinnings of human behavior in the brain in particular and in human biology in general.

Our current knowledge of psychiatric disorders remains limited because of the lack of disease-specific markers and is largely based on observation of concurrent behavioral and psychological phenomena, on response to pharmacological and other treatments, and on data on the familial aggregation of these elements. The task of creating a universal classification of mental disorders is, therefore, a very challenging one that seeks to integrate a variety of findings within a unifying conceptual framework.

ICD-10 System of Classification of Mental Disorders

The International Classification of Diseases (ICD) is the result of an effort to create a universal diagnostic system that began at an international statistical congress in 1853 with an agreement to prepare the causes of death for common international use. Subsequently, periodic revisions were made and, in 1948, when the World Health Organization was formed, the 6th revision of the ICD was produced. Since this date, Member States have decided to use the ICD in their national health statistics. The 6th revision of the ICD for the first time contained a separate section on mental disorders. Since then, extensive efforts have been undertaken to better define mental disorders. Work on the ICD Chapter V for mental disorders has been significantly supported by international work, mainly by the development of the Diagnostic and Statistical Manual (DSM) of Mental Disorders (American Psychiatric Association, 1994). There has been a synchrony between ICD 6 and DSM I, ICD 8 and DSM II, ICD-9 and DSM III, and ICD-10 and DSM IV, with increasing harmony and consistency between the two thanks to the international collaboration between WHO, APA, WPA, and a large network of international collaborative centers. Similarly, work on national classificatory systems, such as the Chinese Classification of Mental Disorders (CCMD) in China, The Latin American Guide for Psychiatric Diagnosis, and the Cuban Glossary of Psychiatry have been standardized with ICD-10 Chapter V, forming a useful internationally comparable yet culturally adapted system.

In the most recent 10th revision of the International Classification of Diseases (ICD-10), the mental disorders chapter has been considerably expanded and several different descriptions are available for the diagnostic categories: The clinical description and diagnostic guidelines (CDDG) (World Health Organization, 1992), a set of diagnostic criteria for research (DCR) (World Health Organization, 1993), diagnostic and management guidelines for mental disorders in primary care (PC) (World Health Organization, 1996), a pocket guide (Cooper, 1994), a multiaxial version (World Health

Organization, 1997), and a lexicon (World Health Organization, 1989). These interrelated components all share a common foundation of ICD grouping and definitions yet differentiate to meet the needs of different users.

In the ICD-10, explicit diagnostic criteria and rule-based classification have replaced the art of diagnosis with a reliable and replicable descriptive scheme that has considerable predictive validity in terms of effective interventions. Its development has relied on international consultation and has been linked to the development of assessment instruments. The mental disorders chapter of the ICD-10 has undergone extensive testing in two phases to evaluate the CDDG (Sartorius *et al.*, 1993) as well as the DCR (Sartorius *et al.*, 1995) and agreement between different assessors as measured by the kappa statistic for most categories was over 0.70, indicating very good agreement. Low agreement categories were later revised so as to improve the reliable use of the classification.

Main Principles and Concepts for Classification of Mental Disorders

The new classification systems have generally greatly facilitated teaching, clinical practice, scientific research, and communication. These improvements depend on better definition of concepts and application of certain principles such as definition of the unit of classification; identification of thresholds between wellness and illness; clinical significance and utility; classification style and other factors. These concepts and principles are briefly described below.

Unit of Classification: Definition of Mental Disorder

While ICD is a classification of diseases (or disorders in the context of mental illness), there is no explicit agreement on the definition of a mental disorder (or disease). Disease in general is now proposed by the WHO to be defined as a set of dysfunction(s) in any of the body systems defined by:

- Symptomatology and manifestations: Known pattern of signs, symptoms, and related findings;
- Etiology: An underlying explanatory mechanism;
- Course and outcome: A distinct pattern of development over time;
- Treatment response: A known pattern of response to interventions;
- Linkage to genetic factors, e.g., genotypes, patterns of gene expression;
- Linkage to interacting environmental factors.

The status of disorder is less well defined and it refers to a similar group of syndromes that share similar features usually without having a clear-cut etiological explanation.

This ambiguity creates a fuzzy boundary between wellness and arbitrarily defined disorder. At the lowest level, a mental disorder is an identifiable and distinct set of signs and symptoms that commonly produce disability, and that the healers in the society claim to be able to ameliorate through various interventions. While practical, such a definition can lead to error; for example, homosexuality was once defined as a mental disorder.

The answer to the question 'What is a disorder?' needs to be evaluated against rigorous scientific standards rather than just from societal or personal points of view. Robins and Guze (1970) in their classic paper proposed five phases for establishing the validity of psychiatric diagnosis: Clinical description, laboratory studies, delimitation from other disorders, follow-up study to show diagnostic homogeneity over time, and family study to demonstrate the familial aggregation of the syndrome. Experience gathered since then shows that some of these criteria lead to contradictory conclusions. For example, if one wants to define schizophrenia by its diagnostic stability over time, the best approach is to define the illness at the very outset by a duration criterion of 6 months of continuous illness, which tends to select for subjects with a poor outcome. In contrast, the familial aggregation of schizophrenia is best demonstrated when the notion of the disorder is broadened to include the notion of schizotaxia – a broad-spectrum notion that views the predisposition to schizophrenia to be characterized by negative symptoms (such as withdrawal, motivation loss, disorganized speech, and blunted effect, etc.) – neuropsychological impairment, and neurobiological abnormalities, and schizophrenia to be a psychotic neurotoxic endpoint in the process. The latter approach suggests that narrowing the definition of schizophrenia using the former strategy may in fact hinder progress in identifying the genetic causes of the disorder (Tsuang *et al.*, 2000).

Threshold for Illness

The lack of a definition of what is a disorder also creates an ambiguity. In many instances, for example, depressive disorders, the distribution of mental disorder symptoms forms a continuum in a population without a distinct threshold. This raises questions on where to set the threshold. Even when clinicians have agreed on an arbitrary expert consensus on the placement of a threshold, there remains a large proportion of so-called subthreshold cases that do not fulfill the criteria for a disorder but suffer from signs of mental disorders and display significant disability (e.g., inability to perform daily activities) (Hasin and Paykin, 1999). A good illustration is subthreshold depression. Perhaps the most common of psychiatric presentations in primary care, subjects with this diagnosis do not meet the diagnostic criteria for any depressive disorder in the classification systems and yet are associated with sufficient distress to lead to a consultation and have an impact on the person's functioning (Pincus *et al.*, 1999). There is a need to understand what establishes normal mood fluctuations in response to life events: Every person may react with sadness to the loss of a loved one, but may come out of grief in time by a homeostatic regulation of the mood. In some people, however, this homeostatic regulation fails and a disorder takes place. It is therefore necessary to know the exact nature and determinants of these events so as to clearly identify the disorder (Kendler *et al.*, 1992).

Clinical Significance

Use of operational descriptions has resulted in augmented numbers of cases identified in the community surveys. Similarly, the numbers of cases in clinical studies identified through research criteria but somehow not diagnosed by clinicians were also increased (Regier *et al.*, 1998; Spitzer and Wakefield, 1999). It has therefore been suggested that the criterion of clinical significance be used to define mental disorders. Clinical significance has two main components: (a) Distress; (b) disability. Distress is expressed by the subjects or their significant relatives in terms of worry, concern, suffering, and pain about the condition. There are many clinical cases, however, in which distress may not be expressed or be explicitly denied. The second component, disability, may usually be associated with diseases (as people who are ill cannot function properly in their daily functions), but not always need to be there (Ustun *et al.*, 1998). For example, a person may have tuberculosis with bacillus-positive status but may not exhibit any functional limitations. Similar examples could be given for HIV infection and other infections, noncommunicable diseases such as diabetes and hypertension, or any type of cancer. In all these conditions, diagnosis is conditional on the presence of a physiological disturbance and does not require any disability to be present. Hence, calling for the existence of disability (i.e., functional impairment in DSM parlance) is controversial because it creates an unequal theoretical position between so-called physical and mental illnesses. This issue remains a key target for further revision of current diagnostic classifications, ICD, and ICF.

The development of the International Classification of functioning, disability, and health (ICF) (World Health Organization, 2001) is an important landmark in this regard. The distinct assessment and classification of disability is a strong theoretical and practical requirement to refine the definition of mental disorders. The separate classification of disease and disability phenomena in ICD and ICF is likely to lead to better understanding the underlying body function impairments for mental disorders and associated disability. In this way, we would be able to describe and delineate the features of mental illness more clearly.

Classification by Syndrome Similarity

In the current mental disorder classifications, disorders are grouped by similarity of their clinical features. All substance-related disorders are grouped together, similarly as psychotic disorders, mood disorders, or anxiety disorders. An important grouping issue is about lumping and splitting. Different users have different needs and views regarding the level of detail of a classification. Usually, for primary care and initial clinical care uses, one needs broad categories of classification that lump relatively similar cases. On the other hand, some users search for even minor differences that may identify different aspects such as response to treatment. Current classification systems are debated in terms of whether the level of detail and the number of diagnostic categories are justified. Also, as scientific knowledge advances, we become aware that the current grouping of classifications may not fully fit neurobiology. For example, obsessive compulsive disorder has been grouped with anxiety disorders even though it has been shown to have a totally different neural circuit (Montgomery, 1993; Lucey *et al.*, 1997; Liebowitz, 1998). Similarly, despite the hair-splitting categorizations of anxiety and depressive disorders with complex exclusion rules, clinical and epidemiological studies indicate high rates of comorbidity and similar psychopharmacological agents prove efficacious in their treatment (Mineka *et al.*, 1998; Boerner and Moller, 1999; Kaufman and Charney, 2000; Kessler *et al.*, 2001). Despite the belief in distinct genetic mechanisms between schizophrenia and bipolar disorders, family studies have shown the concurrent heritability (Kendler *et al.*, 1998). Such examples will inevitably accumulate to identify paradoxes in grouping depending on the appearance or the essence (i.e., the underlying mechanisms).

Atheoretical Approach

The separation of the diagnostic criteria from etiological theories (i.e., what causes mental disorder) was an explicit approach undertaken to avoid being speculative, since these theories about causation had not been empirically tested. However this atheoretical approach has also been severely criticized because if one takes a totally atheoretical and solely operational approach, it may be possible to classify normal but statistically uncommon phenomena as psychiatric disorders, for example, one can propose to classify happiness as a disorder (Kendler *et al.*, 1992). Diagnostic categories have been proposed and accepted merely because of recognizable patterns of co-occurring symptoms rather than because of a true understanding of their distinctive nature that would make them discrete categories within a classification.

Classification Approach: Mind, Brain, or Context?

Recent progress in the cognitive sciences, developmental neurobiology, and real-time *in vivo* imaging of the intact human brain has provided us with new insights into the basic correlates of emotions and cognitions that should inform a new psychopathology. A better understanding of the neural circuitry involved in complex emotional and cognitive functions will accelerate the development of testable hypotheses about the exact pathophysiological basis of mental disorders.

Genetic sciences emphasize the interaction between the genome and the environment. This approach is important in understanding the plasticity of the human brain and how it malfunctions in mental disorders. There is not necessarily a molecular pathology for every mental sign, and there may be multiple paths that may explain the progress of gene expression through central nervous system function to emotional and cognitive constructs.

Progress in the neural sciences is already blurring the boundaries of the brain and mind, yet such a mind–body dualism as expressed in the organic versus nonorganic distinction in the ICD (but not in DSM) does have a utility. It directs the clinician to pay special attention to an underlying physical state as the cause of the mental disturbance. However, the term organic implies an outmoded functional versus structural and mind versus body dualism. Similarly, at the other end of the spectrum, cultural relativism can undermine efforts toward the meaningful diagnosis of mental disorders. The view that stigma and labeling can wrongly define a person as ill implies that mental illnesses are myths created by society. This has resulted in a devaluation of insights that are inherent in a cultural perspective. A similar danger of further dismissing the role of cultural factors in the causation, maintenance, and outcome of mental disorders exists when culture is seen as antithetical to neurobiology.

International Use: Need for Universalism and Diversity

Although some cultural elements have been included in the ICD and DSM, such as culture-bound syndromes, much remains to be done. There is a need to move beyond this because of the role that culture plays in the manifestation of mental disorders. Culture-bound syndromes reflect an extreme view and represent generally rare exotic cases, and provide little if any understanding of the complex interaction between culture and mental phenomena. There is a need for a better cultural formulation of diagnosis and for informed research to address the impact of culture on the explanatory, pathoplastic, and therapeutic processes. Unless typologies are formulated on the basis of careful research, sound theory, and clinical relevance, they are likely to be relegated to the status of historical artifacts.

Etic versus emic approaches

There is a fundamental dilemma with all international crosscultural comparisons: The need to provide an international common language without losing sight of the unique experiences that occur as a feature of living in different social and cultural contexts. There is a need to look for global, universal features of mental conditions, an approach that is driven by analysis and emphasizes similarities rather than differences. This etic approach relies on multigroup comparisons and is often carried out from a viewpoint that is located outside of the system. On the other hand, an emic approach emphasizes the local and specific interpretation that is more bound within culture interpretation. Although the etic and emic approaches are usually presented as opposites, perhaps a balance between the two approaches is in the interest of an international classification. The cultural applicability of international classification warrants careful consideration in future comparative research. For example, WHO's research on drinking norms definitely show differences in terms of thresholds of problem drinking and dependence in wet and dry cultures (Room *et al.*, 1996). Cultural differences in the meaning of mental distress may vary in different ways:

1. In terms of threshold, the point at which respondents from different societies recognize a disorder as something serious;
2. Whether the entities described in international classifications count as problems in all cultures;
3. In causal assumptions about how mental problems arise;
4. In the extent to which there exist culture-specific manifestations of symptoms not adequately captured by official disease nomenclature.

Categorical and Dimensional Models

There are two quite different ways of conceptualizing mental disorders: As dimensions of symptoms or as categories, often by identifying a threshold on the dimension. Clinicians are usually obliged to use categorical concepts, as they must decide who is sufficiently ill to justify treatment. But in our efforts to understand the relationships between social and biological variables, dimensional models are more appropriate (Goldberg, 2000). Dimensional models are more consistent with the polygenic models of inheritance favored for most mental disorders. These models assume that a number of genes combine with one another and interact with the environmental factors to cause the disorder. Persons can thus have various doses of the risk factors that predispose to the illness and depending on the dose, the severity of the manifest condition may vary along a continuum. Such approaches have been shown to provide important clinical advantages with psychotic illnesses (Ustun *et al.*, 1997) and personality disorders.

The Concept of Comorbidity

The concept of comorbidity becomes important when the classification logic posits discrete categories. Comorbidity, the concurrence of more than one diagnosis, does occur in real life and it is more the norm rather than the exception. The phenomenon of comorbidity poses a great challenge to the classification because it can be an artefact of hierarchical rules used in classification systems. Excessive splitting of classical syndromes into subtypes of disorders with overlapping boundaries and indefinite thresholds adds to the confusion. Though the co-occurrence of pathology in different subsystems of the body is indeed possible, it can either be attributed to the same underlying etiological cause affecting different body systems (as is the case, for example, with diabetes causing hyperglycemia, peripheral neuropathy, and nephropathy) or to distinct causes that just happen to co-occur (as is the case with diabetes and a lacerated wound following an injury). Further, the notion of comorbidity can only be accepted when the categories are not mutually exclusive, in order to avoid category errors.

Future of Mental Health Classifications

WHO's network on the family of international classifications has planned for an overall revision of the classification of diseases before 2015. Similarly, DSM has announced a revision by 2012. This period will allow for a more extensive knowledge base to develop and build up mechanisms so that such a knowledge base informs the mental health classifications. In particular, new information on genetics, neurobiology, and epidemiology can be used in an iterative process to update the categories, criteria, and grouping of disorders. A sound epistemological approach could be used to identify the disorder, disease, and disability. It is expected that future classifications should go beyond an expert consensus and reliability. Operationalization and reliability are indeed useful guides for classifications; however, they are not sufficient for validity. An evidence-based review mechanism and focused empirical testing for specific categorizations should be started. Underlying physiological mechanisms should be preferred for disease grouping instead of traditional conventions. Applicability and reliability of the new proposals for classification should be tested in field trials.

The ICD and DSM in their current forms are both descriptive classifications with operationally defined criteria and rule-based approaches to generating diagnoses. The efforts to harmonize the two classifications have left minor differences between the two systems. Currently, both systems are not entirely homologous, but in a large majority of criteria they are identical or differ in a insignificant ways in terms of diagnostic categories and criteria. Differences are most marked in the case of near-threshold, mild, or moderate conditions. Discordance is particularly high with categories such as posttraumatic stress disorder and harmful use or abuse of substances (Andrews *et al.*, 1999; Farmer and McGuffin, 1999; First and Pincus, 1999; van Os *et al.*, 2000). Substantive differences between the ICD and DSM also exist; for example, the ICD separates disability from diagnosis, and the ICD does not put personality disorders or physical disorders in a different axis.

Future classifications will be more than a common language between clinicians. First, the use of computerization in health records will require linkages between clinical symptoms, laboratory findings, and other features of diseases. A number of various domains will have to come together to build classification systems. Such a comprehensive integrated system will require identification of each entity and relations between them as a sound ontology-based system. Different use cases on clinical utility, quality of care, research, administrative reimbursement uses can be defined with different levels of granularity based on such a flexible system. Second, the health information should be shared by all parties, including consumers and providers, which will require more elaborate systems. Consumers and various care providers sharing the same classification system will require different levels of complexity, which is based on the same groupings expressed in different terms. In terms of comparison of views between different users, countries and across-time use of a common international classification is essential. The closer this system comes to the scientific evidence, the more reliable and valid its use between different agents will become.

See also: Population Measurement of Psychiatric and Psychological Disorders and Outcomes.

Citations

American Psychiatric Association (1994) *Diagnostic and Statistical Manual of Mental Disorders*, 4th edn. (DSM-IV). Washington, DC: American Psychiatric Association.

Andrews G, Slade T, and Peters L (1999) Classification in psychiatry: ICD-10 versus DSM-IV. Editorial. *British Journal of Psychiatry* 174: 3–5.

Bentall RPA (1992) Proposal to classify happiness as a psychiatric disorder. *Journal of Medical Ethics* 18: 94–98.

Boerner RJ and Moller HJ (1999) The importance of new antidepressants in the treatment of anxiety/depressive disorders. *Pharmacopsychiatry* 32: 119–126.

Cooper JE (1994) *Pocket Guide to the ICD-10 Classification of Mental and Behavioural Disorders, with Glossary and Diagnostic Criteria for Research.* Edinburgh: Churchill Livingstone.

Farmer A and McGuffin A (1999) Comparing ICD-10 and DSM-IV. *British Journal of Psychiatry* 175: 587–588.

First MB (2004) Clinical utility. *American Journal of Psychiatry* 161(6): 946–954.

First MB and Pincus HA (1999) Classification in psychiatry: ICD-10 v. DSM-IV. A response [editorial]. *British Journal of Psychiatry* 175: 205–209.

Goldberg D (2000) Plato versus Aristotle. Categorical and dimensional models for common mental disorders. *Comprehensive Psychiatry* 41(2 supplement 1): 8–13.

Hasin D and Paykin A (1999) Dependence symptoms but no diagnosis: Diagnostic 'orphans' in a 1992 national sample. *Drug and Alcohol Dependence* 53(3): 215–222.

Kaufman J and Charney D (2000) Comorbidity of mood and anxiety disorders. *Depression and Anxiety* 12(supplement 1): 69–76.

Kendler KS, Neale MC, Kessler RC, Heath AC, and Eaves LJ (1992) A population based study of major depression in women – The impact of varying definitions of illness. *Archives of General Psychiatry* 49: 257–265.

Kendler KS, Karkowski LM, and Walsh D (1998) The structure of psychosis: Latent class analysis of probands from the Roscommon Family Study. *Archives of General Psychiatry* 55: 492–499.

Kessler RC, Keller MB, and Wittchen HU (2001) The epidemiology of generalized anxiety disorder. *Psychiatric Clinics of North America* 24: 19–39.

Liebowitz MR (1998) Anxiety disorders and obsessive compulsive disorder. *Neuropsychobiology* 37: 69–71.

Lucey JV, Costa DC, Busatto GP, *et al.* (1997) Caudate regional cerebral blood flow in obsessive-compulsive disorder, panic disorder and healthy controls on single photon emission computerised tomography. *Psychiatry Research* 74: 25–33.

Mineka S, Watson D, and Clark LA (1998) Comorbidity of anxiety and unipolar mood disorders. *Annual Review of Psychology* 49: 377–412.

Montgomery SA (1993) Obsessive compulsive disorder is not an anxiety disorder. *International Clinical Psychopharmacology* 8(supplement 1): 57–62.

Pincus HA, Davis WW, and McQueen LE (1999) 'Subthreshold' mental disorders. A review and synthesis of studies on minor depression and other 'brand names'. *British Journal of Psychiatry* 174: 288–296.

Regier DA, Kaelber CT, Rae DS, *et al.* (1998) Limitations of diagnostic criteria and assessment instruments for mental disorders: Implications for research and policy. *Archives of General Psychiatry* 55: 109–115.

Robins E and Guze SB (1970) Establishment of diagnostic validity in psychiatric illness: Its application to schizophrenia. *American Journal of Psychiatry* 126: 983–987.

Room R, Janca A, Bennett LA, Schmidt L, and Sartorius N (1996) WHO cross-cultural applicability research on diagnosis and assessment of substance use disorders: An overview of methods and selected results. *Addiction* 91: 199–220.

Sartorius N, Kaelber CT, Cooper JE, *et al.* (1993) Progress toward achieving a common language in psychiatry. Results from the field trial of the clinical guidelines accompanying the WHO classification of mental and behavioral disorders in ICD-10. *Archives of General Psychiatry* 50: 115–124.

Sartorius N, Ustun TB, Korten A, Cooper JE, and van Drimmelen J (1995) Progress toward achieving a common language in psychiatry, II: Results from the international field trials of the ICD-10 diagnostic criteria for research for mental and behavioral disorders. *American Journal of Psychiatry* 152: 1427–1437.

Spitzer RL and Wakefield JC (1999) DSM-IV criteria for clinical significance. Does it help solve the false positive problem? *American Journal of Psychiatry* 156: 1856–1864.

Stengel E (1959) Classification of mental disorders. *Bulletin of the World Health Organization* 21: 601–603.

Tsuang MT, Stone WS, and Faraone SV (2000) Toward reformulating the diagnosis of schizophrenia. *American Journal of Psychiatry* 157: 1041–1050.

Ustun B, Compton W, Mager D, *et al.* (1997) WHO Study on the reliability and validity of the alcohol and drug use disorder instruments: Overview of methods and results. *Drug and Alcohol Dependence* 47: 161–169.

Ustun TB, Chatterji S, and Rehm J (1998) Limitations of diagnostic paradigm: It doesn't explain "need". *Archives of General Psychiatry* 55: 1145–1146.

van Os J, Gilvarry C, Bale R, *et al.* (2000) Diagnostic value of the DSM and ICD categories of psychosis: An evidence-based approach. UK700 Group. *Social Psychiatry and Psychiatric Epidemiology* 35: 305–311.

World Health Organization (1989) *Lexicon of Psychiatric and Mental Health Terms*. Geneva, Switzerland: World Health Organization.

World Health Organization (1992) *The ICD-10 Classification of Mental and Behavioural Disorders: Clinical Descriptions and Diagnostic Guidelines*. Geneva, Switzerland: World Health Organization.

World Health Organization (1993) *The ICD-10 Classification of Mental and Behavioural Disorders: Diagnostic Criteria for Research*. Geneva, Switzerland: World Health Organization.

World Health Organization (1996) *Diagnostic and Management Guidelines for Mental Disorders in Primary Care: ICD-10 Primary Care Version*. Bern, Switzerland: Hogrefe and Huber.

World Health Organization (1997) *Multiaxial Presentation of the ICD-10 for Use in Adult Psychiatry*. Cambridge, UK: Cambridge University Press.

World Health Organization (2001) *International Classification of Functioning, Disability and Health (ICF)*. Geneva, Switzerland: World Health Organization.

Relevant Website

http://www.who.int/classifications/icd/ICDRevision/en/index.html – WHO.

Population Measurement of Psychiatric and Psychological Disorders and Outcomes

T S Brugha and H Meltzer, University of Leicester, Leicester, UK

The measurement of mental and behavioral disorders poses three particular challenges. First, there are no laboratory or similar independent confirmatory diagnostic technologies; instead, the nature of these disorders requires the collection of subjective psychological information on inner states of feeling, thinking, and perceiving, together with, sometimes, reliable information on behavior over time. Second, nearly all measures involve a retrospective element that relies on recall, whereas ideally information should be collected prospectively, requiring a more costly longitudinal element. Third, there is the challenge of achieving external or criterion validity.

This article covers the principles of measurement in psychiatric epidemiology, including discussions around international aspects (e.g., cross-population issues, including excluded groups, and issues of culture), measurement of specific disorders, and application of measurement methods in public health contexts (e.g., surveillance and screening in health settings). Enormous progress has been made in developing and applying such methods, including their use in very large-scale international surveys in recent years. Policy and decision makers can now readily access the information they need but must first understand the potential and limitations of current measurement methods.

It is assumed that the reader of this article is already familiar with basic clinical measurement, epidemiological, and public health concepts. This article points selectively to the ways in which such concepts have been developed in relation to measurement and public mental health. In order to illustrate this with the most up-to-date examples, we refer to survey methods used in Great Britain to collect information for policy on children (Green *et al.*, 2005), adults, and older people (Singleton *et al.*, 2001), but we also refer to more widely known, similar methods used elsewhere in relation to studies of the adult population, including high-quality national surveys in low-income countries. Such surveys have generated not only official government and policy reports but also numerous articles in academic journals. The article begins with a discussion of the nature of mental disorder, study design and measurement issues, procedures and techniques, and the interpretation of findings.

Nature of Mental Disorder

For further reading please see Farmer *et al.* (2002).

Psychopathology

Concepts of psychopathology were first described in the clinical literature on severe mental disorders such as psychosis in the nineteenth century (Farmer *et al.*, 2002). Attempts to define these with a view to their reliable measurement developed in the following century (Wing *et al.*, 1974). Soon after this, work was extended to a wide range of mental and behavioral disorders to support the emergence of detailed mental disorder classification systems (World Health Organization Division of Mental Health, 1992; World Health Organization, 1992, 1993; American Psychiatric Association, 1994).

The psychopathology of mental disorders can be considered in terms of specific mental functions. Emotion

in the form of mood and anxiety is given prominence in such systems with relatively little attention given to other emotions such as anger or happiness (except in the form of inappropriate elation in mania or bipolar disorder). Abnormalities of the experience and perception of reality in the form of psychotic hallucinations is given prominence, together with beliefs that are clearly false and not shared with another person (in contrast to subculturally approved beliefs). Cognitive impairment as seen in mental retardation (also known as learning disability or as intellectual disability) and dementia also receive prominence. Problems due to misuse of psychoactive drugs and their effects on mental functioning have taken greater prominence in recent years. New areas hardly touched on in surveys include developmental, behavioral, and personality abnormalities.

Definition and Classification of Disorders

Until now the official classification systems (American Psychiatric Association, 1994; World Health Organization Division of Mental Health, 1990) have relied exclusively on binary definitions of disorders (Brugha, 2002): either the person has or does not have the disorder. This has been an enormously important and successful development in helping mental disorders to be considered and included in general health policy debates. However, critics have questioned the large number of categories of mental disorder, most of which would not register in surveys of public mental health in the general population anyway. Furthermore, the underlying nature of common mental disorder is likely to be dimensional without obvious cut points representing a diagnostic threshold (**Figure 1**). Dimensional approaches are, however, promised in future revisions of the classification system. Even within the ICD-10 system, depression is described in terms of levels of severity. Subthreshold levels are likely to be given greater prominence in the future in much the same way that clinical medicine increasingly recognizes the significance of lower levels of blood pressure or of serum lipids in terms of prediction of future morbidity. A stepped-care approach to the management of depression that uses these different levels of severity is already officially recommended in Great Britain by the National Institute for Health and Clinical Excellence. This is important for policymakers to consider because it implies that most (but not all) published prevalence tables for depressive disorder do not take into account such clinically significant distinctions.

Purposes of epidemiological methods (epidemiological estimates, modeling determinants, treatment planning, and needs assessment)

It makes sense that any data collection using epidemiological methods should be preceded by a careful

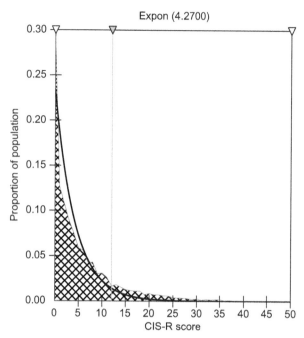

Figure 1 Proportion of population by full range of common mental disorder (CIS-R) scores, and fitted exponential curve. (Goodness of fit (RMS error) test statistic = 0.029E-04.) From Melzer D, Tom B, Brugha T, Fryers T, and Meltzer H (2002) Common mental disorder symptom counts in populations: Are there distinct case groups above epidemiological cutoffs? *Psychological Medicine* 32: 1195–1201.

consideration of the purposes for which they will be used. Yet convention often seems to overtake such considerations.

A key question should be whether the purpose is research, audit, or surveillance. Research should aim to answer a key question and related subsidiary questions and should be designed and planned as such. The purpose of audit is to improve a process or service by examining its functioning against defined objectives and standards; audit should not be carried out without inclusion of a process for correcting flaws in the process or service being audited. Surveillance is similar to audit but is designed to monitor trends in populations over time and to alert decision makers to any changes that require early or urgent action.

A further difficulty may lie in a misunderstanding of the differences between clinical and epidemiological assessment. The measurement of psychiatric disorders in national surveys, which aim to provide population estimates, differs substantially from methods used in judicial and clinical decisions, for example, for benefits, compensation, and need for services. Methods used for assessing individuals, say, for a treatment program, are rarely the same as those required in epidemiology for classifying populations. In the case of the former, detailed and time-consuming assessments by a range of professionals

of contexts such as family situations are justified because such methods are sensitive to individual circumstances and produce results that are equitable between individuals. In surveys, provided that the methods used deal adequately with the majority of people and can be done within a relatively short time, it matters little if a small minority have been classified differently than they would had more detailed procedures been used.

Quality of data

Conclusions regarding epidemiological estimates, the modeling of possible determinants, service planning, and needs assessment all require the use of comparisons. Comparisons have little value or legitimacy if the data employed are not collected reliably. The types of measures available are discussed later in this article. Because it is essential that epidemiological methods are reproducible (reliable), comparison may be either too costly or impractical when purely clinical measures are used. However, it is also important in developing either a new measure or in using an existing measure in a population with different language or culture, that it is generally accepted as representing descriptions used in clinical settings. Small-scale comparisons of epidemiological questionnaires and systematic clinical evaluations have been carried out occasionally in general population samples. At first sight the level of agreement between these appears to be poor and likely to be limited by the uncertain consistency with which clinical assessments can be used outside in the general population where most conditions are less severe and more fluctuant over time. It is reassuring therefore that clinical and epidemiological measures, when compared in clinical settings, can show high levels of agreement.

Design Issues

Study designs can be divided into the experimental and nonexperimental; the former are infrequently used in the collection of information on psychiatric and psychological disorders in the general population. New mental health policies are seldom subjected to the rigors of experimental evaluation in the general population, although where feasible this can be particularly informative. One experimental design variant that may be particularly feasible in practice is the cluster randomized evaluation. Examples are beginning to appear in the mental health field in which the cluster is an organizational unit, for example, a primary care practice, a specialist team: existing and new policies can be compared between randomly allocated cluster units (MacArthur *et al.*, 2002). Another example makes use of the classroom or work team unit, which could be used in prevention policy trials. As in any experiment involving human subjects, ethical considerations arise: interventions can have wanted and unwanted effects, and those participating should be informed. Careful consideration should be given to anticipating possible harm and minimizing its likelihood; experiments are only justifiable when there is genuine uncertainty about the outcome.

A detailed discussion of the use of different designs in psychiatric epidemiology can by found in a chapter by Zahner and colleagues (1995). Here we focus selectively on the factors that are sometimes neglected in the design of studies in the general population. Most first-generation mental health surveys were typically small, based in a local community, and carried out by a small academic team. The past two decades have seen the emergence of adequately powered, large sample size surveys using complex, often clustered sampling methods, systematically developed and tested structured instruments, and specialized 'survey' methods of analysis, carried out by collaborations between professional survey organizations and academic researchers, which are referred to in examples that follow.

Cross-sectional Surveys

This article refers mainly to the use of cross-sectional and longitudinal designs. Great attention is paid in such surveys to ensuring the representativeness of subjects so that inferences are generalizable and can be used, for example, at a national level and sometimes in small area statistics. Because we regard this as a fundamental issue, which is often inadequately handled in surveys other than those carried out by large (generic) survey organizations, we give this particular emphasis here.

The approach taken by one of us to the challenge of sampling children nationally illustrates some of the factors that can and need to be considered. Several methods of obtaining a representative sample of children in Great Britain were considered: carrying out a postal sift of the general population to identify households with children, sampling through schools, using administrative databases, and piggybacking on other surveys. It was decided to draw the sample from administrative records, specifically, the Child Benefit Records held by the Child Benefit Centre (CBC). Parents of each child under 16 living in the United Kingdom are entitled to receive child benefits unless the child is under the care of social services. Using these centralized records as a sampling frame was preferred to carrying out a postal sift of over 100 000 addresses or sampling through schools. The postal sift would have been time consuming and expensive. The designers did not want to sample through schools because they wanted the initial contact to be with parents who then would give signed consent to approach the child's teacher. A two-hour survey was regarded as too long for piggybacking on other surveys.

Use of centralized records (see later also) does have some disadvantages; access to the records can be problematic and the frame may not be accurate or comprehensive. It was realized that some child benefit records did not have postal codes attributed to addresses: 10% in a first survey and 5% in the repeat. The Child Benefit Centre had no evidence that records with postal codes were different from those without. The addresses with missing postal codes probably represent a mixture of people who did not know their postal code at the time of applying for child benefits and those who simply forgot to enter the details on the form. If there are other factors which differentiate between households with and without postal-coded addresses, the key question is to what extent these factors are related to the mental health of children. Because these factors are unknown, one does not know what biases may have been introduced into the survey by omitting the addresses without postal codes.

The survey design dealt with the problem of omission of children in the care of social services by carrying out a separate survey of this vulnerable group even though such children represent only 0.5% of the population in England. Previous research had indicated high rates of mental disorders among this group. Also excluded from the original sample were cases in which 'action' was being invoked, such as occur with the death of the child or a change of address. These are administrative actions as distinct from some legal process concerning the child and hence should not bias the sample in any way.

Small-area statistical estimates are population approximations developed by specialized statistical procedures such as spatial interpolation. They allow policymakers, local planners, and individual users of services to extrapolate census and survey data to specific local areas. Very large survey sample sizes may be used in conjunction with census data allowing linkages between different information sources on economics, health, crime, quality of the environment, and so forth. The estimates obtained may be subject to census (or survey) or modeling error. Trend estimates may not be directly comparable from year to year because of changes in boundaries, data, and methodology. Estimates can be improved by the use of spatially more precise, geographically coded, building identifiers. Alternatively postal code data or an equivalent coding system are essential but will not be available in all parts of the world.

Screening and full assessment

Although in the children survey example all respondents were administered the same set of questions, many surveys employed two-stage or multiphase survey designs. The first stage consists of a self-report questionnaire administered to the full sample by lay interviewers who do not need to have any clinical training. In a second stage, a randomly selected subsample will undergo a more complex and detailed assessment, possibly involving some degree of clinical expertise. The second phase might involve a full clinical assessment of one or more forms of mental disorder, analogous to a second stage of a population dietary survey in which a random subsample of first-stage respondents undergoes a more detailed inventory of all food kept in a household, and of food purchases within a past number of days, which may be carried out by a smaller team of research dieticians.

There are considerable advantages and also disadvantages to both the single and two-phase designs; these are well discussed in the literature (Newman *et al.*, 1990; Shrout and Newman, 1989). The advantages of the single stage approach are as follows:

- Detailed information is collected on all respondents. A sample distribution can be produced on all subscales even though only those with an above-threshold score will have psychopathology.
- With the possibility of a longitudinal element in the survey, there is a large pool of respondents from which to select controls who could be matched on several characteristics to the children who exhibit significant psychiatric symptoms during the first-stage interview.
- A one-phase design is likely to increase the overall response rate compared with a two-phase (screening plus clinical assessment) design.
- A one-stage design reduces the burden put on respondents. Ideally, a two-phase design would require a screening questionnaire to be followed up with an assessment interview administered to the selected respondent. A one-stage design only requires one interview.

One of the advantages of a one-phase over a two-phase design is that it can be carried out in a far shorter time scale. The main disadvantage of a one-stage design is cost. The administration is far cheaper in two-stage designs, although they are likely to have more biases and less precision.

Cohort and Longitudinal Surveys

Cross sectional surveys explore associations between two variables (x and y) whereas prospective surveys allow the researcher to investigate the problem of unknown direction of causality ($x \rightarrow y$; $x \leftarrow y$; $x \leftrightarrow y$). In relation to mental disorder they can also provide invaluable information on the persistence and duration of mental disorder over time in the population (in general the commoner and less severe forms of disorder in adulthood tend to be of short duration rather than long lasting). However, they are not appropriate for examining treatment and service effectiveness prospectively because, if anything, at a

given time, those having treatment are likely to be more severely ill and to have a poorer subsequent health outcome.

In our experience the more common obstacle to successfully carrying out a longitudinal study is a failure to include this element in the design from the beginning of the study, a 'keeping in touch component.' This is essential if the number followed up successfully is to be maximized. In an adequately funded 'keeping in touch' program, respondents are regularly sent reminders and updates, often including personal birthday greetings, on the progress and successful achievement of the study, thus sustaining what can be a considerable commitment on the part of respondents. This of course requires sustained funding over much longer periods some of which could be used to provide incentives.

Informed Consent

According to Martin (2000), the validity of survey research depends crucially on obtaining as high response rates as possible from the sample selected for a survey. However, individuals selected have a right to make an informed decision about whether or not to participate. Martin argues that without personal contact with an interviewer, the conditions needed to obtain informed consent cannot be achieved. Use of opt-out procedures based on a letter (and opt-in procedures to an even great extent) guarantees neither that the information needed to ensure that consent is informed reaches the right person nor that the person has read and fully understood what participation entails. Martin has concluded that truly informed consent can be obtained only if it is sought by an interviewer trained to explain the survey fully and answer all questions. This is analogous to a personal approach to take part in a clinical trial in which informed consent must also be obtained.

The survey research literature and standard survey practice both emphasize the importance of motivating people to agree to take part in surveys by stressing the importance of the survey and of their personal contribution. There is no evidence that such motivation is seen as exerting undue pressure. The voluntary nature of surveys is always explained, and respondents are free to refuse to answer particular questions or to terminate their participation at any stage. Additional safeguards in the case of the longitudinal and panel surveys are that explicit permission is sought to continue at each stage of the survey, so initial consent does not imply consent to every part of the survey process (Martin, 2000).

Case Control Studies

Measures of exposure status can be compared in which disease status is determined at the time of subject selection. This design may be useful in studying rare conditions, events, or exposures. However, unless these are obtained in the same population setting from which controls are drawn, comparisons and resulting estimates may be biased. This design is rarely used in this field.

Information Sources

Types of information sources can be divided into administrative and survey or census. Some very useful studies can be performed by means of existing well-collected administrative data, thus avoiding the high cost of new data collection and using those resources instead for the important tasks of analysis and dissemination.

Administrative Sources

For cultural and legal reasons, administrative authorities will probably have the best data on causes of death such as suicide and homicide. Data can exist in registers of independent organizations, provider services, or of the authority organization itself.

Censuses

Censuses are a similar source of data; the main advantage is that they collect whole-population data. But census sources are limited by the fact that questions on health are rare and virtually unheard of in relation to psychological and mental health. Other disadvantages are that they are carried out relatively infrequently, rely on proxy information (provided by one household member), and rely on another service such as the postal service to convey data.

Surveys

Surveys can be an efficient and relatively low-cost method for obtaining large numbers of observations in a systematic, reliable way and provide powerful methods for addressing questions on health. Such survey data sets are increasingly archived after a period of time and therefore remain available to the wider research community and to policy advisers (see the Relevant Websites section at the end of this article). This is good in that better use is made of such data at little extra cost, but it can have bad effects also, particularly in a complex area such as mental health, unless the original survey designers can contribute the analysis and interpretation of the data in order to obviate serious misunderstandings.

Mental health surveys
Early mental health surveys tended to be carried out on small samples obtained in single communities and were typically conducted by an individual or small academic team. Estimates from these studies carried little precision,

and only substantial effects were demonstrable. Large-scale, statistically more powerful, survey methodologies began to impinge on the field of psychiatric surveys with the Epidemiologic Catchment Area Survey of Mental Disorders (ECA) (Robins *et al.*, 1984), British National Psychiatric Morbidity Surveys (Jenkins *et al.*, 1997) (see Relevant Websites), the National Comorbidity Survey (NCS) (Kessler *et al.*, 1994), and now the WHO World Mental Health Survey (Demyttenaere *et al.*, 2004), all of which have served to transform the field. Not only did this development herald the introduction of new instruments for assessing mental disorders (see below) but it also served to refine sampling and statistical methods used to generate scientific and policy information. Such surveys have probably been more successful in answering questions about effects within subgroups of the population such as those who are economically disadvantaged. They have also been effective in collecting representative data from difficult-to-reach populations, including low-income populations in less economically developed parts of the world. General health surveys and social and economic surveys have also made increased use of measures of mental and physical health and functioning, thus bringing evidence to a much wider community of policymakers and decision makers.

Registers

Disease and service registers have also played a key part, although few countries have been willing to or capable of operating these over sustained periods. Scandinavian countries, most notably Denmark, have made a contribution in this regard to studying, for example, rarer conditions such as bipolar disorder and other specific forms of psychosis within a whole population context. External researchers have also been able to work collaboratively with those responsible for maintaining such registers. The use of such sources must include a careful consideration of the quality of the register's coding of data.

Services

Although services ought to be able to provide information on rarer events and conditions in practice, for example, we have found such sources to be unable to furnish reliable information except, of course, when they are linked to a register that is managed to high scientific standards. A key issue that may underlie this situation is that the purposes for which data are collected and used by a service are likely to be very different from those of scientific or policy researchers. Services may be able to supply information on the use of such services, providing diagnostic coded data (sometimes in close accord with an accepted set of definitions).

Record Linkage

Linking data on respondents or service users across population care sectors and agencies can be of value in ensuring continuity of care, evaluation, and planning of mental health services, depending of course on the aforementioned issue of data quality. Notable research examples have involved linking data on suicide with data on previous service usage. Useful recent examples of the use of record linkage to support services are the Ontario Data Linkage System (Squire *et al.*, 2002) and the Western Australia Linked Database system (Holman *et al.*, 1999).

Measurement Methods

As discussed earlier, we make a distinction in this section between measures suitable for clinical settings and requiring some clinical experience and measures that can be either self-completed or administered by a lay interviewer that are not only less costly to use but are also more feasible to use in the kinds of large-scale general population surveys needed to obtain information that is useful in planning and policy development. Further background reading about these kinds of measures can also be obtained elsewhere (Thompson, 1988; Biemer *et al.*, 1991; Farmer *et al.*, 2002).

Unstructured Methods

When an investigator is beginning to study a new area of research or is beginning to study an understood construct but in a new population or cultural context or setting, it may be prudent to start with qualitative assessments as a first stage in identifying key themes and concepts and in particular the language in which they are expressed.

Once a structured (or semistructured) instrument has been drafted, testing can be enhanced by means of cognitive interviewing (Biemer *et al.*, 1991). After the test respondent answers each question, an interviewer then asks the respondent questions such as: What do you think was meant by that question? What were you thinking when you answered that question? Why did you answer it that way?

Qualitative analytical methods are used to summarize key points emerging from such interviews; questions are revised and further testing is carried out, and so on.

The more structured methods of measurement described further on were developed because of concerns about the use of unstructured measures such as the clinician mental state assessment. Given the all-important consideration of instrument reliability, mentioned previously, we do not propose to give further consideration to unstructured approaches to the assessment of mental health functioning.

Structured Measures

Fully structured measures are completed by study respondents. They can be either directly completed in the form of self-completion, 'paper and pencil' questionnaires although such methods are increasingly computer assisted; (see the Procedures section) or they can be administered face-to-face by a lay interviewer. When an interviewer administers a questionnaire, the interviewer must not impose her or his judgment on the responses to the questionnaire, which must be chosen by the respondent or left blank, unfilled. Considerable ingenuity has gone into the development of such questionnaires in order to gather information on the criteria needed to determine the presence of specified types of psychiatric disorder. Such techniques were first developed within the social survey field in order to collect information on complex social and economic issues. The principles involved began to be used in the field of mental disorders in the 1970s and 1980s. A strength but also a limitation of such interviewer-administered questionnaires is the use of branching rules: when a respondent states that they do not have a particular characteristic (e.g., symptoms of depression in general, being currently unemployed) further questions about depression or about the effects of being unemployed need not be asked. Such methods allow a great deal of information to be collected selectively but are limited by the sensitivity and specificity and positive and negative predictive value of the initial 'screening' or 'sifting' questions.

Self-report questionnaires

Self-report questionnaire can be used at little cost because interviewers need not be directly involved in their administration. A comprehensive listing of such questionnaires can be found in Farmer *et al.* (2002), where rating scales are also described. The best-known examples of such self-report measures for adults are the General Health Questionnaire (Goldberg, 1972), the Short-Form Questionnaire (Ware, 1993), which also assesses physical aspects of health and functioning, and the Strengths and Difficulties Questionnaire for children (Goodman *et al.*, 2000b). These measures have been used in a considerable number of large-scale surveys (including prospective or panel studies), which mainly focus on general health rather than specifically on mental disorder. Also widely used is the Edinburgh Postnatal Depression Scale to screen for perinatal maternal depression (Cox *et al.*, 1987). A promising new measure recommended for identifying more severe forms of mental disorder are the new K6 and K10 Scales (Kessler *et al.*, 2003). A great deal of attention has focused on the psychometric properties of these measures. Unfortunately, their deceptively simple appearance may disguise the enormous work that goes into their development. Therefore, researchers should be very cautious in trying to develop measures of their own, because questionnaire design and development is a highly specialized undertaking.

Structured diagnostic interviews

As already explained, diagnostic interviews extend the concept of self-report further; they either require an interviewer or, in some studies, a computer to administer the interview directly (interviewers will typically also use a computer rather than printed paper to help them correctly follow branching rules). Comprehensive listings are provided by Farmer et al. (2002). The limitations of these useful and efficient interview branching techniques need to be considered. For example, a respondent, perhaps for reasons of social desirability, may deny having symptoms of depression based on stem questions, which might otherwise have been picked up if nonstem questions (for example, about the physical effects of depression and accompanying thoughts) were asked in a nonbranching questionnaire. Therefore, some researchers prefer to use the self-report questionnaire formats that do not include any branching structure.

The first widely used such interview was the Diagnostic Interview Schedule, which later evolved into a series of interviews that carry the common title Composite International Diagnostic Interview (CIDI) (Robins et al., 1988). Although lengthy and highly detailed, this quality has not been detrimental to their widespread use, including in the collection of survey data in low-income countries. However, they are not suitable for measuring severe mental disorders, and there are many different versions of the CIDI, thus limiting comparison between different studies. Less known are similar diagnostic interviews used in the British National Survey Programme (see Relevant Websites). For the child surveys, worth mentioning is a particularly novel solution to the challenge to combine fully structured questions and the use of clinical ratings in the Development and Well-Being Assessment (DAWBA) (Goodman et al., 2000a). The questionnaire used structured interviewing supplemented by open-ended questions. When definite symptoms were identified by the structured questions, interviewers used open-ended questions and supplementary prompts to get parents to describe the child's' problems in their own words. The wording of the prompts was specified. Answers to the open-ended questions and any other respondent comments were transcribed verbatim by the interviewers but were not rated by them. Interviewers were also given the opportunity to make additional comments, where appropriate, on the respondents' understanding and motivation.

A small team of experienced clinicians reviewed the transcripts and interviewers' comments to ensure that the answers to structured questions were not misleading. The same clinical reviewers could also consider clashes of information between different informants, deciding which account to prioritize. Furthermore, children with clinically relevant problems that did not quite meet the operationalized diagnostic criteria could be assigned suitable diagnoses by the clinical raters. There are no other existing diagnostic tools that combine the advantages of structured and semistructured assessments in this way, which is why a new set of measures were specifically designed for this survey. The new measures and their validity are described in more detail elsewhere (Goodman et al., 2000a).

Semistructured

The term 'semistructured' is used to refer to measures that could be considered as lying in between the pre-worded, fully structured measures and largely unstructured qualitative interviews just described. In the sense that it is used here, 'semistructured' refers to a style of interviewing that is flexible and more conversational but critically different in that the interviewer (either the interviewer or others on the research team) has two additional responsibilities: first, the selective framing of supplementary questions in order to add clarification and to respond to the way subjects at first answer and appear to understand questions; and second, sifting through the interview content and deciding on the final ratings. Issues of feasibility, cost, and complexity of the phenomena to be measured will bear on the choice of which approach to use in a study, as discussed earlier.

Diagnostic interviews

Diagnostic interviews are discussed in detail elsewhere (Farmer et al., 2002; Thompson, 1988). As for fully structured diagnostic interviews, all the information needed for the mental disorder classification system is sought (and these interviews also use branching techniques). Because the interviewer is required to provide the judgment of each rating in a semistructured interview as compared to the respondent in a fully structured interview, great care is needed to ensure the consistency of such ratings between interviewers and across time within one study not to mention between studies. Little is known about how successful such efforts are. There is little doubt that such approaches will be very costly in most settings. However, in low-income populations the cost of interviews also may be lower; there may also be advantages arising from the flexible 'clinical' conversational style of such interviews that could serve to minimize misunderstanding among respondents who are perhaps less well acquainted with Western psychological terms. However, these are all conjectural matters for further investigation. Some of the issues are also discussed elsewhere in the wider context of survey measures in general (Biemer et al., 1991).

In a previous section we discussed the DAWBA (Goodman *et al.*, 2000a), which combines a fully structured and a partial semistructured element that has been shown to be reliable in generating DSM-IV and ICD-10 categories. The most widely used such measure in adult mental health surveys is the Structured Clinical Interview for DSM (SCID) (Spitzer *et al.*, 1992). Also used, particularly to elucidate psychotic forms of disorder, is the Schedules for Clinical Assessment in Neuropsychiatry (SCAN) (World Health Organization Division of Mental Health, 1992). Both should be administered by clinically experienced, specifically trained clinicians or by interviewers with greatly extended training that provides such experience (Brugha *et al.*, 1999). The SCAN provides dimensional and ICD-10 and DSM-IV diagnostic outputs and has been translated extensively; the SCID-I provides DSM-IV outputs only and also exists in a number of translated forms.

Rating Scales

Rating scales are similar to semistructured interviews in that the person administering the scale judges the ratings. However, far less guidance is provided on how to collect the data. Such measures were developed in order to efficiently make use of the observations of a clinician, who presumably would already have conducted a mental state assessment, in treating a patient. These approaches have for many years been in widespread use in clinical treatment trials but are rarely used in surveys. Examples can be found in Farmer *et al.* (2002) and Thompson (1988).

Cross-Population Issues

A number of references have been made to considerations that are of importance when measuring mental health in different cultures and language settings. This principle should be extended to consideration of any subpopulation that could be marginalized or excluded, such as prisoners (Brugha *et al.*, 2004) and those with sensory impairment. For example, a version of the DIS interview has been developed for deaf people (Montoya *et al.*, 2004).

Culture and ethnicity

There is a large body of evidence suggesting that the idioms for mental distress vary across different ethnic groups (Sproston and Nazroo, 2002). The implication of possible cultural differences in symptomatic experience is that standardized research instruments will perform inconsistently across different ethnic groups, greatly restricting the validity of conclusions based on their use in surveys. Although there is some evidence of the universality of the major forms of clinical psychopathology (Cheng *et al.*, 2000), this is not universally accepted. Fundamental issues about the transferability of Western psychological and psychopathological

concepts continue to be debated. Invaluable experience of the practicalities and scope for addressing such challenges has come from the International Pilot Studies of Schizophrenia and subsequent research under WHO auspices (Jablensky *et al.*, 1992) and from recent work within the general population survey paradigm of the diverse cultures and languages found in urban Britain (Sproston and Nazroo, 2002), which included detailed qualitative, unstructured assessments carried out in the first language of respondents.

Translation methods and protocols

A great deal of experience has been built up in translating (Sartorius, 1998) and testing instruments in different population and cultural settings. Great emphasis has been placed on the use of both forward- and back-translation. Recent developments emphasize that it is the concepts rather than the words that need to be translated, thus preserving meaning as far as possible. In order for questions to be understood in a way that is comparable within and across populations that rely on different languages and dialects, it is necessary to have a translation procedure that yields equivalent versions of the questions across a variety of settings and cultures.

There are three main problems that occur when trying to standardize the translation process across countries:

- linguistic differences caused by changes in the meaning of words between dialects;
- translation difficulties; and
- differences that arise when applying a concept across cultures.

The conceptual translational method relies on detailed explanations of the terms used in each survey question, as well as the underlying concepts that the questions were intended to measure. This approach differs from the forward-backward method in the 'backward' step, during which rather than translating the question back into the original language, a checker determines whether each question was properly translated such that the intended concepts were actually captured (Robine and Jagger, 2002; Robine and Jagger, 2003).

Measurement of Specific Disorders

As mentioned earlier, mental health survey approaches and programs in a given geographic setting sometimes begin by assessing an overall or 'common mental disorder' outcome that may be dimensional (see **Figure 1**) or based on a categorical case definition. This approach can also be embedded into surveys that assess other aspects of health, economic and social functioning. The influence of clinical psychiatry has led to an expectation of data on specific categories of mental disorder. Most surveys have focused on more common internalizing disorders: anxiety and depression in adults, conduct and emotional disorders in children and young people. Many surveys also attempt to measure rarer and more complex disorders (in terms of diagnostic criteria and their measurement), such as obsessive compulsive disorder and psychosis in adults and attention deficit disorder and developmental disorders in children (e.g., tick disorder and autism). Externalizing disorders involving the use of substances and alcohol are also often assessed; other disorders of behavior, such as personality disorder, are rarely assessed. These expectations are likely to be increasingly questioned in favor of the more practical and parsimonious value of information on severity, complexity *per se,* and persistence over time.

Procedures (Surveys Mainly)

The procedures used in surveys also determine quality, cost, and acceptability. Quality (or accuracy) is the most difficult of these to evaluate. A notable example is that it has been shown that audio computer-assisted self-interviewing (ACASI) administration can yield more information on mental health than that obtained from an interviewer-administered, paper-and-pencil (I-PAPI) mental health module of the CIDI (Epstein *et al.,* 2001).

Face to Face

In face-to-face procedures the respondent is administered the questions by an interviewer who will typically visit the person's home or other agreed-upon place. Although costly, such methods are regarded as of high quality. The researcher has control over the quality of the training and procedures used by interviewers.

Postal

Respondents complete and return a questionnaire by post, usually using a prepaid cover or envelope. Unless additional steps are taken to ensure cooperation, response rates tend to be so low as to make the information provided of limited value, but methods for increasing response rates have been developed. Costs are understandably very low. It may come as a surprise, however, to find that quality can be high, possibly because respondents have time to think more carefully about questions and also because social desirability factors play less of a part (Bushery *et al.,* 1996) than in face-to-face interviews. However, self-completion methods that are fully anonymous are now often included within a face-to-face interview procedure.

Electronic and Digital

Various electronic methods have gradually been introduced; some of these are under active development and likely to become either more sophisticated or drop out of use. In most contexts and cases, costs are lower than for the equivalent interviewer-based approach, although start-up costs may be very high.

Procedures include computer-assisted telephone interviewing, the Internet, interactive voice response over telephone (IVR), and so forth. IVR is a more automated version of telephone interviewing but may be limited by the proportion of the population who subscribe. Telephone interviewing is used widely by commercial organizations in some populations, and this may lead to resistance among some of the public and thus compromise the representativeness of survey findings.

Start-up costs for Internet surveys, although dropping, are still high but then fall to almost zero per unit cost. They may share some of the advantages of accuracy of postal methods. Data can be collected from all over the world (which may be either an advantage or a disadvantage) and is immediately available for analysis. Other computer-administered methods include audio-computer-assisted interviewing (ACASI), in which the respondent may wear ear phones; text to speech (TTS), which may use 'talking heads' (Avatars) that can be specifically gender and culture matched to the respondent; digital recording; and touch screen responses to questions.

Computer adaptive testing (CAT), in which the software calculates and determines the next question to ask in an interview, is probably limited to assessing fairly simple concepts and facts rather than attitudes; when we evaluated such a system in a comparison with a clinical evaluation of neurotic symptoms we found poor agreement (Brugha *et al.,* 1996).

Application of Measurement Methods in Public Health Contexts (e.g. Surveillance and Screening in Health Settings)

Government policy documents are beginning to suggest the use of surveillance methods such as repeat surveys over time in order to evaluate policies and success in implementing health objectives (e.g., England; Department of Health, 1999). National mental health strategies should set realistic targets for improvements in the mental health of the population (Jenkins *et al.,* 2002). The example of a common mental disorder for which there is a range of effective treatments deserves mention. Despite the high prevalence rates of common mental disorders, they have traditionally been underdetected and undertreated. In recent years changes in services should have improved this situation in

Great Britain. A campaign by the Royal Colleges of General Practitioners and of Psychiatrists to increase awareness and the effective treatment of depression led to over half of general practitioners (GPs) taking part in teaching sessions on depression. The pharmaceutical industry successfully encouraged increased prescription of newer antidepressants. The effectiveness of such innovations may be evaluated by monitoring the mental health and treatment of representative samples of the whole population surveyed in 1993 and 2000. However, a recent examination of rates of such disorders in 1993 and 2000, during which rates of treatment increased dramatically, concluded that treatment with psychotropic medication alone is unlikely to improve the overall mental health of the population nationally (Brugha *et al.*, 2005). Similar conclusions have emerged since from the USA (Kessler *et al.*, 2005). Such evidence can be interpreted as pointing to the need to develop effective prevention policies for which surveillance methods would also be essential.

Policy Information and Decision Making

Little is known or understood about how policymakers use information from mental health surveys. Expectations are likely to be shaped by the nature and value of information used in physical health and evidence-based treatments and services, including prevention policies. This may be why information on the prevalence of mental disorders is often sought and provided, although the concept may have little meaning. A surprisingly large number of systematic reviews, often including the use of synthetic methods such as meta-analysis, have appeared in the psychiatric epidemiology literature in the past decade. Policymakers require guidance on the value of such reviews, given the technical difficulties faced in carrying out good-quality studies in this field.

Conclusions

Methods for measuring psychiatric and related psychological disorders and outcomes in populations have advanced considerably, particularly in the past two decades. Some long-standing assumptions have been tested, sometimes with surprising conclusions. Contemporary researchers pay particular attention to consistency and reproducibility of findings, in contrast to an earlier era in which clinical applicability often dominated the choice of the method used. Studies have become much larger and require the input of many more and different disciplines than in the past; this is probably to the good, as it may help render the topic of mental disorder more acceptable and less stigmatizing. Although the field seems new and technologically exciting, old principles are still important:

simplicity and clarity of purpose, an appropriate design, the use of well-tested measures, and the interpretation of findings with a clear understanding of the limitations of the methods used. The measurement of mental disorder now stands equal in importance, in methodological rigor and usefulness, to other major public health topics.

Citations

American Psychiatric Association (1994) *Diagnostic and Statistical Manual of Mental Disorders, Fourth Edition.* Washington, DC: American Psychiatric Association.

Biemer P, Groves RM, Lyberg LE, Mathiowetz NA, and Sudman S (1991) *Measurement Errors in Surveys.* New York: John Wiley & Sons.

Brugha TS (2002) The end of the beginning: A requiem for the categorisation of mental disorder? *Psychological Medicine* 32(7): 1149–1154.

Brugha TS, Teather D, Wills KM, Kaul A, and Dignon A (1996) Present state examination by microcomputer: Objectives and experience of preliminary steps. *International Journal of Methods in Psychiatric Research* 6: 143–151.

Brugha TS, Nienhuis FJ, Bagchi D, Smith J, and Meltzer H (1999) The survey form of SCAN: The feasibility of using experienced lay survey interviewers to administer a semi-structured systematic clinical assessment of psychotic and non psychotic disorders. *Psychological Medicine* 29(3): 703–712.

Brugha TS, Bebbington PE, Singleton N, *et al.* (2004) Trends in service use and treatment for mental disorders in adults throughout Great Britain. *The British Journal of Psychiatry* 185: 378–384.

Brugha T, Singleton N, Meltzer H, *et al.* (2005) Psychosis in the community and in prisons: A report from the British National Survey of Psychiatric Morbidity. *American Journal of Psychiatry* 162(4): 774–780.

Cheng ATA, Tien AY, Brugha TS, *et al.* (2000) Cross-cultural implementation of a Chinese version of the Schedules for Clinical Assessment in Neuropsychiatry (SCAN) in Taiwan. *British Journal of Psychiatry* 178: 567–572.

Cox JL, Holden JM, and Sagovsky R (1987) Detection of postnatal depression. Development of the 10 item Edinburgh Postnatal Depression Scale. *British Journal of Psychiatry* 150: 782–786.

Demyttenaere K, Bruffaerts R, Posada-Villa J, *et al.* (2004) Prevalence, severity, and unmet need for treatment of mental disorders in the World Health Organization World Mental Health Surveys. *Journal of the American Medical Association* 291(21): 2581–2590.

Department of Health (1999) *National Service Frameworks for Mental Health. Modern Standards and Service Models*, pp. 149. London: Department of Health.

Epstein JF, Barker PR, and Kroutil LA (2001) Mode Effects in Self-Reported Mental Health Data. *Public Opinion Quarterly* 65(4): 529–549.

Farmer A, McGuffin P, and Williams J (2002) *Measuring Psychopathology.* Oxford, UK: Oxford University Press.

Goldberg DP (1972) *The Detection of Psychiatric Illness by Questionnaire.* Oxford, UK: Oxford University Press.

Goodman R, Ford T, Richards H, Gatward R, and Meltzer H (2000a) The Development and Well-Being Assessment: Description and initial validation of an integrated assessment of child and adolescent psychopathology. *Journal of Child Psychology and Psychiatry*, JID 0375361, 41(5): 645–655.

Goodman R, Ford T, Simmons H, Gatward R, and Meltzer H (2000b) Using the Strengths and Difficulties Questionnaire (SDQ) to screen for child psychiatric disorders in a community sample. *British Journal of Psychiatry*, JID 0342367, 177: 534–539.

Green H, McGinnity A, Meltzer H, Ford T, and Goodman R (2005) *Mental Health of Children and Young People in Great Britain, 2004.* Hampshire, UK: Palgrave McMillan.

Holman CD, Bass AJ, Rouse IL, and Hobbs MS (1999) Population-based linkage of health records in Western Australia:

Development of a health services research linked database. *Australia and New Zealand Journal of Public Health* 23(5): 453–459.

Jablensky A, Sartorius N, Ernberg G, *et al.* (1992) Schizophrenia: Manifestations, incidence and course in different cultures. A World Health Organization ten-country study [published erratum appears in Psychological Medicine Monograph Suppl. 1992, Nov. 22(4): following 1092]. *Psychological Medicine Monograph Supplement* 20: 1–97.

Jenkins R, Bebbington P, Brugha T, *et al.* (1997) The national psychiatric morbidity surveys of Great Britain – Strategy and methods. *Psychological Medicine* 27(4): 765–774.

Kessler RC, McGonagle KA, Zhao S, *et al.* (1994) Lifetime and 12-month prevalence of DSM-III-R psychiatric disorders in the United States. Results from the National Comorbidity Survey. *Archives of General Psychiatry* 51(1): 8–19.

Kessler RC, Barker PR, Colpe LJ, *et al.* (2003) Screening for serious mental illness in the general population. *Archives of General Psychiatry* 60(2): 184–189.

Kessler RC, Demler O, Frank RG, *et al.* (2005) Prevalence and treatment of mental disorders, 1990 to 2003. *The New England Journal of Medicine* 352(24): 2515–2523.

MacArthur C, Winter HR, Bick DE, *et al.* (2002) Effects of redesigned community postnatal care on women's' health 4 months after birth: A cluster randomised controlled trial. *Lancet* 359(9304): 378–385.

Martin J, Social Survey Division, ONF (ed.) (2000) *Informed Consent in the Context of Survey Research.* London: Office for National Statistics.

Montoya LA, Egnatovich R, Eckhardt E, *et al.* (2004) *Translation Challenges and Strategies: The ASL Translation of a Computer-Based Psychiatric Diagnostic Interview* 4(4): 314–344.

Newman SC, Shrout PE, and Bland RC (1990) The efficiency of two-phase designs in prevalence surveys of mental disorders [published erratum appears in *Psychological Medicine* 1990, Aug. 20(3): following 745]. *Psychological Medicine* 20(1): 183–193.

Robine JM and Jagger C (2003) Creating a coherent set of indicators to monitor health across Europe: The Euro-REVES 2 project. *European Journal of Public Health* 13(3 Suppl): 6–14.

Robine JM and Jagger C (eds.) Euro-REVES (2002) *Report to Eurostat on European Health Status Module.* Geneva, Switzerland: EUROSTAT.

Robins LE, Helzer JE, Weissman MM, *et al.* (1984) Lifetime prevalence of specific psychiatric disorders in three sites. *Archives of General Psychiatry* 41: 949–957.

Robins LN, Wing J, Wittchen HU, *et al.* (1988) The Composite International Diagnostic Interview. An epidemiologic instrument suitable for use in conjunction with different diagnostic systems and in different cultures. *Archives of General Psychiatry* 45(12): 1069–1077.

Sartorius N (1998) SCAN translation. In: Wing JK and Üstün TB (eds.) *Diagnosis and Clinical Measurement in Psychiatry. A Reference Manual for SCAN/PSE-10*, pp. 44–57. Cambridge, UK: Cambridge University Press.

Shrout PE and Newman SC (1989) Design of two-phase prevalence surveys of rare disorders. *Biometrics* 45(2): 549–555.

Singleton N, Bumpstead R, O'Brien M, Lee A and Meltzer H, National Statistics (eds.) (2001) *Psychiatric Morbidity among Adults Living in Private Households*, pp. 154. London: The Stationary Office.

Spitzer RL, Williams JB, Gibbon M, and First MB (1992) The Structured Clinical Interview for DSM-III-R (SCID). I: History, rationale, and description. *Archives of General Psychiatry* 49(8): 624–629.

Sproston K and Nazroo JY (eds.) (2002) *Ethnic Minority Psychiatric Illness Rates in the Community (EMPIRIC) – Quantitative Report*, pp. 210. London: The Stationary Office.

Squire L, Bedard M, Hegge L, and Polischuk V (2002) Current evaluation and future needs of a mental health data linkage system in a remote region: A Canadian experience. *Journal of Behavioral Health Services Research* 29(4): 476–480.

Thompson C (1988) *The Instruments of Psychiatric Research,* 1st edn. Chichester, UK: Wiley.

Ware JE (1993) *SF-36 Health Survey.* Boston, MA: Medical Outcomes Trust.

Wing JK, Cooper J, and Sartorius N (1974) *Measurement and Classification of Psychiatric Symptoms.* Cambridge, UK: Cambridge University Press.

World Health Organization (1992) *ICD-10 Classification of Mental and Behavioural Disorders: Clinical Descriptions and Diagnostic Guidelines.* Geneva, Switzerland: World Health Organization.

World Health Organization (1993) *The ICD-10 Classification of Mental and Behavioural Disorders: Diagnostic Criteria for Research.* Geneva, Switzerland: WHO.

World Health Organization Division of Mental Health (1990) *ICD-10, chapter 5, Mental and Behavioural Disorders (Including Disorders of Psychological Development): Diagnostic Criteria for Research (May 1990 Draft for Field Trials).* Geneva, Switzerland: World Health Organization. (Distribution: limited).

World Health Organization Division of Mental Health WHO SCAN Advisory Committee (ed.) (1992) *SCAN Schedules for Clinical Assessment in Neuropsychiatry,* Version 1.0, pp. 242. Geneva, Switzerland: World Health Organization.

Zahner GE, Chung-Cheng H, and Fleming JA (1995) Introduction to epidemiological research methods. In: Tsuang M, Tohen M and Zahner GE (eds.) *Textbook in Psychiatric Epidemiology*, pp. 23–54. New York: Wiley.

Further Reading

American Statistical Association (1996) How interview mode affects data reliability. *Proceedings of the Survey Research Methods Section, American Statistical Association.* Alexandria, VA: American Statistical Association.

Biemer P, Groves RM, Lyberg LE, Mathiowetz NA, and Sudman S (1991) *Measurement Errors in Surveys.* New York: John Wiley & Sons.

Farmer A, McGuffin P, and Williams J (2002) *Measuring Psychopathology.* Oxford, UK: Oxford University Press.

Green H, McGinnity A, Meltzer H, Ford T, and Goodman R (2005) *Mental Health of Children and Young People in Great Britain, 2004.* Hampshire, UK: Palgrave McMillan.

Shrout PE and Newman SC (1989) Design of two-phase prevalence surveys of rare disorders. *Biometrics* 45(2): 549–555.

Singleton N, Bumpstead R, O'Brien M, Lee A and Meltzer H (eds.) (2001) *Psychiatric Morbidity Among Adults Living in Private Households*, pp. 154. London: The Stationary Office National Statistics.

Sproston K and Nazroo JY (2002) *Ethnic Minority Psychiatric Illness Rates in the Community (EMPIRIC) – Quantitative Report*, pp. 210. London: The Stationary Office.

Thompson C (1988) *The Instruments of Psychiatric Research,* 1st edn. Chichester, UK: John Wiley & Sons.

Wing JK, Cooper J, and Sartorius N (1974) *Measurement and Classification of Psychiatric Symptoms.* Cambridge, UK: Cambridge University Press.

World Health Organization (1993) *The ICD-10 Classification of Mental and Behavioural Disorders: Diagnostic Criteria for Research.* Geneva, Switzerland: WHO.

Zahner GE, Chung-Cheng H, and Fleming JA (1995) Introduction to epidemiological research methods. In: Tsuang M, Tohen M and Zahner GE (eds.) *Textbook in Psychiatric Epidemiology*, pp. 23–54. New York: John Wiley & Sons.

Relevant Websites

http://www.hcp.med.harvard.edu/wmh/ – Department of Health Care Policy, Harvard Medical School.

http://www.nice.org.uk/page.aspx?o=235213 – National Institute for Clinical Excellence, Depression Treatment Guideline.

http://www.dh.gov.uk/PublicationsAndStatistics/Published/Survey/ListOfSurveySince1990/SurveyListMentalHealth/fs/en – Reports of National Surveys of Psychiatric Morbidity, England.

http://www.data-archive.ac.uk – UK Data Archive.

Observational Epidemiology

J L Kelsey, University of Massachusetts Medical School, Worcester, MA, USA

Introduction

Observational epidemiologic studies are those in which an investigator observes what is occurring in a study population without intervening. In an observational study addressing the question of whether physical activity protects against coronary heart disease, an investigator might note at the beginning of a study, and at intervals throughout the study, the physical activity level of the study participants and relate this to the development of coronary heart disease. This contrasts with an experimental (or intervention) study, in which the investigator assigns study participants, preferably at random, either to be exposed or not to be exposed to a particular agent or activity. For instance, an investigator would randomly assign some people to a physical activity enhancement program and others not to be in this program, and then follow them up for development of coronary heart disease. Because of the randomization process, on average those assigned to the physical activity program will otherwise be similar to those assigned to the comparison group. In observational studies, however, physically active individuals might tend to differ in many other ways from inactive individuals. Thus, observational studies, which are the subject of this article, present special challenges when used to learn about disease causation.

Some Uses of Observational Epidemiology

One use of observational studies is to determine the magnitude and impact of diseases or other conditions in populations or in selected subgroups of the population. Such data are useful in setting priorities for investigation and control, in deciding where preventive efforts should be focused, and in determining what type of treatment facilities are needed. Observational studies can be used to learn about the natural history, clinical course, and pathogenesis of diseases. Observational studies may be used to evaluate the effectiveness of therapeutic procedures or new modes of health-care delivery, although randomized trials are usually the preferred method of study for such evaluations. Most commonly, observational epidemiologic studies are used to learn about disease causation, and this application of epidemiology will be emphasized in this article.

Descriptive Studies

Descriptive studies generally provide information about the distribution of diseases and other characteristics without testing specific hypotheses about causation. Often such studies are used to generate hypotheses about causation. Many descriptive studies provide information on patterns of disease occurrence in populations according to such attributes as age, gender, race/ethnicity, marital status, social class, occupation, geographic area, and time of occurrence. Routinely collected data from such sources as cancer registries, death certificates, hospital discharge records, other medical records, and general health surveys are generally used for descriptive studies. This information can be used to indicate the magnitude of a problem or to suggest preliminary hypotheses about disease causation. For instance, in a classic descriptive epidemiologic study, maps of mortality rates of site-specific cancers by county in the United States (Mason *et al.*, 1975) showed that certain geographic areas had particularly high or low mortality rates, suggesting that specific industries or other geographic factors might be responsible for the high rates. In another example, mortality rates from pneumonia in children in the United States have declined markedly since 1939. The steep decline in mortality rates in black children from 1966 to 1982 (**Figure 1**) is hypothesized to have resulted from improved access to medical care for poor children (Dowell *et al.*, 2000).

Other types of descriptive studies are case reports and case series. In a case report, one person with a certain disease and certain exposure is noted. For instance, suppose one young woman with pulmonary embolism is observed to be using oral contraceptives. This one case obviously does not prove that use of oral contraceptives increases the risk for pulmonary embolism, but it might suggest that the possibility of such an association should be considered in more rigorous studies because pulmonary embolism is very rare among young women. In a case series, exposures in several cases with a given disease are noted. A physician might observe that eight out of ten young women with pulmonary embolism were using oral contraceptives at the time the embolism occurred. While 80% may seem a high percentage, oral contraceptives are widely used by young women, and it might be that eight out of ten young women randomly selected from the general population use oral contraceptives. Thus, a case series generally does not provide definitive information because a comparison (or control) group of young women

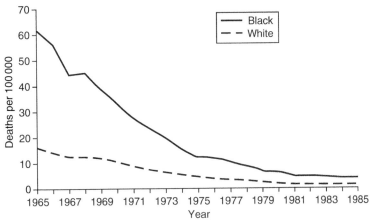

Figure 1 Mortality rates from childhood pneumonia according to race, 1965–85. Reproduced with permission from Dowell SF, Kupronis BA, Zell ER, *et al.* (2000) Mortality from pneumonia in children in the United States, 1939 through 1996. *New England Journal of Medicine* 342: 1399–1407.

without the disease is needed to determine if the 80% figure is in excess of expectation. In a case series from an outbreak of severe viral encephalitis associated with Nipah virus in Malaysia (Goh *et al.*, 2000), some 93% of cases reported direct contact with pigs, usually in the 2 weeks before the onset of the illness. This high percentage is strongly suggestive of transmission from pigs to humans, but a properly designed case-control study (to be described in the next section) would be needed to show this more definitively. A case series of eight patients with vitamin D intoxication in the Boston area was sufficient to indicate that a local dairy was incorrectly and excessively fortifying its milk with vitamin D (Jacobus *et al.*, 1992). In this instance, no comparison group was needed, because even one case was sufficient to raise concern.

Nevertheless, case reports, case series, and other descriptive studies are usually useful only in providing leads for studies designed specifically to test hypotheses. Such hypothesis-testing studies are often referred to as analytic epidemiologic studies.

Analytic Studies

Analytic epidemiologic studies are designed to test causal hypotheses that have been generated from descriptive epidemiology, clinical observations, laboratory studies, and other sources, including analytic studies undertaken for other purposes. Analytic studies seek to determine why a disease is distributed in the population in the way it is. Because analytic studies often necessitate the collection of new data, they tend to be more expensive than descriptive studies, but, if properly designed and executed, generally allow more definitive conclusions to be reached. Common types of analytic observational studies include case-control, cohort, and cross-sectional studies,

as well as some hybrid designs. Ecologic studies will also be briefly described. Although these analytic study designs usually provide more definitive information than descriptive studies, in some instances experimental studies may be needed to demonstrate causality.

Case-Control Studies

These are studies in which the investigator selects persons with a given disease (the cases) and persons without the given disease (the controls). Certain characteristics or past exposure to possible risk factors (e.g., cigarette smoking) in cases and controls are then determined and compared.

Cases are typically people seeking medical care for the disease. Usually only newly diagnosed cases are included in order to be more certain that the risk factor preceded the disease rather than being a consequence of the disease, and so that cases of short duration are appropriately represented.

A useful working concept of a control group has been given by Miettinen (1985): The controls should be selected in an unbiased manner from those individuals who would have been included in the case series if they had developed the disease under study. Thus, the optimal control group depends on the source of the cases, but the relative costs of obtaining the various types of controls and the resources available to the investigator are also taken into account in selecting control groups. Sometimes controls are matched to cases on certain important characteristics such as age and sex (see section titled 'Confounding variables'). These characteristics can also be taken into account in the statistical analysis if no matching was done at the outset or if matching was not fine enough.

If the cases consist of all people developing the disease of interest within a defined population, then the best single control group would usually be a random sample of individuals from the same source population who have not developed the disease. In the United States, controls are frequently identified through random-digit dialing to members of the same community from which the cases arose. In countries with population registries, controls are typically selected from the registries. If cases come from a defined group such as members of a health maintenance organization, controls are generally sampled from among other members of the health maintenance organization.

In a case-control study of the possible protective effect of phytoestrogen consumption against the development of breast cancer (Horn-Ross et al., 2001), breast cancer cases were ascertained from the Greater Bay Area Cancer Registry, which includes all cases of newly diagnosed cancer among residents of the Greater Bay Area. Controls were identified through random-digit dialing of telephone numbers in the same area. A case-control study of the association between blood transfusions and non-Hodgkin's lymphoma (Maguire-Boston et al., 1999) ascertained all cases diagnosed among Olmsted County, Minnesota, residents at the two medical-care providers in the county (Mayo Clinic and Olmsted Medical Center) and sampled controls from other Olmsted County residents who had been enumerated in a special census.

If cases are identified at certain hospitals that do not cover a defined geographic area, it is usually impossible to specify the source population from which the cases arose. In this instance, controls are often chosen from among patients with other diseases admitted to the same hospitals as the cases, since one wants to obtain a source of controls subject to the same selective factors as the cases. It is usually desirable to include as controls people with a variety of other conditions, so that no single disease is unduly represented in the control group. Generally, it is important to exclude potential controls who have had their disease for a long period of time because, like the cases, the presence of their disease may have influenced their exposure to possible risk factors. Such characteristics as physical activity, diet, weight, and medication use may change as a result of many diseases.

The classic case-control studies of Doll and Hill (1952) of the association between cigarette smoking and lung cancer (see **Table 1**) identified cases from several hospitals in England and chose as controls patients admitted to the same hospitals with other diseases who had a similar age and sex distribution to the cases. Although cigarette smoking was very common among both cases and controls, a higher percentage of cases than controls smoked, and when the amount of smoking was taken into account, the cases were much more likely to have been heavy smokers than the controls.

Information on exposure to putative risk factors may be obtained in several ways, depending on the nature of the exposure. Frequently, questionnaires administered to

Table 1 Case-control study of the association between cigarette smoking and lung cancer in males, England

Smoking status	Lung cancer cases	Control group
Smokers	1350	1296
Nonsmokers	7	61
Total	1357	1357
Percent smokers	99.5%	95.5%

Odds ratio $= \frac{1350/7}{1296/61} = 9.1$, 95% confidence interval $= (4.1, 19.9)$
Adapted from Doll R and Hill A (1952) A study of the aetiology of carcinoma of the lung. *British Medical Journal* 2: 1271–1286.

cases and controls by trained interviewers are used, as this is often the only way to find out about past exposures. Existing records may sometimes be used to find out about exposures such as medication use. Physical measurements or laboratory tests on sera or other tissue drawn from cases and controls may also be used, but it must be kept in mind that measurements of some attributes differ after the disease has occurred compared to before the disease developed. Whichever methods are used, it is important that the same measurement methods be used in cases and controls.

Case-control studies can provide a great deal of useful information about risk factors for diseases, and over the years have been the most frequently undertaken type of epidemiologic study. They can generally be carried out in a much shorter period of time than cohort studies (to be discussed in the next section), and under most circumstances do not require nearly so large a sample size. Consequently, they are less expensive. For a rare disease, case-control studies are usually the only practical approach to identifying risk factors.

Nevertheless, certain problems and limitations may affect the conclusions that can be drawn from case-control studies. Among some of the major concerns are that

1. Information on potential risk factors may not be available with sufficient accuracy either from records or the participants' memories;
2. Information on other relevant variables that need to be taken into account to ensure comparability of cases and controls may not be available with sufficient accuracy either from records or from the participants' memories;
3. Cases may search for a cause for their disease and thereby be more likely to report an exposure to a particular risk factor than controls;
4. The investigator may be unable to determine with certainty whether the agent was likely to have caused the disease or whether the occurrence of the disease was likely to have caused exposure to the agent;
5. Identifying and assembling a case group representative of all cases may not be feasible;
6. Identifying and assembling an appropriate control group may be difficult;

7. Participation rates may be low and/or different between cases and controls, causing concern about representativeness and bias.

In view of these potential weaknesses, the case-control study is considered by some to be a type of study that merely provides leads to be followed by more definitive cohort studies. However, decisions about preventive actions often have to be made on the basis of information obtained from case-control studies. Each case-control study should be evaluated on its own merits, since some studies are affected very little by error and bias, while others may be affected a great deal.

Cohort Studies

Prospective cohort studies

In a typical prospective cohort study, individuals without the disease under study at the start of the study are classified according to whether they are exposed or not exposed to the potential risk factor(s) of interest, or according to their level of exposure. The cohort is then followed for a period of time (which may be many years) and the incidence rates (number of new cases of disease per person-time of follow-up) or mortality rates (number of deaths per person-time of follow-up) in those exposed or not exposed (or according to levels of exposure) are compared. A cohort study may also involve measuring exposure status at the beginning of a study and determining how this relates to changes in an attribute (such as blood pressure) over time. Because in most cohort studies people enter and leave the cohort at different times, the total length of time that each cohort member is at risk and under surveillance by the investigator for the outcome of interest has to be taken into account. The sum of the length of time each cohort member is at risk and under observation is the person-time.

Table 2 shows results from a cohort study of whether religiousness is associated with a reduction in mortality rates in the elderly (Zuckerman *et al.*, 1984). Mortality rates over the 2-year period of the study were in fact

Table 2 Cohort study of association between religiousness and mortality over a 2-year period in persons of age 62 years and older

Religiousness	Number of deaths	Person-years at risk	Average annual death rate
Religious	18	418	0.043
Not religious	29	331	0.088

Rate ratio = 0.043/0.088 = 0.49, 95% confidence interval = 0.27, 0.88.
Adapted from Zuckerman DM, Kasl SV, and Ostfeld AM (1984) Psychosocial predictors of mortality among the elderly poor. The role of religion, well-being, and social contacts. *American Journal of Epidemiology* 119: 410–423.

about 50% lower in the religious than in the nonreligious individuals. However, it is still debated whether religiousness itself is beneficial or whether some attribute associated with religiousness (e.g., a healthy lifestyle) is the reason for the lower death rate among religious people.

Cohort studies have a major advantage over case-control studies in that exposures or other characteristics of interest are measured before the disease has developed (or before changes in an attribute take place). On the other hand, cohort studies generally require large sample sizes, long-term follow-up of cohort members, large monetary expense, and complex administrative and organizational arrangements. The outcome of primary interest must be relatively common, or prohibitively large sample sizes will be needed to ensure adequate numbers experiencing the outcome. Therefore, prospective cohort studies are usually initiated under two circumstances: First, when sufficient (but not definitive) evidence has been obtained from less expensive studies to warrant more expensive cohort studies, and, second, when a new agent (e.g., a widely used medication) is introduced that may alter the risk for several diseases. In addition, cohort studies undertaken for one specific purpose are often used to test other hypotheses of interest as well.

Cohorts are sometimes chosen because they are representative of a certain community, such as in the Framingham Heart Study (Dawber *et al.*, 1951), which started in 1948. This study is ongoing and now includes both offspring and grandchildren of the original cohort members. Although the ability to generalize from such studies makes them highly desirable, they are usually expensive and lose a substantial proportion of participants over the course of many years. Furthermore, an exposure of interest may be uncommon in the general population so that selection of a cohort with a higher proportion exposed may be more efficient. People working in a specific industry or occupation are commonly enrolled in cohort studies since (a) they often have exposures of particular interest, (b) are less likely to be lost to follow-up, (c) have a certain amount of relevant information recorded in their medical and employment records, and (d) in many instances undergo initial and then periodic medical examinations. Cohorts from health insurance plans also offer various advantages, including the records that are kept of all patient encounters with the health plan.

A cohort that has provided a great deal of information about risk factors for several diseases in women is the Nurses' Health Study cohort. Nurses were selected not because of any particular occupational exposure, but because it was believed that their cooperation would be good and that they would report disease occurrence with a high degree of accuracy. The first nurses' cohort was established in 1976 and included 121 700 nurses. Following such a large cohort over many years might be prohibitively expensive, except that most of the information is collected through a questionnaire sent through the mail. A cohort study of a second group of nurses was established in 1987.

Retrospective cohort studies

In a retrospective cohort study (also called an historical cohort study), investigators assemble a cohort by reviewing records to identify exposures in the past (often decades previously). Based on recorded past exposure histories, cohort members are divided into exposed and nonexposed groups, or according to level of exposure. The investigator then reconstructs their subsequent disease or mortality experience up to some defined point in time. For instance, cancer incidence during the period 1953–96 was determined in workers who had been employed for at least 6 months in three Norwegian silicon carbide smelters (Romundstad *et al.*, 2001) and then compared to the cancer incidence in the population of Norway over the same time period. A greater number of lung cancer cases was found among the silicon workers than was expected on the basis of lung cancer rates in the general population.

Retrospective cohort studies have many of the advantages of prospective cohort studies, but can be completed in a much more timely fashion; consequently, they are considerably less expensive. However, only when the necessary information on past exposure has been recorded fairly accurately can a retrospective cohort study be undertaken with much likelihood of success. Tracing most of the cohort members must be possible in order to establish whether they developed the disease of interest (or have died). As with prospective cohort studies, a retrospective cohort study is usually feasible only when the outcome of interest is relatively common. Obtaining information on characteristics of the cohort members other than the exposure and outcome of primary interest is also frequently critical, so as to determine whether those with and without the exposure of interest are comparable in other relevant respects (e.g., smoking habits) and to allow statistical adjustment for differences. If such information is not available, interpretation of the study results may be ambiguous.

Cross-sectional studies

In a cross-sectional, or prevalence, study, both the exposure to a hypothesized risk factor and the occurrence of a disease are measured at one time (or over a relatively short period of time) in a study population. Prevalence proportions (numbers of cases of existing disease per population at risk at a given point in time or short period of time) among those with and without the exposure or characteristic of interest are then compared. For a quantitative variable such as blood pressure, the distributions of the variables in the exposed and unexposed are compared.

Cross-sectional studies include all cases of a disease, new and old, at a given point or period in time. Thus, it is

difficult to differentiate cause from effect. For instance, cross-sectional studies reporting higher proportions of smokers among persons with mental illnesses than among others (Lasser *et al.*, 2000) are unable to determine whether smoking predisposes people to mental illness or whether people with mental illnesses tend to take up smoking. Interpretation of cross-sectional studies is generally clear only for attributes that do not change as a result of the disease, such as genotype. In addition, the cases with disease of long duration tend to be overrepresented, since such cases are more likely to be identified at a given point in time than cases who recover or die quickly. Accordingly, any association found between an exposure and a disease may be attributable to survivorship with the disease rather than to development of the disease.

Another use of cross-sectional studies is simply to describe the prevalence of a disease in a population. For such studies to be useful, the individuals studied should be representative of the population to whom the results are to be generalized. Patients seen in tertiary care centers or in the practice of any one physician are seldom representative of all persons in the community with a disease, many of whom may not have sought medical care. Generalizations from such select groups of patients should be avoided.

An example of a cross-sectional study with important public health implications is a study of the prevalence of causes of blindness in a sample of Blacks and Whites in east Baltimore, Maryland (Sommer *et al.*, 1991). Whites were much more likely to have macular degeneration, and Blacks were more likely to have glaucoma. The prevalence of unoperated cataracts was high among middle-aged Blacks and among the elderly in both groups (**Table 3**). The authors suggest that about half of all blindness in this population is preventable or reversible and that certain population subgroups, such as Blacks and the elderly, should be targeted for education and intervention.

Table 3   Cross-sectional study of the prevalence of senile cataract in Blacks and Whites in east Baltimore, Maryland, by age and race

Age (years)	Race			
	Blacks		Whites	
	No. in age group	Prevalence per 1000	No. in age group	Prevalence per 1000
40–49	632	0	563	0
50–59	699	1.4	618	0
60–69	614	4.9	915	0
70–79	349	5.7	631	0
≥80	101	49.5	206	19.4

Adapted from Sommer A, Tielsch JM, Katz J, *et al.* (1991) Racial differences in the cause-specific prevalence of blindness in east Baltimore. *New England Journal of Medicine* 325: 1412–1417.

Hybrid Study Designs

Nested case-control studies

Sometimes it is possible to increase efficiency and maintain the advantages of a cohort study by designing a case-control study within either a prospective or retrospective cohort study. Such a study is often referred to as a nested case-control study. Suppose blood samples from a cohort of 10 000 people free of rheumatoid arthritis at baseline have been frozen and stored. Suppose that after 10 years 200 people have developed rheumatoid arthritis and 9800 have not. The stored sera from the 200 people with rheumatoid arthritis and a sample of, say, 600 of the 9800 people free of rheumatoid arthritis are thawed and analyzed for the presence of some serologic marker. This sampling of nondiseased individuals greatly reduces the cost from what it would be in a traditional cohort study in which sera from all 10 000 cohort members would be tested at the beginning of the study. Nevertheless, the serologic marker was present before the disease developed, thus providing the major advantage of a cohort study. The serologic status of the cases and controls is then compared, as in a traditional case-control study. In a nested case-control study, controls are selected from unaffected cohort members who are still alive and under surveillance at the time the cases developed the disease. Typically, the controls are matched to cases according to age, sex, and time of entry into the cohort. The availability of many banks of stored serum around the world and the current interest in serologic predictors of disease make nested case-control studies an attractive and economical approach, as long as the serologic marker of interest does not undergo degradation over time. Similarly, genetic markers of disease can be examined in a nested case-control study, provided appropriate cells have been properly stored.

In a nested case-control study within the Nurses' Health Study cohort (Hunter et al., 1997), plasma levels of organochlorine chemicals (mostly from pesticide exposure) were measured from the stored sera of nurses who developed breast cancer and a sample of nurses in whom breast cancer had not developed. **Table 4** shows that cases did not have higher levels of either chemical than did controls.

Case-cohort studies

Another hybrid study design being used with increasing frequency is the case-cohort study. A case-cohort study is another method of increasing efficiency compared to a traditional retrospective or prospective cohort study and is particularly useful when the associations between a serologic marker (or other variable) and two or more diseases are of interest. As in a nested case-control study, all cases occurring in a cohort are generally selected for study. However, in a case-cohort study, the comparison

Table 4   Nested case-control study of the associations between plasma levels of 1,1-dichloro-2,2-bis(p-chlorophenyl) ethylene (DDE) and polychlorinated biphenyls (PCBs), in parts per billion, and breast cancer within the Nurses Health Study cohort

Group	DDE		PCBs	
	Number in group	Mean[a]	Number in group	Mean[a]
Cases	236	6.01	230	5.08
Control	236	6.97	230	5.16

Adapted from Hunter DJ, Hankinson SE, Laden F, et al. (1997) Plasma organochlorine levels and the risk of breast cancer. New England Journal of Medicine 337: 1253–1258.
[a]The difference between the means for cases and controls is not statistically significant ($p > 0.05$).

group is a sample of the entire cohort, not just those free of disease, and the cohort members are not matched to the cases. Rather, other relevant variables and the possibility that some cases could be included in the comparison group are taken into account in the statistical analysis.

Cummings et al. (1998) used a case-cohort design within the Study of Osteoporotic Fractures, a prospective cohort study, to determine whether baseline concentrations of certain endogenous hormones predicted the occurrence of hip and vertebral fractures during follow-up. They compared hormone concentrations from stored serum samples of women who developed hip and vertebral fractures during follow-up with hormone concentrations from stored sera of a random sample of women from the same cohort. They found that undetectable serum estradiol concentrations and high concentrations of sex hormone-binding globulin at baseline were associated with increased risks for both hip and vertebral fractures.

Ecologic studies

In an ecologic study, a summary measure of exposure and a summary measure of disease frequency are obtained for aggregates of individuals, such as persons in certain geographic areas or time periods. The purpose is to determine whether the units with the highest (or lowest) frequency of exposure tend to be the units with the highest (or lowest) frequency of disease. For instance, it has long been observed that countries with the highest per capita consumption of beer have the highest incidence rates of rectal cancer. However, there are many other differences among these countries in addition to their beer consumption. Additional analytic studies are needed to determine whether within these countries the individuals who drink the most beer have the highest rectal cancer rates. An ecologic study in the United States (McGwin et al., 2004) reported that states with lower mortality rates from motorcycle accidents were more likely than other states to require a skill test for a motorcycle permit, driver training, a long duration of a learner's permit, three or more learner permit restrictions (e.g., no passengers, no riding at night), and a helmet for motorcycle operators of all ages. This report needs to be followed up by studies to determine whether individuals with these training characteristics are the ones with lower risk of death from motorcycle accidents, taking into account other relevant attributes such as the alcohol consumption of the individuals and the overall safety of the roads in the states.

When appropriate aggregated and individual-level data are available, two or more different levels of aggregation (e.g., state, county, municipality, census tract, block group, block, individual) can be considered in the same study and nested within each other to form a hierarchy of levels, each of which could be contributing to risk for the disease under study. Special methods of statistical analysis, called multilevel analysis or multilevel modeling, are used to try to separate out the contributions of the different levels of aggregation to disease risk.

Selected Epidemiologic Concepts in Observational Studies

Confounding

The possibility of confounding, which is especially likely to occur in observational studies, usually needs to be considered when trying to interpret associations between exposures and diseases. A confounding variable is a variable that (a) alters the risk of the disease or condition under study independent of the exposure or characteristic of primary interest, and (b) is associated with the exposure or characteristic of primary interest in the study population, but (c) is not a consequence of that exposure. Suppose that an investigator finds that coffee drinking during pregnancy is associated with an increased risk for delivery of a low-birth-weight infant. The investigator would have to be concerned that this statistical association between coffee consumption and delivery of a low-birth-weight infant is actually attributable to a tendency of coffee drinkers to smoke cigarettes to a greater extent than non-coffee drinkers, and that it is the cigarette smoking that puts them at an elevated risk for delivering a low-birth-weight infant, not the coffee drinking. In this instance, smoking is considered a confounding variable.

With any study design, information on potential confounding variables can be obtained during data collection and then controlled for in the statistical analysis. Alternatively, in cohort studies, one or more potential confounding variables may be taken into account in the study design by matching unexposed to exposed individuals on the potential confounding variable(s), which then must be taken into account in the statistical analysis by using stratification or regression methods. In case-control

studies, controls may be matched to cases on one or more potential confounding variables, and the matching again taken into account in the analysis. It is possible to match roughly on certain variables in the study design and then control more tightly in the analysis. Measurement of potential confounding variables is highly important, because otherwise they cannot be adequately taken into account in the study design or analysis.

Effect Modification

Effect modification, also called statistical interaction, occurs when the magnitude of the association between one variable and another differs according to the level of a third variable. For instance, the association between obesity and risk for breast cancer varies according to whether a woman is premenopausal or postmenopausal. Among postmenopausal women, obese women are at elevated risk for breast cancer, while before menopause, obese women are not at increased risk for breast cancer and may even be at decreased risk compared to thin women. An area of considerable current interest is whether the effects on disease risk of certain environmental exposures and lifestyle factors are modified by a person's genotype. For example, Hines *et al.* (2001) found that moderate alcohol drinkers as a group were at decreased risk for myocardial infarction compared to non-drinkers. However, an individual's alcohol dehydrogenase type 3 (ADH3) genotype modified this association. Moderate alcohol drinkers who were homozygous for the slow-oxidizing ADH3 allele had greater high-density lipoprotein levels and a substantially decreased risk for myocardial infarction compared to moderate alcohol drinkers of other genotypes. In the statistical analysis, identification of effect modification involves comparing associations between exposures and diseases in subgroups of the population (e.g., in premenopausal vs. postmenopausal women; in those homozygous for the slow-oxidizing ADH3 allele vs. those of other genotypes).

Some Measures of Association and Their Attributes

Relative Risk

In cohort studies, the strength of the association between a putative risk factor and a disease is often measured by what is called a relative risk (or more accurately, a rate ratio or risk ratio; a discussion of rate ratios and risk ratios is beyond the scope of this article). A relative risk is simply the risk (or incidence rate) of disease in one group (usually the exposed) divided by the risk (or incidence rate) of disease in another group (usually the unexposed). A relative risk (or, technically, a rate ratio) of

$0.043/0.088 = 0.49$ can be computed from **Table 2**, consistent with a beneficial effect of religiousness. Before reaching any conclusions, however, one would want to check for confounding by a variety of variables that are associated with religiousness and life expectancy, such as smoking habits, alcohol consumption, and many other attributes.

Odds Ratio

In case-control studies, risks and incidence rates usually cannot be determined because the investigator has selected the study population based on the presence or absence of disease and does not know disease frequency specifically in the exposed and unexposed. Therefore, relative risks cannot be computed. Rather, the odds ratio is calculated. In an unmatched case-control study, the odds ratio is estimated by the ratio of exposed to unexposed among cases divided by the ratio of exposed to unexposed among controls. In a case-control study in which controls are individually matched to cases, the odds ratio is estimated as the ratio of the number of case-control pairs in which the case is exposed and not the control to the number of pairs in which the control is exposed and not the case. It can be shown that for all but the most common diseases (i.e., more than 10% of the exposed or unexposed population affected), the odds ratio is a good approximation to the relative risk and can be interpreted in a similar manner. In the case-control study described above of the association between smoking and lung cancer (**Table 1**), the odds ratio of $\frac{1350/7}{1296/61} = 9.1$ indicates that the odds of lung cancer in smokers is more than nine times that in nonsmokers. The odds ratio in the study mentioned previously of the association between phytoestrogen consumption and breast cancer was 1.0 for the highest quartile of consumption versus the lowest quartile, suggesting no association, either negative or positive, between phytoestrogen consumption and breast cancer.

Standardized Ratios

The standardized mortality ratio (SMR) and the standardized incidence ratio (SIR) are generally used when disease rates in the cohort under study are being compared to disease rates in a reference population, such as the general population of the geographic area from which the cohort was selected. The SMR (or SIR) is the ratio of observed number of deaths (or incident cases) in the cohort to the number of deaths (or incident cases) that would be expected, for example, on the basis of age- and gender-specific death (or incidence) rates in the general population. The SIR of 1.85 (74 observed cases/39.9 expected cases) for lung cancer incidence in male Norwegian silicon carbide smelter workers (Romundstad

et al., 2001) indicates that there are almost twice as many lung cancer cases among the smelter workers as would be expected based on the age- and time-period-specific incidence rates in the male population of Norway.

Confidence Interval

A confidence interval should be presented along with estimates of the relative risk, odds ratio, or other parameter in order to give a range of plausible values for the parameter being estimated. A 95% confidence interval of 1.46–2.75 around a point estimate of relative risk of 2.00, for instance, indicates that a relative risk of less than 1.46 or greater than 2.75 can be ruled out at the 95% confidence level, and that a statistical test of any relative risk outside the interval would yield a probability value less than 0.05.

Attributable Fraction

Provided that the association between a risk factor and a disease is causal (see the section titled 'Guidelines for Assessing Causation from Observational Studies' below), the attributable fraction provides a rough indication of the proportion of disease occurrence that potentially would be eliminated if exposure to the risk factor were prevented. It should not, however, be confused with the proportion of cases caused by the exposure or the probability of causation. The attributable fraction can be calculated either for exposed individuals only or for the population as a whole. In a cohort study, the attributable fraction for the exposed can be computed as

$$\frac{(\text{Risk for exposed} - \text{Risk for unexposed})}{\text{Risk for exposed}}$$

or, equivalently

$$\frac{\text{Relative risk} - 1}{\text{Relative risk}}$$

The attributable fraction for the population can be computed as

$$\frac{(\text{Risk for entire population}) - (\text{Risk for unexposed})}{\text{Risk for entire population}}$$

or, equivalently

$$\frac{\text{prevalence of exposure in population} \times (\text{Relative risk} - 1)}{1 + (\text{prevalence of exposure in population}) \times (\text{Relative risk} - 1)}$$

In case-control studies of uncommon diseases, the odds ratio can be substituted for the relative risk to provide a good approximation to the attributable fraction that would be computed using the relative risk.

It is important to note that in the presence of confounding, other formulae must be used to estimate attributable fractions.

Measurement Error

Inaccurate measurement can lead to erroneous conclusions. The possibility of measurement error is of concern for most variables considered in observational epidemiologic studies. Exposures such as diet and physical activity are almost always measured by questionnaire, and their measurement can entail a great deal of error. Measurement of some diseases such as arthritic disorders and psychiatric disorders is difficult because of the frequent absence of definitive diagnostic criteria.

The validity or accuracy of a measurement refers to the average closeness of the measurement to the true value. Reliability or reproducibility refers to the extent to which the same value of the measurement is obtained on the same occasion by the same observer, on multiple occasions by the same observer, or by different observers on the same occasion. Precision refers to the amount of variation around the measurement or estimate; a precise measure will have a small amount of variation around it, but may or may not be valid. Measurement error is said to be differential if the magnitude of error for one variable differs according to the actual value of other variables, and nondifferential if the magnitude or error in one variable does not vary according to the actual value of other variables. In a 2×2 table (e.g., exposure present or absent, disease present or absent), nondifferential misclassification always causes the relative risk or odds ratio to be closer to 1.0 than the true value, provided that errors in measurement of the two variables are independent. Dependent, or differential, misclassification, on the other hand, can cause associations to be overestimated or underestimated, depending on the circumstances.

When measurement error occurs for a potential confounding variable, adjusting for the confounding variable in the analysis will not entirely remove its effect. When both the exposure and confounder are measured with error, effects are less predictable. Also, when estimates are made from tables larger than 2×2, there are circumstances under which even nondifferential measurement error can cause an association to appear larger than it really is.

Common Sources of Bias in Observational Epidemiologic Studies

Bias refers to the tendency of a measurement or a statistic systematically to underestimate or overestimate the true value of that measurement or statistic. Bias can arise from many sources in observational epidemiologic studies. It can affect estimates of disease and exposure frequency and the magnitude of associations between exposures and diseases. Biases from uncontrolled confounding and from measurement error were described in previous sections. Some other common sources of bias are described in the following sections.

Information Bias

This is systematic error in measuring the exposure or outcome such that data are more accurate or more complete in one group than in another. Interviewer bias, recall bias, and reporting bias are examples of information bias.

Interviewer bias is systematic error occurring when an interviewer does not collect information in a similar manner for each group being compared. For example, if an interviewer believes, whether subconsciously or not, that a certain drug increases the risk for breast cancer, in a case-control study the interviewer might probe more deeply into the medication history of cases than controls.

Recall bias is systematic error resulting from differences in the accuracy or completeness of recall of past events between groups. In a case-control study, mothers of infants whose children are born with a congenital malformation may think back and remember events during the pregnancy more thoroughly than mothers of apparently healthy infants.

Reporting bias is a systematic error resulting from the tendency of people in one group to be more or less likely to report information than others. In a case-control study, cases with certain diseases might be more likely to deny that they had used alcohol than controls.

Selection Bias

This is systematic error occurring as a result of differences between those who are and those who are not selected for inclusion in a study or who are selected to be in a certain group within a study. Examples of selection bias are ascertainment bias, detection bias, and response bias.

Ascertainment bias is systematic error consequent to failure to identify equally all categories of individuals who are supposed to be represented in a group. For example, a specialty hospital may include mostly very sick or complicated cases who are not representative of all cases.

Detection bias is systematic error resulting from greater likelihood of some cases being identified, diagnosed, or verified than others. For instance, a diagnosis of pulmonary embolism may be more likely to be made in oral contraceptive users than in non-users because the oral contraceptive users may be more likely to have a lung scan for chest pain. As a result, an association between oral contraceptives and pulmonary embolism might result at least in part from greater likelihood of disease detection.

Response bias is systematic error resulting from differences between those who do and do not choose to participate in a study, and between those who remain in a cohort study and those who do not. In a study to estimate disease incidence or prevalence, even though a sample is scientifically selected, if a substantial proportion of those who are selected do not participate, the sample is likely to give biased results. In a study trying to estimate the prevalence of a disease, for instance, those with serious disease may be too sick to participate, and busy people may have little interest in participating. Accordingly, very ill and very busy people may be underrepresented in the study. If people who are sicker are less likely to return for follow-up visits in a cohort study, information on disease status of those who do continue to participate will not be representative of the disease status of all persons who were originally enrolled in the study.

Guidelines for Assessing Causation from Observational Studies

Because most epidemiologic studies are observational, conclusions about the likelihood of causation often have to be made on the basis of observational studies, despite their limitations and potential biases. In recent years, counterfactual, graphical, and structural equation models have begun to be applied to the analysis of possible causal relationships. Although beyond the scope of this article, these models are likely to see increasing applications in observational epidemiology in the future.

Over the years, epidemiologists have developed practical guidelines to be used as tests of whether a causal association exists. Not all criteria need to be fulfilled in all instances, nor are all equally important or always applicable. However, taken together, they provide some guidance about whether an association between a given exposure and disease is one of cause and effect.

- Strength of association: The measure of association (e.g., relative risk) should be elevated (or decreased for a protective factor), indicating that the exposed are at increased risk of disease compared to the unexposed. The higher the relative risk, the more likely the association is to be causal. As a rough rule of thumb, a relative risk or odds ratio of 2 suggests a moderate elevation in risk, and a relative risk of 3 or more is considered strong.
- Ruling out alternative explanations: Once it has been determined that an association between an exposure and disease exists, other explanations for the observed association, such as methodological deficiencies and confounding, should be carefully considered and tested against any available data or background information.
- Dose–response relationship: If increasing dose or length of exposure is associated with increasing risk, then the case for causality is considerably enhanced. The absence of a dose–response relationship, however,

does not disprove causality since other patterns, such as a threshold effect, could also exist.
- Removal of exposure: If the presence of an exposure increases risk of disease and removing the exposure reduces risk, the likelihood of a causal association is increased.
- Time order: It should be clear that the exposure caused the disease and not that the disease caused the exposure. This issue is especially relevant in cross-sectional studies, in which prevalent cases and exposures are considered simultaneously. Time order is unique among the causal guidelines in that if the disease can be shown to have preceded the exposure, the exposure cannot have caused the disease.
- Predictive ability: Tentative hypotheses regarding causation that can be shown to predict future occurrences better than alternative hypotheses provide strong support for causality.
- Consistency: If associations of similar magnitude are found in different populations by different methods of study, the likelihood of causality is increased, since all studies are unlikely to have the same methodological limitations or idiosyncrasies of the study population.
- Biologic plausibility: When a new finding fits well with current knowledge of the biology of a disease, it is more plausible than if a whole new theory must be developed to explain the finding. Another way of enhancing biologic plausibility is through laboratory experiments. However, what occurs in a laboratory or in animals may have limited applicability to free-living humans.
- Coherence of evidence: The various relationships and findings should make biologic and epidemiologic sense.
- Confirmation in experimental studies: When available, the results of well-designed experiments in which exposures are assigned at random are very convincing because the only factor on which groups differ, except by chance, is the exposure of interest. However, in many circumstances, exposures cannot be ethically or practically assigned at random. In addition, experiments on carefully selected people may have limited relevance to the general, free-living population.

It should be apparent that decisions on the likelihood of causality are of necessity partly judgmental. What one person may believe is a causal association, another person may not. Lilienfeld (1957) divided the degree of evidence for causation into three levels (**Table 5**). At the first level, the evidence is considered sufficient for further study. For instance, studies suggesting that the risk of certain cancers is increased by high levels of exposure to electromagnetic fields fall into this category. At the second level, the evidence is considered sufficient to warrant public health action, even if the causal association has not been definitively established. Many people would put the

Table 5   Levels of evidence for causation

Level 1	The evidence is sufficient to warrant further investigation
Level 2	The evidence is sufficient for recommending preventive action
Level 3	The evidence is sufficient to say that a causal inference has been proved; this causal hypothesis is included in our body of scientific knowledge

Adapted from Lilienfeld A (1957) Epidemiologic methods and inferences in studies of non-infectious diseases. *Public Health Reports* 72: 51–60.

evidence that a healthy diet protects against certain cancers at this second level. At the third level, the evidence is so strong that the causal association is considered part of the body of scientific knowledge. The evidence that smoking causes lung cancer or that the human immunodeficiency virus causes AIDS is at this level of certainty.

Conclusion

Observational epidemiology plays an important role in learning about disease causation. Major concerns of epidemiologists undertaking observational epidemiologic studies include using the best sources of data, employing the proper study designs, selecting appropriate study populations, using good methods of measurement, quantifying the magnitudes of associations, controlling for confounding, and detecting effect modification. In practice, it is often not possible to meet all these objectives to the extent desired because people may choose not to participate in a study, optimal measurement may not be feasible, and a variety of other problems may arise. It is important to recognize the effects of these inadequacies in various situations because specific inadequacies can affect study results in different ways.

It should be readily apparent that conclusions drawn from observational epidemiologic studies, as with other types of scientific inquiry, are often not final. Results generally require confirmation from additional epidemiologic or laboratory studies, experimental studies, or ascertainment of the effect of removal or modification of the suspected risk factor. What was believed to be a causal association may later be found to be attributable to uncontrolled confounding, and an association thought to be attributable to uncontrolled confounding may turn out to be causal. A causal agent in one population may not operate the same way in another population. The best method of measurement at one point in time may later be supplanted by a better method. In any one study, a reported association may have occurred by chance, especially when many possible associations are being examined.

Thus, it is essential to keep an open mind as new knowledge accumulates about disease causation from epidemiologic, laboratory, and other types of studies and as attempts are made to replicate the results of even the most carefully executed individual studies. In this way, knowledge about disease causation gradually evolves.

See also: Clinical Epidemiology; Demography, Epidemiology and Public Health; Genetic Epidemiology; Social Epidemiology; Surveillance of Disease.

Citations

Cummings SR, Browner WS, Bauer D, *et al.* (1998) Endogenous hormones and the risk of hip and vertebral fractures among older women. Study of Osteoporotic Fractures Research Group. *New England Journal of Medicine* 339: 733–738.

Dawber TR, Meadors GF, and Moore FE Jr (1951) Epidemiological approaches to heart disease: The Framingham Study. *American Journal of Public Health* 41: 279–286.

Doll R and Hill A (1952) A study of the aetiology of carcinoma of the lung. *British Medical Journal* 2: 1271–1286.

Dowell SF, Kupronis BA, Zell ER, *et al.* (2000) Mortality from pneumonia in children in the United States, 1939 through 1996. *New England Journal of Medicine* 342: 1399–1407.

Goh KJ, Tan CT, Chew NK, *et al.* (2000) Clinical features of Nipah virus encephalitis among pig farmers in Malaysia. *New England Journal of Medicine* 342: 1229–1235.

Hines LM, Stampfer MJ, Ma J, *et al.* (2001) Genetic variation in alcohol dehydrogenase and the beneficial effect of moderate alcohol consumption on myocardial infarction. *New England Journal of Medicine* 344: 549–555.

Horn-Ross PL, John EM, Lee M, *et al.* (2001) Phytoestrogen consumption and breast cancer risk in a multiethnic population: The Bay Area Breast Cancer Study. *American Journal of Epidemiology* 154: 434–441.

Hunter DJ, Hankinson SE, Laden F, *et al.* (1997) Plasma organochlorine levels and the risk of breast cancer. *New England Journal of Medicine* 337: 1253–1258.

Jacobus CH, Holick MF, Shao Q, *et al.* (1992) Hypervitaminosis D associated with drinking milk. *New England Journal of Medicine* 326: 1173–1177.

Lasser K, Boyd JW, Woolhandler S, *et al.* (2000) Smoking and mental illness: A population-based prevalence study. *Journal of the American Medical Association* 284: 2606–2610.

Lilienfeld A (1957) Epidemiologic methods and inferences in studies of non-infectious diseases. *Public Health Reports* 72: 51–60.

Maguire-Boston EK, Suman V, Jacobsen SJ, *et al.* (1999) Blood transfusion and risk of non-Hodgkin's lymphoma. *American Journal of Epidemiology* 149: 1113–1118.

Mason TJ, McKay FW, Hoover R, *et al.* (1975) *Atlas of Cancer Mortality for US Counties: 1950–1969* Washington, DC: US Department of Health Education, and Welfare. DHEW Publication No. (NIH) 75–750.

McGwin G Jr, Whately J, Metzger J, *et al.* (2004) The effect of state motorcycle licensing laws on motorcycle driver mortality rates. *Journal of Trauma* 56: 415–419.

Miettinen OS (1985) The "case-control" study: valid selection of subjects. *Journal of Chronic Diseases* 38: 543–548.

Romundstad P, Andersen A, and Haldorsen T (2001) Cancer incidence among workers in the Norwegian silicon carbide industry. *American Journal of Epidemiology* 153: 978–986.

Sommer A, Tielsch JM, Katz J, *et al.* (1991) Racial differences in the cause-specific prevalence of blindness in east Baltimore. *New England Journal of Medicine* 325: 1412–1417.

Zuckerman DM, Kasl SV, and Ostfeld AM (1984) Psychosocial predictors of mortality among the elderly poor. The role of religion, well-being, and social contacts. *American Journal of Epidemiology* 119: 410–423.

Further Reading

Austin H, Hill HA, Flanders WD, *et al.* (1994) Limitations in the application of case-control methodology. *Epidemiologic Reviews* 16: 65–76.

Friedman GD (2004) *Primer of Epidemiology,* 5th edn. New York: McGraw-Hill Inc.

Gordis L (2000) *Epidemiology,* 2nd edn. Philadelphia, PA: WB Saunders Company.

Greenland S (2000) Causal analysis in the health sciences. *Journal of the American Statistical Association* 95: 286–289.

Greenland S (2001) Ecologic versus individual-level sources of bias in ecologic estimates of contextual health effects. *International Journal of Epidemiology* 30: 1343–1350.

Kelsey JL, Whittemore AS, Evans AS, *et al.* (1996) *Methods in Observational Epidemiology,* 2nd edn. New York: Oxford University Press.

Koepsell TD and Weiss NS (2003) *Epidemiologic Methods. Studying the Occurrence of Illness.* New York: Oxford University Press.

Last JM (ed.) (2001) *A Dictionary of Epidemiology,* 4th edn. New York: Oxford University Press.

Rothman KJ and Greenland S (1998) *Modern Epidemiology,* 2nd edn. Philadelphia, PA: Lippincott Raven.

Szklo M and Nieto FJ (2000) *Epidemiology, Beyond the Basics.* Gaithersburg, MD: Aspen Publishers.

Health Surveys

J H Madans, National Center for Health Statistics, Hyattsville, MD, USA

Published by Elsevier Inc.

Information on health status, risk factors, health insurance, and health-care utilization is used to plan, conduct, and evaluate public health programs, to inform policies, regulations, and legislation, and to conduct research to better understand the determinants and consequences of health and health care. Much of this information is collected through health surveys. Although some surveys focus on only one aspect of health, others are multipurpose and attempt to gather at least some information on the range of factors that define health so that the interconnections among these factors can be studied. Although surveys may differ in content, sample design and data collection methodologies, the general issues that guide survey development apply to most health surveys.

How to Measure Health

Health is as much a social as a biologic concept. There is no question that the biologic aspects of health are of great importance to individuals and to society, but how these objective aspects of health affect social functioning is perhaps even more important. In addition, although the biologic aspects of health lend themselves to objective measures, the social aspects present a much greater challenge. Characteristics of the environment and the individual affect how objective health is perceived and reported. The same objective health states can have very different impacts on an individual's ability to function and perform social roles. Health is affected by socioeconomic factors and in turn affects those factors. Some health surveys attempt to address all aspects of health; others focus in greater depth on only one aspect. The universes from which the samples are drawn, the methods used to collect the information, and the health and health-related information obtained will wary depending on the specific objectives of the survey.

Content of Health Surveys

The information collected on health surveys can be divided into three general types: (1) health status; (2) determinants or correlates of health and risks to health, including health behaviors; and (3) health-care utilization. In addition, information is also collected on demographic and socioeconomic factors that affect health. Each of these subjects is complex and multidimensional. Health status has many components, which range from physiologic structure and function to the ability to participate in a range of social activities. Risk factors also are varied and include exposure to environmental contaminants, economic and social characteristics, and individual behaviors. Health care can affect the incidence, development, and impact of health conditions. To obtain information on all of these topics, a range of survey mechanisms is used, but each mechanism is subject to known, and often uncontrollable, measurement error. It is usually necessary to piece together information from different sources to get a full picture of health.

Conditions and Diseases

Health status is sometimes equated with having one or more physical, psychological, or mental diseases or conditions. A variety of approaches can be used to measure disease incidence and prevalence, including reporting of a diagnosis by a health-care provider, reporting of symptoms (if an appropriate symptom battery exists), medication use, and direct diagnostic testing. Additional information of interest related to conditions includes date of onset, the use of health-care services, and the impact of the condition on the individual's ability to function. Condition severity is often inferred from the type of medications or health-care services used or the nature of the functional impact of the condition. Information on conditions that is obtained through interviews reflects an individual's knowledge of his or her health status, which in turn is a function of the receipt of appropriate health care and adequate communication between a health-care professional and a patient. This is particularly true when condition prevalence is based on having received a diagnosis from a health-care professional. Surveys that include direct physical exams, however, have the advantage of allowing for the measurement of previously undiagnosed conditions.

Sources of Information

Interview surveys provide a major source of information on conditions and disease. One issue that must be addressed is the number of conditions to be included in the questionnaire. Condition checklists can be used to obtain information on a great number of conditions, but in most cases, only a minimal amount of information on any given condition is collected. In addition, long checklists are difficult to administer and may result in reporting errors. However, the use of comprehensive lists does allow for the ascertainment of comorbidities. An alternative is to obtain more detailed information on a select group of conditions. Criteria such as the prevalence of the condition or the potential impact on the individual or the health-care system are used to select target conditions such as heart disease, diabetes, cancer, pulmonary diseases, depression, and arthritis.

Another way to limit the amount of information that needs to be collected is to focus on more serious conditions. Some surveys do this by limiting their focus to conditions that result in the receipt of medical care or in activity restriction such as missing work or school. This provides a somewhat more concrete referent for the questions being asked, which should result in improved data validity and reliability. However, limiting the definition of health problems to those that result in behavior such as seeking care or restricting activity is more appropriate when ill health is primarily the result of acute conditions for which onset is clear and there is a closer association between the condition and the care-seeking behavior. As a result of the 'epidemiologic transition,' acute conditions have given way to chronic conditions as the major sources of morbidity. Chronic conditions are more difficult to

diagnose, and longer periods are spent in the disease state both prior to and after diagnosis. This complicates the collection of self-reported condition information because respondents have difficulty recalling the onset of symptoms or diagnoses made many years prior to the survey.

Requiring that health-care use or activity limitation be present when identifying conditions also makes it difficult to investigate social correlates of health status, since the definition incorporates a social dimension. Access to sick leave or affordable medical care may be limited by social or economic factors. Persons who do not demonstrate the required behaviors because of these social factors will not be considered as having a health condition. This can result in bias if the data are used to measure the condition's prevalence or impact or to investigate disparities across subgroups.

Examination surveys provide a complementary mechanism for obtaining information on conditions. The results of the physical exam, and of blood and other tests, can be used to objectively measure health status. For example, information on diagnosed hypertension or diabetes can be obtained from an interview, but information on undiagnosed conditions must be obtained from objective tests. However, if a condition is controlled by medication, the objective test will not provide information on diagnosed cases. Information on diagnosed and undiagnosed conditions is needed for a complete accounting of the health condition.

Surveys of providers (hospitals, office-based private physicians, managed-care organizations, hospital outpatient departments, emergency departments, ambulatory surgery centers, and long-term care facilities) are generally used to obtain information on health-care utilization and the health-care system, but information in the administrative and medical record can be used to study conditions that are associated with medical care.

Provider-based surveys are particularly important for obtaining information on rare conditions that would not be picked up in population-based surveys. Although information is collected on all conditions for which health care is obtained, the nature of the information available is limited to that which would routinely be obtained from medical records. Information on the condition can be abstracted from the record and then coded, or the codes can be taken from summaries or billing records. The amount of information available affects the accuracy with which codes can be assigned. Payment considerations can affect what is entered into the record and the coding process. These constraints need to be considered when analyzing this type of data. In addition, the event (e.g., the discharge), rather than the person, is the unit of analysis. For example, although it is possible to estimate the number of hospital stays associated with hip fracture from a survey of hospital stays, it is not possible to estimate the number of persons with hip fracture even if one could assume that all persons with hip fracture were admitted to the hospital. An enhancement to healthcare surveys would be to follow patients after the healthcare encounter.

The development and adoption of electronic health records has the potential of changing how provider-based surveys are conducted. Currently, information is usually obtained from discharge summaries or billing records. If more detailed information is needed, it is necessary to abstract information from the medical record, a method that is costly and subject to bias, as information is not entered into records in a structured and standardized way. Electronic health records have the potential not only to facilitate the retrieval of information but also to standardize the information made available, thus improving the quality of that information.

Cause of death statistics obtained from vital registration systems also provide essential information on medical conditions. Although not error free, a great deal of effort is put forth to standardize the collection and coding of cause of death. International standards (WHO, 2004) have been developed which provide coding rules and specifications, and these are updated periodically to reflect advances in medical science.

Measuring Function and Disability

Physical, cognitive, emotional, and social functioning are important components of health status. Although disease states are more closely related to the biologic aspects of health, functioning is dependent on both the biologic and social realms. Information on functional status can be ascertained through objective tests but is most often obtained through direct reporting by the individual or a proxy. Information on functional status encompasses a wide range of activities from the very basic such as raising an arm to the more complex such as working and going to school. Obtaining information on functioning is complicated by the fact that performance is affected not only by physiologic abilities but also by the environment (which includes the physical environment and the use of assistive devices). A person's ability to walk may be impaired by a condition that leads to weakened muscles, but with the use of braces or a wheelchair, along with appropriate accommodations in the physical environment (e.g., ramps), that individual is mobile and able to carry out appropriate social roles. For some purposes, information is needed on functional ability without the use of assistance of any type. In other cases, functioning ability as measured by usual performance is important. Although functional limitations in a given domain can result from a range of impairments and conditions and it is not necessary to know the specific causes to evaluate functional status, information on the conditions causing the limitation is often collected. This information is needed to fully understand causal processes and to plan targeted interventions. Age at onset and changes in functioning ability over time are also often used to characterize functional status.

Although the concept of functioning is central to health, the measurement of functioning presents complex problems in collecting data. Since functioning involves all aspects of life, obtaining complete information on functioning would require an extensive effort to collect data. In addition, since functioning results from the interaction between abilities and the environment, a full evaluation would require independent documentation of the component parts. Following good survey practices, specific questions would be needed to assure standardized responses. However, no health survey is comprehensive enough to obtain all the necessary information. As a result, information is usually collected on a limited number of functioning domains using questions that are general rather than specific in nature and that use unstated rather than explicit standards against which respondents compare their own functioning. The less explicit the standard, the more likely the response will be affected by external factors and the less likely that the data will be comparable across population groups. For example, no explicit standard is provided by a question that asks subjects if they are limited in the kind or amount of work they can do. Responses to this question will be affected by the kind of work that the individual thinks he or she should be doing as defined by his or her own expectations and by the requirements set by government agencies such as disability programs as well as by more objective states of health. This is less of a problem if one is interested in monitoring the impact of health on work. However, it is much more of a problem if the aim is to understand and monitor a more objective measure of health. As a result of these complexities, a large number of questionnaire batteries have been developed to measure functioning. Some use only a few questions, focus on the more complex social roles, and do not differentiate between different aspects of functioning (physical, cognitive, emotional, or behavioral). Others are quite lengthy and obtain detailed information on a wide range of activities both with and without assistance.

Survey data on functioning are used to study disability from a policy and programmatic perspective. Disability is an umbrella term that encompasses physiological impairments; limitations in physical, cognitive, mental, and psychological functioning; and restrictions in the ability to participate in daily life. This requires information on characteristics of the individual but also on characteristics of the environment and the interaction between the two. Historically, statistics on disability have been a function of the specific conceptual definition used and the way the concepts were operationalized in the data collection process. As a result, disability statistics have not been comparable across time, place, or population subgroup or easily interpretable. Recent work has focused on clarifying the various aspects of disability (including aspects of functioning, as previously mentioned) and developing standard data collection methods that will produce a range of statistics that can be used for different purposes.

Many health surveys are limited to the noninstitutionalized population and therefore do not include those segments of the population in poorest health or with the highest level of functional limitations: those in long-term care settings. Special studies of these populations can be carried out, and there should be some attempt to combine results from the noninstitutionalized and long-term care populations. Changes in the delivery of long-term care with the expansion of transitional establishments have made this an even more important issue for survey designers.

Overall Health Status and Summary Measures of Health

As previously noted, health status is a multidimensional concept. This complex construct requires multiple indicators and methodologies for adequate measurement. However, there is a strong desire on the part of policymakers and researchers for an overall measure of health in order to more easily characterize and monitor the health status of a population and for use in cost–benefit and cost-effectiveness analyses. There is also increasing interest in developing basic health status indicators comparable to the economic indicators currently in use. These indicators would be used to monitor the effects of public policy and to identify areas in which interventions are needed. An overall health measure is very appealing in this context. Such a measure could take a variety of forms. A single question can be used to obtain information on overall health status. An example of such a question is the request for the respondent to rate his or her own health or the health of another person as excellent, very good, good, fair, or poor. Respondent-assessed general health status is a popular summary indicator of health status. This measure has been shown to be highly correlated with other measures of health status and is predictive of mortality and admission to long-term care facilities. However, this measure also has limitations when used to monitor change over time, one of the primary uses of health status indicators. The means by which individuals evaluate the various aspects of health have been shown to be affected by contextual parameters. Implicit in self-perceived health status is the individual's evaluation of his or her health status against some unstated standard. Societal norms act to define the standard, but the norms and the standards change in response to a variety of conditions and can change over time. For example, another measure of overall health, reported limitation of activity, has been shown to be affected by the criteria used by government agencies

in determining eligibility for disability benefits, which influence how individuals evaluate their health. Thus, observed changes in the indicator may not reflect changes in underlying health status but rather reflect changes in broader societal trends that affect how individuals evaluate their health.

Alternatively, summary measures can be constructed by using information on diagnosis of a disease or condition, symptoms such as pain or fatigue, and physical, cognitive, emotional, and social functioning. Health surveys that collect information on the widest possible range of health-related factors offer the opportunity to develop multiple summary measures that can be used for different purposes. Measures of health states can also be combined with measures of life expectancy to create measures of healthy life expectancy. Examples of this kind of measure include disability-free life years, disability adjusted life years, healthy life expectancy, and years of healthy life. Constructs such as these combine measures of the different aspects of health into a single number by using a conceptual model that views health as a continuum. The health states are assigned weights that represent the values that either society as a whole or individuals place on that health status. Various methods have been used to determine the values of the different health states. These measures are used to modify duration of life and may be multiplied by the number of years in that state.

Determinants of Health

Health surveys generally include measures of risk factors, health behaviors, and non-health determinants or correlates of health such as socioeconomic status. The range of measures that can be included is wide and varies by survey. Age, gender, and race/ethnicity are the basic demographic variables that are included in health surveys. Socioeconomic determinants of health include education, income, geographic region, and urbanicity of residence. Strong health differentials are found across these variables, and public programs are designed to eliminate these health disparities. However, the relationship between these measures and health is often complex. Social factors can act as causal agents or they can be affected by health. For example, low income can result in poorer health status, but poor health status can also affect earning capability and income. In order to identify causal relationships between determinants and outcomes, longitudinal designs are needed. The causal pathways are more easily teased apart if health surveys can include a broader array of potential determinants of health (biologic, psychological, and social).

Tobacco use, alcohol use, diet, and physical exercise are common health behaviors that are included in health surveys. As in the case of health status, these concepts present difficult measurement challenges. Diet is particularly difficult to capture in the survey context. Respondents have difficulty remembering what they ate and in what quantities. Obtaining valid information on behaviors such as diet, smoking, and exercise requires significant survey time. There is also a tendency for respondents to underreport negative behaviors such as smoking, and this is even more of a problem for surveys that obtain information on illegal activities such as drug use. Survey procedures have been developed to improve reporting of health behaviors such as maximizing privacy to encourage accurate reporting and developing aids to enhance memory.

Health-care Utilization

The use of the health-care system is a major dimension of health. Information on utilization and related characteristics such as health insurance are collected from person-based surveys and through surveys of administrative records. In person-based surveys, respondents are asked to recall the number of contacts they have had with various health-care providers and the nature of the provider and the contact. Information on the receipt of particular services, such as immunizations or mammography, is also obtained. This is often difficult for respondents and the reporting of contacts with the health-care system drops off considerably when the recall period extends beyond two weeks. To address this recall problem, some surveys ask respondents to keep detailed diaries of their medical care contacts, obtain the name of the provider, and then contact the providers (with the subject's permission) to verify the self-reported information. Information on utilization can also be obtained from surveys of providers. More accurate information on the nature of the contact, including the reason for the contact and the services provided, can be obtained in this way. Surveys of providers can also address the structure of the health-care system itself and how the characteristics of the system affect access to care and the cost of care.

The ability to assess quality of care is becoming more and more important. Utilization data can address this issue, but there are serious methodological challenges. Many data systems do not contain the needed information or enough specificity to be able to address quality issues. Moreover, there are many differing opinions on how best to measure quality. More in this area is progressing and data systems are attempting to collect information that will address the issue of quality and appropriateness of care (Agency for Healthcare Research and Quality, 2006).

General Design Issues

Sample Design

Health surveys either can obtain information directly from individuals (the subject or an informant) or can rely on administrative records. A wide range of sampling methodologies, sampling frames, and data collection strategies are used depending on survey objectives and the characteristics of the area in which the survey is done. Countries that have universal health care with centralized administrative systems can use designs that would be inappropriate in countries with less well-developed or decentralized health-care systems. The simplest sampling scheme is a simple random sample of a population obtained from a complete and up-to-date list such as from a census of the population or a centralized health-care system. In the case of surveys of persons, if such lists do not exist, area sampling can be used with clustering to reduce costs. In order to be able to report information on subpopulations of interest as defined by geography and/or demographic, socioeconomic, or health characteristics, designs often include oversampling of these groups to provide adequate sample size for analysis. It is often necessary to incorporate screening into designs to achieve this objective.

Many health surveys limit their population of interest. For example, it is common for health surveys to only include the noninstitutionalized population. The dramatic differences in the living conditions of the institutionalized and noninstitutionalized populations make it difficult to design survey methodologies that would apply in all situations. The military population is also often excluded from general health surveys. The scope of the universe needs to be clearly defined, especially if populations that differ in their health status are omitted – such as persons residing in nursing homes.

When obtaining information directly from the population is inefficient or would result in either poor data quality or high costs or both, an alternative is to sample from existing records that were created for other purposes. Information on health-care utilization for specific conditions is more easily obtained from hospital or provider records than from a population sample, given the relative rarity of the phenomena of interest. The vital statistics system can also be considered a census of administrative/legal records for the purpose of describing the health of the population. Administrative systems, in addition to providing basic health information, are often used as sampling frames for population-based surveys. They are very attractive for this purpose, as they eliminate the need to identify members of the population who have the characteristics of interest.

Longitudinal Designs

Most health surveys use cross-sectional designs which provide data for the calculation of population estimates and are most appropriate for monitoring changes in health over time. A cross-sectional design is not appropriate for investigating causal patterns or for documenting transition probabilities from one health state to another where change at the individual level needs to be measured. Longitudinal studies are expensive and more complicated to field but are needed to study causal patterns and transitions. A less expensive alternative is to transform cross-sectional studies into longitudinal studies by linking information from mortality or health-care-provider records to the survey data. Cross-sectional surveys also can form the baseline cohorts for future active longitudinal follow-ups. These longitudinal activities present extensive opportunities for understanding the relationship between risk factors and disease outcome, as well as the natural history of disease.

Mode of Data Collection

Information can be obtained either by mail, phone, in-person interview, or by some combination of modes, depending on the ability of the researchers to contact the population using these means. The latter two modes can also incorporate computer-assisted technologies, and the use of the Internet for the administration of health surveys is being investigated. Computer-assisted telephone and personal interviewing have allowed for increasing levels of complexity of survey administration. Errors associated with keying and coding have been replaced by errors associated with programming. The use of these technologies has resulted in the need for longer lead times prior to fielding a study but has reduced the time from the end of data collection to the availability of results.

Each mode of data collection has strengths and weaknesses. More complex questions can be used for interviewer-administered in-person interviewing, since the interviewer is available to provide standard explanations and can use the social interaction aspects of the interview to establish a relationship with the respondent. These surveys are the most expensive on a per case basis, and when the subject matter is sensitive, the presence of the interviewer can bias responses (although this can be alleviated by the use of computer-assisted techniques in which the respondent listens to the question on a headset and enters responses directly into the computer). Mail and Internet surveys usually use simpler, more direct questions and, although cheaper, have response rate and coverage problems, as do phone surveys that are done through random digit-dialing (RDD). A growing problem for RDD surveys is the increasing prevalence of households with cell phones only. RDD surveys have not included cell phones in their frameworks because the respondent would be responsible for charges and the concern that respondents might be participating while driving. The percentage of households in this category is growing and can affect the generalizability of RDD results.

Selection of Respondents

In general, obtaining information directly from the survey subject provides more reliable and valid health data. However, this is not universally true and depends on the nature of the information sought and the characteristics of the subject. For example, although accurate information on risk behaviors among adolescents can probably only be obtained from the adolescent in a private environment, adolescents are not good reporters of health-care utilization or household income. Even more problematic is the situation in which a health condition does not permit a subject to respond for himself or herself. Eliminating the subject from the survey would seriously bias the results, so a proxy respondent is often used. Although necessary, the use of proxy respondents does introduce a source of error into health surveys, particularly longitudinal surveys. Obtaining information on the relationship of the proxy to the subject, as well as the conditions leading to the use of a proxy, can reduce this error. There are other areas in which the subject is not a good reporter of the needed information. For example, information on the characteristics of an insurance plan is usually better obtained from the insurer rather than the person holding the insurance. Finally, reliable assessment of specific types of morbidity, risk factors, and mortality requires direct measurement through physical examination or access to administrative records from health-care providers.

Question Development

A major advancement has been the development and application of cognitive methods for questionnaire construction. Drawing from the field of cognitive psychology, cognitive research laboratories have been established and can investigate how respondents perceive and answer questions. Another fruitful area of research involves studying the behavior of both interviewers and respondents within the social context of the interview situation. A more structured approach to the errors found in health surveys can enhance data quality. The results of such research will lead to improved design that reduces error but can also lead to ways to adjust for known errors in the analysis and interpretation of results.

Data Linkage

The increase in electronic as opposed to paper files has greatly expanded the opportunities for linking data from various sources. Ecological or contextual information about the geographic area in which survey respondents reside can now be linked to the survey data. This has the advantage of allowing researchers to incorporate variables defined for different units of analysis into their investigations of complex problems. Survey data can also be augmented with administrative data from mortality files and from health-care providers. In addition to enhancing the amount of information available for analysis and reducing survey costs, this often leads to data of improved quality.

When survey data are linked to other sources of information on the respondent, permission to do the link must be obtained from the sample person. This is often required by research ethics review boards and by the organization responsible for the data to be linked, especially if it is considered private data (e.g., medical records). Concerns about privacy and confidentiality have made some respondents unwilling to allow this linkage and to provide the information to facilitate the link. Persons who do not allow the linkage become nonrespondents on the linkage information. It is possible to use standard techniques to adjust for nonresponse if the rates are not too high, but as rates increase the linked data will be of limited usefulness.

International Comparability

There is great interest in comparing health status and health-care systems across countries. Variation in disease rates across countries can be used to understand disease etiology. Policymakers and directors of health programs can use the experiences of other countries to devise strategies to improve health status. Perhaps most important, the health status of populations in other countries provides a standard by which domestic characteristics can be evaluated. However, there are many reasons for observed international variation in health, and many of them do not reflect true differences in health. As already discussed, health is a complex phenomenon with a large social component. International comparisons often reflect cultural differences rather than objective measures of health. These cultural differences can relate to social, economic, or environmental factors but also relate to basic differences in how subjects respond to questions. Work is under way to identify ways to design data collections that minimize the influence of cultural factors that are unrelated to the intent of the data collection.

Informed Consent, Privacy, and Confidentiality

For ethical reasons and in order to obtain high response rates and valid information, most health surveys closely guard the information provided by respondents. In some cases, the requirement to protect confidentiality is legislatively mandated. This is particularly important for health surveys, given the personal nature of the information collected. Confidentiality is protected by not releasing

data that could identify a respondent. Most survey sponsors subject files that are to be released for public use to rigorous disclosure review, but the risk for inadvertent disclosure has increased in recent years. It is no longer necessary to have access to large mainframe computers to use survey data that are provided on the Internet or on CD-ROMs. In addition, databases that are not related to the survey data but can be used to identify individuals in the survey data files are more available and more easily accessible. It is the potential linking of survey data to these external databases that increases the risk of disclosure, and the risk increases with the amount of information that is available. The ability to link external data to survey responses presents an analytic breakthrough, as the utility of survey data can be greatly increased through the appropriate linkages; however, this ability also greatly increases the risk of disclosure, especially when the linkages are done in an uncontrolled and inappropriate way. The increased sensitivity to issues of privacy in many countries, especially as related to health care, is affecting how confidential data are being protected. There has been a decrease in the amount of data that can be released as public use files, especially data that are collected by national statistical offices under strong promises of confidentiality. Other mechanisms are being developed so that access to data can be maximized while protecting confidentiality. The use of special use agreements, licensing, and research data centers are examples of these approaches.

See also: Biostatistics; Measuring the Quality of Life of Children and Adolescents; Systematic Reviews in Public Health.

Citations

Agency for Healthcare Research and Quality (2006) *2006 National Healthcare Quality Report.* Rockville, MD: U.S. Department of Health and Human Services, Agency for Healthcare Research and Quality. AHRQ Pub. No. 07-0013.
World Health Organization (2004) *International Statistical Classification of Diseases and Related Health Problems.* 10th rev. 2nd edn. Geneva, Switzerland: WHO.

Further Reading

Biemer PP, Groves RM, Hyberg L, Mathiowetz N, and Sudman S (eds.) (1991) *Measurement Errors in Surveys.* New York: Wiley.
Bradburn NM and Sudman S (1979) *Improving Interview Method and Questionnaire Design.* San Francisco, CA: Jossey-Bass.
Cannel CF, Monquis KH, and Launent A (1977) A summary of studies of interviewing methodology. *Vital and Health Statistics* (Series 1, No. 69).
Fowler FJ (1995) *Improving Survey Questions.* Thousand Oaks, CA: Sage.
Groves RM and Couper MP (1998) *Nonresponse in Household Interview Surveys.* New York: Wiley.
Groves RM, Fowler FJ, Couper MP, Singer E, and Tourangeau R (2004) *Survey Methodology.* New York: Wiley.

Korn EL and Graubard BI (1999) *Analysis of Health Surveys.* New York: Wiley.

Lessler JT and Kalsbeek WT (1992) *Nonsampling Error in Surveys.* New York: Wiley.

Madans JH (2002) Health surveys. In: Baltes P and Smelser N (eds.) *International Encyclopedia of the Social Sciences* 10: pp. 6619–6627. Amsterdam, The Netherlands: Elsevier.

Madans JH and Cohen S (2005) Health Surveys. *Health Statistics in the 21st Century: Implications for Health Policy and Practice.* London/New York: Oxford University Press.

Sirken MD, Herrmann DJ, Schecter S, and Tourangeau R (eds.) (1999) *Cognition and Survey Research.* New York: Wiley.

Relevant Website

http://www.cdc.gov/nchs/ – National Center for Health Statistics.

Clinical Trials

W R Harlan, National Institutes of Health, Rockville, MD, USA

Published by Elsevier Inc.

Introduction

Clinical trials are prospective tests of the effects of interventions in humans in which the assignment of intervention (treatment) is made by the investigator usually according to a protocol. These studies are designed to provide reliable estimates of beneficial and harmful effects on health outcomes and inform society, healthcare providers, and policy makers regarding treatment decisions. The randomized controlled trial provides the gold standard of evidence regarding preventive, diagnostic, and therapeutic approaches and is critical in developing guidance for treatment (Gibbons *et al.*, 2003). Clinical trials of treatments are required by regulatory authorities worldwide for licensure of new drugs, biologicals, and devices because this study design provides for unbiased testing of efficacy and safety. Although not required for marketing, trials are commonly used to establish the effectiveness of surgical and radiological procedures, behavioral interventions (including diet), combined treatments, and treatment paradigms.

James Lind is widely credited with conducting the first controlled trial in 1753 that found the addition of lemons to the diet of British sailors would prevent scurvy (Lind, 1753). In the ensuing 200 years, observational, rather than experimental, studies predominated and guided treatment recommendations until the middle of the twentieth century when clinical trials became the standard for determining treatment effectiveness. Currently, tens of thousands of clinical trials are being conducted worldwide and over 100 000 reports have been published. While many aspects of trial conduct continue to change, there are core principles and practices that underpin clinical trials. These best practices are followed in planning, conducting, monitoring, analyzing, and interpreting trials.

This article is intended to provide a brief review of trial components and the application of these principles. The description follows the sequence of trial development and the publication of results. It is intended to assist in reading and understanding reports of trials and to provide the rationale behind the design and conduct of studies. Because good reporting of studies guides careful planning and analysis, references are made to the evolving Consolidated Standards for Reporting Trials (CONSORT) recommendation and definitions (Altman *et al.*, 2001). Some aspects of trial planning are sketched only briefly in published reports but the rationale is discussed in greater detail here. Several texts provide detailed coverage of design, conduct, and analysis and are listed in the Further Reading.

Trial Development

Rationale for Conducting a Clinical Trial

Clinical trials are conducted to answer specific questions regarding efficacy and safety of interventions. When planning or reporting a trial, the investigators should provide a concise explanation of the specific question(s) being addressed, the rationale, and the background of evidence supporting the need for a study. In general, trials are needed when there is uncertainty about the effects, beneficial or harmful, of the intervention, and the expected difference has importance for health. Importantly, the question should be addressed within ethical and safety limits. If the effects are clearly apparent and statistically supported from observational studies, it would be inappropriate to initiate a trial. The relationship between smoking and lung cancer is very strong and based on numerous studies (odds ratios of 12 or greater); there is no reason to conduct a trial of smoking cessation versus no cessation. It would not add to the evidence on which recommendations not to smoke are made. Such a trial would be unethical as it places the nonintervened group at inordinate risk and unlikely to receive any benefit. However, there is a continuing need to compare different smoking cessation strategies and in this instance all groups receive an active treatment. The need for a trial may not always be obvious especially when a treatment has widespread and often long-term acceptance. Postmenopausal hormone treatment was generally accepted for over 50 years and used by about a third of U.S. women, but there was no reliable evidence for a balance of benefit over harms. When tested in a large randomized controlled trial, the public 'conventional wisdom' for a predominance of benefit was overturned (Anderson *et al.*, 2004) and the widespread use declined. Because clinical trials are developed to resolve uncertainties associated with moderate or small treatment differences, the public health utility may be underrated. However, application of modest effects over large populations can have profound public health consequences.

The initial step in trial development is describing the questions to be addressed in the context of previous studies and unresolved questions. This requires review of the information available from previous studies, both observational and interventional. Reviews should be conducted systematically and often can use meta-analysis or statistical aggregation of results from prior trials. This review can clarify the populations to be recruited, the potential magnitude of interventional effect, the most effective dose or approach to application, the competing treatments or interventions, and the potential harms that might be associated with the trial. From this summarization, the investigators are prepared to formulate the question(s) in specific terms, select an appropriate study design, and develop a detailed protocol. The background and rationale section of a published report provides a synopsis of this review.

Protocol

Creation of the experimental protocol is essential to any investigative work but is critical in clinical trials, especially multicenter studies that require many investigators to follow a common plan of study.

The document characteristically contains detailed specifications of all of the methods to be used from recruitment through treatment management, outcome measurement, and statistical analysis. The organizational structure for the collaboration is described as is the handling of data, usually by a designated data management group. Protocol development is done by investigators and may have the assistance of study sponsors. Following approval by the collaborating investigators, the protocol is reviewed and approved by an ethics review committee

and by the data and safety monitoring group. These approvals must occur before the first participant is enrolled. The trial should be registered in one of the global trial registries (see the section titled 'Relevant Websites'). This provides prospective disclosure of the essential elements of the trial to potential participants, to other investigators, and to those who might want to compile all the evidence for treatment guidance (Zarin *et al.*, 2007).

Adherence to the protocol by investigators is usually monitored by the data management center and by the data and safety monitoring committee. While the protocol represents the rules of the road for the study and should be referred to when questions arise, it remains a 'living instrument' that can, and often does, undergo modifications in the course of the trial. The modifications can be clarifications to ambiguous definitions or major alterations in the trial including treatment changes or elimination of an arm of the study. Major changes in protocol must be reviewed and approved by the ethics committee and by the data and safety monitoring committee before further enrollment and treatment can continue. The protocol for a study is not currently made public during the study but is filed with the sponsor and may become available on study completion. A brief synopsis of the protocol is provided in the 'Methods' section of a published report.

Ethical and Safety Oversight

In a clinical trial, special responsibilities fall to investigators and overseers of research because the assignment of treatment is made according to an experimental protocol rather than by a caregiver or patient preference. Trials are conducted to advance knowledge for future management and the individual subject may not benefit and could be harmed from his or her participation. The subjects should have an altruist motivation. The investigators have an obligation to design a study that does not inordinately disadvantage participants while carefully assessing efficacy and harms that will reliably inform future treatment. These potential benefits and harms must be carefully explained to potential subjects who indicate acceptance through informed consent. A review of the ethics is conducted by a review group independent of the investigators or sponsors. When subjects are to be randomly assigned to different treatments it is important for the investigators and monitoring groups to consider whether the compared interventions are in 'clinical equipoise' (Freedman, 1987). This term is used to indicate that experts consider that there is reasonable uncertainty about the clinical superiority of the compared treatments and that the subjects assigned to the groups will not be inordinately disadvantaged by the assignment.

The investigators and sponsors have an obligation to participants to ensure that the efficacy and harms of the treated groups are monitored and that the study is conducted with integrity. The participants should be protected from continued exposure if the study objectives have been achieved sooner than expected or the harms exceed potential efficacious results. Continuation of the study beyond this point exposes participants to risks without providing additional information. There is a further need to assure integrity of the study by ensuring adherence to the protocol and achieving reliable collection and analysis of data. All studies should have data and safety monitoring conducted by an independent group. This group reviews and approves the protocol before study, reviews major protocol changes, and develops a plan for monitoring the study progress. It periodically reviews data on recruitment and retention and aggregated data on efficacy and harms during the course of the study. The committee may make these assessments with the treatment assignments masked or with the treatment assignments disclosed. The monitoring committee generally makes decisions regarding continuing or stopping in confidential meetings and communicates its decision to the sponsor and responsible ethics review committees. The independence of the committee members protects the participants' interest from influence by sponsors and investigators. Monitoring of trials involves difficult decisions but is critical to the ethical conduct of a study (see Ellenberg *et al.*, 2002).

Study Design

The study design is selected to accomplish the objectives of the trial and is outlined in the published report. The single group design is used in early exploratory phases of investigations, and is often categorized as Phase 0, Phase 1, or Phase 2 by national regulatory authorities such as the U.S. Food and Drug Administration (FDA). These early studies are the first trials in humans and follow preclinical studies in animals. They are designed to determine the pharmacokinetics and safety of interventions, principally drugs, and whether changes in biologic parameters might alter disease processes. The sample sizes are small, varying from 10 to about 100 with increasing numbers as successive experiences and changing dose exposure provide data about potentially efficacious biologic and biochemical changes and an acceptable level of harmful effects. The earliest exploratory studies can be conducted with healthy volunteers, or in the case of life-threatening cancers and rare disorders, in volunteers with these conditions. All enrolled subjects receive the intervention. Measurements of biochemical and physiologic variables are made before administration of the test material and at intervals after administration. Varying doses may be used to determine dose levels that produce desirable effects without unacceptable harms. Promising early phase materials move to testing in larger groups and to parallel group

studies comparing interventions. These early phase studies represent an important and stringent barrier to further development; the overwhelming majority of study compounds do not progress to further confirmatory trials. Treatment trials for rare conditions with serious prognoses may always be conducted as single group studies relying on comparisons of before and after changes and historical experience to determine efficacy.

Confirmatory and comparative trials (late Phase 2, Phase 3, and Phase 4 in regulatory parlance) commonly use parallel group design with assignment of a study treatment to one group or arm (**Figure 1**) and comparative treatment(s) – either placebo or an active comparative – treatment in the other. The intermediate changes from baseline and the clinical outcomes are compared across arms. The sample sizes vary from several hundred (Phase 2 and 3) to thousands (Phase 4) depending on the requirements for statistical comparison of outcomes. Participants are recruited and enrolled according to the criteria for inclusion and exclusion and if eligible and willing to participate are assigned to a treatment group. Baseline measurements are made and are compared to measurements made during the course of the treatment. The parallel group design is the most common model for comparing two or more treatments. The regulatory approval of drugs or devices depends on demonstration of efficacy and safety of a tested intervention using this design. The conduct and analysis are considered further in a subsequent section of this article.

Cross-over design provides for comparison of treatments, either active or placebo, but each participant receives both treatments at different time periods. After baseline measurements, subjects are assigned, preferably randomly, to receive one of two treatments during an initial treatment period. Measurements of baseline, mediating, and outcome variables are made before, during, and at the conclusion of this period. After a washout period to allow dissipation of the initial treatment effect, each group crosses over to the alternative treatment. Measurements are made during the washout period (a second baseline) and at the same intervals during the second period. This approach effectively doubles the sample size from a simple parallel group design and matches the groups on important variables, because each subject receives both treatments. While efficient, this approach has some important limitations. The conditions being treated should remain stable through both periods of the study so there is no time-dependent change in the measured outcome. Such a change might be attributed to the treatment but, in fact, represented a variation in the study condition. For example, depression may resolve over 6 to 8 weeks in about 40% of those treated with placebo, and comparisons should not be made through this period of spontaneous resolution. Participants must complete both periods of the crossover to be included in analysis so minimizing attrition becomes

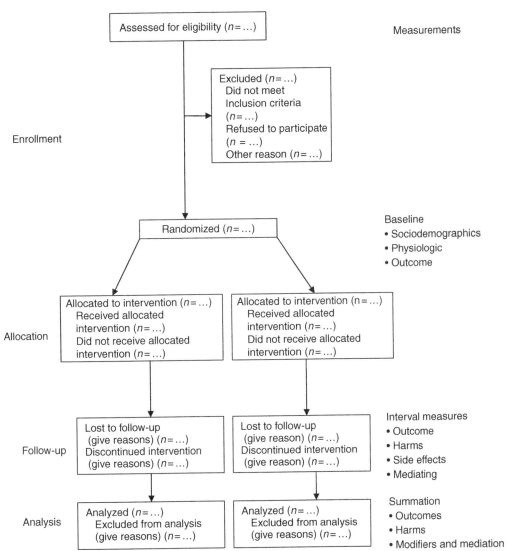

Figure 1 Scheme of participant flow and measurements in randomized trials. Participant flow in a parallel design, randomized controlled trial. Measurements to be made during the course of study are shown on right side. Adapted from Altman DG, Schulz KF, Moher D, *et al.*, and CONSORT (Consolidated Standards of Reporting Trials) Group (2001) The revised CONSORT statement for reporting randomized trials: Explanation and elaboration. *Annals of Internal Medicine* 134: 663–694.

important. The washout period before the crossover must be sufficiently long to provide for a dissipation of the effects of the initial regimen. Measurement of blood chemistries at the end of the washout can be helpful in determining the return to baseline. However, learned behaviors such as dietary changes may not be easily discarded or replaced resulting in persistent but difficult-to-measure effects that carry over into the second period.

Factorial design tests two or more interventions, their combinations, and a control for their effects against common outcome(s). A 2×2 factorial design would have four groups when testing interventions 'A' and 'B.' The treatment assignment can be randomized and the resultant four treatment groups would be: A, B, AB, and control. The outcomes are measured for each of the four groups and compared. This is an efficient design for testing two interventions that might affect the same primary outcome. The attribution of effects on the treatment groups depends on knowing the interactions between the interventions (e.g., A vs. B). If there is no interaction between A and B then the AB group can be combined with both A and B to increase sample size for A versus control and B versus control. An interaction occurs when the effect of the two combined treatments is different (greater or lesser magnitude) from each individually. An interaction might be anticipated if the two interventions operate through the same or similar mechanisms and are additive or multiplicative. Whether the interaction is important is determined statistically, but the power to find an interaction is less than the power to find a difference between any intervention and control, as the available sample sizes for comparisons are less. Careful planning is required to anticipate potential or proven interactions and is preferred to post hoc tests of interactions. Interactions are less likely when the biologic mechanisms of the interventions are different and less likely to facilitate or compete with each other.

Other Design Variations

The basic designs can be varied to suit particular questions or issues that arise. This presentation will only illustrate variations that are more frequently used.

Withdrawal of intervention(s) can be used when there is a desire to know whether the treatment remains active or necessary after initial and perhaps continuing therapeutic success has been demonstrated. For example, when and for whom could medication be discontinued after several years of drug or behavioral treatment? This can be tested by randomly discontinuing treatment in a group of successfully managed patients while continuing treatment in another group. Randomized discontinuation of successful therapy requires careful attention as withdrawal might result in rapid clinical deterioration.

Cluster randomized design is used to test public health or community interventions (Rosen *et al.*, 2006). If an intervention is to be tested in a population and the intervention(s) might spill over or contaminate the comparison group(s) because of shared learning or resources, then the intervention and comparison groups must be sufficiently isolated to avoid cross-contamination. This is especially an issue for behavioral interventions and for prevention studies. For example, interventional trials in school children often involve classroom, school, and parental activities that could not be isolated for individual students. It would be necessary to cluster the intervention to schools or even school districts, if policy interventions within a school are likely to contaminate the comparison group. Similarly, trials of complex regimens requiring special skills or training can only be provided by practitioners who would be unwilling or unable to provide the treatment regimens with equal fidelity. Therefore, the treatment groups might be clustered to the specially prepared practitioners and participants to the treatment regimens.

Sample Size, Recruitment, and Enrollment

The protocol and the report of the trial should provide information on critical elements. A trial should provide a valid estimate of the effect of the intervention to inform future management of health and disease. Determining adequate sample size is an important consideration for planning or interpreting comparative studies designed to confirm differences between interventions. It is important to verify that a significant difference exists, if there is truly

a difference, and to be sure that a difference could be detected if it exists. The power of the study is the probability that a clinically important effect could be detected if it truly exists (Cohen, 1992). Power is a function of sample size and the magnitude of interventional effect (i.e., effect size). The effect size to be tested should be sufficient to lead to adoption of the more favorable treatment. When the magnitude of effect is large, smaller sample sizes are required to find statistically significant and clinically important effects. Small effect sizes might be detected with statistical significance in studies when very large sample sizes are available, but the small biologic differences might not have any clinical importance. It is important for the investigators to consider what degree of biologic or clinical difference is likely to lead to a change in treatment and use this level in planning. When comparing two or more active treatments, it is often important to determine whether a tested treatment is equivalent or not inferior to another treatment. The non-inferiority difference between treatments to be exceeded is set at a level that might result in adoption of the new treatment. Noninferiority trials are common in comparing treatments that have been demonstrated to have superiority over placebo (Piaggio *et al.*, 2006).

The information for determining sample size includes expected event rate for the control group (and its variability), the difference in outcomes to be detected between the comparison groups, and estimates of the attrition from the groups during study. The event rates can be estimated from other studies, including observational studies, but should be adjusted for the healthier status of the trial volunteers. Allowance should be made for the potential loss of subjects. The expected effect size for a randomized comparison can be suggested by previous trials, but it should be appreciated that effect sizes estimated from nonrandomized and poorly designed studies usually provide overestimates and can lead to sample sizes inadequate to test the hypothesis. In general, studies are designed with sample sizes to provide a power of 80% or greater and to be able to detect significant differences at the 0.05 (two-sided) level.

Interventions

A broad spectrum of preventive, diagnostic, and treatment approaches can be tested by clinical trials. Drugs, biologics, diagnostic tools (e.g., mammography), surgery, manipulative approaches (e.g., acupuncture), behavioral treatments (e.g., diet, cognitive behavioral therapy), and treatment regimens requiring multiple simultaneous or sequential treatments have been successfully assessed in clinical trials. Recently completed and current trials can be found in registries of clinical trials (see the section titled 'Relevant websites'). Regardless of the type of intervention, there should be a clear specification of the quantity (or dose) of the treatment, the timing of application (and repetition), and assurance of the uniformity and quality of application over time. Additionally, changes in treatment that would be permitted or additional permitted interventions should be specified, along with whether such changes should be counted as adherence to the protocol, or, conversely, whether they constitute a protocol violation. Standardized training for therapists may be needed to ensure consistent application. This requires particular attention when manipulative or behavioral therapy is being used because the therapist may pursue a personal variation of the principal therapeutic approach, either improving or diminishing the result.

Determining the dose, both strength and frequency, regardless of the type of the intervention may require preliminary studies in which the dose is varied and responses of intermediate markers are assessed. This is especially important when efficacy and safety can depend on age and gender. Rules for and frequency of monitoring anticipated side effects and harms are usually stated in the protocol.

Adherence to treatment can be prespecified with the intention that a particular level of adherence is necessary for response. Monitoring of intermediate measures responsive to the intervention can assist in determining adherence by disclosing changes in these intermediates. For example, in studies of the effects of cholesterol-lowering agents on cardiovascular disease, one would expect the serum cholesterol (an intermediate) to decrease with adherence to the active agent but not in the placebo group. Adherence to mediation sufficient to alter a key mediating measure is assumed to be necessary to test the intervention against the more distal clinical outcome of cardiovascular disease.

To establish efficacy of an unproven treatment, it is common to use a placebo or sham treatment in one arm and to compare the responses for effectiveness. A placebo is an inactive intervention disguised to plausibly resemble the active intervention and is delivered with similar frequency and attention to dosing and measurement of effect. In some conditions, notably depression, about 40% of patients will respond with a positive outcome to placebo treatment and the putative active treatment must have a significantly greater effect. For drugs, placebos can be produced to have remarkably similar characteristics of appearance, texture, and taste as the active medication. For manipulative procedures, such as acupuncture, a needle inserted very superficially or at an incorrect site might be used as a placebo for a needle inserted to the correct depth at the correct site. The confidence of the therapist and his or her interaction with the patient is very important as the placebo effect is related to patient expectation of improvement. The use of 'sham surgery' as a placebo comparison is controversial because of the risks inherent in undergoing anesthesia and 'postoperative'

care. However, sham surgery was performed as a placebo control for a surgical ligation of the internal mammary arteries to relieve angina. The sham-treated patients received as much symptomatic benefit as the patients receiving ligation and this failure to prove a therapeutic effect led to abandonment of the procedure and subsequent health and economic benefits. There are examples in which those receiving placebo have fared better than those on active treatment. In a study of antiarrhythmic agents, patients received an appropriate antiarrhythmic or a placebo to prevent death, presumably from an arrhythmia. The trial was stopped early by the monitoring board when a strong excess of death was observed in the actively treated patients compared to those receiving placebo. The clinical use of antiarrhythmic agents changed remarkably thereafter. In other situations, it is deemed unethical to use a placebo control and place the placebo-treated patient at a disadvantage. In this situation, the comparator might be an established treatment or 'active control.' When this approach is used, it is important to recognize that the study will only test the difference (or similarity) of the new intervention to an accepted intervention and not disclose that the new intervention has efficacy greater than no treatment. If the established treatment has questionable efficacy, then the new equivalent treatment could have a similar questionable efficacy. The appropriateness of using a placebo intervention or active control requires thoughtful consideration regarding risks and benefits to participants and to the interpretation of the results.

Outcomes

The outcomes of a clinical trial represent the bottom-line assessment of interventional effect and measure the capability of the intervention to change important aspects of human health or disease. For single group, early phase studies, the outcomes are physiologic changes whereas for later phase, confirmatory studies the outcomes are principally clinical. Outcomes are classified as primary or secondary. The primary outcome is the principal measure for which the study is designed and conducted. The statistical power and the sample size are predicated on finding a difference in primary outcomes across the comparison groups. Usually there is one primary outcome and it is measured by the most reliable and clinically relevant measurement method. The outcome and the measurement methodology are prespecified in the protocol. The methods for assessing outcomes should be validated in observational and interventional studies and should ideally measure aspects of health having prognostic importance and for which treatment might improve prognosis. Composite outcomes can be developed from a variety of clinical outcomes and used to capture different manifestations of disease. For example, angina, myocardial infarction, and heart failure may be combined in a composite primary outcome for treatment or prevention of coronary heart disease if the intervention is hypothesized to affect all manifestations. If the intervention is presumed to be specific to one of these outcomes, then that single outcome should be measured, thus the other manifestations become secondary.

Other outcomes that are prespecified before study initiation are secondary outcomes. Estimates of the likelihood of finding significant differences in secondary outcomes can be made, but the sample size is usually not changed to accommodate them. When secondary outcomes are prespecified, attention to measurement is warranted so as to avoid posttrial estimates of interventional effect that are based on less than the best assessments. Secondary outcomes often clarify the mediators and mechanisms underlying the primary effect and can inform the development of further studies through generation of testable hypotheses.

The measurement and timing of measurement must be clearly defined in the protocol. The most objective and reliable methods should be used, but the measurements should have clinical and public health utility that will lead to application of the proven interventions. When special training is required for measurement or when adjudication of conflicting assessments is necessary the methodologic approach requires description. The assessor of outcomes, whether investigator or designated evaluator, might have to rely on measures requiring personal judgment or subjective assessment. If the perceptions of the evaluator can influence outcome measurement, it is important to 'blind' the evaluator to treatment allocation. Similarly, the participant may be biased in reporting outcomes or symptoms based on allocation to a particular treatment, thus blinding the participant to treatment assignment minimizes biased reporting.

Allocation of Treatments, Randomization, and Blinding

Patients are most commonly allocated to treatment arms by a process of random assignment for most studies with two or more treatment arms (see **Figure 1**). Random allocation balances the treatment groups with respect to measured and unmeasured variables and effective randomization ensures that the groups receiving the intervention have essentially identical characteristics. This maximizes the likelihood that the effects on outcomes can be attributed to the treatment or intervention and not to differences in the treatment groups. Therefore, random allocation of treatments is a critical feature in minimizing bias and maximizing treatment attribution. To mitigate investigator bias in allocation, the allocation is best conducted independent of the researchers. There should be minimal likelihood that the investigator or

participant could anticipate the next allocation. Truly random sequences can be generated and are preferable to predictable or haphazard sequences. A scheme that generates sequences centrally can provide blocks of randomly sequenced allocations to clinics discouraging 'guessing' of the next allocation to be made based on the last assignment. The information regarding assignment can be conveyed from the central generation by computers or opaque envelopes provided at the point of randomization.

Randomization is done only after verification that the subject is eligible for the study and has agreed to participate and to be randomly assigned to treatment. This means that informed consent has been obtained and measurements have been recorded that meet enrollment criteria. These requirements can be included in a computer program that releases the random assignment only after eligibility and consent are confirmed. When clinics are likely to enroll different numbers of participants, the randomization can be blocked to increase the likelihood that each clinic will have relatively equal numbers of each group assignment. Randomization is critically important to balancing the subjects across arms. To confirm the balance across arms, baseline demographic, physiologic, and biochemical measures across subject groups are compared in analysis.

In multicentered studies, it is useful to assure that there is an adequate representation in each center of participants with important variables related to outcome. Among these are age and other prognostic determinants. The randomization can be stratified by the variable(s) one wishes to balance. After stratifying the variables, then the randomization provides an equal chance that the variables will be balanced even though clinics may recruit from different populations. These permutations of randomization improve the statistical comparisons during analysis.

Concealment of the treatment assignment (i.e., masking) is important to minimize biases in management and evaluation or reporting of outcomes. Several groups can be blinded to treatment assignment. These include: investigators, participants, evaluators of outcomes, and those analyzing or monitoring the outcomes. There may be situations in which the investigator or therapist must know treatment to make adjustments to treatment or avoid progression of harmful effects. The therapist or a medical monitor can be unblinded but the evaluator should be blinded. To determine whether blinding has been successful, the participants and evaluator can be asked their perception of the treatment assignment at the conclusion of the study.

In some studies, particularly late phase studies testing management variations or safety issues, the subjects may be randomized but the allocation of treatment is disclosed and the study is termed an open randomized trial.

After completion of the randomized period of study, observations of the groups can be extended without repeating randomization to provide long-term data on effectiveness or safety. However, the groups may not remain in the treatments originally assigned and the specificity of effects to the treatment is decreased. Also, the subjects may be randomized again to new treatments based on the earlier responses and the sequential treatments evaluated.

Conduct and Reporting of Trials

Recruitment and Enrollment

Specific criteria are described for recruitment of the study population and include conditions for risk status and clear description for inclusion and exclusion. Specifications for inclusion might include age, health, disease status, and prior treatment. Recruitment of the study population represents a major task. Studies having over 50 participants often require multiple clinics to recruit and randomize the numbers needed for adequate sample size. Multicenter trials require unambiguous definition of eligibility. Only individuals meeting criteria can be considered for enrollment. A participant can be enrolled if he or she meets the criteria and provides informed consent. It is informative to characterize those responding to recruitment, their eligibility, and whether they are ineligible or unwilling to participate. The information bears on the generalizability of the study results as it allows characterization of the population volunteering for the study and how this may differ from those eligible for the study.

Participant Follow-up and Measurements

After randomization, the comparison arms are considered to be equivalent in characteristics that affect outcomes. This sets the stage for being able to attribute differences in outcome to the tested interventions. However, important differences between the treatment arms may occur during the follow-up. These differences can occur nonrandomly and differentially affect differences in outcomes across the arms.

The repeated observations and clinic visits during the postrandomization follow-up are critical in accounting for these changes, as well as measuring outcome efficacy and treatment harms. **Figure 1**, adapted from the CONSORT flow diagram for a randomized parallel group design, provides a scheme to account for participants during the course of study from enrollment through analysis. This format is used in reporting of trials in leading journals and allows for comparison of participant numbers in each of the treatment groups and displays graphically treatment assignment, withdrawals, lost to follow-up, and those analyzed for outcomes.

Participants may choose not to continue the assigned treatment and withdraw or the investigators may discontinue treatment because of measured harms. Participants may fail to return or seek other care. The sequence of measurements is indicated on the right side of **Figure 1**. Measurements are made at prespecified intervals from prerandomization and baseline through the period of follow-up on treatment and to the assessment of final outcomes. Both efficacious outcomes and harms are tabulated as well as the time of occurrence. The data are compiled by a data management center for monitoring reports on progress and for subsequent analysis of results. The sponsors, investigators, evaluators, and patients are usually not privy to the aggregated data on efficacy and harms as knowledge of these data could bias recruitment, conduct, and continuance of the trial. The independent data monitoring group reviews periodic reports from the data center and determines discontinuance and integrity of the trial.

Adverse Events and Harms

Clinical trials make important contributions to assessment of harmful effects of interventional agents and strategies. The assessment of adverse events is a primary concern in Phase 1 and 2 trials (exploratory) of new agents and their discovery is a major cause for not pursuing further development. The frequency and magnitude of harmful effects are critical in efficacy (Phase 3 and 4) trials and in large postapproval trials comparing competing interventions over extended periods. Large studies with long follow-up periods can disclose serious harms that are relatively frequent and require long follow-up and careful recording to be detected. The capability of detecting serious, but relatively infrequent, adverse events is limited in many moderate-sized studies and it may not be possible to find statistically significant differences in a single trial. Consider that serious events occurring with a frequency of 1 in 500 persons exposed would be detected only 4 times when the sample size of those exposed is 2000. The sensitivity is limited but the specificity is good because the exposure is controlled by treatment assignment, improving attribution of the effect to the intervention. Harms should be assessed throughout the study and reported fully, even if the frequency in an individual study does not achieve statistical significance. If the rate of harms is not significant in a single study, the aggregation of harms data from multiple studies may achieve statistical significance and thereby guide treatment. More prevalent harms and side effects of a less serious nature can be reliably compared in larger studies and provide estimates of benefits and harms. Many interventions are associated with competing efficacy and harms. The careful assessment of each dimension can aid in choosing and directing treatment. An example is preventive use of hormonal therapy in postmenopausal women in which reduction of coronary heart disease and osteoporoses are potential benefits, but breast cancer, thrombophlebitis, and stroke are harms. The net effect when these risks and harms were studied was significant excess of harms over benefits leading to a recommendation to avoid long-term preventive use of hormones. A more complete discussion of recording of harms and useful definitions is available in the CONSORT statement on harms (Ioanidis *et al.*, 2004).

Analysis

The primary and secondary outcomes are compared across the treatment groups. Because the groups are assumed to be equivalent at randomization, the differences in outcomes are attributed to the differences in treatment if there are not losses in groups that are not random (see **Figure 1**). All participants who received at least one treatment are included in analysis in the groups to which they were originally assigned even though participants may be lost from the groups for various reasons. This is an intention-to-treat analysis and is generally favored as the principal analysis because it avoids the bias associated with nonrandomized loss of participants. For example, subjects may withdraw or be withdrawn from their treatment assignment because of failure to control the condition or for intolerable symptoms or adverse effects from the condition or the treatment. Without an intention-to-treat approach, this nonrandom loss would bias the results because only participants responding to treatment or experiencing no adverse events might remain for comparison, yielding incorrect estimates of efficacy and harms. An additional analysis of 'as treated' or 'per protocol' participants can be performed using those who continue or adhere to treatment. While this may be useful if noncompliance to treatment is common, it is a less rigorous test of treatments.

Baseline levels of demographic, biochemical, and clinical characteristics are compared across groups to determine whether randomization balanced the treatment groups with respect to known and measured variables.

The measured outcomes to be compared can be quantitative, categorical, or time-to-event (survival). Quantitative changes, such as serum cholesterol response to diet or drugs, are compared across groups using comparisons of mean differences in final levels or differences between baseline and final measures or both. Multiple logistic models can control for variables that could influence the differences.

Categorical outcomes such as mortality from cancer or heart disease or clearly defined nonfatal events are compared using the differences in odds ratios across treatment groups. The denominators for each treatment group are the number randomized to each treatment and the numerators are the number of events for each group using the intention-to-treat principle. Proportional hazard models can be used to account for moderating variables.

Time-to-event analysis can be used to determine the time course of response to treatments and help to identify when the treatment response occurs and the course of changes in response over the duration of the study. Statistical significance is determined for the treatment differences.

The primary outcomes are the first consideration in analysis. Prespecified secondary outcomes should be analyzed with the understanding that the sample size may not provide adequate statistical power to find significant differences, as the sample size with adequate power for finding differences was determined for the primary outcome(s) only. When multiple comparisons are made, adjustment should be made to the level of significance to reflect the increased likelihood of chance findings.

Interpretation

The questions addressed in clinical trials are specifically stated in terms of the interventions, populations, and conditions studied. The results and the interpretation are specific as well. The results apply to the conditions studied and the stage or severity, the intervention and its dose and duration, the outcomes measured, and the demographics of the population enrolled in the study. If well conducted, the results have good internal validity but extrapolation beyond the study intervention and populations is limited. Generalizations are improved if the populations are representative of the broader group of affected persons and the exclusion criteria and recruitment have not constrained trial enrollment. It is important that the findings be interpreted in the context of other relevant studies. It has been suggested that discussion and interpretation of clinical trials in published reports should include a review or meta-analysis of all related studies. This would place the reported study in context with other trials and observational studies and provide for discussion of the implications for and limitations of treatment. The total body of evidence regarding an intervention is often evaluated in additional analyses using systematic reviews and meta-analysis. These allow integration of all relevant information into the evidence base on which recommendations are made.

On one hand, when the differences in outcomes are significant, either beneficial or harmful, the interpretation is generally straightforward. On the other, failure to find a significant difference does not prove that there is truly no difference. The planning and conduct may not be able to find a difference. For example, sample size might have been inadequate to detect a significant difference or the conduct of the study and resulting dropouts or losses may have biased toward the null. If differences are found that are not statistically significant, it is useful to compute the sample size that might have found a significant difference as a guide to future studies.

Reporting

There are scientific and ethical reasons that all clinical trials should be reported. From the ethical perspective, the participants were subjected to risk and inconvenience with the expectation of increasing societal knowledge about the treatment and with the hope that the trial might improve treatment for others. Failure to report the findings is a breach of this trust. Society, either directly or indirectly, has paid for these studies and reporting of data is a responsibility. Further, data from trials, even if not productive of significant differences, can inform planning of future studies or be included in meta-analysis.

Trials providing clear evidence for efficacy find a receptive audience in journals that are eager to publish such reports. Similarly, trials that report an excess of harms, particularly serious adverse events, receive journal attention and publication. Successful trials describe significant and important differences whether efficacious or deleterious. However, not all trials provide clear-cut answers for a variety of reasons. If the totality of evidence is to be compiled to guide treatment then all relevant data should be made publicly available. It has been suggested that clinical trials registries have a reasonably complete listing of all initiated trials and should also capture trial results and provide a complete record of all trials whether published or not.

Future Directions

Clinical trials are complex, resource-intensive, and require attention to myriad details to achieve valid and useful results. The investment is small in comparison to the gains in evidence that improve medical care and public health. The number, size, and scope of clinical trials continue to increase exponentially. Increasing reliance on the methodology for evidence-based decisions and the proliferation of new treatments requiring validation are important drivers of this increase. There is a need to increase and broaden subject participation as well as increase efficiency. Developing designs that allow efficiencies without compromising scientific principles or introducing biases is increasingly important. Adaptive designs are being pursued that allow for modifications of sample size or outcomes. It is important that these adaptations are overseen by independent monitors and do not permit the sponsors or investigators to change the study to achieve a biased outcome. Improving public trust is critical in improving support for trials. Registration and reporting of all clinical trials can avoid duplication of studies, increase scientific scrutiny, improve quality, and demonstrate the utility to public health and medical care.

See also: Biostatistics; Concepts of Health and Disease; Meta-Analysis; Systematic Reviews in Public Health.

Citations

Altman DG, Schulz KF, Moher D, *et al.* and CONSORT (Consolidated Standards of Reporting Trials) Group (2001) The revised CONSORT statement for reporting randomized trials: Explanation and elaboration. *Annals of Internal Medicine* 134: 663–694.

Anderson GL, Limacher M, Assaf AR, *et al.* Women's Health Initiative Steering Committee(2004) Effects of conjugated equine estrogen in postmenopausal women with hysterectomy: The Women's Health Initiative randomized controlled trial. *Journal of the American Medical Association* 291: 1701–1712.

Cohen J (1992) A power primer. *Psychological Bulletin* 112: 155–159.

Freedman B (1987) Equipoise and the ethics of clinical research. *New England Journal of Medicine* 317: 141–145.

Gibbons RJ, Smith S, and Antman E (2003) American College of Cardiology; American Heart Association clinical practice guidelines: Part 1: Where do they come from? *Circulation* 107: 3101–3107.

Ioanidis JP, Evans SJ, Grotzhe PC, *et al.* (2004) Better reporting of harms in randomized trials: An extension of the CONSORT statement. *Annals of Internal Medicine* 141: 781–788.

Lind J (1753) *A Treatise of the Scurvy.* Edinburgh: Kincaid and Donaldson.

Piaggio G, Elbourne DR, Altman DG, Pocock SJ, and Evans SJ CONSORT Group (2006) Reporting of noninferiority and equivalence randomized trials: An extension of the CONSORT statement. *Journal of the American Medical Association* 295: 1152–1160. Erratum in: *Journal of the American Medical Association* 296: 1842.

Rosen L, Manor O, Engelhard D, and Zucker D (2006) In defense of the randomized controlled trial for health promotion research. *American Journal of Public Health* 96: 1181–1186.

Zarin DA, Ide NC, Tse T, Harlan WR, West JC, and Lindberg DAB (2007) Issues in the registration of clinical trials. *Journal of the American Medical Association* 297: 2112–2120.

Further Reading

Elbourne DR and Campbell MK (2001) Extending the CONSORT statement to cluster randomized trials. *Statistics in Medicine* 20: 489–496.

Ellenberg S, Fleming T, and DeMets D (2002) *Data Monitoring Committees in Clinical Trials: A Practical Perspective.* New York: John Wiley.

Emanuel EJ, Wood A, Fleischman A, *et al.* (2004) Oversight of human participants research: Identifying problems to evaluate reform proposals. *Annals of Internal Medicine* 141: 282–291.

Friedman LM, Furberg CD, and DeMets DL (1998) *Fundamentals of Clinical Trials,* 3rd edn. New York: Springer Science.

Hampton T (2006) Are placebos in advanced cancer trials ethically justified? *Journal of the American Medical Association* 296: 265–266.

Mermert CL (1986) *Clinical Trials: Design, Conduct and Analysis.* New York: Oxford University Press.

Moher D, Schulz KF, and Altman DG (2001) The CONSORT statement: Revised recommendations for improving the quality of reports of parallel-group randomised trials. *The Lancet* 357: 1191–1194.

Simon SD (2006) *Statistical Evidence in Medical Trials: What Do the Data Really Tell Us?* New York: Oxford University Press.

Van Spall HG, Toren A, Kiss A, and Fowler RA (2007) Eligibility criteria of randomized controlled trials published in high-impact general medical journals: A systematic sampling review. *Journal of the American Medical Association* 297: 1233–1240.

Relevant Websites

http://clinicaltrials.gov – Clinical Trials, a service of the U.S. NIH, developed by the National Library of Medicine.
http://www.clinicalstudyresults.org – Clinical Study Results.
http://www.consort-statement.org – The CONSORT Group.
http://www.cancer.gov – Comprehensive Cancer Information, National Cancer Institute.

http://www.controlled-trials.com – Current Controlled Trials, Clinical Trial Search.
http://www.isrctn.org – The ISRCTN Register.
http://www.jameslindlibrary.org – The James Lind Library.
http://www.plosclinicaltrials.com – PLoS Hub for Clinical Trials.
http://www.who.int/ictrp/en – WHO International Clinical Trials Registry Platform.

Surveillance of Disease

I Arita and M Nakane, Agency for Cooperation in International Health, Kumamoto-city, Japan
T Nakano, National Mie Hospital, Mie, Japan

Historical Development

In civil society, police and security systems are alert to abnormal incidents that may cause hazards in communities, nations, and perhaps the world. The information discovered and assembled by this system is transmitted to an authority responsible for setting up measures to eliminate the cause of hazard. The human body provides immunological surveillance, the body's defenses that recognize foreign materials or malignant cells; thus surveillance information helps the body's immunological mechanism destroy such foreign materials or cells.

In the early twentieth century, information gathering on infectious diseases and other hazards to humans was developed in parallel with the development of microbiological technology and epidemiology. The data thus collected were analyzed and the results were distributed to systems and individuals responsible for control actions. Epidemiological surveillance was the beginning of a new era of infectious disease control. In recent years, surveillance activities have been expanded from infectious diseases to chronic diseases and automobile accidents and other injuries; in addition, long-term data collection such as vital statistics and surveillance of health-related social or economic activities have been surveyed systematically. In this article, we discuss surveillance systems and activities on which public health control action is based.

Around the mid-twentieth century when infectious diseases were a major problem and menace to public health, two medical experts attempted to set up surveillance as an essential component of public health practice. Alexander Langmuir, from the Centers for Disease Control and Prevention (CDC), developed systematic surveillance mechanisms for infectious diseases and associated control programs. In 1963, he outlined surveillance as: (1) systematic and active collection of pertinent data of target disease(s); (2) assessment and practical report of these data; and (3) the timely dispatch of such reports to individuals responsible for formulation of action plans. It is important to note that surveillance would not be useful unless data are known and acted upon by individuals responsible for initiating action plans. A surveillance system, in principle, does not include the control measures within its system. A surveillance system is better if it is independent from the control system, because experience has shown that on some occasions, disease prevalence was artificially modified by individuals who were responsible for control measures and sought to gain seemingly better results than what was actually occurring. In the 1960s, Karel Raska, Communicable Disease Division at the World Health Organization (WHO) headquarters, further expanded the system's definition, including epidemiological research in surveillance activities. He promoted a surveillance study, for example by strengthening smallpox surveillance and approving special research funds to the newly intensified eradication program in 1967; malaria surveillance was intensified when the effectiveness of malaria control was demonstrated with investigation of malaria prevalence rates in patients using or not using mosquito nets.

In the area of public health practice, we may need to rethink the boundary of surveillance systems. It may be wise not to expand it to a broad investigation or epidemiological research, which certainly interests many researchers or health officers but does not lead to practical public health action to reduce immediate hazard or risk. Thus, the surveillance tool as a public health action may be further refined and solidified.

The latest challenge in surveillance has been in terrorism, exemplified when a terrorist group attacked facilities in the United States, Spain, and England in recent years. Anthrax was also used as a bioweapon in the United States. Surveillance against bioterrorism with smallpox virus, *Bacillus anthracis*, and other agents is now being developed in the West.

Surveillance Methods

Target Disease

The target diseases for surveillance are key to defining the sensitivity, specificity, effectiveness, and efficiency of the systems used. Fever and rash diseases such as measles and chickenpox or neurologic diseases such as poliomyelitis or meningococcal meningitis may be discovered or suspected readily by surveillance and allied workers: Such reportable diseases require clinical and laboratory confirmation by experienced workers. Certain principles underlie identification of target diseases.

Usually surveillance systems aim at a particular disease or only a limited number of diseases. Those who work for surveillance should have clear ideas of clinical pictures, mode of transmission and its infectivity. Further, it is advisable to know probable frequency or prevalence of such diseases and if possible, the inhabitants attitudes' to the diseases. It is important to note that some populations may feel it is necessary to conceal the patient's presence in the family. On the other hand, populations may be pleased to collaborate with surveillance, willingly reporting the target diseases. Sometimes, the target disease can be reported to surveillance workers only as symptoms, such as jaundice (for hepatitis B), acute flaccid paralysis (poliomyelitis), and confirmation can be made after reporting.

The Surveillance System

The surveillance system usually is set up as a distinct section or organization within the national or regional health service system and has an independent function as described in the previous section. The method or function may consist of the two main functions discussed in the next sections.

Community-Based Surveillance

The main reporters are villagers or town inhabitants or health workers in a dispensary or private clinic contacting or seeing the patients with the target diseases. It is important that there be a public relations campaign through radio, television, the press, etc. to encourage reporting the disease to the nearest health center or some designated office, which will transmit the report to the supervisory level, as shown in **Figure 1**.

Hospital-Based Surveillance

The main reporters in this system are hospital physicians who diagnose the diseases. This system functions in parallel with community-based surveillance, but is also important in finding rare diseases or diseases that are difficult to identify by the public because of their rare

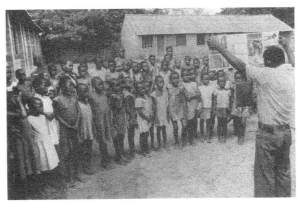

Figure 1 Community-based surveillance needs to be understood by the community. A surveillance information officer is explaining the disease and why it should be reported.

occurrence and/or because the clinical manifestation is difficult to recognize. The advantage of this system is that if hospitals are fully cooperative, surveillance coverage is good. The hospital may need to assign a physician to take responsibility for such reporting. Needless to say, the hospital administration should be fully informed and understand the importance of such surveillance.

Nosocomial or hospital-induced, infection is a special surveillance target within hospitals to be handled by a special hospital committee. The hospital administration should be aware of the occurrence of nosocomial infections and work to develop its control.

Passive or Active Surveillance

Both community- and hospital-based surveillance systems are in principle passive. If the health service controlling the surveillance report urgently needs a special report, it can organize active surveillance in which special teams are formed to make house-to-house or hospital-to-hospital visits to determine the occurrence of the disease either through direct communication with community members or hospital personnel and seeing the patients or examining the hospital records or the patients on location.

Special Surveillance

Effective surveillance requires innovative ideas to augment its sensitivity.

Rewards

Surveillance efficacy often depends on the public's interest in reporting the disease. Reward is, in certain circumstances, a useful method for a health service to express the importance of reporting to the public. For example, a reward system was utilized to encourage reporting in

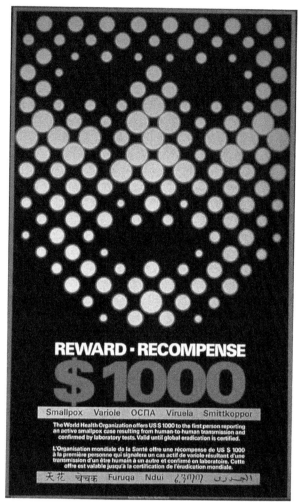

Figure 2   WHO's poster in mid-1978, publishing the reward of US$1000 for finding a case of smallpox.

of occurrence such as influenza that may become pandemic or a dangerous pathogen requiring immediate action for public health measures in high-risk areas.

Measures to Handle Incomplete Surveillance Reports

Incomplete surveillance reports include mistaken reports due to the incompetence of technical personnel, active concealment of disease occurrence, or the combination of these two causes. Although these look like anecdotal episodes or events during surveillance, they often considerably influence the success or failure of control measures, which require high-quality surveillance data.

Particularly if such incomplete surveillance reports are made intentionally by health authorities, the results may become disastrous. Examples include the smallpox epidemic in the Horn of Africa during the last phase of the global smallpox eradication program in 1976–77, and the early phase of epidemics of severe acute respiratory syndrome (SARS) in East Asia, which subsequently formed a pandemic on other continents. How should such incomplete surveillance reports be treated? No standard remedy has been found so far. There have been trial and error attempts such as practical dialogue, development of collaborative research, political pressure and recommendation from a higher authority, and emphasis on moral obligation. Experience has shown that such incomplete surveillance reports from health services in the area or nation concerned often cause disastrous results that end in failing to control the epidemics thus incorrectly reported.

Laboratory Diagnosis and Surveillance System

Surveillance requires the collaboration of laboratories to confirm the diagnosis if initial reports are based on clinical diagnosis alone. Laboratory diagnostic measures may not be needed in some instances. For example, if there is a large number of cases with similar clinical manifestations, laboratory testing of only cases that are representative of the outbreaks may be satisfactory, provided that missing the correct diagnosis of other cases does not pose significant risk in developing control measures. This may be applicable to determining containment of outbreaks with vaccination in the case of measles outbreaks, a hepatitis A outbreak, etc.

The interval between the time the specimen is taken and the time when laboratory results are available to the surveillance office should be carefully determined, depending on the type of specimen testing such as serology, isolation, and specific tests such as strain differentiation. The reliability of the testing technique should always

many countries such as India and Somalia during the smallpox eradication program (1967–80). In 1978, when a probable world last case was discovered in Africa, WHO encouraged people or medical personnel throughout the world to report (**Figure 2**). The announcement was followed by many smallpox reports from West Africa, Indonesia, even Heathrow and Kennedy airports. All such reports were investigated by the WHO team with negative results.

Nil Report

Surveillance certainly receives positive reports of the target diseases, but often it is also important to receive nil reports indicating positive assurance that the disease did not occur during a particular time period such as a week. In other words, regular nil reports indicate that sensitive surveillance is continuing. The nil report is useful to see the situation of specifically suspected areas be assured with periodic assessment of the laboratory technique and testing the suitability of reagents by a reference laboratory.

For surveillance of specific diseases such as poliomyelitis, measles, or influenza, international reference laboratories have been designated by WHO. In addition, national reference laboratories can be set up for collaboration by the individual government as the need arises. **Figure 3** shows the special collection kits that were used for safe and easy handling of specimens during the WHO smallpox eradication program (1967–80). Some nations that do not have the appropriate laboratory facilities may be assisted by nearby reference laboratories, often through an arrangement with WHO. Safe measures for transportation of infectious specimens and infectious substance label are shown in **Figure 4**.

Collation of Surveillance Data by Time, Place, and Person

Surveillance data collected and confirmed for its accuracy may be sorted by three major elements throughout the process at peripheral and central levels.

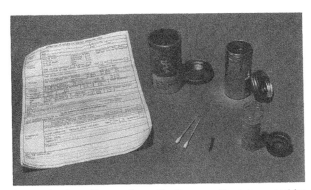

Figure 3 Surveillance of specific diseases: Container used for smallpox specimen. Transportation of dangerous pathogens or specimens requires special double container to ensure safety.

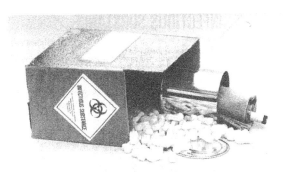

Figure 4 Example of packaging of an infectious substance. Note infectious substance label on the box.

Time

Specimen collection date and patient dates reflecting information such as date of occurrence, course of clinical picture, etc. are necessary. Standard tabulation includes case serial number and deaths by week number 1 to 51 or 52. Monthly or daily records are also used, but weekly records are convenient, since the WHO Weekly Epidemiological Record (WER) and the US CDC Morbidity and Mortality Weekly Report (MMWR), etc. use week number for easy reference. Usually, the date of occurrence of the disease is the important date. The date of receipt of the report at health services is recorded to indicate the efficacy of the reporting system in some geographical areas.

Place

It is important to record the geographical areas where cases occurred or were discovered. Usually the place where the case occurred is important because there is the risk of spread. The movement of patients before the onset of the disease and during the course of the disease is also important to estimate the source of infection as well as the potential spread of the disease. In today's rapidly developing travel, the movements of patients are very rapid and distant, suggesting rapid transmission of the pathogen across the continents, as seen in the SARS pandemic in 2002–03.

Person

In addition to the information mentioned above, important patient information includes gender, age, occupation, and the patient's movement and activities during the incubation period and the estimated time and place in relation to the exposure to the patient of the infectious source, whether human, animal objects, or other sources.

This information is sorted and collated to form a report that will be sent to the system or individuals who plan and initiate control measures. Additionally, the information is further analyzed with simple statistical methods or elaborated mathematical methods (**Figure 5**). **Figure 6** shows co-relation between HIV prevalence and malaria mortality. These are discussed elsewhere. It is important to stress that simple raw data from sensitive surveillance are very useful for planners to initiate strategy formation.

Salient Surveillance Experiences: How It Works

International Sentinel Surveillance

Sentinel-based surveillance may help to improve weaknesses by monitoring an area's situation more closely and directly. For example, global surveillance on certain diseases may have certain weaknesses because adequate

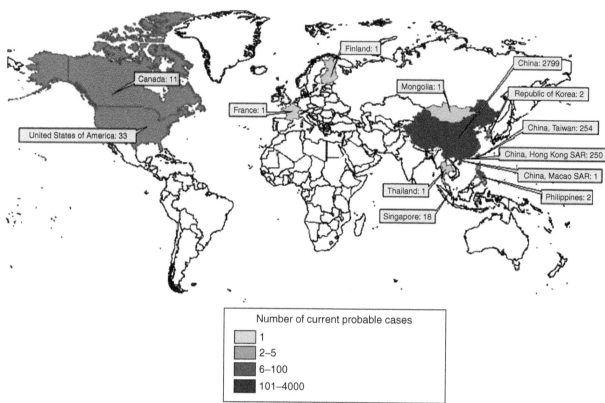

Figure 5 Number of severe acute respiratory syndrome (SARS) probable cases on 19 May 2003.

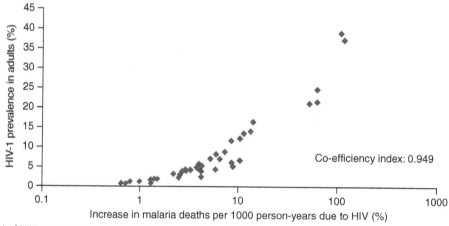

Figure 6 Impact of HIV on malaria deaths in sub-Saharan Africa, 2004. From Arita I (2006) HIV/AIDS research and development. *Lancet Infectious Diseases* 6(3): 124–125.

information is not available from areas because of political unrest, disinterest, poorly developed infrastructure, etc. The Agency for Cooperation in International Health (ACIH), a Japanese nongovernmental organization, has developed a voluntary sentinel surveillance system for selected target diseases, covering South America, Africa, and Asia. Its aim is to add more disease information and thus contribute to global epidemiological surveillance headed by WHO. The AGSnet (Alumni for Global

Surveillance network) was organized in 1998. It consists of selected experts and managers who participated in several infectious-disease courses that were sponsored by the Japan International Cooperation Agency (JICA) and organized by ACIH. As of May 2006, the group consisted of 59 sentinel sites in 32 countries (**Figure 7**). Sentinels are divided into three categories: Hospitals and clinics, laboratories, and blood transfusion centers. Feedback from ACIH consists of selected epidemic information in the media and WHO and various surveillance articles published by medical journals. Despite a limited geographical coverage, the system seems to supplement disease information being obtained by global surveillance, as described in **Table 1**. The system has found unreported infectious diseases of international importance, including cholera, plague, and influenza. The surveillance data on prevalence of hepatitis B and C, HIV, and syphilis in blood donors from blood transfusion centers is unique, not usually available in the global surveillance network. It should be noted, however, that such a network in no way replaces or negates the need for strong national surveillance and alert and response mechanisms.

Smallpox Eradication and Its Surveillance System

The intensified smallpox eradication program was initiated in 1967 and succeeded in identifying the last chain of natural transmission in 1977 and the continuing program certified that the world was free of smallpox in 1980.

The first task of the program was to provide effective reporting of cases from the village/town level through the district to the national level and then the WHO regional level and finally to WHO HQ level.

In practice, the surveillance was divided into two areas: Smallpox-endemic countries (30 countries) and smallpox-free countries (or smallpox-imported countries).

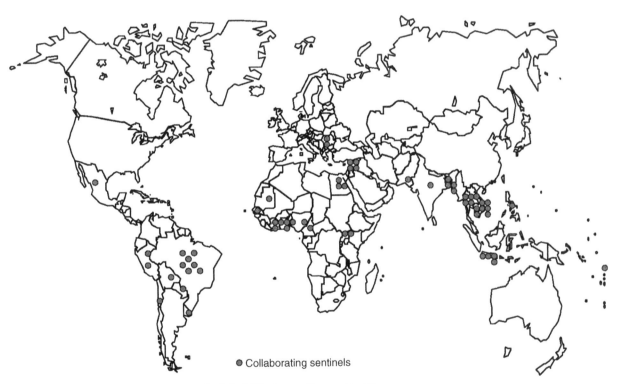

● Collaborating sentinels

Figure 7 Distribution of collaborating sentinels in AGSnet surveillance network.

Table 1 Number of outbreak episodes reported by surveillance systems of WHO, ProMED, and AGSnet during the period from January to December 2002

	WHOWER[a]	*WHO OVL*	*ProMed*[b]	*AGSnet Sentinels*[c]	*No. of same information*
Cholera	116 (58 countries)	22 (19 countries)	51 (28 countries)	15 (6 countries)	3
Measles	1 (1 country)	2 (2 countries)	11 (8 countries)	23 (8 countries)	0
Influenza	69 (43 countries)	1 (1 country)	1 (1 country)	15 (7 countries)	1
Plague	1 (1 country)	3 (3 countries)	9 (7 countries)	1 (1 country)	0
Dengue fever	0	0	40 (25 countries)	21 (4 countries)	3

[a]Weekly Epidemiological Record.
[b]ProMed is an Internet-based reporting system to provide up-to-date news on disease outbreaks around the world, more than 20 000 members.
[c]Including the suspected cases.

The former had a less effective system with significant problems of unreported cases and the latter had accurate reports; both operated following the International Health Regulation, which makes smallpox reporting obligatory, where smallpox occurrence in a smallpox-free nation should be regarded as a national emergency for immediate report and containment measurers. In both groups, also, the global program insisted that national health services and WHO should have the report weekly, including nil reports from endemic nations.

The measures to keep this principle workable specifically in the smallpox-endemic group are listed hereafter.

1. Smallpox has no subclinical infection and its clinical manifestation is distinct. This increased the sensitivity of surveillance greatly. The picture cards, termed smallpox recognition cards, were invented by the Indonesian

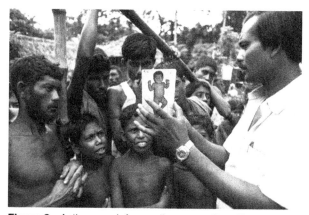

Figure 8   Active search for smallpox case. Surveillance officer showing smallpox recognition card to villagers in South Asia. Smallpox was known to villagers because of its typical clinical picture. Hence, this method is effective as far as villagers want to collaborate.

surveillance program as shown in **Figure 8**. Villagers immediately understood what disease was being searched for and that it had to be reported to the surveillance agent. The method was used in the entire smallpox eradication program.

2. This clear clinical manifestation did not require laboratory diagnosis procedures when the disease was known to be endemic (**Figure 9**). Only when the disease became rare was laboratory confirmation needed. This greatly simplified the surveillance procedures.

3. As mentioned earlier, rewards were offered to the public who reported suspected smallpox and when it was confirmed by laboratory diagnosis.

4. In India, despite their intensive national vaccination program with the target of 100% coverage of the entire population for more than 5 years, transmission continued (**Figure 10**). Then the prime minister instructed all the health center staff (more than 200 health centers) to stop work for 1 week once a month and go to the villages to actively search for smallpox cases, and if found, immediately vaccinate the population of only the village where the case was found. This special campaign, termed the autumn campaign, started in September 1973 and the final case occurred in May, 1975. The evidence showed how surveillance combined with focused containment was effective. Since then (as of June 2006), there has been no smallpox case in India for a population of one billion.

During the 2-year certification period, every surveillance method was employed to search for hidden foci in the previously smallpox-endemic countries and their adjacent countries, with special house-to-house visit surveillance. Two years were determined to be the necessary period of such surveillance, based on the fact

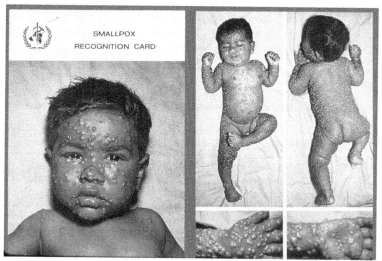

Figure 9   Clinical manifestation is typical for smallpox. Hence, usual report does not need laboratory confirmation. It is only needed to confirm the freedom of case.

that it was known that 9 months had been the longest period between a false date of a last case and a true date of a last case in Africa. For safety, the 9 months were doubled to roughly 2 years.

In sum, the effectiveness of smallpox surveillance was proved by the fact that since the last case's date of onset (October 26, 1977) in Somalia, there has been no occurrence of smallpox to date (as of 2006) except for the laboratory-infected case in the United Kingdom in 1978.

Surveillance of Influenza Pandemics

As of June 2006, when this article was written, the world was close to a new influenza pandemic since the world experienced the last major pandemics in 1918, 1957, and 1968. This new threat is characteristic, with possible devastating effects on the world's population with its severe pathogenicity to humans, perhaps comparable to the 1918 pandemic.

Furthermore, in view of an increased world population (two billion in 1918, six billion in 2006) as well as the increased speed and frequency of travel, once a pandemic occurs, the virus will spread rapidly throughout the world, possibly reaching all continents in less than 3 months. To prepare for such a pandemic virus, continuous global surveillance of influenza should be the key. WHO issued a series of recommended strategic actions for responding

to the influenza pandemic threat and, based on these, each national authority has been preparing the National Influenza Pandemic Plans, as illustrated in **Table 2**.

Recognizing the event

Epidemiological signals, such as an increase in the number of persons with unexplained respiratory illness with high mortality in an area over a short period of time, are likely to be the most sensitive and reliable indicators of a suspected pandemic event. Surveillance should focus on hospitals and communities with occurrences of respiratory infections and pneumonia. This may also be related to epidemics in poultry or bird populations, as will be discussed in the next section. Following detection of a cluster of suspected cases, an investigation should be started to characterize patients by person, place, and time and investigate the source or reservoir. Laboratory testing of samples to identify the causative agent should ideally be completed within 48 h following detection of the cluster.

Surveillance of animal influenza

WHO issued the *WHO Manual on Animal Influenza Diagnosis and Surveillance* in collaboration with the World Organization for Animal Health (OIE: Office International des Epizooties). The aims of surveillance in lower animals such as pigs and birds are intended to complement the human surveillance network, to understand the ecology of

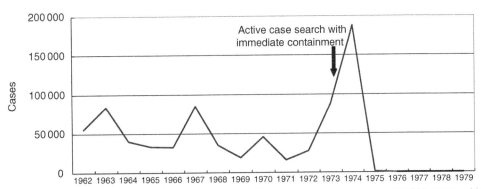

Figure 10 Number of smallpox cases reported by year for India. Active search discovered some 200 000 cases, which otherwise were not reported to the program. Thus, containment was more effective. The campaign resulted in a sharp incidence increase in 1973 and 1974. The transmission was interrupted in 1975.

Table 2 Current phase of alert in the WHO Global Influenza Preparedness Plan as of November 2007 (number 3 as circled)

Interpandemic phase	Low risk of human cases	1
New virus in animals, no human cases	Higher risk of human cases	2
Pandemic alert, new virus causes human cases	No or very limited human-to-human transmission	③
	Evidence of increased human-to-human transmission	4
	Evidence of significant human-to-human transmission	5
Pandemic	Efficient and sustained human-to-human transmission	6

From http://www.who.int/csr/disease/avian-influenza/phase/en/index.htm. (accessed November 2007).

influenza viruses that are relevant to human and animal health, and to determine the molecular basis of host range transmission and spread in new hosts.

Notification to national health authorities

Local health authorities should respond with a high level of suspicion and notify national health authorities as soon as preliminary information suggests that the cluster of cases is either unusual or different.

Reporting to WHO

Under the 2005 International Health Regulations, the national health authority should notify WHO within 24 h of detection of an epidemiological/virological signal suggestive of sustained human-to-human transmission of a new influenza virus. The national authority is requested to provide WHO with all relevant information, including the clinical, epidemiological, and laboratory data and the actions undertaken to contain the outbreak. Following the initial notification, the national authority should continue to report to WHO in a timely manner.

As of 4 July 2006, WHO had reported 229 cases including 131 deaths throughout the world since 2003. While the risk assessment with surveillance will continue (assuming the human pandemic has not yet occurred), it is essential for the world research efforts to concentrate on the geographical areas of risk where the favorable mutation of the virus is likely to occur, regardless of national boundaries. This tentatively includes East Asia, known to have a large concentration of the world avian population. Multi- and bilateral organizations are anticipated to join such efforts, which may lead to swift preventive vaccine production.

Polio Eradication Surveillance

WHO global eradication of poliomyelitis was launched in 1988 with the target year of 2000, but in 2005, 2000 cases were reported in 16 nations in Africa and South Asia. Intensive surveillance and mass vaccination of children under 5 years are continuing.

Acute Flaccid Paralysis Surveillance

All acute flaccid paralysis (AFP) cases under 15 years of age should be reported immediately and investigated within 48 h. Because the causes of flaccid paralysis include not only poliomyelitis but also other diseases such as Guillain-Barré syndrome and transverse myelitis, AFP surveillance takes human power, time, effort, and skill to sort out true poliomyelitis cases. In China and elsewhere, hospital-based surveillance was useful for searching for patients by checking the medical records in the hospitals. To cover the problem nationwide, investigation was needed for all medical institutes, including large hospitals in urban areas and dispensaries in rural areas. In Africa's

rural areas, where health facilities are sparse, community-based surveillance is conducted to detect polio cases. It is useful to have support from community leaders, such as senior members of the community and faith healers.

Laboratory surveillance

For confirmation, two stool specimens should be collected 24–48 h apart and within 14 days of the onset of paralysis; viral isolation is performed in a laboratory. As poliovirus is excreted in feces during the acute period of illness, it is desirable to take samples at the early stage (less than 14 days from the onset of paralysis). The temperature should be carefully controlled during transportation of specimens (2–10 °C with refrigeration). The results of laboratory diagnosis should be reported to the proper clinical/public health facilities without delay so that necessary action can be taken.

Surveillance performance

AFP surveillance requires the following criteria: (1) one case per 100 000 children under 15 years of age (in 2006, WHO augmented this one AFP case to two cases because the recent intensified surveillance has resulted in two to three AFP cases when the surveillance was intensified due to reduced number of polio cases); (2) two adequate specimens collected from at least 60% of detected AFP cases; and (3) all specimens processed in a WHO-accredited laboratory. Currently, it is anticipated that this surveillance system will continue in the foreseeable future until WHO recommends discontinuing it.

Measles and Rubella Surveillance

Measles is the most transmissible viral disease. Until the vaccine was introduced in 1963, practically every child got measles. The primary purpose of measles surveillance is to detect, in a timely manner, all areas in which measles virus is circulating, but not necessarily detect every case. This requires the notification mainly of health units and timely case investigation of all suspected measles infections. Laboratory investigation for anti-measles IgM antibodies of suspected measles cases is important to confirm or exclude measles virus infection. A single serum specimen collected within 28 days of rash onset is used for the diagnosis. In previously vaccinated persons, there may be a small increased risk of not detecting an IgM response to measles when specimens are collected more than 2 weeks after rash onset due to the increased rate of IgM decay. There is some increased sensitivity if the sample is taken on or after day 3 of rash onset (though taking the sample at first contact is recommended).

Measles surveillance may need to be community-based in areas where health units are nonexistent. It may be necessary to establish a system and procedures for collecting and testing blood samples from cases of acute fever and rash (AFR). Some other diseases whose main symptoms include fever or rash, such as rubella and parvovirus B19 infection, exist. In the surveillance of AFR, these patients are also reported and blood specimens are taken.

Surveillance of Ebola Virus Hemorrhagic Fever

Since the 1976 discovery of the disease in Central Africa, the disease has been the focus of national and international surveillance because its spread has increased through recent frequent travel in Africa as well as intercontinental travel. Ebola is often characterized by the sudden onset of fever, intense weakness, muscle pain, headache, and sore throat. This is often followed by vomiting, diarrhea, rash, impaired kidney and liver function, and in some cases, both internal and external bleeding. Specialized laboratory tests on blood specimens detect specific antigens and/or genes of the virus. Antibodies to the virus can be detected, and the virus can be isolated in cell culture. For patient management, supportive care is to be given. No specific treatment or vaccine is yet available.

Surveillance is aimed at early detection of cases in order to avoid possible spread of the disease. Suspected cases should be isolated and strict barrier nursing techniques implemented. Contact tracing and follow-up of people who may have been exposed to Ebola through close contact is essential. All hospital personnel should be briefed on the nature of the disease and its routes of transmission. Communities affected by Ebola should make efforts to ensure that the population is well informed, both about the disease itself and about necessary

outbreak containment measures, including burial of the deceased. People who have died from Ebola should be promptly and safely buried. As the primary mode of person-to-person transmission is contact with contaminated blood, secretions, or body fluids, any person who has had close physical contact with patients should be kept under strict surveillance. Ebola surveillance is a typical model that surveillance and containment are highly interrelated.

Surveillance of Noncommunicable Diseases

Public health surveillance has been extended not only to areas of communicable diseases but also surveillance of noncommunicable diseases. Although deaths caused by communicable diseases account for half of the total deaths in low-income countries, the proportion of deaths by chronic diseases has been significant, changing and increasing as the world economy changes (**Figure 11**). A few examples of how surveillance has elucidated analysis of the status and risk of specific noncommunicable diseases are given in the next sections.

Surveillance on risk factors for noncommunicable diseases

WHO developed the stepwise approach to surveillance of noncommunicable disease risk factors, termed STEPS (STEPwise approach to chronic disease risk factor surveillance), as part of a global surveillance strategy, aiming to monitor emerging patterns and trends worldwide and contain and reduce noncommunicable diseases. The STEPS approach is based on the concept that noncommunicable disease surveillance systems need to be simple, focusing on a minimum number of risk factors that predict disease, before placing too much emphasis

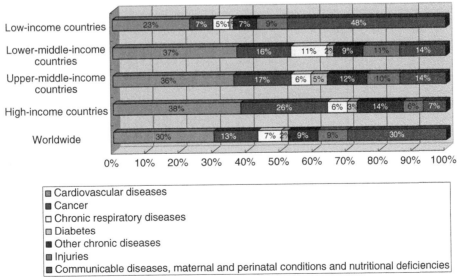

Figure 11 Proportion of deaths of chronic diseases. From World Health Organization (2007) *Preventing Chronic Diseases: A Vital Investment*. WHO Global Report. http://www.who.int/chp/chronic_disease_report/en/ (accessed October 2007).

on costly disease registries that are difficult to sustain over the long term, especially in low- and middle-income countries. STEPS is a sequential process, starting with the gathering of information on key risk factors by the use of questionnaires (sociodemographic features, tobacco use, alcohol consumption, physical inactivity, and fruit and vegetable intake); then, taking simple physical measurements (height, weight, waist circumference, and blood pressure); and lastly, collecting blood samples for biochemical assessment (measurement of lipid and glucose levels).

Epidemiological surveillance research on stroke and cardiovascular diseases

In Hisayama Town (population 7000), Japan, three cohort studies were conducted targeting residents aged 40 years or over in 1961, 1974, and 1988 after screening examinations. The cohort populations have been undergoing longitudinal observations by repeated health examinations (follow-up rate, 99%). When the subjects died, autopsy examinations were performed (mean autopsy rate, >80%). First, it aimed to study the prevalence of stroke and its risk factors, but later the study was expanded, targeting stroke, cardiovascular diseases, cancer, senile dementia, diabetes, and lifestyle-related diseases. The fourth study has been started, adding the molecular epidemiological study to find the genomic risk factors. The results have been reflected in national policy formation on the prevention.

Cancer registries

Cancer registries are part of the surveillance system. Population-based registries provide information on incidence cases and incidence trends, whereas hospital-based registries provide information regarding diagnosis, stage distribution, treatment methods, and survival. For example, in Japan, cancer occurrence is monitored through population-based and hospital-based cancer registries by the Japanese Association of Cancer Registries in collaboration with 34 prefectural governments, supported and maintained by the Research Center for Cancer Prevention and Screening, National Cancer Center. Hospitals and clinics are encouraged to report the occurrence to the prefectural government, which summarizes and analyzes their reports.

Surveillance of Accidents and Self-Inflicted Injuries

Injuries constitute a major public health problem. According to WHO data for 2000, an estimated 5 million people die each year as a result of some form of injury, comprising almost 9% of all deaths worldwide. Road traffic and self-inflicted injuries are the leading causes. The costs of injury mortality and morbidity are immense in terms of lost economic opportunity, demands on national health budgets, and personal suffering. Nevertheless, few countries have surveillance systems that generate reliable information on the nature and frequency of injuries. Aiming to collect better information and, in turn, to develop effective prevention programs, the WHO, in collaboration with the U.S. CDC, produced manuals on how to set up surveillance systems for collecting, coding, and processing data. In active surveillance, injury cases are sought out and investigated; injured persons are interviewed and followed up. For example, active surveillance of child abuse cases would involve identifying and locating cases through a variety of sources, such as police reports, social agencies, and educational authorities. It might involve seeking out the abused children, their parents, and/or the appropriate authorities, conducting interviews and follow-up. In passive surveillance, relevant information is collected in the course of doing other routine tasks. For example, doctors are routinely required to fill out death certificates for legal purposes, but it is possible to extract information entered on those certificates to obtain data on deaths from injuries. Forms filled out by doctors or nurses for medical insurance purposes can also be used for surveillance purposes. Other potential sources of data on fatal injuries include autopsy/pathology reports and police reports, and on severe nonfatal injuries, trauma registries, and ambulance or emergency medical technician records. In Japan, the statistics on fatal and nonfatal injuries, including accidents and suicide, are available based on police reports, the Population Survey Report, and death certificates. In addition to a hospital-based surveillance system, community-based surveys may provide a complement to capture further reports on injury events and deaths in the community. Those treated outside the formal health sector or those with minor injuries that do not necessarily require hospital attention might be missed by a hospital-based surveillance system, so that community-based surveys are one way of obtaining injury events within a community. Surveillance on this type of health hazards will become an important surveillance function in today's world, depending upon the level and extent of the health hazard in individual nations (**Figure 12**).

Global Surveillance Network

International surveillance on epidemic diseases or diseases of international importance has been carried out by different organizations under WHO's Global Outbreak Alert and Response Network (GOARN) (**Figure 13**).

The office covering GOARN is situated in WHO headquarters in Geneva and every week through the electronic network dispatches assorted surveillance data to all nations and individual institutions for their review and necessary action (**Figure 14**).

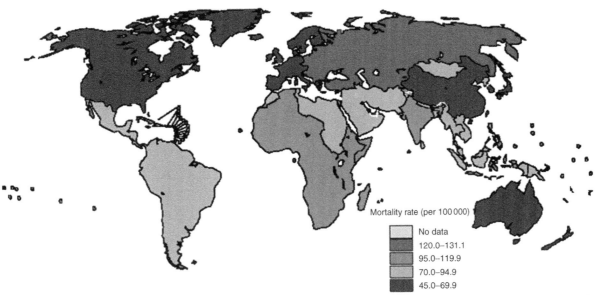

Figure 12 Global injury-related mortality. From World Health Organization (2002) *The Injury Chartbook: A Graphical Overview of the Global Burden of Injuries.* http://whqlibdoc.who.int/publications/924156220x.pdf (accessed October 2007).

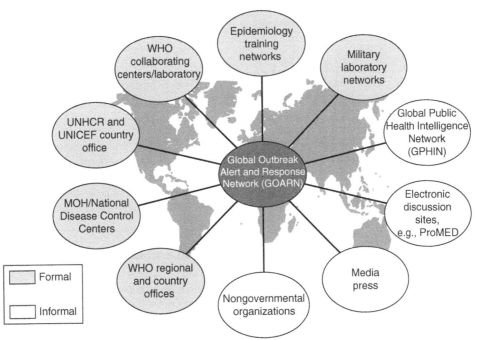

Figure 13 Global surveillance of communicable diseases: Network of networks. As growing importance of worldwide surveillance on emerging and re-emerging diseases, surveillance networks have been developed by WHO and various organizations, research centers, and NGOs.

In 2005, WHO and the member states renewed the International Health Regulations whose purpose is "to ensure the maximum protection of people against the international spread, while minimizing interference with world travel and trade." The diagram of the surveillance system is shown in **Figure 15**.

This purpose certainly requires a well-organized surveillance network, as shown in **Figure 14**. The diseases that veillance network, as shown in **Figure 14**. The diseases that

the system would handle are shown in **Figure 15**. In 2006, the World Health Assembly (WHA) further amended the International Health Regulations (IHR) to strengthen surveillance on the possible avian influenza pandemic.

The performance of international surveillance has been significantly affected by the unprecedented technology development in the last and this century. For example, electronics technology has prompted the real-time

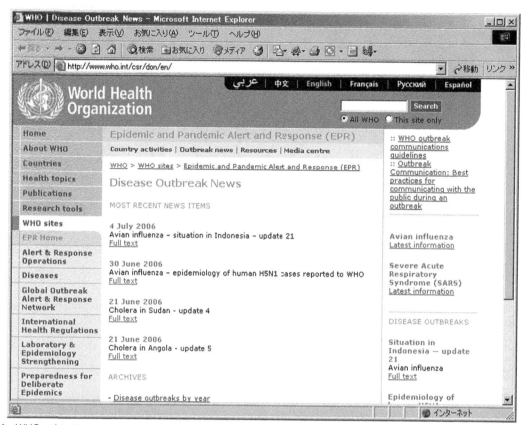

Figure 14 WHO epidemic and pandemic alert and response. From World Health Organization (2006) Disease Outbreak News. http://www.who.int/csr/don/en (accessed October 2007).

reporting and molecular biology has led to the discovery of the pathogen source in distant or unthinkable circumstances such as the spread of polio virus or SARS virus cases. On the other hand, a rapid increase in the global population (4 billion at the end of the nineteenth century, 6 billion at the end of the twentieth century) and increasing frequency of travel by air, sea, and land accelerates disease transmission. The situation is further worsening by expanding inequality. Of 6 billion people in the world, 1.5 billion (15%) live at a level of poverty of $1–2 per day (**Table 3**). Thus, in sub-Saharan Africa, for example, extreme poverty and the prevalence of severe diseases cause a vicious cycle and pose a threat to neighboring geographical regions. The situation makes conducting surveillance ineffective and complicated, coupled with the inadequacy of health services under the strain of limited resources and in some areas of political unrest. In these circumstances, the importance of global collaboration to strengthen area-wide surveillance was increasingly recognized in the late twentieth century and early in this century.

The surveillance system mentioned above requires the collaboration by all WHO member states. WHO Assembly, as necessary, reviews and makes recommendations on how the member states and experts concerned contribute to the effective performance of international surveillance

in different geographical regions. It is important to note that the surveillance activities in areas of extreme poverty require substantial cooperation from rich nations. Such cooperation contributes in turn to the development of effective global surveillance.

Ethical and Legal Aspects of Surveillance

Surveillance activities often involve surveillance workers handling communities, people, and institutions in terms of health hazard investigation, collection of technical as well as originally private information, and publication of the collected information. It is important that the purpose of surveillance should be known or fully explained as needed to the community or individuals so that surveillance teams can obtain needed information with good cooperation on the part of the community or individuals. When it is planned, surveillance should ensure that individuals' and agencies' right to privacy will not be violated. In some cases, however, this is not simple, because the right to privacy and the right to know scientific information conflict.

See also: Ethics of Health Promotion; Ethics of Public Health Research.

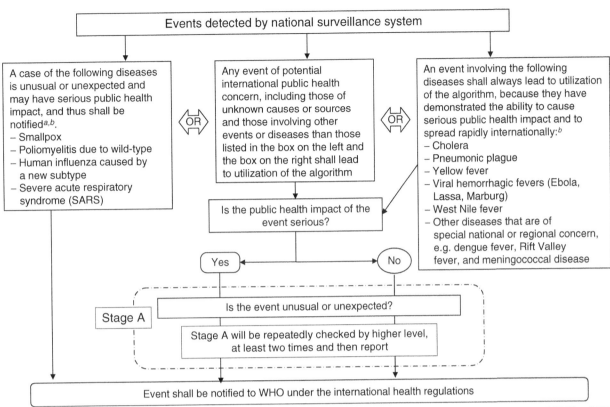

Figure 15 Notification system of events that may constitute a public health emergency of international concern, as of 23 May 2006. [a]As per WHO case definitions. [b]The disease list shall be used only for the purposes of these Regulations. From World Health Organization (2005) Third Report of Committee A–Fifty-Eighth World Health Assembly, 23 May 2005 (modified). http://www.who.int/gb/ebwha/pdf-files/WHA58/A58_55-en.pdf

Table 3 World Bank estimates of absolute poverty, 1990 and 2001

Number of poor: 1 million	$1.08/day 1990	$1.08/day 2001	$2.15/day 1990	$2.15/day 2001
East Asia	472	284	1116	868
South Asia	462	428	958	1059
Latin America	49	50	125	128
East Europe and Central Asia	2	18	58	94
Middle East and North Africa	6	7	51	70
Sub-Saharan Africa	227	314	382	514
World	1218	1101	2690	2733

Extreme poverty – people who can spend only one or two dollars per day for their survival are increasing in Middle East and certain areas of Asia and Africa. They are very numerous in South Asia and sub-Saharan Africa. Any health measures are a luxury. From The World Bank Group (2004) Millennium Development Goals. http://www.developmentgoals.org/Poverty.htm#povertylevel (accessed October 2007).

Further Reading

Arita I, Nakane M, Kojima K, Yoshihara N, Nakano T, and El-Gohary A (2004) Role of a sentinel surveillance system in the context of global surveillance of infectious diseases. *Lancet Infect Diseases* 4(3): 171–177.

Dowdle WR, Hopkins D, and Hopkins DR (eds.) (1998) *Dahlem Workshop on the Eradication of Infectious Diseases*. London: John Wiley.
Fenner F, Henderson DA, Arita I, *et al.* (1988) *Smallpox and Its Eradication*. Geneva, Switzerland: World Health Organization.
Heymann DL and Rodier GR (1998) Global surveillance of communicable diseases. *Emerging Infectious Diseases* 4(3): 362–365.
Teutsch SM and Churchill RE (2000) *Principles and Practice of Public Health Surveillance*. 2nd edn. New York: Oxford University Press.
The World Bank Group (2004) Millennium Development Goals. http://www.developmentgoals.org/Poverty.htm#povertylevel (accessed October 2007).
World Health Organization (1999) *WHO Recommended Surveillance Standards*, 2nd edn. WHO/CDS/CSR/ISR/99/2/EN, Geneva, Switzerland: World Health Organisation.
World Health Organization (2002) *The Injury Chartbook: A Graphical Overview of the Global Burden of Injuries*. http://whqlibdoc.who.int/publications/924156220x.pdf (accessed October 2007).
World Health Organization (2007) *Preventing Chronic Diseases: A Vital Investment*. WHO Global Report. http://www.who.int/chp/chronic_disease_report/en/ (accessed October 2007).

Relevant Websites

http://www.polioeradication.org/– Global Polio Eradication Initiative.
http://www.who.int/csr/en/– World Health Organization, Epidemic and Pandemic Alert and Response.
http://www.who.int/csr/ihr/en/– World Health Organization, International Health Regulation (2005).
http://www.who.int/wer/en/– World Health Organization, Weekly Epidemiological Record.

Emerging Diseases

J D Mayer, University of Washington, Seattle, WA, USA

Introduction

Emerging and re-emerging infectious diseases have been major features of contemporary societies. Indeed, there is evidence that history has been characterized by the constant interplay of humans and pathogens (McNeill, 1977). However, it is impossible to say when the terms 'emerging infection' or 'emerging infectious diseases' were first used to describe new infectious diseases, or diseases that meet the criteria that are described in this article. The belief in the 1960s that the threat of infectious diseases had been eliminated in developed countries was unfounded. A broader view of history would have demonstrated this. One possible reason for the optimism is that the 1960s was a decade of optimism in general. In the United States, social programs were instituted to address inequities; humankind had not only orbited the Earth, but landed on the moon; the gains of science and technology were impressive; economic expansion was equally impressive; poliomyelitis had been all but eliminated in the United States; and the sense of 'control' was widespread.

Beyond the borders of the United States, however, in Africa, Asia, Latin America, and elsewhere, malaria proved to be a huge challenge to life, although its prevalence was decreasing, and diarrheal diseases continued to take their toll, particularly among the young. Transportation links created the potential for transmission of infection between tropical regions and developed countries such as the United States. The potential for new diseases to emerge in the United States was there, and it took just a few years until this happened, catching the medical and public health communities by surprise.

Definitions of 'Emerging' and 'Re-emerging' Disease

In discussions of emergence, both 'emerging infections' and 'emerging infectious diseases' are commonly found. While the two are closely related, they are not synonymous. An infection does not necessarily represent a state of disease. 'Infection' suggests that an agent (usually a microbe) has become resident in the host. Usually that agent is replicating in the host. However, the host need not show any sign of disease, in the sense that it can conduct its normal activities without hindrance. 'Disease' is a state in which the normal functioning of the host is impaired, and both signs and symptoms are present – indeed, they are what limit normal function. An infectious disease is therefore a disease that is due to a pathogen.

Emerging Diseases

What, then, is an emerging infection, or an infectious disease? There has been some implicit variation in the literature. However, a general definition was articulated by Morse in the first volume of a then-new journal, *Emerging Infectious Diseases*:

> We can define as emerging infections that have newly appeared in the population, or have existed but are rapidly increasing in incidence or geographic range. (Morse, 1995: 7)

Thus, emerging infectious diseases are clinically significant diseases that are due to pathogens that have either appeared *de novo*, or are being experienced in a region with greater intensity, or for the first time.

Some authors have used a more specific definition of emerging to diseases and have specified five types of emerging diseases: (1) diseases that arise *de novo*, (2) diseases that are newly recognized, (3) diseases that have not previously existed in a specific area, (4) diseases that had not yet made a species jump to humans until the present, and (5) diseases that are increasing in prevalence. There are other definitions as well. The simplest definitions are frequently the most useful, and thus Morse's definition will be used in this article.

Resurgent (Re-emerging) Diseases

Re-emerging infectious diseases are frequently thought of as being closely related phenomena to emerging infectious diseases. Whereas emerging diseases denote diseases that are being experienced for the first time in a given location, re-emerging diseases are diseases that are reappearing in regions from which they have disappeared. Usually eradication is due to deliberate efforts on the parts of government and public health agencies. For example, malaria control programs following the end of World War II were instrumental in the elimination of malaria from some areas of the world, such as Italy and Spain. Sometimes, malaria eradication was eliminated as part of multisector development programs. For example, the Tennessee Valley Authority, created during the 1930s primarily for flood control, hydroelectric power, and economic development, also had an explicit aim of malaria control. This resulted in the drainage of most swamps, and the elimination of malaria from this part of the United States.

Just as malaria was disappearing from many regions in the 1950s, the next decade saw the resurgence of malaria, and the global prevalence of malaria has been increasing ever since. There are multiple reasons for this. These include anopheline spp. resistance to DDT, banning of DDT because of suspected environmental effects, and the development of resistance to chloroquine. Malaria, then, is a re-emerging disease. Another is tuberculosis. In many societies, TB had been nearly eliminated, but with the appearance of HIV/AIDS, immunocompromised individuals were much more susceptible to TB reactivation. TB, therefore, is also considered to be a re-emerging disease.

The New Realization of the Threat of Infectious Diseases

The public and the medical and public health communities gradually came to realize that their complacency over the potential threat of infectious diseases was misplaced, and that new and emerging diseases constituted one foci of concern over health threats to the public. This change in attitude came gradually, and can be thought of as a series of historical 'moments,' each of which refocused attention on infectious diseases. While it is impossible to be exhaustive here, this section takes a roughly chronological approach in describing the events that led the public and professional communities to realize that infectious diseases had not been 'conquered.'

Legionellosis (Legionnaires Disease)

The Bicentennial of the United States was celebrated in 1976, and there were many gala events around the nation in July. One was the meeting of the Pennsylvania Chapter of the American Legion. The events surrounding this meeting were the first to bring the attention of both the population and the broad scientific and medical communities to the argument that infectious diseases in the United States had been 'conquered,' and both alarmed the public and aroused the curiosity of the scientific and medical communities because this appeared to be a new disease. Indeed, before legionellosis was identified and antimicrobial treatment identified, legionellosis was called a 'monster disease.'

Over 220 members of the American Legion who had attended the meeting developed an unusual respiratory illness, and it became clear that it was of bacterial etiology, although it was initially thought to be viral, due to its close clinical resemblance to influenza. Approximately 34 people died as a result of this outbreak. However, two things remained unclear. First, the pathogen could not be identified with conventional methods, and second, no common source of exposure could be identified initially, although the fact that the number of incident cases followed a typical epidemic curve suggested very strongly that there was some sort of common exposure to the pathogen. The news media seized upon this medical 'mystery,' and the public knew that they were dealing with an unknown infectious disease. This constituted a historical moment in contemporary American history, because it had been decades since something like this had happened. Six months later, the bacterium was finally identified.

Legionella was not a new bacterium. Stored samples from outbreaks as early as 1943 tested positive for *Legionella* spp. However, the bacterium had not been identified in these outbreaks because it had not yet been described and characterized. In retrospect, most renowned is an outbreak that occurred in Pontiac, Michigan in 1968, although the symptoms were milder than in the *Legionella* outbreak in Philadelphia. In fact, mild legionellosis with a nonpneumonic form is often called 'Pontiac fever.'

This is not the place to review the epidemiology, pathophysiology, and clinical aspects of legionellosis in depth. Briefly, though, it usually has an acute onset, and is usually caused by *Legionella pneumophila*, although other species are also pathogenic. In fact, there are 40 species of the genus, and numerous serotypes. Epidemiologically, *L. pneumophila* is by far the dominant species in human disease. The major reservoirs are bodies of freshwater, and the main mode of transmission is through small droplets that are inhaled from the environment. In the Philadelphia outbreak, the source was finally traced to the air conditioning system in the hotel in which most attendees were lodged; the attendees were inhaling small particles in certain parts of the building. Dozens of subsequent outbreaks have been traced to similar mechanisms. These have been not only air conditioners but also shower heads, aerosolizers in sinks, and whirlpools. Virtually anything that aerosolizes fresh water is a potential mechanism by which legionellosis may be transmitted.

Symptoms of classic legionnaires disease are nonspecific and include fever, malaise, headaches, and myalgias. Frequently, rigors will develop, as will a productive cough (in about half the cases). Dyspnea (shortness of breath) is almost invariably present, and chest pain is common, as is a relative bradycardia for the elevated temperature. There are a number of abnormalities in laboratory tests, and chest films are markedly abnormal. A urine antigen test is available for one serotype, so laboratory diagnosis must frequently rely on more complex and time-consuming laboratory methods such as DFA. Sputum cultures or cultures from bronchoalveolar lavage have been the mainstay of laboratory diagnosis.

Since laboratory methods do not show a definitive diagnosis until a minimum of 3 days following onset, diagnosis is usually made on clinical grounds, and treatment is initiated based upon index of suspicion. Erythromycin proved to be effective in 1976, and other macrolides (azithromycin, clarithromycin) are highly effective. Tetracycline and doxycycline are frequently used, as are the fluoroquinolones, such as levofloxacin. In hosts who are not immunocompromised, the prognosis is generally positive.

There is no doubt that legionellosis was an emerging disease when it was first identified. Its particular significance lies in its historical context – in the fact that this was the first occurrence that began shaking the optimism of the 1960s and early 1970s that infectious diseases had been conquered, and also in the fact that the etiology of an obviously infectious syndrome with a reasonably high case fatality ratio remained unknown for a number of months.

Toxic Shock Syndrome

Chronologically, the next event to bring infectious disease to the attention of the public was another emerging infectious syndrome. In late 1979 and 1980, a number of women in the United States became seriously ill with a syndrome characterized by high fever, shock, rash, hypotension, and capillary leak. This syndrome had been first described as such 2 years earlier, although in retrospect it had been noted in the medical literature in the 1920s. The 1978 paper identified toxic shock syndrome in males, females, and children – and the females were both menstruating and not menstruating. The 1980 outbreak was associated with menstruating women, many of whom were using superabsorbent tampons. Although this was a major risk factor in the 1979–80 outbreak, much of the public and many physicians were under the erroneous impression that toxic shock syndrome (TSS) was necessarily associated with menstruating women who were using superabsorbent tampons. Although TSS is not necessarily associated with menstruating women, this does remain a risk factor in the epidemiology of TSS.

As with legionnaires disease, TSS was a rare disease, yet the public's perception of it was out of proportion to its true prevalence – the risk was exaggerated. This is something that social scientists have called the 'social amplification of risk' in the context of new events that are potentially dangerous, but that nonetheless carry with them a low risk. Amplification takes place as a result of media coverage, and as a result of intrapsychic processes that tend to amplify the threat of novel threats when the locus of control over the event is external to the individual. During the outbreak of toxic shock syndrome, newspapers were full of stories about TSS and the sometimes deadly consequences of developing the syndrome. These were frequently on 'page 1 above the fold' and

necessarily caught the attention of the public. The same was true of television news.

Once this outbreak of TSS appeared to be concentrated in one single group – menstruating women using superabsorbent tampons – the general public's fear of TSS began to diminish, and the federal government mandated the withdrawal of those tampons from the market. The number of incident cases began a rapid decline, and was back to baseline of about 100 cases per year by 1985. Some reports demonstrated that there was a decrease in the use of all tampons – not just superabsorbent tampons.

It was already known in 1980 that toxic shock syndrome was caused by staphylococci (specifically, *S. aureus*). In these cases, treatment is threefold: removal of the tampon, indwelling tampon, or other hypothesized environmental cause; aggressive fluid resuscitation; and rapid use of antistaphylococcal antibiotics.

Other bacterial species can cause toxic shock syndrome. In rare cases, other *Staphylococcus* species have been associated with toxic shock syndrome, and because they are coagulase-negative, they are difficult to treat. At this time, coagulase-negative staphylococci constitute the most common cause of hospital-acquired bacteremia. This sometimes results in endocarditis, and usually the only effective treatment is surgical valve replacement, particularly in the case of those who have had earlier valve replacement. Aggressive antibiotic therapy is occasionally effective.

Should toxic shock syndrome be considered to be an emerging disease? It certainly was in 1980, when the public was so concerned with its appearance. Now, in 2007, 29 years after it was first described, this label is more questionable. What was most significant about toxic shock syndrome, however, was its historical significance. It followed the outbreak of legionnaires disease so closely that it turned the public's attention, once again, to infectious diseases, and to infectious diseases that had been unknown. It also reminded the biomedical community that infectious diseases had not been conquered. The issue at the time was whether legionnaires disease and toxic shock syndrome were anomalies, whether the assumption of the conquest of infectious diseases had clearly been erroneous, or whether these two outbreaks were harbingers of a new stage in 'epidemiologic history' – a historical period during which emerging infections would become common and would catch the attention of the public, the public health community, the medical community, and government agencies. The public health and medical communities were divided on this. It would soon become clear, however, that the latter would hold true – that emerging infectious diseases would come to the forefront of public health, epidemiology, and the medical community. In the cases of legionnaires disease and TSS, the social amplification of risk exaggerated perceived threats. Nonetheless, the public became more attentive to infection. Two other phenomena would solidify this attention. One was the appearance of HIV/AIDS in the United States, and the other was public attention that was drawn to hemorrhagic fevers, mostly in Africa.

HIV/AIDS

The details of HIV/AIDS are covered elsewhere in this encyclopedia, and there will be no attempt here to duplicate this material. Rather, this discussion concentrates on the significance of HIV/AIDS.

When HIV/AIDS first appeared in several urban areas in the United States in 1981, it appeared to be an anomalous syndrome. It was not called 'AIDS' until 1982, when the Centers for Disease Control (CDC) gave the syndrome that label. In the same year, researchers at CDC also linked one of the pathways of transmission to blood and blood products, causing a great deal of public concern – if it was possible to contract AIDS through a frequently used medical practice, it had the potential of affecting millions of people. Until then, AIDS was thought to be restricted to the gay community. In 1983, blood banks were warned by the CDC that blood and blood products could definitely transmit AIDS, and surgeons and other medical personnel began rethinking the criteria necessary for transfusion. By 1983, it was clear that the exponential increase in the number of incident cases was a definite trend. In 1983 and 1984, two teams discovered that the pathogen causing AIDS was viral, and although it had a different nomenclature at first, there was a great deal of relief that the causal agent had been discovered. It is an interesting study in the sociology of science to analyze the competing claims by Luc Montagnier at the Institut Pasteur and Robert Gallo in the United States concerning their respective claims that they discovered HIV. It is now clear that Montagnier discovered the virus.

Shortly after the virus was discovered and characterized, an antibody test was developed to detect HIV *in vivo*. This was quickly used to screen blood products as well as to detect HIV in individuals. Whereas some people decried the slowness of the U.S. government's response to HIV, the time from the first presentation of a group of males with Kaposi's sarcoma or oral thrush until the antibody test for a recently identified virus was only 3 years. Granted, the president of the United States, Ronald Reagan, had not even mentioned AIDS, and funding was less impressive than it could have been, but the time was quite short. The real challenge with HIV has been to find an effective vaccine, or to find a 'cure,' although antivirals have been effective in suppressing viral load in the majority of cases since 1995–96.

The prevalence and mortality data are well-known. The best estimates are that globally, over 40 million people are living with HIV/AIDS, and approximately 22 million have died of HIV/AIDS. Currently, about 19–20 million of those living with HIV/AIDS are women, and in developing countries, particularly in sub-Saharan Africa, HIV/AIDS is becoming, increasingly, a disease of women. Currently, approximately two-thirds of those living with HIV/AIDS are in sub-Saharan Africa, but the increasing prevalence and incidence of HIV/AIDS in Asia – and particularly, in India and China – are making East Asia and South Asia regions of tremendous concern. This is because each country has over 1 billion people, and the prevalence rates do not have to be high to result in large numbers of infected people.

The global significance of HIV/AIDS is that it, by itself, has altered demographic trends, and the political economy of nations and regions, not to mention the human suffering that this disease has exacted. In Botswana and Swaziland, for example, the gains in life expectancy during the 20th century have not only been completely reversed, but the life expectancy at birth is lower now than it was at the beginning of the 20th century. In the context of this article, HIV/AIDS is an emerging infectious disease *par excellence*. A generation ago, it was literally unheard of. Now in all developed countries and in many developing countries, HIV/AIDS shapes many behaviors, is responsible for significant stigma, is feared, and causes a significant percentage of deaths. Globally, HIV/AIDS is the fourth leading cause of death, although in many parts of Africa, it is the leading cause of death.

HIV/AIDS is an emerging infectious disease because of the historical rapidity with which it moved from an unknown localized zoonotic complex in West and Central Africa to the most prevalent infectious disease in the world. While the scientific evidence suggests that there were a number of species jumps of both HIV-1 and HIV-2 that occurred in Africa, these were so localized and the societies isolated enough from the rest of the world that HIV went unnoticed. Thus, it appeared as though the disease went from nonexistence to a major pandemic in a matter of a few years. And there is another major significant dimension. Since HIV/AIDS appears to have originated in Africa – 'out there,' away from Northern Europe and North America – some have argued that HIV/AIDS acquired a certain nefariousness – a disease emerging from the dark, foreign, isolated jungle – the stereotypical cauldron of new diseases.

Hemorrhagic Fevers

Viral hemorrhagic fevers have been in the public eye since 1969, when there was a major outbreak of a hemorrhagic fever in the Jos Plain of Nigeria. The disease came to be called Lassa fever, caused by an arenavirus (Lassa) that seemed particularly undesirable to the public. The virus is named after the town in which this outbreak occurred. Like all hemorrhagic fevers, including dengue in some cases, one of the characteristics of Lassa fever is that it can disturb the clotting/coagulation mechanism, resulting in disseminated intravascular coagulation (DIC) and diffuse hemorrhage. The 1969 outbreak was publicized in the United States through the news media, perhaps because it was an 'exotic' or newsworthy event, and once again, the social amplification of risk was responsible for exaggerated fears of 'what if it spreads here?' That this outbreak occurred in sub-Saharan Africa, which, in the eyes of the North American public, may have been thought to be all 'jungle' (the Jos Plain is not rain forest) probably also contributed to the amplification of risk.

Serologic tests demonstrate that exposure to Lassa virus is common in West Africa. For example, in parts of Nigeria, seroprevalence is positive in 21% of those tested; in Sierra Leone, the figure varies from 8–52% depending on the region (Richmond and Baglole, 2003). It is now known that humans are dead-end hosts, and that the rat species *Mastomys natalensi* is the natural host. These rats are extremely common throughout sub-Saharan Africa. People become infected by inhaling aerosols from rat excreta, and risk is increased by eating them, which is a very common practice in West Africa.

Modern modes of travel have allowed infected individuals who are either symptomatic or asymptomatic at time of entry to travel to other continents, where they require treatment for Lassa fever. These cases have not been numerous, but cases have appeared in the United States and Japan, as well as in several European countries. This has caught some clinicians unprepared, since they were not trained in tropical medicine and were unaware of how to diagnose or manage a viral hemorrhagic fever.

The prevalence rate of Lassa fever is much higher than was initially thought. In one series, Lassa fever accounted for 30% of adult deaths in Sierra Leone, and as many as 16% of hospital admissions (Richmond and Baglole, 2003). Following the outbreak in 1969, it took some time to investigate adequate treatment protocols, but now, aggressive fluid replacement and the use of antivirals – particularly ribavarin – are the treatments of choice.

Ebola hemorrhagic fever and closely related Marburg virus are both single-stranded RNA viruses, as are other viruses that cause hemorrhagic fevers. Ebola and Marburg are Filoviruses; Ebola virus is actually a genus and there are four species. It was first described in the Sudan in 1976, and estimates are that mortality from this virus has now exceeded 1000 people. The case fatality ratio exceeds 50%, and may be as high as 90% in some cases. Transmission is different than Lassa fever. It is usually through direct contact with blood and bodily secretions from individuals who are ill with Ebola fever, or from nonhuman primates who are also infected. Evidence points to bats as the natural reservoir of Ebola virus, but this is not certain. In several studies, however, bats have been shown to be infected by the virus (Leroy *et al.*, 2005). This is highly suggestive, but it is not conclusive proof.

Like so many other viral hemorrhagic fevers, the symptomatology of Ebola is very nonspecific and typical of viral syndromes in general. The clinician needs to have a high index of suspicion. At this point, the only certain treatment is supportive, and from a public health point of view, quarantine is of the utmost importance, since Ebola fever is so contagious. This was well-documented by the news media in the outbreak in Kikwit, Democratic Republic of the Congo (DRC, then Zaire) in 1995. This was so well-documented that once again it led to exaggerated perceptions of risk, with overtones of the 'exotic disease' from sub-Saharan Africa and its possible spread to the United States.

Recent advances in understanding the pathogenesis of Ebola and the role of proinflammatory cytokines has led to the use of some recombinant products that block the progression of the inflammatory cascade to DIC in some animal models. Nonetheless, this approach has not been used in humans as of 2007.

There are three notable points that need to be mentioned concerning Ebola. First is that it appears to be increasing in prevalence in Africa. This may be because detection is better and the disease has been better described, both epidemiologically and pathophysiologically. Second is that there is significant concern that Ebola virus could be used as a biological weapon. It has thus been placed on the highest level (Category A) of potential biological weapons by the CDC. Finally, Ebola, more than any other emerging infectious disease, typifies in the mind of the public the sort of dangerous, threatening disease risk that is associated with tropical areas, the 'jungle,' and the threats that are associated with a more interconnected world.

Bovine Spongiform Encephalopathy

Bovine spongiform encephalopathy (BSE), or 'mad cow disease' in nontechnical terms, is another infectious disease that focused public awareness on emerging infections. The pathogen in this case was unusual not only in the sense that it had not been described elsewhere, but also because the whole class of pathogens – prions – have been very rare. Like another neurologic disease, kuru, BSE turned out to be due to a prion. Essentially, prions are very simple since they are just unusually folded and self-replicating proteins. They cannot even be described as organisms. The source of the prion is not known, although many speculate that it is somehow derived from sheep infected with scrapie.

In 1986, an unusual disease seemed to be affecting cattle in the United Kingdom, and by the end of the year, over 175 000 cattle had died because of spongiform encephalopathy. Since it was apparent that the disease was contagious, over 4 million cattle were intentionally slaughtered to limit contagion and ensuing effects on the cattle industry.

By the mid-1990s, there was a clear epidemiologic association between BSE and a variant of a neurodegenerative disease in humans that had been described in the middle of the 20th century: Creutzfeldt-Jakob disease (CJD). However, there were some notable differences between CJD and the disease that was affecting humans in the 1990s. The median age of this new syndrome was much younger than in classical CJD; the median duration of survival from onset of symptoms was longer than in classical CJD; and pathological differences and differences on MRI were apparent with this new variant. Accordingly, the CJD associated with BSE first was named 'new variant Creutzfeldt-Jakob disease' or 'nvCJD;' as time progressed, nvCJD was renamed 'variant CJD' or 'vCJD.'

Although there were very few cases of vCJD in the UK human population, the threat of this disease was great according to public perception. According to the World Health Organization (WHO), as of November 2002, there had been 129 cases of vCJD in the United Kingdom, six in France, and one each in several other countries (WHO, 2002). Nearly all of those with vCJD died or would die within 3 years.

Because of the realistic fear of contagion, several steps have been taken to limit the spread of vCJD. Feeding practices for cattle have changed so that it is no longer legal to feed animal protein that might contain any tissues proximal to the central nervous system to other cattle. In the United Kingdom, there was a ban on cattle over 30 months old from entering the commercial food supply. In the United States, individuals who have lived in the United Kingdom or who have spent more than 6 months in the United Kingdom are banned from being blood donors on the assumption that they might have consumed infected beef during their stay(s) in the United Kingdom. A ban was instituted on importing cattle and cattle feed from the United Kingdom, and, occasionally, from Canada, in an attempt to prevent BSE from spreading to the United States (Kuzma and Ahl, 2006). While the number of incident cases of vCJD and BSE have decreased in a typical epidemic curve pattern, the effects of the BSE 'scare' have been tremendous. The very credibility of the UK government was threatened. The whole cattle and meat industries were severely hurt. On the other hand, surveillance techniques and understanding of cattle food chains were vastly improved.

SARS

Severe acute respiratory syndrome (SARS) proved to be of great import in both the public awareness of emerging infectious diseases and in the testing and real-time construction of both domestic and international systems of public health surveillance and response. It was particularly important in terms of public awareness because it spread very rapidly on the international and intercontinental scales.

SARS apparently began as a few cases of a viral pneumonia in Guangdong province in southeastern China in late 1992. However, this was not immediately apparent to the global public health communities because it was not publicized by the Chinese government. What catapulted SARS to international attention in the media and in the public health community was the appearance and rapid increase of incident cases in Guangdong in February 2003 (Zhao, 2007).

SARS spread rapidly to Hong Kong, where contact tracing eventually identified one night in a specific hotel where the index case stayed as being the epidemic focus. The index case infected at least 16 others who were in the hotel at one time or another during that night.

SARS spread from Hong Kong to other areas of Hong Kong and to Singapore, Vietnam, and Canada (Toronto, Ontario). The spread of all these cases has been traced to airplane travel, followed by localized spread by an index case.

A case definition was developed based upon clinical presentation, which typically consisted of fever, initially, followed by lower respiratory signs and symptoms, sometimes resulting in acute respiratory distress syndrome and respiratory distress typical of acute lung injury as a response to the inflammatory cascade.

Just over 8000 cases were identified worldwide, and 774 died, for a case fatality ratio just <10%. A disproportionate degree of contagion occurred in intensive care units and areas of hospitals in which hospital personnel were exposed to respiratory excretions; close proximity – within 1 m – to an infected patient who was undergoing endotracheal intubation was the single greatest risk factor for contracting SARS.

Local measures to control the spread of SARS consisted largely of quarantine and containment. In China, for example, separate quarters for SARS patients were constructed very rapidly. In Singapore, arriving and departing passengers were required to pass through automated temperature detectors, and anybody with a fever was required to undergo further medical evaluation. The same was true at most points of entry in most developed countries. Since most cases were contracted in hospitals and health facilities, rigorous contact control procedures were instituted, and in some cases, hospitals were closed to visitors and new admissions.

The identification of the pathogen causing SARS constitutes a textbook example of how international cooperation in science and public health may occur when the willpower is there and the scientific capability exists. By mid-March 2003, many leading laboratories with advanced virologic capabilities had agreed to cooperate in a network that was coordinated by the World Health

Organization. Within 2 weeks, a pathogen was identified as a novel coronavirus, using a combination of methods: molecular polymerase chain reaction, culture, and electron microscopy, and shortly thereafter, the criteria of Koch's postulates were met. Thus, the evidence was quite clear that the new coronavirus was the pathogen. The virus was named the SARS coronavirus, or, almost always, SARS coV.

The ecology of SARS was not understood as quickly as the pathogen was identified. Some features were identified within a number of months. First was the phenomenon of superspreaders, which is a concept that previously had received scant attention. In this case, it became apparent that a small number of individuals spread SARS to a disproportionately large number of people. It is not clear whether this is because of behavioral factors, host–pathogen interaction, or environmental factors. What is fairly clear is that were it not for superspreaders, the epidemic would not have affected nearly as many people as it did. This is because the R_0, or number of people who one individual could infect, was inflated by superspreaders. Thus there was a domino effect of contagion.

In 2007, bats were identified as the reservoir of SARS coV. There had previously been some speculation about bats being the reservoir, but there was no solid evidence, and the reservoir had been a mystery. Some had suggested that proximity of people to avian species could possibly be a factor in the pathogenesis of SARS, because of the importance of this process in avian influenza. However, this turned out not to be the case with SARS.

SARS is a prototype of an emerging infectious disease (Berger *et al.*, 2004). There is no evidence that SARS coV existed in the human population prior to the outbreak of late 2002–03. The specific syndrome surprised the public health and medical communities, yet its general features did not, and the emergence of new diseases had been a familiar concept since the U.S. Institute of Medicine report of 2002. At the same time, the rapidity of the appearance of SARS and its very rapid spread at every scale fueled public apprehension, and even hysteria in some cases.

Avian Influenza

Evidence exists that history has been punctuated by relatively regular influenza epidemics and pandemics. The rapidity of epidemic spread, leading to pandemics, is largely determined by the velocity of the prevailing transportation modes. Severe epidemics and pandemics are caused by genetic shift, whereby the viral genome expressing surface antigens (hemagglutinin and neuraminidase) undergoes relatively major change. Relatively minor epidemics occur because of genetic shift, in which the surface antigens undergo minimal yet detectable changes in their configuration. Following genetic shift, people have minimal immunity to the virus, and are susceptible.

In one sense, each year influenza constitutes an emerging infection, because the precise genome of the influenza viruses and the surface antigens undergo change. Similarly, whenever a pandemic occurs, influenza represents a more significant emerging infection. On the other hand, influenza represents a disease entity that is not new to the population. Thus, it is a matter of semantics whether to consider influenza to be an emerging infection.

Avian influenza may constitute the next serious pandemic threat. It has been known for decades that genetic reassortment occurs in southeastern China because of the proximity of humans, avian species, and swine. An unusual number of influenza epidemics appear to arise there. However, the concern over avian influenza arises from a slightly different situation.

It has been known for some time that no less than 24 influenza subtypes – different configurations of surface antigens – can infect aquatic bird species. It has been well-established that several of these subtypes can infect humans, although recent experience suggests that all subtypes that circulate in avian species may have the potential to infect humans. This is one of the reasons that has given rise to concern over the possibility of an avian influenza pandemic. This theoretical concern moved closer to reality in Hong Kong in 1997, when one influenza strain (H5N1) was transmitted directly from poultry to humans. This took place in 'wet markets' – markets in which live poultry are densely packed, and where people co-mingle with their intended purchases. The transmission in 1997 appears to have been limited: Only 18 cases were confirmed. However, the case fatality ratio was high. Six of the 18 people died.

Transmission also occurred with another strain – H9N1 – in 1999, and in 2001 and 2002 there was widespread transmission and mortality among chickens in Hong Kong. Because of a concern over possible transmission to humans, and because of the devastating economic potential in the poultry industry, containment of this epidemic in poultry was partly obtained by the slaughter of millions of chickens and other poultry.

Avian influenza viruses have shown some propensity, since 1997, for transmission to humans. So far, human cases of influenza that have been identified as avian strains have been limited to approximately 200, and these have all been in Asia. Human-to-human transmission has been implicated in only a few cases. If this is the case, what is the concern over avian influenza?

Because of the tendency for influenza viruses to mutate, many virologists and epidemiologists predict that there is a high likelihood that a mutation could occur that would facilitate human-to-human transmission of H5N1 and other avian subtypes that have been transmitted to humans. If this occurs, then there is little doubt that this strain would spread rapidly among the human population, and would spread locally, nationally, and between continents in a manner similar to SARS. Other epidemiologists and virologists are more circumspect in their predictions, and argue that the probability of a mutation that would increase the propensity of avian influenza to spread from human to human is unknown. A minority of authorities argue that the probability is low. Thus, in assessing the overall threat of avian influenza, the crucial question is whether the virus will spread readily from human to human. At this point (mid-2007), it is unknown whether this will occur. However, it is prudent public health policy to bolster surveillance systems, and governments are stockpiling neuraminidase inhibitors, which are medications that can moderate the course of influenza if taken early in the course of clinical disease, or sometimes prevent the onset of symptoms if taken prophylactically. Similarly, there has been great emphasis on vaccine development and stockpiling.

Attempts to Understand Emerging Infections

In response to growing public concern over emerging infectious diseases, both domestically and internationally, as well as to both interest and concern in the medical and public health communities, a major conference on emerging viruses was held at Rockefeller University in 1989. The conference was cosponsored by several government agencies. The conference participants reached many conclusions, but two of them were that emerging infections had become a major focus for scientific research and that emerging infectious diseases had become and would remain a major public health challenge for the United States. Accordingly, the Institute of Medicine of the National Research Council of the United States took a proactive role and sought funding for a major study of emerging infections. The study was funded by a number of government units, and in early 1991, a high-powered committee met in Washington for the first time to:

> identify significant emergent infectious diseases, determine what might be done to deal with them, and recommend how similar future threats might be confronted to lessen their impact on public health. (Institute of Medicine, 1992: vi)

The committee issued a report in 1992 that quickly became a standard scientific and policy reference on emerging infectious disease. *Emerging Infections: Microbial Threats to Health* was the first major comprehensive discussion of how emerging infections arise, and how they might be addressed by the public health community. The committee also identified the six 'factors' or causes of emergence.

Briefly, the factors that this committee identified were the following: human demographics and behavior; technology and industry; economic development and land use; international travel and commerce; microbial adaptation and change; and the breakdown of public health measures. It is notable that five of these six factors are social factors that are consequences of changes in society. Even microbial adaptation and change, such as the development of antimicrobial resistance as a response to selective pressure, has a large behavioral dimension. This is partly a response to a technical innovation – the development of antimicrobials – and partly a response to a behavior – the prescribing of those antimicrobials. Of course, one dimension of this factor is the nonselective and improper prescribing of antimicrobials. This has several dimensions: The prescription of antibiotics when none are needed, the prescription of broad-spectrum antibiotics when narrow-spectrum antibiotics are sufficient, the free availability of antibiotics in many developing countries on the street and in pharmacies where no prescription is needed, and the free use of late-generation antibiotics in the food industry to promote the growth of cattle, chickens, and other animals intended for human consumption. So, in fact, all of the six factors of emergence are social and behavioral in nature.

Social Causes of Emerging Infectious Diseases

It is ironic that despite the fact that both Institute of Medicine reports concluded that the major causes of emergence have been social, there have been very few social analyses of emerging infections. For example, *Emerging Infectious Diseases*, a new journal founded in 1995 in response to the growing importance of emerging infections, has an explicit aim of including a social understanding of emerging infections in its contents, yet there have been very few articles written by social scientists in this journal, and very few articles with any social content have been published. The main point is that the overwhelming understanding of emerging infections has been 'biomedical.' This is not a criticism of either the journal or of any field in public health or medicine. In large part, this is the result of the sociology of knowledge and science. For whatever reason, few social scientists have become involved in research on emerging infections, whereas the same cannot be said about chronic diseases.

Some researchers have asked the question of why emerging infectious diseases are emerging now and in the societies where they are emerging, and have sought a more contextual understanding of emerging infections. David Bradley asks a very penetrating question:

> [A]ttaching a microbiological label to an outbreak...does not answer either the micro-scale questions such as "why

is there an outbreak here, now, of this size, affecting these people?" nor does it answer the macro-questions such as "why are there more (or fewer) outbreaks this decade than last?" Nor does it answer the question "what drives the overall worldwide trends in such problems?" (Bradley, 1998: 1)

For example, a number of individuals have argued that emerging infections may represent another stage in the epidemiologic transition.

Our understanding of emerging infections has not been totally devoid of social analysis. Inequality and poverty have become a major focus for the social analysis of health and disease. The argument is that through a complicated series of pathways that are yet to be fully understood, both poverty and inequality result in poor health status. This has not been applied extensively to emerging infectious diseases, although Paul Farmer's (1999) insightful work has been applied to emerging infections. In his critical analysis of emerging infection, Farmer asks, "Emerging for whom?" In other words, the diseases that Westerners might label as emerging may have been present or endemic in poorer societies for a long time:

> If certain populations have long been afflicted by these disorders, why are the diseases considered "new" or "emerging"? Is it simply because they have come to afflict more visible – read more "valuable" persons? This would seem to be an obvious question from the perspective of the Haitian or African poor. (Farmer, 1999: 39)

In other words, Farmer argues, the concept of emerging infectious diseases is one of epistemology – the theory of knowledge. How do emerging diseases come to be categorized as 'emerging'? By implication, many of these diseases have been present in poorer societies for a long time.

The evidence affirms this. HIV was probably present in small foci in Central Africa for decades to centuries; Ebola was similarly endemic in West Africa for an unknown period, as was Lassa fever. What is novel about the past few decades is greater interconnection between places, allowing diseases, and news of diseases, to spread; better methods of detection; and changing settlement geographies that have brought people into different forms of contact with animal reservoirs. The root cause of the infectious disease emergence is human action, both intentional and unintentional. Most of this action is the result of cumulative individual acts on a mass scale. For example, the mass urbanization of society in poorer countries is the sum of millions of individuals who move from rural to urban areas. This is largely the result of the perceived economic opportunities in urban areas, and the 'push' factor of lack of opportunity in rural areas. Yet, taken together, millions of individual moves result in urbanization, and this urbanization facilitates the spread of diseases by the respiratory route, the fecal–oral route, and many other modes of transmission.

Policy in IOM Report

The Institute of Medicine Committee also developed a set of policy recommendations. These concentrated in two areas: the need for vastly increased resources for interdisciplinary training in infectious diseases because of the depleted workforce resources in this area; and the need to develop new surveillance and public health response systems, since the committee had determined that emerging infections did, indeed, constitute a major public health threat to the United States.

This report was issued with a great deal of publicity. The U.S. public's attention was already focused on emerging infectious diseases as a result of legionnaires disease, viral hemorrhagic fevers, and toxic shock syndrome. Now there was a major quasi-governmental report by a group of the nation's leading scientists who issued the sobering conclusion that:

> even with unlimited funds, no guarantee can be offered that an emerging microbe will not spread disease and cause devastation. (Institute of Medicine, 1992: 169)

Predictions Realized

Part of the Institute's report identified specific microbes and diseases that could possibly threaten public health in the future. Three of these were *E. coli* 0157:H7, cryptosporidiosis, and hantavirus. The report was prescient, because within a few years there were serious outbreaks of all of these. In 1993, which was the year after the IOM report was issued, there was a major outbreak of cryptosporidiosis on the south side of Milwaukee, Wisconsin. It caused diarrhea, ranging from mild to severe, in over 400 000 people. *Cryptosporidium parvum* is a protozoan parasite; evidence in animal models is that ingestion of even one oocyst can result in severe gastrointestinal symptoms. In humans, as few as 12 oocysts can produce these effects (King and Monis, 2007). It is impervious to usual methods of water treatment, and only recently has an effective medication become available. The Milwaukee outbreak was probably due to groundwater absorption of cattle feces, subsequent runoff due to both heavy rains and snow melting, transport of the oocysts to river tributaries, and movement of the oocysts into Lake Michigan, which serves as the water supply for the south side of Milwaukee. The filtration plant for that water was ineffective in eliminating the oocysts. Many of these events are putative, but together they constitute a logical chain. Meanwhile, research is still proceeding on the ecology of cryptosporidiosis. Understanding is progressing, but it is still incomplete.

E. coli 0157:H7 was also mentioned in the IOM report as being an emerging disease. In January 1993, the Washington State Department of Health ascertained that an outbreak of 0157:H7 was occurring in the state, and this outbreak was associated with having eaten at Jack in the Box fast-food restaurants. Subsequently, it became apparent that the epidemic was not limited to Washington, but also included Idaho and Nevada.

The epidemiologic investigation of this outbreak was intricate, and implicated a chain of events. First, because meat inspection in the United States was inadequate, one theory is that *E. coli* 0157:H7 from the bowels of cattle had gotten into meat that was sent to market when cattle were slaughtered, and the bowel was probably nicked or severed. Another is that under stress, cattle defecate over one another, and fecal matter from one cow can contaminate the hides of other cattle. Second, when this meat was ground into hamburger, it increased the surface area of the meat by several orders of magnitude, thereby allowing the pathogen a great deal of exposure. Third, once this hamburger meat was shipped to Jack in the Box restaurants, it appears that hamburgers were being systematically undercooked, below industry standards. This allowed the *E. coli* to survive and enter the hosts' systems. The consequences of such infection can be severe, and were in 1993, with those who were symptomatic frequently suffering from bloody diarrhea, fever, cramps, and, in the worst case, hemolytic uremic syndrome. The pathogenesis of this disease was only partially understood in 1993, but understanding is more complete in 2007.

The third disease that was mentioned in the IOM report that occurred shortly after its publication was hantavirus. In May 1993, in the Four Corners area of Arizona, New Mexico, California, and Utah, several males who were otherwise in good health developed a sudden serious respiratory disease that was thought to be a rapidly progressing acute respiratory distress syndrome, since this was the immediate cause of death. However, it was noted that these cases had formed a cluster, and investigators tried to find some sort of common source to explain a possible environmental exposure to explain this serious and sometimes fatal syndrome. Though hantavirus had never been described in the United States, serologic tests in patients showed a surprising seropositivity to hantavirus. It was apparent that this was the pathogen that had caused the dozen deaths associated with the outbreak. The chain of events that led up to the outbreak is now fairly clear. Winter 1993 was unusually warm in the Four Corners area as a result of El Nino, and the spring was also unusually rainy. These two conditions led to the rapid and plentiful growth of pinon trees, which provided food for a number of rodents. There is consensus that the

deer mouse (*Peromyscus maniculatus*) population increased by an order of magnitude. Testing demonstrated that about 30% of the mice that were trapped after this epidemic were infected with hantavirus, and studies demonstrate that households from which infected individuals came were far more likely to have heavy rodent infestations than were households of controls. More rigorous studies eventually showed that transmission occurred from rats to humans, and that many of the cases, in this instance, were associated with crawling under houses and other places in which rodent exposure was likely to occur.

Emerging Infections Reconsidered: Second IOM Report

By 2000, many of the predictions of the first Institute of Medicine report (1992) had been realized, and understanding of emerging infectious diseases had improved. There was greater focus on globalization as a process of disease spread, and the attacks on the World Trade Center and Pentagon on September 11, 2001 focused attention on terrorism. A new Institute of Medicine committee was formed to consider the nature of microbial threats and emerging diseases, and the report of this committee was issued in 2003 (Institute of Medicine, 2003). This report represented a rethinking of the factors of emergence, and presented a more nuanced understanding of the causes of emerging diseases, most of which were still social at one level or another. Bioterrorism ('intent to harm') was specifically mentioned as a factor of emergence, as was lack of political will. Policy recommendations for surveillance, response, and training were more detailed than in the 1992 report, and there was a more urgent tone to the need to respond to emerging threats.

In this report, the emphasis on biological and social interaction was strong:

> Genetic and biological factors allow microbes to adapt and change, and can make humans more or less susceptible to infections. Changes in the physical environment can impact on the ecology of vectors and animal reservoirs, the transmissibility of microbes, and the activities of humans that expose them to certain threats. Human behavior, both individual and collective, is perhaps the most complex factor in the emergence of disease. Emergence is especially complicated by social, political, and economic factors...which ensure that infectious diseases will continue to plague us. (Institute of Medicine, 2003: 2)

Antimicrobial Resistance

Increasing resistance to antibacterials, antivirals, and other antimicrobials is frequently grouped under the heading of 'emerging infections.' Resistance is certainly a

constantly growing and very major public health problem, but this is of importance to emerging infections
only in the sense that diseases that were once highly
treatable with first- and second-generation antimicrobials
are no longer treatable by them. The selective pressures
exerted by antimicrobials have made numerous pathogens resistant to even the newest antimicrobials due to
mechanisms that are now understood. For example, many
respiratory pathogens are no longer treatable by β-lactam
antibiotics since their β-lactam rings are cleaved by
β-lactamases. There are fluoroquinolone-resistant strains
of *Neisseria gonorrhoeae*, resistant strains of *Staphylococcus
aureus*, and so on.

The problem is most severe in hospitals, where severe
infections once responsive to vancomycin are now resistant to this glycopeptide. Several new antimicrobials have
been developed, in part to address vancomycin resistance,
but resistance to these medications developed within a
few years of their introduction.

Thus, antimicrobial resistance is both a community
problem and a hospital problem. There is great concern
over multiple drug-resistant tuberculosis, which is defined as tuberculosis that is resistant to two first-line medications, and extensively resistant tuberculosis, which has a
more complex definition specifying several medications.
There is not space in this article to explore antimicrobial
resistance in greater depth.

Summary

The relationship between people and pathogens has been
an integral part of history, and will continue to be.
The progress in the diagnosis, detection, and clinical
management of infectious diseases has been substantial.
Indeed, Fauci (2001) has gone so far as to argue that:

> The successful diagnosis, prevention, and treatment of
> a wide array of infectious diseases has altered the very
> fabric of society, providing important social, economic,
> and political benefits.

Nonetheless, infectious diseases, aggregated together,
constitute the second leading cause of death worldwide,
and in many regions, they account for the dominant cause.
Moreover, emerging diseases will continue to emerge,
because of constantly changing social and demographic
conditions, as well as selective pressures. The prototypical
emerging infectious disease, HIV/AIDS, has an uncertain
future in the long run. Perhaps a vaccine will be developed that will be inexpensive, and perhaps distribution
systems will be developed that will transport the vaccine
to points of demand. Perhaps antiretrovirals will become
extremely inexpensive, and perhaps the failure rate for
antimicrobials of 30% will be overcome. However, it
is unlikely under present conditions that all of these

improvements will occur. Thus, the future of HIV/AIDS
is more sobering.

The same is true of antimicrobial resistance. In an age
of optimism when antimicrobials were developed and used
successfully – perhaps the first 30 years of antimicrobial
use – concern over resistance was minimal. However,
the fact that organisms adapt to changing environmental
conditions and threats is something that has not been
realized only recently. The inevitability of adaptation
is undeniable, and the only way to meet the challenges
of resistance is through a combination of appropriate antimicrobial use (including the use of narrow-spectrum
antibiotics as soon as possible in the clinical course of
an individual) and the development of new antimicrobials,
as well as new understanding in the physiology and genetics of microorganisms, which might lead to the development of new technologies in addressing the pathogenic
basis of disease.

See also: Epidemiology of HIV/AIDS and its Surveillance.

Citations

Berger A, Drosten C, Doerr HW, *et al.* (2004) Severe acute respiratory
    syndrome (SARS): Paradigm of an emerging viral infection. *Journal of
    Clinical Virology* 29: 13–22.
Bradley DJ (1998) The influence of local changes in the rise of infectious
    diseases. In: Greenwood B and de Cock K (eds.) *New and Resurgent
    Infectious: Prediction, Detection, and Management of Tomorrow's
    Epidemics*, pp. 1–12. Chicester, UK: John Wiley.
Farmer P (1999) *Infections and Inequalities: The Modern Plagues.*
    Berkeley, CA: University of California Press.
Fauci A (2001) Infectious diseases: Considerations for the 21st century.
    Clinical Infectious Diseases 32: 675–685.
Institute of Medicine (1992) *Emerging Infections: Microbial Threats to
    Health in the United States.* Washington, DC: National Academy
    Press.
Institute of Medicine (2003) *Microbial Threats to Health.* Washington,
    DC: National Academy Press.
King BJ and Monis PT (2007) Critical processes affecting
    cryptosporidium oocyst survival in the environment. *Parasitology*
    134: 209–223.
Kuzma J and Ahl A (2006) Living with BSE. *Risk Analysis* 26: 585–588.
Leroy E, Kumulungui B, Pourrui X, *et al.* (2005) Fruit bats as reservoirs of
    Ebola virus. *Nature* 438: 575–578.
McNeill W (1977) *Plagues and Peoples.* New York: Doubleday.
Morse SS (1995) Factors in the emergence of infectious diseases.
    Emerging Infectious Diseases 1: 7–15.
Richmond JK and Baglole DJ (2003) Lassa fever: Epidemiology, clinical
    features, and social consequences. *British Medical Journal* 327:
    1271–1275.
WHO (2002) Variant Creutzfeldt-Jakob disease. http://www.who.int/
    mediacentre/factsheets/fs180/en/ (accessed October 2007).
Zhao GP (2007) SARS molecular epidemiology: A Chinese fairy tale of
    controlling an emerging zoonotic disease in the genomics era.
    Philosophical Transactions of the Royal Society B 362: 1063–1081.

Further Reading

Garrett L (1995) *The Coming Plague: Newly Emerging Diseases in a
    World out of Balance.* New York: Penguin Books.

Greenwood B and de Cock K (eds.) (1998) *New and Resurgent Infections: Prediction, Detection, and Management of Tomorrow's Epidemics.* Chicester, UK: John Wiley and Sons.

Institute of Medicine (2002) *The Emergence of Zoonotic Diseases: Understanding the Impact on Animal and Human Health.* Washington, DC: National Academy Press.

Mascie-Taylor N, Peter J and McGarve ST (eds.) (2004) *The Changing Face of Disease: Implications for Society.* Boca Raton, FL: CRC Books.

Morens DM, Folkers GK, and Fauci AS (2004) The challenge of emerging and re-emerging infectious diseases. *Nature* 430: 242–249.

Weber JT and Courvalin JT (2005) An emptying quiver: Antimicrobial drugs and resistance. *Emerging Infectious Diseases* 11: 791–793.

Whitman J (ed.) (2000) *The Politics of Emerging and Resurgent Infectious Diseases.* New York: St. Martin's Press.

Wilson ME, Levins R and Spielman A (eds.) (1994) *Disease in Evolution: Global Changes and Emergence of Infectious Diseases.* New York: New York Academy of Sciences.

Relevant Websites

http://www.cdc.gov – Centers for Disease Control and Prevention.
http://www.cdc.gov/ncidod/EID/index.htm – *Emerging Infectious Diseases Journal.*
http://www.fas.org/promed/ – Program for Monitoring Emerging Diseases (ProMED).
http://www.who.int – World Health Organization.

Re-emerging Diseases

M E Wilson, Harvard Medical School/Harvard School of Public Health, Boston, MA, USA

Introduction and Definition of Re-emerging Infections

During the past 50 years remarkable gains have been achieved with the control of many infectious diseases. At the same time, new and previously unknown pathogens have emerged, and some, like HIV, have spread globally killing millions of individuals, disrupting societies, and reshaping the demographics of countries and regions. In addition, infectious diseases previously thought to be under control have re-emerged in many parts of the world. For purposes of this discussion, re-emerging infections are defined as those that have one or more of the following characteristics: increase in number of cases; expansion of current foci of infection or appearance in new geographic areas; appearance of infections in populations previously unaffected; and increase in severity of illness or mortality. This article explores the mechanisms through which infections re-emerge and the multiple factors in the world today that facilitate the re-emergence of infections. Several specific infections are used as examples to illustrate key points. A discussion of the characteristics of infections that are most likely to re-emerge in the future and a framework for preventing re-emergence of infections, and thereby mitigating their consequences, concludes the article.

Mechanisms for Re-emergence

Multiple Factors Involved

Infectious diseases are dynamic; unless eradication of a microbe is achieved, which is rare, the interactions between microbes and humans undergo constant change and evolution. Microbes, with their rapid replication time, have the capacity to adapt to change much more rapidly than humans. At a fundamental level, infections that have been controlled re-emerge because: the microbe has changed, moved, or become more abundant; the host lacks or loses immunity (or capacity to respond to infection) or is not treated; or contacts between microbe and host increase. Although this may sound simple, multiple factors – biological, socioeconomic, demographic, and environmental – influence this dynamic relationship.

The convergence model (**Figure 1**) illustrates the broad context and interlocking domains of determinants in which infections emerge or re-emerge. Although the interactions between the human host and microbe are at the center of the process, other factors interact with each other and affect host, microbe, and their interactions. Disease emergence is often complex with multiple interacting factors involved. The model aptly depicts the central area of overlap as a black box, illustrating gaps in our understanding of many of the elements and how they interact.

For an infection to be defined as re-emerging, it must be recognized and characterized. It is important to acknowledge that many infections persist, reappear, and spread silently. Unless adequate clinical and laboratory facilities exist to accurately diagnose infections, they may go undetected or be categorized as a viral illness or flu. Microbes that cause infections that produce clinical signs and symptoms (such as fever and cough, fever and diarrhea, fever and muscle aches) similar to those of many common infections – such as influenza, tuberculosis (TB), salmonellosis, dengue fever, and malaria – may not be identified, especially in resource-poor settings where clinical

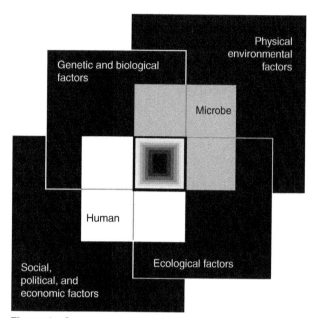

Figure 1 Convergence model. Reproduced from Smolinski MS, Hamburg MA, and Lederberg J (eds.) (2003) Microbial threats to health: Emergence, detection, and response. Institute of Medicine of the National Academies. Washington, DC: The National Academies Press.

laboratory support is absent or limited. Microbes that cause unusual clinical findings (e.g., vesicular skin eruption in monkeypox), high mortality (e.g., yellow fever), or produce large outbreaks (e.g., dengue fever and dengue hemorrhagic fever [DHF]) may be more likely to be identified.

Re-emerging infections are caused by all classes of pathogens (i.e., viruses, bacteria, fungi, helminths, protozoa) and involve pathogens with different modes of transmission (e.g., direct person-to-person transmission, airborne, vectorborne, food- and waterborne) and different sources (e.g., another human, animal reservoir, soil and water). Typically multiple factors will have contributed to the re-emergence of a specific infection. These may vary by time or geographic region. Populations and regions vary in their vulnerability to the re-emergence of infections and capacity to intervene promptly, so to some extent re-emergence may be specific to time, place, and population. Because of the extensive linkages in the world today through trade and travel, re-emergence of an infection may have broader implications and pose greater risk to distant populations than it might have a few decades ago.

Changes in the Pathogen

The types of changes in a pathogen that can contribute to the re-emergence of an infection include development of resistance to antimicrobial agents that were previously effective, acquisition of new virulence factors or

emergence of strains that are more virulent or transmissible, and emergence and spread of strains against which available vaccines are ineffective. Examples of each follow.

Resistance, virulence, and transmissibility

Resistance of a microorganism to an antimicrobial drug refers to the capacity of an organism to survive in the presence of that drug in therapeutic concentrations. Microbes can also be characterized by their resistance to killing by physicochemical conditions (e.g., heat, cold, acid, other) that may be relevant for survival in the environment, but these attributes are not discussed in this section. Virulence is a quantitative measure of pathogenicity of an organism or its likelihood of producing disease. Transmissibility refers to the ease of spread of a microbe from one host to another. These are three separate attributes that are not necessarily linked. For example, the H5N1 virus, the influenza strain currently circulating in avian populations, has shown resistance to the adamantane group of antiviral drugs. It is highly pathogenic in chickens and humans (and some feline species) causing high mortality in those species. In contrast, some infected ducks excrete the virus without showing symptoms of infection. As of early 2007, it is poorly transmissible from human to human, but highly transmissible in chicken populations. In general, many of the viruses that cause the common cold are highly transmissible from person to person but cause only mild illness.

Resistance

Increasing resistance of microbes to antimicrobials is occurring globally and involves microbes that cause millions of human deaths annually, including *Staphylococcus aureus*, *Streptococcus pneumoniae* (the cause of pneumococcal pneumonia and meningitis), *Mycobacterium tuberculosis* (the cause of TB), malaria parasites, influenza viruses, and human immunodeficiency syndrome viruses (HIV), among others.

Increasing resistance among some bacteria was initially localized primarily to tertiary care hospitals (e.g., methicillin-resistant *S. aureus*) but has now moved into the community and around the world. Increasing resistance is found among antimicrobials used to treat all types of infections, including viral, bacterial, fungal, and parasitic infections. In some instances, alternative agents are available for treating resistant infections, but alternative drugs may be more toxic, less effective, unavailable because of limited supplies, or expensive. High cost alone can mean many populations will be unable to have access to effective treatment, rendering infections operationally untreatable. In addition, resistance of arthropod vectors (e.g., mosquitoes) to pesticides has complicated the control of vectorborne infections, like malaria and dengue.

Bacteria can become resistant through mutations or by acquiring genetic material from related or unrelated bacterial species through horizontal exchange. Genetic changes in bacteria can occur in the absence of antimicrobials, but the presence of antimicrobials puts selective pressure on microbial populations. Resistant organisms may be able to flourish when an antimicrobial agent kills off other organisms that may compete for resources and may become the predominant population. Resistance traits are transferred to the progeny and potentially to unrelated strains of bacteria. The broad and indiscriminate use of antimicrobials has contributed to the rising resistance, but even appropriate use of antimicrobial agents puts pressure on microbial populations. In addition, certain clones or strains of resistant bacteria may become widely disseminated. With penicillin-resistant *S. pneumoniae*, for example, only 10 clones were shown to be responsible for 85% of invasive disease by this organism in the United States in 1998 (Corso *et al.*, 1998). Travel and social networks may be important in the spread of resistant (or virulent) clones.

S. aureus resistant to methicillin has expanded in geographic range, but until recently only five major clones were responsible for most of the worldwide problem. The microbe spread initially in defined groups with close contact – for example, children in child care facilities, athletes, intravenous drug users, prison inmates, and military recruits – then the organism disseminated into the general community. This may have been facilitated by special virulence factors of the organism that favored its survival (Furuga *et al.*, 2006).

Resistance as a single factor cannot fully explain the re-emergence of TB or malaria, for example, but presence of resistance has contributed to increasing morbidity and mortality in some populations and makes control more complicated and costly.

Virulence

A previously uncommon but more virulent strain of *Clostridium difficile*, a cause of colitis that can be severe, has emerged to cause multiple outbreaks with substantial mortality in hospitals in North America and Europe. It produces 16–23 times more toxin than other strains of *C. difficile*, which may account for its increased virulence. It is also resistant to fluoroquinolones, and their wide use may have favored its emergence (McDonald *et al.*, 2005).

An unusual example of a change in virulence has occurred in the attenuated live poliovirus vaccine. In rare instances (0.4–3 per million children vaccinated), the vaccine virus, which replicates in the gastrointestinal tract of the recipient, reverts to full neurovirulence. Not only can the vaccine-derived neurovirulent virus cause paralysis in the vaccine recipient, but vaccine-derived virus can also circulate in populations. Circulation of virulent vaccine-derived virus, in some instances with associated outbreaks of paralytic polio, has been documented in China, Egypt, Haiti, Madagascar, and the Philippines. Paralytic polio that has re-emerged in areas where circulation of wild poliovirus had ceased in some instances has

been caused by vaccine-associated poliovirus (Kew *et al.*, 2002). In other areas, wild poliovirus has been reintroduced from areas where polio persists in the human population. Geographic areas that appear to be at highest risk for circulation of vaccine-associated poliovirus are those with low vaccine coverage. Immunodeficient individuals (especially those with hypogammaglobulinemia) have been found to be long-term excreters of vaccine-derived poliovirus (in feces), one for at least 20 years (MacLennan *et al.*, 2004). This remains a concern in making decisions about when it might be possible to stop using oral poliovirus and killed polio virus vaccines.

Strains, serotypes, serogroups, subtypes

Microbes often exist as many different subtypes, serotypes, serogroups, or strains. This antigenic variation means persons who are immune (by natural infection or immunization) to one strain of an organism, may be susceptible to another. A previously uncommon serogroup of *Neisseria meningitidis* W135 (cause of meningococcal meningitis and sepsis) caused outbreaks among pilgrims to the Hajj in Saudi Arabia in 2000 and spread internationally. Because of previous outbreaks of meningococcal infections among the pilgrims (and subsequently their contacts in their countries of residence), Saudi Arabia started requiring all visitors to the Hajj to produce a certificate of vaccination against meningococcal disease upon entry into the country. Most visitors received a meningococcal vaccine active against serogroups A and C, the serogroups responsible for most epidemics of meningococcal disease in the past. It was in this context that meningococcal infections re-emerged in the pilgrims in the spring of 2000, caused by serogroup W135. About 240 cases were reported in Saudi Arabia. In all, more than 400 cases in pilgrims and their contacts were identified in at least 14 different countries. Analysis of isolates from patients in France and the UK using multilocus sequence typing, DNA fingerprinting, and other techniques showed that they were indistinguishable from isolates from Saudi Arabia. Pilgrims who became infected could carry the W135 meningococcal clone and transmit infection, even if they did not develop symptoms. Of note, the vaccine used in the United States was a quadrivalent vaccine active against serogroups A, C, Y, and W135. Although the risk of disease was low in recipients of the quadrivalent vaccine, recipients could still become carriers of the outbreak strain as the vaccine does not prevent carriage (Dull *et al.*, 2005). Saudi Arabia now requires pilgrims to the Hajj to have a vaccine active against W135. During February 2002, an epidemic caused by W135 began in Burkina Faso. By May more than 12 500 cases had been reported to the World Health Organization (WHO).

Dengue virus, a mosquito-transmitted flavivirus, is widespread in tropical and subtropical regions of the world and is expanding in geographic range and severity. Four different serotypes of dengue viruses cause disease in humans:

DEN-1, DEN-2, DEN-3, and DEN-4. Infection with one dengue serotype is followed by only brief immunity to the other serotypes. Subsequently, if individuals are infected with a different dengue serotype, they are at increased risk (perhaps 100-fold greater) for severe disease, manifested as dengue hemorrhagic fever or dengue shock syndrome. In studies from Thailand, no cases of DHF were observed in patients with primary dengue infection, whereas 1.8–12.5% of those with a secondary infection developed DHF. The appearance of a new dengue serotype in a population that already has previously experienced high rates of infection with a different serotype may be followed by an outbreak of DHF. Infections that occurred a decade or more earlier may remain immunologically relevant and predisposed to severe illness. It is also becoming clear that dengue viruses vary in virulence, and introduction of a more virulent strain may be followed by particularly severe outbreaks.

Abundance

The presence (or absence) and abundance of many organisms is linked to the physicochemical environment, directly – for example, through temperature, rainfall, humidity, soil or water characteristics, pH, nutrients, and so on – or indirectly, for example, through the presence or abundance of arthropod vectors (e.g., mosquitoes), intermediate and reservoir hosts (such as rodents), and vegetation. Coccidioidomycosis, caused by a soil-associated fungus, is found in arid and semiarid areas with alkaline soils in regions with hot summers and short, moist winters. Humans become infected by inhaling airborne arthroconidia. Growth of the fungi in soil is linked to temperature and rainfall. Outbreaks in the southwest United States have been correlated with the amount of rainfall over preceding months. The sequence of heavier than usual rainfall followed by prolonged drought in association with hot and dusty conditions favors dispersal of the fungus in a form that can be inhaled. But several other factors have also contributed to increasing cases of coccidioidomycosis in the U.S. southwest (Kirkland and Fierer, 1996). This area is one of the most rapidly growing parts of the United States; many new residents have moved from nonendemic areas, and thus lack immunity to the fungus. The area has become a popular place for retirement (**Figure 2**); persons more than 65 years of age have the highest incidence of infection of any age group. The HIV-infected population, another vulnerable group, has also grown in size. Land development, including construction, increases dust and potential exposures. Off-road vehicle use, which has become more common, also creates dust that can disperse the fungus. So although coccidioidomycosis is a 'place' disease that is influenced by geoclimatic conditions, the demographic shifts, human activities, and land development in the area have been important forces in the increase in cases. This disease would not have re-emerged if humans had not entered into and altered this environment.

An infection with a rodent reservoir host, such as hantavirus infection, can increase in response to geoclimatic

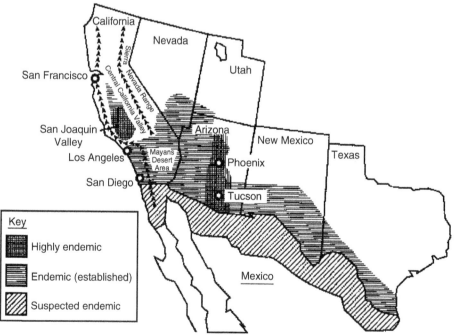

Figure 2   Distribution of coccidioidomycosis. Reproduced from Kirkland TN and Fierer J (1996) Coccidioidomycosis: A Reemerging infectious disease. *Emerging Infectious Diseases* 2(3): 192–199.

conditions (Hjelle *et al.*, 2000). The El Nino–Southern Oscillation (ENSO) has been associated with increased precipitation in the southwestern part of the United States. In this instance, the increased rainfall is associated with an expansion of the deer mouse population, presumably because of an expanded food supply for the mice, which are infected with the virus and excrete it in saliva, urine, and feces, typically without showing symptoms. Rodent populations can increase more than 10-fold in a year. More rodents mean more virus and more potential opportunities for human–rodent excreta contact and human infections.

Changes in the Human Host

Improved sanitation and increase in clinically apparent hepatitis

As noted above, presence of antibodies because of past infection with one dengue serotype can predispose to more severe infection if exposure to a different serotype occurs. However, many infections are followed by long-lasting, sometimes lifelong, immunity. When infection with hepatitis A occurs in young children, infection is often mild or asymptomatic and often not diagnosed. With increasing age, severity of infection increases, and the case-fatality rate may be 2% or higher in persons 65 years and older. Paradoxically, as availability of clean water and good sanitary facilities have improved in many countries, outbreaks of hepatitis A are now occurring, whereas they were unknown in the past when virtually everyone was infected and immune by age 5 years. By shifting upward the age at which individuals are infected, the virus causes acute, often severe clinical illness. Some countries that did not previously have visible hepatitis A outbreaks are now seeing large outbreaks in young adults.

Outbreaks of vaccine-preventable infections

Infections that have been prevented by immunization programs can re-emerge if immunization programs and other supports fail. After having been largely controlled for several decades, diphtheria re-emerged in the Russian Federation in 1990 and spread to all of the newly independent states and Baltic states of the former USSR (Dittmann *et al.*, 2000) (**Figure 3**). Between 1990 and 1998, more than 157 000 cases and 5000 deaths were reported by countries of the former Soviet Union. Diphtheria, an acute bacterial infection caused by the toxin-producing bacterium *Corynebacterium diphtheriae*, which spreads from person to person through close contact, has a case fatality rate of 5–10%. Infection can be prevented by immunization with diphtheria toxoid; when infection occurs, mortality can be reduced by treating with diphtheria antitoxin. Universal childhood immunization was introduced in the 1940s and 1950s; developing countries also achieved high levels of immunization after the Expanded Program on Immunization (EPI) in the 1970s. Even before 1990, serologic studies had shown a substantial percentage of adults lacked immunity to diphtheria. Adults in the former Soviet Union who were in the 40–49-year-old age group in the 1990s had the lowest levels of immunity. They had lived during a time when diphtheria was largely controlled by immunization, so had not been exposed to natural infection. Most had never received any doses of vaccine since childhood, as adult booster doses were not recommended at that time. Toxigenic strains of diphtheria from Afghanistan were introduced into a refugee population. Infection spread first to large urban centers and then along major transportation routes to other cities and towns, and finally to rural areas. The spread was facilitated by the presence of large numbers of displaced persons. The proportion of cases in persons more than 15 years old was 64–82% in some areas. Relatively few cases occurred in

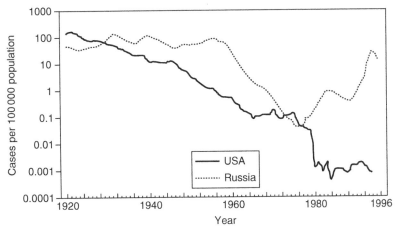

Figure 3 Diphtheria incidence – United States and Russian Federation, 1920–1996. Reproduced from Vitek CR and Wharton R (1998) Diphtheria in the former Soviet Union: Reemergence of a pandemic disease. *Emerging Infectious Diseases* 4(4): 541.

adults aged 50 years or more, presumably because of past exposure to diphtheria, which was still occurring when they were children. The highest incidence and death rates were in individuals between the ages of 40 and 49 years. At the outset of the epidemic, the case fatality rate exceeded 20%, probably due to delayed treatment and lack of diphtheria antitoxin.

Multiple factors contributed to the massive outbreak as analyzed by Dittmann and colleagues (2000). Among those identified were: less intensive immunization, use of lower potency vaccine, antivaccine campaigns in some areas, deterioration of the health-care infrastructure, delay in outbreak control, and lack of adequate supplies for prevention and treatment in many areas. Other countries were also affected by the outbreak as cases were imported into several European countries and the United States. Most countries today do not routinely give diphtheria toxoid to adults; in many countries 30–60% of adults may be susceptible to diphtheria, which is a phenomenon created by the vaccine era and vaccine policy of giving vaccine primarily to young children.

Increased risk of infection because of altered immune response

Tuberculosis

The appearance of and spread of infection with HIV has had a profound effect on the burden from many other infectious diseases, most notably TB. The interaction between HIV/AIDS and TB is bidirectional, with each making the other worse. Infection with *M. tuberculosis* upregulates HIV replication, increases viral load, accelerates the decline of CD4 count, leads to more rapid progression of HIV, and increases the risk of death. The impact of HIV on TB is to increase the risk of primary infection, increase risk of rapid progression, increase likelihood of reactivation in those with latent infection, and increase the risk of reinfection. About one-third of humans are infected with *M. tuberculosis*, though infection is latent and asymptomatic in the majority. In most individuals the likelihood that TB infection will progress to active disease is only 5–10% over a lifetime. In persons co-infected with HIV and TB the risk of developing active TB may be as high as 10% per year. In areas where the incidence of TB was already high, the spread of HIV infection has led to an increase in incident cases of TB. Although the spread of HIV infection is not the only reason for re-emergence of TB in many areas, it is an important one – and one that has made control of TB much more difficult.

Data collected during the first half of the twentieth century on TB mortality showed notable increases in TB deaths during World War I and World War II, including in some countries that were not occupied (see **Figure 4**). This was an era before specific antituberculosis drugs

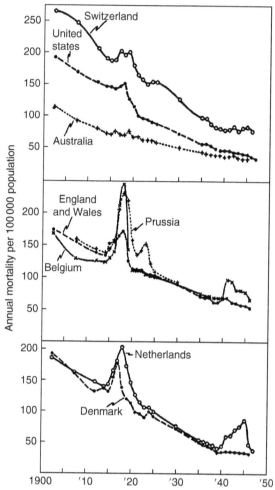

Figure 4 Tuberculosis mortality, 1900–1950. Reproduced with permission from Dubos R and Dubos J (1987) *The white plague: Tuberculosis, man, and society*. Piscataway, NJ: Rutgers University Press.

were available. Increases in mortality were thought to relate to poor nutrition (especially limited protein supply), crowding in dark dwellings, and stress. Of note, Denmark was not occupied and did not take part in the armed conflict, yet TB mortality rose starting in 1915 (**Figure 4**). The rise in TB coincided with a drop in meat consumption, as meat was exported to England to support the war. Submarine attacks interrupted exportation from Denmark in 1917, making meat available for local consumption – and TB mortality fell (**Figure 4**).

Even today with good drugs available for the treatment of TB, social, political, and economic factors can influence treatment and outcome. TB has been a problem in disadvantaged populations, including inmates in prisons and homeless populations. Gustafson and colleagues (2001) described events in Guinea-Bissau, West Africa, where armed conflict, starting in 1998, limited access to TB treatment. This was followed by an increase in the mortality rate ratio (MR) (3.21) among those being treated for TB and was most pronounced among those who were HIV infected (MR 8.19).

Contacts between Host and Microbe

Many factors can lead to an increase in contact between host and microbe. The outbreaks of infectious diseases, such as shigellosis, cholera, and measles in refugee camps and in other displaced populations, indicate how rapidly infections can spread when basic supports, such as clean water, adequate sanitary facilities, and immunization, are unavailable (Goma Epidemiology Group, 1995).

Hepatitis C

Although a serologic test to identify persons infected with hepatitis C virus (HCV) was not developed until 1989, the infection had been described based on its clinical and epidemiologic features, and by the absence of antibodies to other common infections, including hepatitis A and hepatitis B. Before the wide use of tests to screen donated blood, hepatitis C was the most common blood-borne infection following blood transfusions. Although hepatitis C is found worldwide, prevalence varies widely. Seroprevalence in Egypt has been reported to be in the range of 20% in blood donors, one of the highest prevalence rates anywhere in the world. Prevalence varies by age and geographic region, but is higher in Egypt than in neighboring countries. The HCV subtypes in Egypt are mostly the same, suggesting epidemic spread throughout the country. Children have a low prevalence of infection and people living in desert areas have the lowest prevalence. Investigators have tried to find plausible explanations for these observations.

Schistosomiasis, a parasitic infection that requires snails as an intermediate host, is widespread in the Nile Delta and Nile Valley. After it was discovered in 1918 that injections with an antimony salt could kill schistosomal flukes residing in humans, use of parenteral antischistosomal therapy (PAT) became widespread. Because the drug could be administered only by injection and multiple injections (12–16) were required, mass treatment campaigns were organized to deliver the drug. Sterilization procedures of reusable injection equipment were likely to have been omitted in some instances or were inadequate. When effective oral therapies for schistosomiasis became available in the 1970s and 1980s, they replaced PAT. Investigators who have analyzed the prevalence of HCV antibodies by age and geographic region have found a significant association between exposure index for PAT and HCV prevalence rates. This suggests that the mass campaigns to treat schistosomiasis may have effectively spread HCV to a significant portion of the Egyptian population (Frank et al., 2000). Although initial infection with hepatitis C may be mild or asymptomatic, infection becomes persistent in 50–80% of those infected. The burden of disease related to infection, progression to cirrhosis or development of hepatocellular carcinoma, comes years or decades after infection was acquired. Unsafe injection equipment can be a source of infection in any country, but the prevalence of infection is less than 2–3% in most countries.

Although safer, more effective treatment for schistosomiasis is now available, schistosomiasis has increased in some communities in Egypt, Senegal, Cote d'Ivoire, and elsewhere following the building of dams (N'Goran et al., 1997). Dams can have potential economic and health benefits, but have also been associated with increases in vectorborne infections (see the following section).

Malaria

Malaria continues to kill a million or more, mostly young children in Africa, each year, and saps the strength and productivity of individuals in endemic areas by causing fatigue, episodic fevers, and anemia. Although in the overall area of the globe where malaria is endemic the disease has decreased by half in the last century, demographic changes have resulted in an increase of 2 billion people living in areas with malaria risk (Hay et al., 2004). The intensity of transmission has also increased in some regions. Some reasons for increase in malaria include insecticide resistance of the mosquito vector and breakdown in control programs, increase in resistance of the malaria parasite to the inexpensive, older antimalarial drugs (e.g., chloroquine), and population movements (both movement of nonimmune populations into malarious areas and also migration of malaria-infected persons into regions infested with competent malaria vectors and climatic conditions compatible with malaria transmission). Co-infection with malaria and HIV also appears to have adverse consequences, though not of the magnitude noted with HIV and TB. HIV infection is associated with an increased risk of parasitemia and clinical malaria in adults and increased risk of treatment failure. HIV-infected pregnant women have more frequent and higher-density malaria parasitemia than do uninfected women; infants born to women infected with both malaria and HIV have a three- to eightfold higher risk of postnatal death than infants born to mothers with either infection alone. Malaria in HIV-infected persons also leads to increased viral load, which returns to baseline with prompt treatment of malaria.

Because malaria is transmitted by a mosquito vector – environmental factors, including temperature, humidity, rainfall, and land use – can also influence abundance and location of mosquito vectors. A study in northwestern Ethiopia linked an increase in malaria transmission to intensified maize cultivation. Maize pollen, eaten by mosquito larvae, can influence the insect's size and development. In many villages, maize was planted in fields less than 2 meters from houses. The predominant variety planted, chosen for its high yield, matured late, with pollen dispersal extending into the peak period of mosquito larval development (Kebede *et al.*, 2005).

In the Peruvian Amazon in South America malaria prevalence increased sharply in the 1990s at a time of population migration and growth as well as extensive deforestation. Researchers gathered data from 56 different study sites that varied by type of vegetation and human population density. They captured mosquitoes that landed on human volunteers in the evening hours to assess whether deforestation was associated with increased biting rate of *Anopheles darlingi*, the primary vector of falciparum malaria in that region. They found that human-biting rates were consistently higher in deforested areas, with the *A. darlingi* biting rate more than 278 times higher in deforested areas than in areas that were predominantly forested (Vittor *et al.*, 2006).

Dams built to provide irrigation for crops can also provide water for breeding of mosquito vectors. In a longitudinal study of communities living near dams and control communities at similar altitude but beyond the flight range of mosquitoes that might breed in standing water created by dams, researchers found that malaria was significantly more common in communities near the dams (14.0 episodes in 1000 child months vs. 1.9 in control villages) (Ghebreyesus *et al.*, 1999).

Introduction of a mosquito species that is a more efficient vector for malaria transmission can also lead to an increase in transmission. An example of this occurred when *Anopheles gambiae* was introduced into Brazil, probably by way of boats that made mail runs between Dakar, Senegal and Natal, Brazil. *A. gambiae* larvae were first identified in March 1930 and subsequently spread along the coastal region and 200 miles inland into the Jaguaribe River valley. Although malaria was endemic in this area, the local mosquitoes were not efficient vectors, so the human burden from malaria was low. The establishment of the highly efficient vector, *A. gambiae*, was followed in the late 1930s by explosive malaria outbreaks with more than 100 000 cases and about 20 000 deaths in this population with low levels of immunity. A massive campaign to eradicate *A. gambiae* was successful, but the event illustrated the key role of the type of vector present in malaria transmission.

Movement through trade

Movement of microbes through travel and trade continues to lead to outbreaks in unexpected places and populations. In many instances, transmission cannot be sustained and the infection dies out. Infections that are transmitted from person to person can potentially be carried to any country, as has been observed with HIV. Influenza, though never absent, re-emerges every year in temperate climates during the colder months to cause epidemics. The severity of the epidemics depends on the extent of change in the virus (genetic drift or shift), and to some extent on use of vaccine in the population, and closeness of match between the vaccine virus and circulating virus. Traveling, infected humans introduce the virus into new geographic areas, where it can spread rapidly because it is highly transmissible. The H5N1 avian influenza that has caused massive die-offs in poultry and other birds, since it was first identified in 1997 in Hong Kong, can also be carried by migratory birds to new countries and continents (Rappole *et al.*, 2000). Legal and illegal movement of poultry and trade involving pet birds and fighting cocks are other routes of spread.

Dengue and mosquito vectors

Humans are the main reservoir for dengue virus (primates are not significant in its epidemiology in most areas). They spread it into new geographic areas by traveling while infected (virus in bloodstream) and being bitten by mosquitoes competent to permit the replication of the dengue virus to levels in which it can be transmitted via mosquito saliva when it bites a nonimmune host many days later (typically a week or two for the extrinsic incubation period). Dengue has increased in geographic reach and severity and is now present in most tropical and subtropical areas of the world. Several factors are contributing to its re-emergence, with the increased travel of humans being an essential but insufficient reason. Much of global travel is by plane, allowing travelers to reach anywhere in the world within the incubation period of dengue fever, typically 4–7 days (full range is 3–14 days). The most important dengue vector is *Aedes aegypti*, and it now infests most tropical and subtropical areas. It thrives in urban areas and is able to breed in discarded plastic cups, flowerpots, and used tires and enters homes and prefers a human host. The greatest volume of population growth today is occurring in urban areas in low latitude regions, and in areas infested with a competent vector and linked to the global community via travel and trade. More and more urban areas in tropical regions have reached the population size (estimated to be 150 000 to 1 million) needed to sustain the ongoing circulation of dengue virus.

Of note, presence of a competent vector and a climate that is warm enough to permit the virus to become infective in mosquitoes is not sufficient to lead to outbreaks of dengue fever. The mosquito vector must have access to the human population. Presence of screens and air conditioning can limit transmission as a study by Reiter and colleagues (2003) showed, which looked at two urban areas (Laredo, Texas and Nuevo Laredo in Mexico) with similar climate and separated only by the Rio Grande River. *A. aegypti* was present in both areas. In a serosurvey, residents in Mexico were significantly more likely to have antibodies indicating recent or remote dengue infection than were residents across the border in Texas. Absence of air conditioning was significantly associated with dengue antibodies. Poor housing is also associated with increased exposure to mosquitoes, and the absence of piped water can also increase risk of exposure to mosquitoes because water storage vessels kept in the household can serve as good breeding sites for mosquitoes.

Mosquitoes are also moved around the world on ships, airplanes, and other vehicles. In some instances, the species can become established in a new geographic area. *Aedes albopictus*, the Asian tiger mosquito, was introduced into the United States in 1985 in used tires imported from Asia and within 12 years had spread to at least 25 states. It has also recently been introduced into many areas in Latin America. It was the primary vector responsible for the outbreak of dengue fever that occurred in Hawaii in 2001–02 and is also competent to transmit West Nile and other viruses that can cause severe disease in humans.

Monkeypox

Monkeypox, a viral infection that resembles smallpox, was first recognized in captive primates in 1958 and first identified in humans in 1970 in the Democratic Republic of the Congo. Infections that occurred earlier were probably diagnosed as smallpox because of similar clinical findings. Only after smallpox had been eradicated from this area and surveillance for smallpox-like infections was instituted was this virus identified. Unlike smallpox, whose only host is the human, monkeypox is a zoonosis, though human-to-human spread can occur. It is not as easily transmitted as smallpox among humans, and transmission is usually not sustained beyond 2–3 generations. Although primates, including monkeys, can be infected, other animals, perhaps squirrels and other rodents, are thought to be the reservoir hosts for this virus. The virus is found in tropical rain forest areas of west and central Africa. Because vaccination with vaccinia virus gives partial protection against monkeypox, some investigators have speculated that monkeypox might increase after the eradication of smallpox and cessation of the vaccination.

No one expected monkeypox to appear in North America in 2003, though in retrospect public health officials should not have been surprised. Exotic animals, such as the Gambian giant rat, imported from Ghana had been housed by distributors with prairie dogs sold as pets in the United States. At least 37 human monkeypox infections were documented in pet dealers and owners and veterinarians. Humans became sick after contact with sick prairie dogs. No humans died; in African outbreaks mortality has ranged from 4–22%, perhaps because of greater virulence of the virus subtype. There have been no additional cases since 2003 or any evidence that the virus has become established in prairie dogs or other animal populations in the United States.

Characteristics of Infections Likely to Re-emerge

Infections caused by microbes that have an animal reservoir (especially wild animal) or are found in the environment (soil, water, vegetation) are difficult to contain and to keep under containment with currently available tools. Even if an effective vaccine is available, as there are for the flaviviral infections, Japanese encephalitis and yellow fever, elimination of the agent is not feasible in most instances. Unless high levels of immunization are maintained or the vector (or contact with the vector) can be eliminated, risk of resurgence will remain. Even with vaccine-preventable diseases that do not have an animal or environmental reservoir, sustained, global control has been difficult to attain. Measles, for which a highly effective vaccine exists, still causes outbreaks, though endemic circulation has been eliminated in large areas of the world. As long as the infection persists anywhere and people travel, risk of reintroduction will persist.

The logical conclusion is that infections will continue to re-emerge in the foreseeable future because elimination almost never occurs and currently available tools (such as vaccines, vector control, education and change in behavior, screening blood and tissues, antimicrobial drugs, surveillance) are imperfect or incompletely or inconsistently applied. While efforts to control disease are taking place, microbes continue to evolve in ways to favor their continued existence in today's world. The combination of population size, density, mobility, vulnerability (e.g., AIDS, aging, immunosuppressed populations), and location (increasingly in low latitude urban areas often without good infrastructure) provides the milieu in which continued episodes of re-emergence are likely.

See also: Emerging Diseases; Epidemiology of HIV/AIDS and its Surveillance; Factors Influencing the Emergence of Diseases.

Citations

Corso A, Severina EP, Petruk VF, Mauritz YR, and Tomaz A (1998) Molecular characterization of penicillin-resistant Streptococcus pneumoniae isolates causing respiratory disease in the Untied States. *Microbiology and Drug Resistance* 4: 325–337.

Dittmann S, Wharton M, Vitek C, *et al.* (2000) Successful control of epidemic diphtheria in the states of the former Union of Soviet Socialist Republics: Lessons learned. *Journal of Infectious Diseases* 181(supplement 1): S10–S22.

Dull PM, Abdelwahab J, and Sacchi CT (2005) *Neisseria meningitidis* serogroup W-135 carriage among U.S. travelers to the 2001 Hajj. *Journal of Infectious Diseases* 191: 33–39.

Frank C, Mohamed MK, Strickland GT, *et al.* (2000) The role of parenteral antischistosomal therapy in the spread of hepatitis C in Egypt. *The Lancet* 355: 887–891.

Furuya EY and Lowy FD (2006) Antimicrobial-resistant bacteria in the community setting. *Nature Reviews Microbiology* 4: 36–45.

Ghebreyesus TA, Hile M, Witten KH, *et al.* (1999) Incidence of malaria among children living near dams in northern Ethiopia: Community based incidence survey. *British Medical Journal* 319: 663–666.

Goma Epidemiology Group (1995) Public health impact of Rwandan refugee crisis: What happened in Goma, Zaire, in July, 1994? *The Lancet* 354: 339–344.

Gustafson P, Gomes V, Vieira CS, *et al.* (2001) Tuberculosis mortality during a civil war in Guinea-Bissau. *Journal of the American Medical Association* 286(5): 599–603.

Hay SI, Guerra CA, Tatem AJ, Noor AM, and Snow RW (2004) The global distribution and population at risk of malaria: Past, present, and future. *Lancet Infectious Diseases* 4: 327–336.

Hjelle B and Glass GE (2000) Outbreak of hantavirus infection in the Four Corners region of the United States in the wake of the 1997–1998 El Nino-southern oscillation. *Journal of Infectious Diseases* 181: 1569–1573.

Kebede A, McCann JC, Kiszewski AT, and Ye-Ebiyo Y (2005) New evidence of the effects of agro-ecologic change on malaria transmission. *American Journal of Tropical Medicine and Hygiene* 73(4): 676–680.

Kew O, Morris-Glasgow V, Landaverde M, *et al.* (2002) Outbreak of poliomyelitis in Hispaniola associated with circulating type 1 vaccine-derived poliovirus. *Science* 296: 356–359.

Kirkland TN and Fierer J (1996) Coccidioidomycosis: A reemerging infectious disease. *Emerging Infectious Diseases* 3(2): 192–199.

MacLennan C, Dunn G, Huissoon AP, *et al.* (2004) Failure to clear persistent vaccine-derived neurovirulent poliovirus infection in an immunodeficient man. *The Lancet* 363: 1509–1513.

McDonald LC, Killgore GE, Thompson A, *et al.* (2005) An epidemic, toxin gene-variant strain of Clostridium difficile. *New England Journal of Medicine* 353(23): 2433–2441.

N'Goran EK, Diabate S, Utzinger J, and Sellin B (1997) Changes in human schistosomiasis levels after the construction of two large hydroelectric dams in Central Cote d'Ivoire. *Bulletin of the World Health Organization* 75(6): 541–545.

Rappole JH, Derrickson SR, and Hubalek Z (2000) Migratory birds and spread of West Nile virus in the Western Hemisphere. *Emerging Infectious Disease* 6(4): 319–328.

Reiter P, Lathrop S, Bunning M, *et al.* (2003) Texas lifestyle limits transmission of dengue virus. *Emerging Infectious Diseases* 9(1): 86–89.

Vittor AY, Gilman RH, Tielsch J, *et al.* (2006) The effect of deforestation on the human-biting rate of Anopheles darlingi, the primary vector of falciparum malaria in the Peruvian Amazon. *American Journal of Tropical Medicine and Hygiene* 74(1): 3–11.

Drucker E, Alcabes PG, and Maarx PA (2001) The injection century: Massive unsterile injections and the emergence of human pathogens. *The Lancet* 358: 1989–1992.

Gubler DJ (2002) Epidemic dengue/dengue hemorrhagic fever as a public health, social and economic problem in the 21st century. *Trends in Microbiology* 10(2): 100–102.

Guernier V, Hockberg ME, and Guegan J-F (2004) Ecology drives the worldwide distribution of human diseases. *Public Library of Science Biology* 2(6): 740–746.

Levy SB and Marshall B (2004) Antibacterial resistance worldwide: Causes, challenges and responses. *Nature Medicine Supplement* 10(12): S122–S129.

Martens P and Hall L (2000) Malaria on the move: Human population movement and malaria transmission. *Emerging Infectious Diseases* 6(2): 103–109.

Smolinski MS, Hamburg MA and Lederberg J (eds.) (2003) *Microbial Threats to Health: Emergence, Detection, and Response. Institute of Medicine of the National Academies.* Washington, DC: The National Academies Press.

Sutherst RW (2004) Global change and human vulnerability to vector-borne diseases. *Clinical Microbiology Review* 17(1): 136–173.

Taubenberger JK, Reid AH, Lourens RM, *et al.* (2005) Characterization of the 1918 influenza virus polymerase genes. *Nature* 437: 889–893.

Webby R, Hoffmann E, and Webster R (2004) Molecular constraints to interspecies transmission of viral pathogens. *Nature Medicine Supplement* 10(12): S77–S81.

Wilson ME (1995) Travel and the emergence of infectious diseases. *Emerging Infectious Diseases* 1: 39–46.

Wilson ME (1995) Infectious diseases: An ecological perspective. *British Medical Journal* 311: 1681–1684.

Wilson ME (2003) The traveller and emerging infections: Sentinel, courier, transmitter. *Journal of Applied Microbiology* 94: S1–S11.

Relevant Websites

http://www.cdc.gov/ncidod/EID/index.htm – CDC, Emerging Infectious Diseases.

http://www.cdc.gov – Centers for Disease Control and Prevention (CDC).

http://www.nas.edu – The National Academies.

http://www.nap.edu – The National Academies Press.

http://www.promedmail.org – ProMED mail for the International Society for Infectious Diseases.

http://www.who.int/wer/en – World Health Organization (WHO).

Further Reading

Connolly MA, Gayer M, Ryan MJ, *et al.* (2004) Communicable diseases in complex emergencies: Impact and challenges. *The Lancet* 364: 1974–1983.

Factors Influencing the Emergence of Diseases

A M Kimball, University of Washington, Seattle, WA, USA

Background

In 1991, the U.S. Institute of Medicine published the report of a multidisciplinary working group to (1) identify significant emerging diseases, (2) determine strategies to deal with them, and (3) recommend actions to confront future threats and to lessen their impact on public health (Lederberg *et al.*, 1992). The group embraced a global rather than U.S.-specific frame of reference and elected to avoid a disease-specific description for an approach based on factors of emergence. Factors of emergence are defined as "...specific forces that shape infectious disease emergence [which] operate on different elements in the process of emergence," (p. 47, *ibid*). The original six factors examined were: human demographics and behavior, technology and industry, economic development and land use, international travel and commerce, microbial adaptation and change, and the breakdown of public health measures. The report provided examples of how these factors work and on which emergent infections they apparently operated.

A follow-up report, *Microbial Threats to Health: Emergence Detection and Response* was published in 2003 (Smolinski *et al.*, 2003). Additional factors of emergence were examined in this report: human susceptibility to infection, climate and weather, changing ecosystems, poverty and social inequity, war and famine, the lack of political will, and intent to harm. Thus the original six factors grew to 13. While enriching the discussion and description of emergence, this proliferation of factors also created overlapping domains within factors; for example, climate and weather are an integral physical science aspect of ecosystems, the failure of political will is integral to the neglect of public health systems, and so forth. From an analytic point of view, the need for in-depth study of factors and how they actually work has become critical for scientific insight into public health protection.

Interplay of Man-Made Factors

This description of factors of emergence will focus on their interplay and how they work where they are most understood: (1) human pressures on the ecosystem and changes in land use, (2) globalization of markets for food animals concurrent with the growth of global trade and commerce, and (3) antimicrobial resistance that leads to microbial change and adaptation. Every factor linked to emergence is essentially created or caused by humans. Some factors are more feasible to correct than others. One is the increasing burden on the Earth's limited resources. Another is the new ecosystem of sorts that we have created through burgeoning trade and travel – a world of high mobility and porous boundaries. Also, food production practices intensify as global commerce accelerates. Finally, we have a growing array of medical practices with unknown consequences, such as xenotransplantation and widespread antibiotic use (see **Figure 1**).

Exhausting Our Ecospace?

Typically, diseases emerge when a pathogen moves from another vertebrate species to humans. The mechanisms of crossover are largely unknown, but some factors seem to

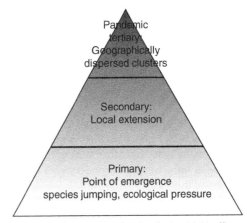

Figure 1   The prevention pyramid.

facilitate the process: poor sanitation, encroachment of humans on animal habitats, maintaining food animals in crowded conditions, and extensive use of antimicrobials. The rapid acceleration of poultry agriculture in Southeast Asia has converted avian influenza into a growing number of human cases – 371 at current count. An offshoot, cockfighting, includes behaviors that contribute to further infection, such as humans sucking blood and mucus from the beaks of injured birds. Early in the HIV epidemic, a transmission between monkeys or apes and humans was thought to have occurred. Whether this was through exposure between hunters and their primate prey in the rainforests or through bush meat consumption or another route remains a mystery.

Most new pathogens that have emerged over the last 20 years have done so in response to ecological pressure rather than natural evolutionary change in the microbes. Ecological changes, such as new agricultural practices, urbanization, globalization, and climate change, seem to drive microbes from animals into their new human hosts (Slingenbergh *et al.*, 2004). Again, the drivers are largely the product of human activity. Despite this certainty, little definitive work has been done to determine the threshold of each factor in the emergence of new human pathogens. For example, while most international authorities agree that the intensified poultry industry is related to the emergence of fatal avian influenza outbreaks in Europe and Asia little is known about how, why, or at what point this RNA virus jumps from birds to humans.

Influenza: A Recurring Emergence

At the microbial level, recent studies of the highly fatal 1918 influenza virus suggest that the neuraminidase portion of the virus was responsible for its contagiousness in humans. Scientists believe that the 1957 pandemic influenza emerged after the virus moved from ducks to pigs or chickens that were infected at the same time by a human virus. After the viruses exchanged bits of genetic material during their reproduction in the pigs and chickens, the new virus was equipped to infect humans. However, because of the state of science in 1957, this information has always been tentative. In fact, it is now believed that the 1918 influenza virus was avian in origin, and did not go through the mixing bowl of a pig or another land-based animal before infecting humans. Intensive study of the virus causing Asian avian influenza is now underway. The virus has already hopped the species barrier in 371 recorded human cases, causing 235 human deaths.

At the macro level, we do not know the threshold number at which a safe density of poultry becomes unsafe. How many birds per square meter can be handled safely? How many are too many? What role do ducks migrating from farm to farm play in disease transmission? The U.S. Department of Agriculture (USDA) stipulates that no more than ten chickens can be housed per square meter. Contemporary practice in the United States is for ten chickens to inhabit a 3-square-foot space for their entire lives, often with their beaks and talons removed to prevent injury. Practices using dense poultry habitat are correlated with the susceptibility of birds to highly pathogenic avian influenza. That susceptibility, thought to be related to stress and crowding, has been demonstrated all over the world (Slingenbergh *et al.*, 2004) (**Figure 2**).

It appears that Asia has seen relatively little increased productivity in chickens despite a rapidly increasing density of the agricultural population on both small farms and large industrial-scale enterprises. This mixture of large and small enterprises in close proximity has served as a potent combination for the outbreak of avian influenza. The small farms probably served as the first points of illness, but the large commercial farms played a critical role in extending the outbreaks through high-volume traffic of vulnerable fowl populations and products over large geographic areas.

A New Environment, New Rules?

Extensive scientific work has been done suggesting that the human community is outstripping the planet's ability to accommodate it. While not yet as crowded as chickens on factory farms, with 6.2 billion human inhabitants, the Earth's balance within natural systems is increasingly affected by anthropogenic (man-made) activity. In his landmark 1993 book *Planetary Overload: Global Environmental Change and the Health of the Human Species,* Anthony J. McMichael outlines the human-generated stress on natural systems. He posits that food will become increasingly scarce for the human community. The macro-ecologic effects of human activity on climate, water, food, agriculture, pollution, and human health are well described, but the systematic link between the macro (what we can see) and what is occurring on the micro level remains an important area of research. To address the emergence of new pathogens, we need more precise knowledge about the mechanisms that form the critical pathway to emergence.

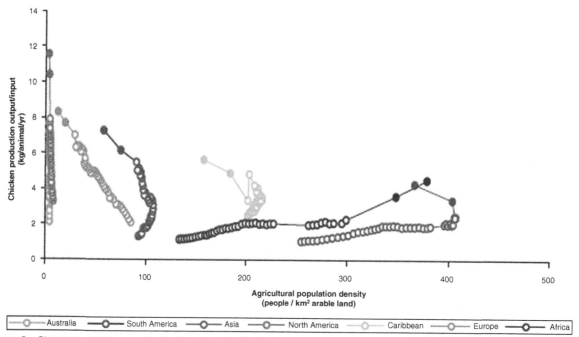

Figure 2   Change in chicken meat output/input and agricultural population density grouped by continent between 1961 and 2001 (empty circles) and predictions for 2015 to 2030 (full circles). Reproduction from Slingenberg JL, Gilbert M, *et al.* (2004) Ecological sources of zoonotic diseases. *Scientific and Technical Review* 23: 467–484, with permission of OIE Publications Service.

While there is a finite amount of space on the surface of Earth, we have, in some sense, created a new dimension of space – the mobile environment. In considering environment, increasing emphasis has been placed on the built environment for humans. For example, the roads and pavement have hardened the land and created challenges for disposing of water and human pollutants. Buildings are studied for their effects on human health, from second-hand smoke to sick-building syndrome.

New man-made spaces also have been created in the pursuit of trade and travel. How they act on the life processes of microbes and affect infection is yet to be described. But we are beginning to see some telltale signs. Human travel, for instance, seems to have the potential to affect seasonal disease patterns. Many biological aspects of life appear to be seasonal – births, deaths, numerous chronic diseases, and, of course, infectious diseases all peak during certain times of the year. At least this is the case in temperate climates, where the phenomena have been the most extensively studied. Seasonal effect is a well-described aspect of infectious disease, including respiratory infections, such as colds and flu, and more serious infections, such as pneumonia. Interestingly, this seasonality has remained a constant even as humans have modified their natural environment in remarkable ways – building shelters, designing heating and cooling systems, and inventing new protective clothing, for example. This well-described but poorly understood phenomenon has enabled us to plan vaccine development and prevention efforts at certain times of the year in anticipation of upcoming outbreaks. When people travel between hemispheres, where the seasons are reversed, they can introduce viruses off-season, potentially throwing off this historically reliable rhythm of vaccines and prevention.

Another illustration of the influence of human mobility on the microbial world is the transportation, via food products, of a pathogen from one region, where it may be endemic, to another, where it is not. In processing, shipping, packaging, and preparing food, we bring into our homes and our digestive systems food and microbes from thousands of miles away. We experience some of this microbial traffic as illness, when microbes pathogenic to humans infect us. Microbes that we know because they make us ill are an exceedingly small percentage of the microbes moving around. Our new man-made ecological space of mobile microbes impacts the rapidly evolving microbial world, but what that impact is remains a mystery.

Evolution of Microbes

We must not limit the potential ecological adaptability of microbes or lose sight of their abundance because currently the number of known human pathogens is limited.

Recognizing that most commensal microorganisms, provided that they are in the right environment, can become human and animal pathogens of concern helps us approach the issue holistically. Microbes, beneficial or detrimental, are an integral part of the ecosystem. Land-use changes might increase, decrease, or completely replace existing microbes with others. The strong need to use multidisciplinary approaches when examining land-use change becomes apparent when considering that more than half the recognized human pathogens are zoonotic.

In the last two decades, we have witnessed an increased emergence and resurgence of human diseases in many parts of the world. Some of the infectious diseases include HIV/AIDS, tuberculosis, malaria, *E. coli* O157:H7, H5N1, Ebola hemorrhagic fever, cholera O139, West Nile, Lyme borreliosis, cryptosporidiosis, and Ross fever. Changes in land use as a result of deforestation, reforestation, irrigation systems, urbanization, and crowding have been identified as the major players in the emergence of diseases. These land-use changes allow humans to encroach and settle in a new environmental niche with known and novel pathogens. **Table 1** illustrates the diversity of infectious agents suspected or linked to known changes in landscape. The majority of these infectious diseases are either vector-borne or zoonotic. The spread of pathogens is aggravated by factors that support the introduction and eventual transmission of these and many other infectious agents, including lack of access to health care, population growth, changes in human behaviors, microbial adaptation, urbanization and crowding, and travel.

Changes in Land Use

The increased demand for more food, lumber products, and living space are some of the main factors that have dramatically increased the way we change land to fit our daily needs. The question of what land-use changes, if any, have been responsible for the emergence of diseases is summarized in this article. At the same time, looking solely at ecological changes, whether human-induced or not, and the emergence of human diseases would oversimplify the complex relationships between ecological changes, microorganisms, and human and animal diseases.

Humans have made significant changes to the Earth's landscape. Human history is a record of forests cleared for agriculture, streams redirected for irrigation, cities built, urban dwellings created, roads, dams, and bridges constructed, and other ecological changes. As the population increases, the speed of ecological changes dramatically increases. Humans, sometimes unaware, and at other times fully aware, of the consequences are rapidly altering the basic foundations of the environment that sustains us. According to the World Health Organization's (WHO) Millennium Ecosystem Assessment report, humans have

Table 1   Agents and infectious diseases with suspected or known links to landscape change

Vector-borne and/or zoonotic	Soil	Water	Human	Other
Dengue	Melioidosis	Schistosomiasis	Asthma	Hemorrhagic fevers
Lyme disease	Anthrax	Cholera	Tuberculosis	
Yellow fever	Hookworm	Shigellosis	Influenza	
Rift Valley fever	Coccidioidomycosis	Rotavirus		
Japanese encephalitis		Salmonellosis		
Onchocerciasis		Leptospirosis		
Trypanosomiasis		Cryptosporidiosis		
Plague				
Filariasis				
Meningitis				
Rabies				
Leishmaniasis				
Kyasanur forest fever				
Hantavirus				
Nipah virus				

Adapted from Patz JA, Daszak P, and Tabor GM (2004) Unhealthy landscapes: Policy recommendations on land use change and infectious disease emergence. *Environmental Health Perspectives* 112: 1092–1098.

made more significant ecological changes in the last 50 years than in any other comparable time period. These landscape changes inevitably have increased our access to new ecological niches. Changes in ecology or climate not surprisingly bring about both beneficial and detrimental organisms that cause diseases in humans and animals. Of course, the type and incidence of infectious disease depends on the particular ecosystems affected, type of land-use change, disease-specific transmission dynamics, sociocultural changes, and the susceptibility of human populations.

Ecological Changes

Numerous, simultaneous, and continuous ecological changes make it difficult to characterize its complexity. Ecological changes for agriculture rank highest for impact to public health and are implicated as a major factor in the emergence of diseases. The volume of agricultural impact on public health and spread of disease can only be appreciated by understanding that agriculture occupies about half of the world's land and uses more than two-thirds of the world's fresh water. Changes in land use directly and indirectly linked to agricultural activities include deforestation/reforestation, irrigation, monocropping, construction of roads and dams, macro and micro climate change, and erosion.

Deforestation/Reforestation

The rate of deforestation worldwide is estimated at about 40 million acres per year. In other words, a land area roughly equivalent to the state of Pennsylvania is destroyed each year. Vector-borne diseases are the most sensitive to climate and weather changes, with malaria one of the most climate-sensitive. Deforestation has increased

the burden of malaria in some countries by exposing land to sunlight and creating pools of water that are known to favor the breeding of malaria-transmitting mosquitoes, anopheles gambiae. An increase in the prevalence of malarial infection in the New Guinea Highlands, an area previously malaria-free, has been linked to a rapid increase of anopheline populations after forest clearance and other local developments. Similar trends have been documented in several other countries, including Kenya, Madagascar, Uganda, and Rwanda. Of course the increase in malarial infection in the last two decades is not solely due to deforestation but rather is concomitant with increases in anti-malarial drugs, resistance to insecticides, the breakdown of public health services, and the change in demographics. It is very hard to tease out the net increase in the rate of infections as a result of deforestation.

Yellow fever, a viral disease of primates transmitted by the bite of infected mosquitoes, is also classified as an important reemerging disease, with 34 sub-Saharan countries at risk. Like malaria, the increased transmission of yellow fever as well as dengue, another viral pathogen, are influenced by similar ecological changes, including clearing land for agriculture, logging, building roads, and mining. Deforestation creates a suitable environment for mosquito breeding and increases soil erosion. Flooding can increase the transmission of diseases from runoff and from disturbing breeding grounds and habitats. Soil erosion has been linked to an increase in human infection by helminths and pathogenic microbes.

Lyme disease is another vector-borne disease that arose from reforestation and people's proximity to animal reservoirs. Lyme disease was first recognized in the United States in 1975 in the town of Old Lyme in southeastern Connecticut. It occurred in a new residential development where the deer population had provided the sustenance for the vector *Ixodes dammini*, which were infected by *Borrelia burgdorferi*. Lyme disease illustrates the interrelationship between microorganisms, biodiversity, and change in land use. It also provides us with a timely example of the complexity of the determinants of diseases and how they come to be human pathogens. Once again, as a result of ecological changes, there was a loss of biodiversity and changes in the host communities, increasing the risk of infection by vector-borne diseases.

Irrigation and dams

Some studies have linked the use of irrigation systems to the increase in breeding sites for malaria and other mosquito-borne diseases. A recently published article by Klinkenberg *et al.* (2005) quantified the incidence of malaria in Accra, Ghana where irrigation is practiced. They found a higher rate of malarial infection in communities around the urban agricultural sites than in the control group (16.6% vs. 11.4%, respectively). Similarly, building dams causes an increase in the mosquito population. For example, Rift Valley fever is a disease transmitted by mosquito that has surged in Africa as a result of the construction of dams. Dams, by preventing the flushing of snail vectors, increased the prevalence of schistosomiasis in the region. Still bodies of water are particularly well suited for breeding snail vectors. For example, construction of the Aswan Dam in Egypt resulted in a shift from predominantly *S. haematobium* to *S. mansoni*.

The Senegal river basin water and environmental management project, which was a joint project of four West African countries (Guinea, Mali, Mauritania, and Senegal), constructed the Manantali and Diama dams. Despite an improvement in water availability and electricity supply, the dams resulted in proliferation of aquatic weeds and higher incidence of schistosomiasis and malaria. These examples illustrate that ecological changes can alleviate the risk of exposure to novel pathogens by creating a suitable environmental niche for mosquito-breeding sites. As a consequence, humans have increased their risk of acquiring new or previously recognized pathogens. The problem is that our understanding of the global microbiological population is less than limited, and we are unable to see the risk to humans and animals as a result of the ecological changes.

Roads

One of the outcomes of deforestation is the construction of roads. Access roads increase the opportunity for animal–human interactions. As a result, hunters, loggers, and others who often frequent the wilderness have a higher risk of contracting a novel pathogen by being in a new environmental niche. The increase in wild meat (bushmeat) trade in parts of central Africa has been attributed to the increase in access roads.

Among the approximately 177 newly emerged human diseases, about 58% are zoonotic. This underscores the influence of human–animal interactions on the emergence of diseases and recognizes that most emerging zoonotic disease outbreaks result from ecological changes. Some known human infections, such as influenza, tuberculosis, and measles, are zoonoses originally introduced to humans from other species. Strong evidence exists indicating that the emergence of HIV-1 and HIV-2 in humans results from transmission of simian immunodeficiency virus (SIV) strains from distinct, naturally infected nonhuman primate hosts. Nipah virus, a newly recognized zoonotic disease found in Malaysia, results from bat–human interactions. Nipah virus demonstrates that infectious diseases do not have boundaries. The infection of people with Nipah virus in Malaysia was traced to disruption of bat habitat in Indonesia that forced bats to migrate to Malaysia. The spread of Nipah virus to humans was aggravated by humans' close vicinity to dense populations of farmed pigs. Other similar examples – the epidemic of Japanese encephalitis in Sri Lanka resulting from pig husbandry; rabies resulting from the spread of raccoons in New York; Lyssaviruses resulting from human–bat interaction in Thailand and Australia – are some examples of emergence and reemergence of diseases caused by human–animal interaction.

Many gaps exist in our understanding of how zoonotic agents are maintained in nature or how they respond to environmental changes exacerbated by overcrowding, living close to animals, and exposure to new microorganisms with potential to become human pathogens. Emergence of zoonoses is likely to persist as long as human–animal interactions increase, particularly interaction caused by destruction of, or encroachment into, wildlife habitat (particularly through logging and road building).

Extending Production Chains

Production of food and biological products has changed dramatically over the last 20 years. In the 1930s, our food came from local farms. Quality and supply of produce and products were often uneven. Good years followed bad years. Not any longer. Production chains extend thousands of miles and often across continents for biological products we eat, such as meat, eggs, and milk, and increasingly for biological products we use as pharmaceuticals.

Globalization and consolidation of agribusiness corporations have changed the playing field. Bovine spongiform encephalopathy demonstrates an aspect of the phenomena. The United Kingdom's beef industry had historically been a relatively stable one when fragmented among many smaller farms across the British Isles. To protect this industry, the government maintained a tariff on the imports of competing products from abroad. With the explosion of global trading in beef after World War II, coincident with refrigerated transport, and the movement toward global free trade, the United Kingdom negotiated a timetable under the General Agreement on Tariffs and Trade to scale down tariffs on beef, which heightened competition in the United Kingdom's beef industry and increased pressure for more efficient and less costly production methods.

Against this backdrop, innovation in rendering was introduced into the slaughterhouses of the United Kingdom. The rendering or processing of carcasses of cows and other animals after the edible and usable bits of flesh and meat have been cut away has been done for centuries. And for decades, United Kingdom farmers used the meat and bone meal (MBM) from rendering as a protein source for beef cattle. Historically, the rendering process was similar to pressure cooking – applying very high temperatures for very long times so eventually even the bones broke down into powder. It was an expensive, fuel- and time-consuming process. When a new cold vacuum extraction method of rendering was introduced requiring lower temperatures (i.e., less energy) and less time, it seemed a win–win situation considering the increasing pressure on the United Kingdom's beef industry in the face of global competition. But some time after the new rendering practice was introduced into the United Kingdom, the prion disease known as mad cow disease emerged. The new process, it was discovered, was not effectively disinfecting for prions. Existence of prion disease was unknown prior to its dramatic emergence, first in cows and then in people. The context is important to appreciate. Somehow the streamlining of the rendering process played a role. British scientists tested the new process by deliberately introducing animals with mad cow disease and assaying the resulting MBM product. They found that the newer rendering process does not remove the infection, whereas the older process did.

Xenotransplantation: Technology as a Factor in Emergence

With more than 50 000 Americans waiting for organ transplants in the United States, the demand for new parts is outstripping the supply. Animals seem to many like the logical next source of transplants, and scientific work is underway to access this source. In the United States, the Food and Drug Administration (FDA) has not licensed animal transplants. But other countries have, and they are attracting what the press calls medical tourists.

The truth is that scientists remain largely ignorant of the ecology at the microbial level despite their swagger. Another truth is that there is a nascent industry in xenotransplantation just waiting for the green light from the

FDA. When an organ from a pig or baboon is transplanted into a human, four things happen: (1) the human defenses recognize the foreign material and mount a defense, (2) this vigorous immunological battle that would normally cause the rejection of the foreign material is treated with a variety of powerful drugs to stop rejection, and the patient becomes immunosuppressed, (3) any viruses or prions in the animal donor immediately become residents in the human donor, and (4) the new organ slowly begins to pick up the physiological functions of the organ it has been brought in to replace. Clearly, the second and third parts of this scenario introduce potentially dangerous conditions for disease transmission.

Some very strong, compassionate arguments exist for xenotransplantation: There are not enough organs available for transplant, and people with kidney or liver failure or pancreatic crises can wait years for a donor. The wait is difficult and can be life-threatening. Renal dialysis, for example, which replaces the function of a working kidney, makes patients feel increasingly ill as they undergo repeated treatment. According to Matching Donors, a Massachusetts-based nonprofit organization that matches donors with recipients, an estimated 17 people die each day waiting for transplants in the United States alone.

The pig has become the preferred candidate for donating organs to humans. Primates, the other most promising potential candidates, are expensive to acquire and keep, more likely to provoke ethical objections, and are perceived as risky because HIV is a simian (monkey) virus. Pigs can be bred to genetically erase their foreignness to humans by manipulating the genetic coding for the glycoproteins on their cells. Their organs are about the right size to fit the human body. However, pigs also carry new porcine (pig) retroviruses. Recall that HIV is a retrovirus, albeit of a different type. These retroviruses are actually embedded in their genetic material, so although pigs can be bred in sterile surroundings, there is no way to remove retrovirus agents from their makeup. They are, in the language of microbiology, endogenous.

Much work is ongoing to overcome the various obstacles to using pigs as donors for human organs. The problem of the endogenous retroviruses caused the FDA to halt early clinical trials in the United States. But scientists are working hard to study the risks and how to overcome them. In India, caution is not as pronounced, and pig-donated organs are transplanted into humans there. Those humans may return to the United States to recover, and presumably, seek medical care if and when they become ill, potentially exposing other patients. If there are risks from pig retroviruses, eventually they will be known, but the incubation period may be as long as the decade of quiet infection that precedes clinical AIDS in those with HIV. Potential risks lurk on two biological fronts. One concern is that the retroviruses from the pig could infect the human host and, in turn, the infected person's contacts and community. Another is that the retroviruses might incorporate genes from the human (0.1% of the human genome contains endogenous retrovirus sequences) and the resulting mixed organism would prove infectious to the human and that human's contacts and community.

A final area of concern, which is general for animal organ donation to humans, is the transfer of antibiotic-resistant infections from the animal. Animals of many types are receiving antibiotics in great volumes in their feed and treatments. While guidelines are very strict for how donor animals for human organ transplantation trials are raised in nations carrying out such experiments (including the United Kingdom and Australia), the guidelines in other countries may not be strict. So medical tourists who travel in search of the cheaper transplant bear close watching, and their close contacts should be made aware of the potential risks of unknown infections.

Microbial Change: Antibiotic Selective Pressure

Another type of emergent threat has a clearer path: evolution of resistant microbes in response to exposure to antibiotics. Antibiotics act as a selective pressure for resistance by killing off the susceptible microbes in each generation, leaving only those that have developed a strategy to resist them. Since microbes reproduce so often, this pressure assures the emergence of a fair number of resistant microbes in a relatively short period of time.

The selective power of microbes in response to antibiotics has been well demonstrated, starting with a classic experiment conducted by microbiologist Stuart Levy and his colleagues in the latter half of the 1970s:

> In the mid-1970s, we performed a study that involved raising 300 chickens on a small farm outside Boston. We provided 150 newly hatched chicks with oxytetracycline-laced feed and another 150 without. We followed the effect of the antibiotic-laced feed on the animals and people on the farm. As we began the study, the control group had little or no resistant organisms. In the group receiving low levels (200 ppm) of oxytetracycline, tetracycline resistance began to emerge among the fecal *Escherichia coli*. What was surprising was that, within 12 weeks, we detected as much as 70% of all *E. coli* with resistance to more than two antibiotics, including ampicillin, sulphonamides, and streptomycin. The resistances were all on transferable plasmids that emerged following use of just tetracycline.   (Levy, 2002: 27)

While antibiotics were designed to fight off infections in sick people and animals, they were approved for use as growth promoters for animals in the United States in 1949 and in the United Kingdom in 1953. Meanwhile, in the 1960s, scientists began to understand that the presence of antibiotics in the microenvironment of bacteria caused transferable antibiotic resistance. This means that populations of microbes not only become resistant to the antibiotic over time, but also can pass the new, adaptive characteristic resistance to other microbes – their biological extended family, as it were. Antibiotics fed to animals are not deactivated in the animals' digestion process. In fact, they remain largely biologically active when they are excreted by the animals on fields, into waterways, or elsewhere. Other vertebrates, including humans, begin to be colonized with the resistant organisms, if they share an environment with animals in which the resistant strains are developing. In areas where animals and humans are crowded together with poor access to sanitation, this aspect of antibiotic usage in animals becomes even more dangerous.

Campylobacter and *Salmonella* are the two best known microbes. They have been shown to acquire new resistance while in animals and to transfer that resistance to humans through the consumption or handling of contaminated meat. In the case of *Campylobacter*, the practice of intensive poultry production plays a role. Most chickens are colonized by *Campylobacter* – they carry them in their gut. The chickens are not sickened by these microbes; the *Campylobacter* are part of the normal gut flora. When chickens are raised in very close proximity, with thousands in a single facility, they are more prone to disease, as we have seen with the avian influenza virus. They also are more prone to bacterial disease. Thus, chickens are often treated with antibiotics, including fluoroquinolones, a particular type of antibiotic that is important in treating human infections. According to the U.S. Centers for Disease Control and Prevention, the rate of resistance to this important class of antibiotics in human infections with *Campylobacter* rose from 13% in 1997 to 19% in 2001. In Minnesota, fluoroquinolone-resistant strains were isolated from 14% of chicken products in retail markets. When molecular-level comparisons were made, these strains exactly matched those isolated from human infections in the surrounding communities.

But the use of antibiotics as growth promoters is not confined to resource-challenged regions. In fact, it has been a long-standing practice in the United States, where a host of microbes have developed resistance, most likely as a result of the drugs in food animals, including *Salmonella*, *Campylobacter jejuni*, and *Escherichia coli*. A number of other industrialized nations have been more diligent about monitoring and curbing the use of antibiotics in animals. The European Union has prohibited lacing the feed of animals with antibiotics that might also be useful in human disease, with the intent of preserving the effectiveness of such antibiotics as long as possible. The scientific evidence for this move is powerful and comes largely from the United Kingdom, Denmark, and Germany, where scientists have carefully monitored feed practices and resistance patterns over the last decade. Research suggests the bans can lead to a corresponding drop in drug-resistant bacteria. One study showed that rate of resistance to the antibiotic avoparcin declined in Germany and Denmark after that drug was prohibited for use as a growth promoter (Witte, 2000). Scientists studied the disease patterns by using molecular genetic techniques to fingerprint specific gene groups that characterize both animal and human resistance to particular bacteria. These characteristic patterns were then tracked in different populations of animals and humans to trace the changes in their frequency of occurrence. Research demonstrated that the decline in resistance was correlated in time with the proscription of the use of avoparcin as a growth promoter and that the decline in the characteristic gene cluster took place in numerous animal and human systems coincidentally.

Antibiotics in Humans: Are Prescriptions Useful?

In many developed countries in Europe and North America, antibiotic prescription authority has been vested in health-care workers since the mid-1900s, and usually is limited to physicians or nurse practitioners. In many other countries, antibiotics are available from pharmacists without a prescription. The U.S. CDC and many state health departments have launched programs to educate the public and physicians about prudent use of antibiotics. Antibiotics are, of course, only useful in infections where bacteria (or mycobacteria, such as tuberculosis) are involved. They have no effect whatsoever on human infections caused by viruses. Viruses cause the majority of infections seen by doctors, including sore throats, cough, fever, and diarrhea. However, when patients come to the doctor, they expect to be treated, not just advised to rest, take fluids and "two aspirin and call me in the morning." This is even more the case in the current health-care practice milieu in the United States, where visits with health-care providers are difficult to schedule, short, and expensive. Patient demand for antibiotics is a major driver of inappropriate use.

What role does sanitary practice play in the transmission to humans? What are the critical variables in keeping cages clean, providing safe water to poultry, or clean and safe feed? What is the compromise between the most efficient and profitable poultry-raising practices and safety among poultry workers? When the Food and Agriculture Organization of the United Nations (FAO) discusses restructuring the increasingly intense poultry industry in Southeast Asia, the optimal design of that restructuring is not clear – we have no scientific blueprint

to follow. The United States' experience with avian influenza, in fact, suggests that USDA guidelines do not prevent the disease in poultry.

We have quantitative tools we can use to answer some of these important questions. A group of scientists recently analyzed the impact of the livestock revolution on the ecology of infectious diseases. The revolution, or the growing demand for animal protein, has been incited by Earth's increasing human population and the rising incomes of growing urban populations. This demand is met in Asia primarily with poultry, much of which is raised in crowded conditions just outside urban centers. Slingenberg and his colleagues (2004) outline four major areas of risk in this process that need to be carefully considered in terms of the emergence of new infections:

1. production intensification;
2. the host metapopulation, which means a population that experiences microbial traffic and, therein, experiences the spread of disease (in this case, the poultry);
3. the transmission pathways other than those within the animal population, in other words, the entire food chain from feed to live animals, processing, marketing/distribution, food preparation, and consumption; and
4. the nature of the pathogen, that is, its virulence and the ease with which it spreads.

While crops can only be intensified within the bounds of arable land, the livestock revolution is not so constrained. A key feature is the "severance of the traditional links between the amount of available local land and feed resources" (Slingenbergh *et al.* 2004: 470). Poultry intensification in Latin America, the Near East, North Africa, East Asia, and South Asia is taking place close to the exploding markets of the urban megacities. It is estimated that by 2015, half of the world's human population and 35% of the global meat production will be in Asia. Working with data from the FAO on the agricultural population and chicken meat output, the scientists plotted the information on a graph (**Figure 2**).

Bringing ecological science into the study of how microbes change or adapt within their microscopic world is the study focus of evolutionary biologist Paul Ewald and his colleagues. They have posited that a microbe's mobility is linked with its virulence (how seriously ill it can make us). The argument is that the basic value of ecological fitness is central for populations of microbes. This is simply the ability to pass their genetic material from one generation of their species to the next through replication. If the microbe can easily move from host to host, that is, if it is highly infectious, it invests more energy moving in mobile hosts and less on developing high virulence. On the other hand, some species, such as anthrax, lie in wait for extended periods of time and then immobilize their hosts by making the host moribund or dead, counting on the immobilized host to serve as a point of infection for other hosts. Ewald has coined the term 'cultural vectors' to describe transmission that takes place independent of typical mechanisms such as flagellae, which allow the microbe to swim, or mosquitoes, which transport the microbe to another host (Kimball, 2006). These strategies have developed within the plethora of microbe species over thousands of years of evolution.

The emergence of mad cow disease raises three key points: (1) changes in production and processing of products based on animal or human material can spark the emergence of new human infectious pathogens, (2) production changes can be hastened in a global marketplace in which increased efficiency in production is reward by providing a competitive edge or more profit, and (3) the new agent can be distributed globally before the problem is fully recognized and public health measures are implemented. As these rising resistance rates indicate, one obvious strategy to prevent the emergence of drug-resistant strains is to limit the antibiotic exposure of microbes living in humans and food animals. Possible strategies would include limiting or discouraging the use of antibiotics by veterinarians, pharmacists, physicians, and the public through legislation and/or international policy and law. But this is actually not at all straightforward in today's world. The use of antimicrobials to fight disease in humans and animals and promote growth in animals is a well-entrenched practice.

In the United States alone, an estimated 23 000 000 kg (50 000 000 lbs) of antibiotics are used annually. While surprisingly little information is available about the usage of antibiotics in food animals in most countries, WHO estimates that roughly half of all antimicrobials produced are used to treat humans, and most of the rest are used in animal feed – primarily for pigs and poultry – to either fend off infection or enhance growth (WHO, 2002). The practice has become even more important with the rise of intensive agriculture, in which animals are kept in crowded conditions that make them more vulnerable to infectious diseases.

Subtherapeutic use of antibiotics in these settings not only reduces outbreaks of illness but also has been shown to increase the overall weight of the animal by 4 or 5%, which adds to productivity and eventually to profitability. The tension between ecological caution and business profit is noted in a recent report by the U.S. General Accounting Office:

> While antibiotic use in animals poses potential human health risks, it also reduces the cost of producing these animals, which in turn helps reduce the prices consumers pay for food. Antibiotics are an integral part of animal production in the United States and many other countries where large numbers of livestock are raised in confined facilities, which increases likelihood of disease.
> (U.S. General Accounting Office, 2004: 1)

The degree to which the drugs are used as growth enhancers (rather than to combat disease in sick animals) is subject to debate. According to the Animal Health Institute, an industry group that represents U.S. antibiotic manufacturers, some 10.2 tons of antibiotics a year are used on the 8 billion food animals produced annually in the United States – 87% of which is for "treating, controlling and preventing disease". In contrast, the Union of Concerned Scientists, an environmental group, in 2001 estimated that U.S. animal producers administer 12 300 tons of antibiotics a year for nontherapeutic (i.e., growth-enhancing) purposes.

National legislation and guidelines for antibiotic use in animal husbandry vary among countries, as does the level of surveillance. In the 1990s, amid growing concerns about the emergence of drug-resistant bugs, the WHO identified the issue as one of global public concern. In 2001, WHO, together with the Food and Agriculture Organization of the United Nations and the Office International des Epizooties (World Organization for Animal Health), drafted a set of global principles to address the use and abuse of antimicrobials in animals. Included was a strategy to ban drugs that are important for treating human illnesses for use as growth promoters in animals.

But as the WHO initiative acknowledges, given the world market, any successful effort will have to be global in scope. The strategy that WHO disseminated in 2001 is not a regulation but a series of recommendations "to both persuade governments to take urgent action and then to guide this action with expert technical and practical advice" (WHO, 2001). As a nonbinding recommendation, the strategy may fail to galvanize sufficient international action, particularly in areas that are strapped for public health resources. Indeed, a workshop in 2002 examining the degree to which the recommendations were implemented found significant gaps. The workshop summary concluded:

> The extent of implementation of the Global Strategy was very variable, both across and within Regions. Where priority interventions were in place, in many instances these were nominal only, since compliance was not enforced.   (WHO, 2002: 1)

Among the obstacles identified were limited resources, unregulated use of antimicrobials in food-producing animals, and "lack of inclination to enforce existing regulations."

In most developing countries, where agricultural exports are a potential source of critically important foreign currency, few regulatory barriers exist for using antibiotics as growth promoters, and those that do exist are weakly enforced. In many cases, veterinary services have transitioned in recent decades from the government to private hands, and the livelihood of veterinary workers now depends on the ability of farmers to pay for services. If a practice such as subtherapeutic use of antimicrobials is judged potentially profitable, chances are it will continue relatively undisturbed.

As of 2006, all antibiotics were, in principle, banned from use for growth promotion in European Union member countries. Many producers and others have questioned the science behind these bans. Indeed, some have called for a quantitatively based formal risk assessment. But others point out that conducting such an assessment would require waiting until the potential negative health consequences had played out in terms of human therapeutic failures (Witte, 2000). Then, once deaths or other health consequences had begun to occur, we could count them and do calculations to demonstrate risk. Awaiting this outcome when the science from the bench, the lab, and numerous animal systems is clear seems unconscionable. Thus the precautionary principle moved the European Union to implement the ban.

As the recent GAO (the U.S. General Accounting Office) report indicates, the European Union's impending implementation of more stringent bans of antibiotics is being watched closely by the United States as a potential source of future trade embargoes (U.S. General Accounting Office, 2004). The United States is beginning to benchmark its own system of monitoring the problem with efforts in other countries, particularly the European Union. But as the report also points out, to date, public authorities in the United States have lacked sufficient access to reliable industry information on the use of antibiotics, making it difficult to assess the current situation and what actions may be appropriate. Here science has no gap in its knowledge. The risks of increasing antibiotic resistance are clear. However, in terms of information needs for policy, the GAO report states flatly that:

> Although they have made some progress in monitoring antibiotic resistance, federal agencies do not collect the critical data on antibiotic use in animals that they need to support research on the human health risk.
>
> (U.S. General Accounting Office, 2004: 7)

So at present, the United States, a major meat exporter in the world marketplace – with exports of $2 billion in 2002 – appears to lag behind the global community in this aspect of food safety, running a risk of trade embargoes that eventually could drive it to regulate the practice without key information from industry practice.

Around the world, in developed as well as developing countries, the research base and national policies regarding antibiotic use are uneven. While there is no reason to believe that the biology and ecology are fundamentally different with regards to the use of antibiotics as animal growth-promoting agents in Europe, Asia, or Africa, national policy makers historically have made decisions based only on studies related to their own particular situations. Meanwhile, on a daily basis, additional resistance is being stockpiled through the consumption by humans of resistant strains of pathogenic microbes. As noted earlier, these antibiotics do not disappear from the environment when their use is halted. While information from Europe indicates that resistant strains will become sensitive again when the selective pressure of antibiotic use is removed, that information is not nearly as complete or compelling as it should be to justify the persistence of risky practices in animal husbandry. Antibiotic residues and active compounds are not only found in the food we eat. Increasingly they are found in groundwater and in the soil, begging a serious question: Is there a point where we have accumulated enough active antibiotics in the human environment to permanently alter the equilibrium of nature? Is this prospect a real threat to us?

In other developed countries, antibiotics are often not controlled by prescription. In most Asian, Latin American, and some European countries, they are available from pharmacists over the counter, without a doctor's prescription. This has become an issue in antibiotic resistance. It might best be apparent in the case of tuberculosis. Tuberculosis is a slow-moving but devastating infection that begins in the lungs. It requires long-term treatment (6 months to a year) with three active antituberculosis drugs. In some countries, such as the Philippines, compounds available in pharmacies to treat cough may contain one active antituberculose agent mixed with vitamins. This will help with symptoms, but not cure the infection. Instead, as we have seen, resistant organisms will be selected and thrive in the patient. Most of the drug-resistant tuberculosis seen in Seattle and other U.S. West Coast cities occurs in people from countries where this is standard practice.

Creating prescription authority and regulation of antibiotic use internationally is not a simple matter. The majority of pharmaceutical corporations are transnational in their marketing and production. Like their counterparts in the meat industry, they have financial incentives to avoid government regulation of their product sales. While industry has increasingly come to understand that widespread, inappropriate use of antibiotics will shorten the effectiveness of their products, that inevitability is likely to occur well beyond the life of the drugs' marketing plans, so this consideration may not be as central to decision making as safety would dictate. Misaligned financial incentives also are evident in the Asia Pacific region. Physicians in the region have historically been marketed with financial incentives to prescribe antibiotics. Drug salesmen, known as detailers, call and visit physicians in practice to promote their products. In Asia, some hospital systems actually compensate physicians according to the number of prescriptions they write. This has resulted in profound overuse of antibiotics and, consequently, very effective selection for drug resistance in a number of medical centers.

In developed countries where consumers are able to purchase drugs, incentives exist for drug producers to limit the regulations they work under and to promote the drugs they produce. In the past decade, the United States has seen the emergence of direct marketing to the consumer. This trend includes high investment by pharmaceutical companies in media advertisement campaigns to promote certain brand names of drugs. This trend has not included direct marketing of antibiotics to consumers, rather focusing on the promotion of pain relievers, antidepressants, medications for sexual dysfunction, antihistamines, and cold remedies. This relatively new media approach includes medications available by prescription only, often advising the public to "ask your doctor" for the pill by name.

Primary Prevention: An Ongoing Challenge

The actual emergence of new microbes is difficult to prevent. In the case of antibiotic-resistant organisms, the selective pressure is well known and characterized, and yet it is apparently difficult to remove. The promiscuous use of antimicrobials in humans and animals seems destined to continue in the near term, and thus laws of nature suggest the emergence of new resistant microbes will also continue. Similarly, medical forays into xeno-transplantation and other procedures with unknown risks for disease emergence are inevitable. Meanwhile, the human population will continue to grow and increasingly tax the planet's resources. International travel and trade will continue to expand, all the while tweaking the microbial world in unexpected ways. The challenge of preventing the emergence of new microbes is daunting, and our resources and knowledge for doing so are limited. Factors of emergence provide an outline for additional interdisciplinary research that needs to be done to provide more scientific insight into this phenomenon. As we await such insight, the one clear fact is that emergence is continuous and, if anything, is continuous at a quickening pace.

See also: Emerging Diseases; Epidemic Investigation; Surveillance of Disease.

Citations

Kimball AM (2006) *Risky Trade: Global Trade; Infectious Disease in the Era of Global Trade.* Aldershot, UK: Ashgate.

Klinkenberg E, McCall PJ, Hastings IM, et al. (2005) Malaria and irrigated crops, Accra, Ghana. *Emerging Infectious Diseases* 11(8).

Lederberg J, Shope RE and Oaks SC (eds.) (1992) *Emerging Infections: Microbial Threats to Health in the United States.* Washington, DC: National Academies Press.

Levy SB (2002) The 2000 Garrod lecture: Factors impacting on the problem of antibiotic resistance. *Journal of Antimicrobial Chemotherapy* 49: 25–30.

McMichael JA (2001) *Human Culture, Ecological Change, and Infectious Disease: Are We Experiencing History's Fourth Great Transition?* Malden, MA: Blackwell Science.

Patz JA, Daszak P, and Tabor GM (2004) Unhealthy landscapes: Policy recommendations on land use change and infectious disease emergence. *Environmental Health Perspectives* 112: 1092–1098.

Slingenbergh JI, Gilbert M, De Balogh K, et al. (2004) Ecological sources of zoonotic diseases. *Scientific and Technical Review* 23: 467–484.

Smolinski MS, Hamburg MA and Lederberg J (eds.) (2003) *Microbial Threats to Health: Emergence Detection and Response.* Washington, DC: National Academies Press.

U.S. General Accounting Office (2004) *Antibiotic Resistance: Federal Agencies Need to Better Focus Efforts to Address Risk to Humans from Antibiotic Use in Animals.* Washington DC: GAO.

Witte W (2000) Selective pressure by antibiotic use in livestock. *International Journal of Antimicrobial Agents* 16(supplement 1): S19–S24.

Woolhouse MEJ and Gowtage-Sequeria S (2005) Host range and emerging and reemerging pathogens. *Emerging Infectious Diseases* 11(12).

World Health Organization (2001) *Use of Antimicrobials Outside Human Medicine.* Geneva, Switzerland: World Health Organization.

World Health Organization (2002) *Implementation Workshop on the WHO Global Strategy for Containment of Antimicrobial Resistance.* Geneva, Switzerland: World Health Organization.

Further Reading

Colwell R, Patz JA, and Patz R (1997) *Climate, Infectious Disease and Health: An Interdisciplinary Perspective.* Washington, DC: American Academy of Microbiology.

Morse S (2004) *Emerging and Reemerging Infectious Diseases: A Global Problem Interview with Stephen S. Morse.* Washington, DC: Action Bioscience.

Nadakavukaren A (1990) *Man and Environment: A Health Perspective.* Washington, DC: Waveland Press.

World Bank Group (2005) *Environment Matters: Annual Review 2005.* Washington, DC: The World Bank Group.

World Health Organization (2004) Ecosystems and human well-being: Health synthesis. *A Report of the Millennium Ecosystem Assessment.* Geneva, Switzerland: World Health Organization.

Risk Factors for Cardiovascular Diseases

K Jamrozik, University of Adelaide, Adelaide, SA, Australia
R Taylor and A Dobson, University of Queensland, Brisbane, QLD, Australia

Introduction

Collectively, cardiovascular diseases (CVDs) are the leading cause of death of *Homo sapiens* in the late twentieth and early twenty-first centuries (World Health Organization, 2002). While they constitute a diverse group of conditions (see **Table 1**), the subgroup related to atherosclerosis is easily dominant as a cause of death globally, as well as being a leading cause of morbidity throughout at least the developed world. The atherosclerotic group includes (1) ischemic heart disease (IHD), presenting clinically as angina pectoris, acute myocardial infarction (AMI), and acute coronary syndrome (ACS); (2) cerebrovascular disease (CeVD), presenting clinically as transient ischemic attack and stroke; (3) abdominal aortic aneurysm (AAA); and (4) peripheral arterial disease (PAD), presenting clinically as intermittent claudication and gangrene. In developed countries, IHD is one of the major causes of heart failure (Braunwald, 1997) and therefore many cases of heart failure in such communities are ultimately due to atherosclerosis. Because atherosclerotic 'cardiovascular disease' is so important, in developed countries the phrase cardiovascular disease is understood as referring to the consequences of atherosclerosis unless it is specifically qualified in some other way. That usage will be followed here.

With one notable exception, the absence of a relationship between diabetes mellitus and AAA, the risk factors for atherosclerosis are the same, regardless of the specific anatomical arterial territory affected. That said, it is useful to divide the risk factors for atherosclerosis into three broad groups, according to their implications for prevention (see **Table 2**). This article provides a brief review of the unmodifiable or fixed factors, those not amenable to change,

before considering in greater detail the relationships between the major modifiable factors and the risk of CVD, and particularly the evidence that altering the levels of these factors results in a reduction in that risk. The next part of the article addresses the group of other modifiable factors, several of which are important determinants of one or more of the major modifiable factors, while others have complex epidemiological relationships with cardiovascular risk. The known risk factors for atherosclerosis explain at least 75% of cases of IHD and offer enormous scope for preventive interventions, at both individual and whole-of-population levels (Beaglehole and Magnus, 2002). The article therefore concludes with a section addressing a possible approach to reducing the burden of cardiovascular disease in a given community, derived from the seminal work of Geoffrey Rose (Rose, 1981). After more than 50 years of intensive scholarly enquiry, more will be gained, and more quickly, by systematically applying what we already know about how atherosclerotic CVD might be prevented than by searching for additional modifiable factors (Beaglehole and Magnus, 2002).

Fixed, Unmodifiable Factors

A large proportion of any individual's absolute risk of CVD, his or her chance of suffering a significant clinical event related to atherosclerosis in the near future, is determined by a set of factors that he or she cannot change.

Age

The risk of a major cardiovascular event rises with age, in an accelerating fashion. Of the four principal conditions,

Table 1   Selected categories of cardiovascular disease

Subgroup	Example
Atherosclerotic cardiovascular disease	Ischemic heart disease, cerebrovascular disease, abdominal aortic aneurysm, peripheral arterial disease
Congenital heart disease	Tetralogy of Fallot
Primary cardiomyopathy	Hypertrophic obstructive cardiomyopathy
Secondary cardiomyopathy	Alcoholic cardiomyopathy
Primary myocarditis	Coxsackie B infection
Autoimmune cardiac disease	Rheumatic heart disease

Table 2   Risk factors for atherosclerosis

Fixed unmodifiable factors	Major modifiable factors	Other modifiable factors
Age	Smoking	Overweight and obesity
Male sex		Diet: Fat, salt, fish
Ethnicity	Blood pressure	Stress
Family history	Blood cholesterol	Personality
Clinically evident cardiovascular disease	Lack of physical activity	Alcohol
	Diabetes mellitus	Oral contraceptive pill
	Homocysteine	Hyperuricemia
		Hypothyroidism

ACS alone has a notable incidence in the working age group (20–64 years). The median age at which a first-ever stroke is experienced is usually beyond 70 years, and both AAA and PAD are conditions of old age, although the latter may be brought forward by diabetes mellitus.

Male Sex

At any given age, men are at higher risk of CVD than women. The increase in cardiovascular risk with age is smooth in males but accelerates around the time of the menopause in women before slowing once more. In the working age group, the male excess of AMI is three- to fourfold (Tunstall-Pedoe, 2003), although this gap narrows considerably in old age. Rates of stroke in males always exceed those in females, but absolute numbers of events are more similar because of the greater longevity of women and the rapid increase in risk with age. AAA is a rare condition in women, by a factor of about seven. The male excess of PAD is at least partly due to historical differences in smoking habits between the sexes.

Ethnicity

The concept of ethnicity combines both biological (including racial) and cultural aspects which differ both within and between populations. The MONICA Project, coordinated by the World Health Organization over a decade from the early 1980s (Tunstall-Pedoe, 2003), confirmed the long-known and obvious international differences in mortality from CVD and demonstrated that they reflected major differences in the incidence of cardiovascular events. However, the project was largely confined to Caucasian populations and had limited representation from both the United States and the UK where there are significant non-Caucasian populations living under relatively good economic conditions. Results from multiracial studies in both these countries show that ethnic differences in modifiable risk factors explain a significant proportion of the ethnic differences in mortality from CVD.

Family History

Family history has long been associated with an individual's cardiovascular risk. Leaving aside rare conditions such as familial hypercholesterolemia, this relationship almost certainly has some genetic basis, but shared environment and behavior in early life and persistence of some of these habits into adulthood are also likely to be important.

Clinically Evident Cardiovascular Disease

Clinically evident CVD in one major arterial territory is a strong marker of the risk of a major cardiovascular event affecting another. Thus, even among survivors of a stroke, acute coronary events rather than recurrent strokes are the leading cause of death, and men with AAA have a considerably stronger history of AMI than those without aneurysms (Jamrozik et al., 2000).

Major Modifiable Factors

Although part of an individual's risk of CVD is determined by factors that cannot be changed, attention to the major modifiable risk factors for CVD can appreciably reduce the risk of experiencing a major cardiovascular event.

Traditionally smoking, blood pressure, and blood lipids have dominated thinking about major modifiable and independent risk factors for CVD, but lack of physical activity has equal standing with members of this trio. Some authorities would also include diabetes mellitus in the set but, while its importance as a determinant of risk is clear, the evidence that this contribution can be reduced, even by the best metabolic control of diabetes, is distinctly limited. Homocysteine, a sulfur-containing amino acid derived principally from meat, has attracted a lot of attention as a further modifiable risk factor.

Of the four major modifiable factors, smoking and physical activity are obviously under the direct control of the individual, while the other two, blood pressure and blood lipids, are related to diet and relative body weight and hence are also largely determined by personal behavior, though less directly. The latter factors are more proximal to events at the vascular endothelium where the lesions of atherosclerosis are initiated and propagated. In addition, because blood pressure and blood lipids are amenable to pharmacological intervention, this has made it easier to demonstrate, via randomized controlled trials, that changes in these factors are followed relatively quickly by changes in the incidence of the clinical endpoints related to atherosclerosis. However, the observational epidemiology for all four risk factors indicates clearly that each has a "continuous and graded relationship" (Stamler et al., 1986) with risk of CVD. In turn, this means that dichotomizing the population into hypertensive versus normotensive, for example, potentially results in large numbers of individuals ignoring advice regarding lifestyle and behavior that, if followed, could materially reduce their risk of CVD.

The relative importance of the major modifiable factors differs across the different arterial territories (**Table 3**) and to some extent across populations. Smoking and diabetes are especially significant in the genesis of PAD, while blood pressure is most closely associated with the risk of stroke. Like the other factors, lack of physical activity has some bearing on risk of major clinical events across each of the arterial territories.

Table 3   Relationship of major modifiable risk factors to various manifestations of cardiovascular disease

Factor	Ischemic heart disease	Cerebrovascular disease	Abdominal aortic aneurysm	Peripheral arterial disease
Smoking	+++	+++	+++	+++++
Blood pressure	+++	++++	++	+
Cholesterol	++++	?	+	−
Inactivity	+++	++	++	++
Diabetes	+++	+++	−	++++

The number of + signs reflects the strength of positive associations; − signs indicate that no association has been consistently demonstrated; ? denotes an uncertain relationship.

Smoking

There is a strong relationship between smoking and all manifestations of CVD, and the risk rises with both level of consumption and duration of smoking. In the case of IHD, the relative risk for current smokers compared with never smokers is inversely related to age, such that it exceeds tenfold in mid-adulthood and falls progressively into old age. This pattern is consistently apparent but has not been fully explained. Even so, because background risk rises steeply with age, the smaller relative risk experienced by smokers in older age still translates into a sizeable increase in absolute risk and large numbers of additional, and avoidable, events.

Although every reputable medical and scientific organization that has reviewed the evidence agrees that smoking is a major cause of CVD, the biological mechanism underlying the relationship remains uncertain. Carbon monoxide, of which there are large amounts in tobacco smoke, is known to increase the permeability to lipids of the vascular endothelium, and numerous others of the four thousand chemicals in tobacco smoke affect physiological systems that are potentially relevant to the development of atherosclerosis (Leone, 2007). The same mechanisms are likely to explain the significant excess risks of IHD in nonsmokers passively exposed to tobacco smoke.

Importantly, the excess risks of IHD and CeVD associated with current smoking decrease rapidly once an individual gives up the habit, such that the risk returns almost to that of an otherwise equivalent lifelong non-smoker within a few years (Doll et al., 2004). Curiously, the significant increase in risk of AAA related to smoking appears to persist for several decades after quitting (Jamrozik et al., 2000), although this question has not been studied anywhere near as extensively. The data on risk of PAD in ex-smokers are inconsistent, with some reports suggesting only a limited reduction of risk, but it is widely accepted that cessation of smoking significantly improves the prognosis once clinical manifestations of PAD, such as intermittent claudication, are apparent.

Blood Pressure

The levels of both systolic and diastolic blood pressure show continuous, graded relationships with cardiovascular risk (MacMahon et al., 1990). The notion of hypertension is therefore a clinical short-cut designed to help doctors identify those at greatest absolute risk of developing CVD. Recognizing this, the World Health Organization and the International Society of Hypertension have progressively lowered the levels of blood pressure used to define the upper limit of clinical acceptability. The fundamental point is clear – the lower one's blood pressure, the lower the risk of CVD – and messages about determinants of blood pressure levels such as diet (less salt, more fruit and vegetables, maintaining weight in the ideal range) and lifestyle (adequate physical activity, keep any consumption of alcohol within moderate limits) are applicable over virtually the entire population.

Blood Lipids

Like blood pressure, blood cholesterol shows a continuous and graded relationship with cardiovascular risk, and more specifically, coronary risk (Stamler et al., 1986). Thus, apart from the familial condition, the notion of hypercholesterolemia is really a matter of clinical convenience. Serum triglycerides are also related to the risk of both IHD and stroke (Asia Pacific Cohort Studies Collaboration, 2004).

Just as there has been debate, from time to time, as to which measure of blood pressure (systolic, diastolic, or pulse pressure) carries most predictive significance, so there has been extensive discussion of which lipid subfraction or the ratios of which subfractions define the risk of major coronary events most precisely. Aside from the fact that an individual's level of low-density lipoprotein cholesterol (LDL cholesterol) is directly related to his or her coronary risk, while that of high-density lipoprotein cholesterol (HDL cholesterol) is inversely related to that risk, it has required very large studies to demonstrate statistically significant differences in the prognostic importance of the various lipid subfractions, suggesting that the clinical impact of choosing one from another verges on marginal.

Of greater practical importance are the observations that the level of HDL cholesterol is increased by physical activity and consumption of alcohol at moderate levels, while the level of LDL cholesterol is lower among those who keep their weight in the ideal range and who eat less fat, and especially less saturated fat, which is mainly of animal origin. These data lend themselves to practical advice from health professionals to individual patients and to population-wide health promotion activities. Physical activity and achieving and maintaining weight-for-height in the recommended range are key messages because only 20% of blood cholesterol is exogenous in origin. For most people, higher levels of total and LDL cholesterol represent intrinsic metabolic responses to imprudent choices regarding behavior and lifestyle rather than direct consequences of the amount of fat in their diets.

Where an individual's level of cholesterol remains a matter of clinical concern, even after he or she has lost weight, begun to exercise more, and reduced the amount of fat consumed, pharmacological treatment can help to reduce the level of cholesterol and the associated coronary risk. This approach is supported by a series of large and well-conducted randomized controlled trials.

Interestingly, the same trials that demonstrated the beneficial effects of statins on coronary risk also consistently showed a reduction in stroke events among those participants taking one of these drugs as compared with a placebo (Baigent et al., 2005). Thus, there is Level I evidence implicating high blood cholesterol as an important risk factor for stroke, a relationship that observational epidemiology has been slow to reveal. It is now evident that a high level of cholesterol is associated with an increased risk of occlusive stroke but a decreased risk of primary intracerebral hemorrhage, relationships that will have been obscured when all types of stroke are considered together. As noted in **Table 3**, the level of blood cholesterol is only weakly linked to the risk of AAA and has not consistently been linked to the risk of PAD.

Lack of Physical Activity

In an early and now classic study, Jerry Morris demonstrated that conductors on double-decker buses in London had lower rates of coronary events than did the drivers of the buses, a finding that could not be attributed to preexisting vascular disease. Despite the possibility that physical activity was a potential explanation for this difference, lack of physical activity has been the least investigated of the major, independent, modifiable risk factors for CVD. To be fair, collecting data on frequency, intensity, and duration of physical activity at home, work, and during leisure time is far more difficult than asking about smoking habits or measuring blood pressure or blood cholesterol.

Studies of physical activity in other occupational groups and leisure time physical activity demonstrated reduced coronary risk in those who undertook physical activity regularly, leading to a landmark report from the Surgeon General of the United States, published in 1996

(National Center for Chronic Disease Prevention and Health Promotion, 1996).

Recommendations regarding physical activity have evolved over time as the evidence has accrued. For many years, people were encouraged to undertake periods of vigorous activity lasting 20 min each at least three times weekly. This advice was based on studies of competitive athletes and reflected a pattern of exertion necessary to cause a progressive increase in maximal uptake of oxygen, indicating gains in cardiorespiratory fitness. Blair's group at the Cooper Institute in Texas was among the first to demonstrate beneficial effects on cardiovascular health – lower risks of both IHD and stroke – as well as general health associated with more moderate levels of regular physical activity (Blair et al., 2001). Their work has been particularly influential in reformulating advice about physical activity such that current recommendations are for at least 30 minutes of moderate physical activity, in bursts of at least 10 minutes each, on most days of the week. For individuals who choose walking as part of their response to this advice, the appropriate level of exertion is usually defined as walking at a pace where the degree of breathlessness is just sufficient to make it difficult to hold a normal conversation.

In terms of benefits to cardiovascular and general health, more is better appears to hold across a wide range of levels of physical activity, although the dose–response relationship eventually tends to a plateau. Paffenbarger's studies of Harvard alumni demonstrate clearly that one cannot bank the benefits of physical activity undertaken early in adult life; initially active individuals who then become inactive show higher cardiovascular risk than those who remain persistently active, while the opposite transition, from inactive to active, is clearly associated with reductions in risk compared with that experienced by otherwise similar individuals who remain sedentary (Paffenbarger et al., 1984).

Diabetes Mellitus

Diabetes is an important risk factor for occlusive cardiovascular disease, even if not for AAA. To the extent that most cases of diabetes are of adult-onset type, and that this proportion is only likely to increase with the epidemic of overweight and obesity now occurring in many parts of the world, much of the burden of CVD associated with diabetes is theoretically avoidable through prevention of type 2 diabetes. However, as the UK Prospective Diabetes Study has demonstrated, once diabetes has developed, even tight metabolic control of hyperglycemia does not reduce the incidence of large-vessel cardiovascular disease, that is, of events related to occlusion of the coronary, major cerebral, and lower limb arteries (UK Prospective Diabetes Study, 1998). Thus, diabetes once developed may not be a modifiable risk factor for major cardiovascular events.

Homocysteine

That individuals with the rare metabolic defect known as familial hyperhomocystinemia show a vastly elevated incidence of CVD has sparked considerable interest in whether homocysteine plays any role in the genesis of atherosclerosis. Indeed, by the mid-1990s there was already a large body of observational epidemiology implicating homocysteine as a significant independent risk factor for CVD affecting each of the coronary, cerebral, and peripheral arterial territories (Boushey et al., 1995). Like the relationships of CVD with each of smoking, blood pressure, blood cholesterol, and physical activity, this relationship appears continuous and graded, with no threshold level of homocysteine below which there was no association evident. Homocysteine is toxic to vascular endothelium and therefore may be responsible for the initial disruption of endothelial physiology that sets in train the complex series of events leading to atherosclerosis.

Part of the attraction of homocysteine as a significant risk factor for CVD lies in the ease with which levels can be lowered safely and effectively by treatment with folic acid and B vitamins. Ongoing trials may help to provide a definitive answer regarding the utility of treatment with B vitamins for reducing risk of CVD.

Other Modifiable Factors

Numerous other characteristics of individuals have been associated with an increased risk of CVD. From one perspective, once the fixed and major modifiable risk factors are taken into account, the contributions of many of these factors are rather modest. From another perspective, many of these factors cause increases in risk due to changes in modifiable risk factors; for example, diet affects overweight and obesity, which in turn affect blood pressure. Thus from a population perspective these upstream factors may provide the best opportunities for prevention.

Overweight and Obesity

Overweight and obesity have only limited independent contributions to cardiovascular risk, probably because their principal effects relate to their contributions to higher levels of blood pressure and blood lipids. Thus clinical intervention on the two biomedical factors should always include efforts to achieve and maintain a body mass index in the range of 20–25 kilograms per meter (of height) squared. In practical terms, this translates roughly into maintaining a body weight below height in centimeters minus 100. Debate continues as to whether

ranges of recommended weight for height should be modified for non-European, and especially Asian, populations (Misra et al., 2005). From a population perspective, the growing epidemic of excess body weight can be expected to increase risk of CVD, and controlling this epidemic is a major public health goal in many countries.

Diet: Salt, Fat, Fish, Fruit, and Vegetables

Dietary salt and fat are also direct upstream factors for raised blood pressure and blood lipids, and, like overweight and obesity, offer obvious targets for intervention. In this regard, it is often not appreciated that meat that appears lean to the naked eye still contains a large amount of saturated fat and that many residents of the developed world would experience only benefits and no adverse effects on their health were they to consume less meat.

Vegetarians have lower blood pressure and lower rates of CVD than omnivores, but which aspect or aspects of the vegetarian diet confers these benefits has proved difficult to identify. In part, a higher intake of fruit and vegetables results in beneficial increases in the potassium:sodium ratio in the diet, with consequent reductions in blood pressure, but vegetarians also consume more fiber and frequently follow a more prudent lifestyle.

The observation that Inuit people experienced far less CVD than one might expect among people whose traditional diet contained so much fat and so little fruit and vegetables eventually led to the identification of the significance of long-chain poly-unsaturated fatty acids for vascular health. These omega-3 compounds have a variety of effects on the vascular endothelium and platelets (as well as other physiological systems) and are now widely available over the counter as dietary supplements. Of greater practical import, however, is the significant body of evidence suggesting that a greater intake of fish would bring benefits to cardiovascular health (Schmidt et al., 2005).

Stress

In this discussion, a distinction is drawn between stress, meaning events and factors external to the individual that may cause some distress, and personality, meaning the intrinsic characteristics of the individual that may shape his or her response to such stimuli. People can often cite anecdotes that suggest that an acute emotional or physical stress has precipitated a heart attack or stroke. The more formal scientific literature does demonstrate a relationship between cumulative exposure to life events that independent observers agree are potentially stressful and significant illnesses of many kinds, but the association of major cardiovascular events with single specific instances such as news of a sudden, unexpected bereavement, is much less clear (Hemingway and Marmot, 1999).

Depression is associated with CVD but the direction of causation is not well understood and so the implications for prevention or treatment of CVD are unclear (Bunker et al., 2003).

There has also been extensive research into the relationship between occupational position and CVD, in part stimulated by the well-established social gradient at least of IHD. The Whitehall studies of British civil servants have been the leading investigations in the field. They suggest that limited latitude to control the pace and pattern of one's work is associated with greater coronary risk (Hemingway and Marmot, 1999). However, it is difficult to assess if such studies have fully accounted for confounding by more proximal risk factors. Additionally, a response to these findings probably lies more in the realm of organizational management than clinical medicine or public health.

Personality

The time-urgent, competitive, easily angered type A personality enjoyed a long vogue as a potential marker of cardiovascular risk, especially while white collar occupational groups continued to experience a high rate of coronary events. That epidemiological picture has since undergone a radical change, with people of lower socioeconomic position now being at greater risk of CVD in many developed countries. The focus on personality as a cardiovascular risk factor has also faded because of the difficulties in classifying individuals' personalities reliably. There is also only limited evidence that personalities can be changed, although new ways of responding to the stresses of everyday life can be learned, and the evidence that attempting to do so results in a meaningful reduction in cardiovascular events is scant indeed.

Alcohol

Consumption of alcohol shows a J-shaped relationship with cardiovascular risk, such that lowest rates of events are observed among individuals who regularly consume one to two alcoholic drinks (10–20 g of alcohol) daily. There are somewhat higher risks in complete abstainers, and progressively increasing risks in those who consume alcohol at higher levels than those mentioned (McEdluff and Dobson, 1997), whether on a regular basis or as binges. Drinking alcohol raises levels of HDL cholesterol and both acute and regular heavy intake are associated with higher levels of blood pressure.

Oral Contraceptive Pill and Hormone Replacement Therapy

Because estrogens are prothrombotic, there are theoretical reasons for predicting that women taking exogenous estrogens in the form either of oral contraceptive pills (OCPs) or hormone replacement therapy (HRT) would have an increased risk of occlusive cardiovascular events. This prediction was certainly fulfilled for first-generation OCPs, which had relatively high levels of estrogen. It is likely that modern, lower-dose contraceptive pills carry a smaller relative risk, and the absolute risk of an acute coronary event or stroke in a woman taking OCPs has always been small, because the background risk of such events in women of reproductive age is very small indeed.

HRT stands to mitigate many of the metabolic changes consequent on menopause that are likely to increase cardiovascular risk. Formal proof of the hypothesis that HRT would also reduce the incidence of major cardiovascular events is still awaited, because one large trial testing this prediction was suspended prematurely once it became clear that women taking HRT also had a significant increase in the risk of thromboembolic cardiovascular events and of developing breast cancer (Writing Group for the Women's Health Initiative Investigators, 2002). Subsequent reports have tended to confirm that HRT increases risk of CVD (Vickers et al., 2007).

Socioeconomic Position

While the incidence of IHD originally showed a positive relationship with socioeconomic position, that association has now been reversed so that the least well-off have the highest rates of CVD in Western developed countries, although this transition is occurring later in developing countries. Important variations in the social distributions of many of the other behavioral risk factors for CVD almost certainly contribute to this picture and, given the available evidence, strategies to modify those factors are likely to reduce social gradients in cardiovascular health much faster than interventions to reduce disparities in economic circumstances.

Other Risk Factors

There is a considerable literature on hyperuricemia as a marker of cardiovascular risk, and it is well recognized that hypothyroidism is associated with an increased risk of CVD. There is also reasonable evidence for other putative risk factors (Marmot and Elliott, 2005).

Multiple Risk Factors

From a population perspective, there is ample evidence that the combined effects of multiple risk factors contribute to differences in rates of CVD between countries and changes in risk factor levels are related to changes in rates of CVD events (Tunstall-Pedoe, 2003).

While the statistical relationships between risk factors and the experience of CVD are complex, patients, clinicians and public health authorities can find these matters easier to discuss in terms of summary numbers for relative risk. As a great oversimplification, each of smoking, hypertension, and inadequate physical activity doubles an individual's risk of a major cardiovascular event, and hypercholesterolemia and diabetes increase risk by up to three times, each of these comparisons being with individuals who do not have the relevant risk factor. Where more than one risk factor is present, the effects multiply, such that an inactive smoker with high blood pressure has approximately eight times the risk of experiencing a major cardiovascular event compared with a physically active, normotensive nonsmoker.

While this approach facilitates discussion between patients and their clinicians, it ignores the graded relationships between each of the major modifiable factors and cardiovascular risk and also omits the individual's fixed factors from the consideration. Thus, there has been a concerted move in recent years to encourage a more all-encompassing assessment of individual patients and population groups, the results of which are usually expressed in terms of absolute cardiovascular risk. This is the probability that a given individual will experience a major cardiovascular event in the next decade, given his or her sex and age and existing levels of each of at least smoking, blood pressure, and blood total cholesterol (Smith *et al.*, 2004). Relative risk, comparing smokers with non-smokers, for example, can be somewhat misleading; the numerical multiplier might be large, but if it is applied to a low background risk such as the incidence of CVD in women in the reproductive age group, the resulting absolute risk is still modest. By contrast, as well as being more comprehensive, the approach based on absolute risk fosters concentration of intervention efforts on those likely to gain most (Smith *et al.*, 2004).

The presence of multiple risk factors also comes into play in the concept of the metabolic syndrome. This refers to a clustering of abdominal obesity, high blood pressure, abnormalities of lipid profiles, and insulin resistance, but this is an evolving area, with multiple definitions of the syndrome available. Apart from identifying a possibly sizeable subgroup of the population at particularly high risk of CVD, it is not yet clear what advantages the label of metabolic syndrome offers for clinical management of cardiovascular risk over and above attention to each of the principal elements of the cluster of risk factors.

Practical Steps for Prevention of Cardiovascular Disease

It has now been over 25 years since Geoffrey Rose first identified the inherent limitations in the high-risk strategy, used alone, for improving the health of the population and suggested that mass strategies aimed at whole communities had potentially greater impact (Rose, 1981). The

Table 4   Components of a prudent lifestyle

- No smoking
- 30 minutes of moderate physical activity on most days
- Body mass index in the range 20–25 kg/m^2
- Up to 20 g alcohol daily; no binge drinking
- Consumption of meat <4 times weekly
- Two servings of fruit and five of vegetables daily
- No addition of salt during preparation or consumption of food
- Consumption of fish at least twice weekly
- Avoidance of full-fat milk
- Use of margarine rather than butter

goal for public health is therefore to achieve population-level reductions in the major modifiable risk factors by shifting the risk factor distribution to the left through primary prevention (the population approach) as well as secondary prevention in individuals at elevated risk. Much can be achieved through population-level interventions, such as tobacco control using education, legislation, and taxation. Nevertheless, the development and implementation of effective mass strategies for the prevention of CVD (and noncommunicable diseases more generally), and specifically strategies that address multiple risk factors, remains a challenging problem. **Table 4** lists ten behaviors for which there is a varying degree of epidemiological evidence of an association with lower rates of morbidity and mortality, principally from CVD and common cancers. For some of these, such as not being a smoker, there is ample evidence that the imprudent counterpart has a causal association with ill-health. For others, such as type of milk consumed, the significance may lie in indicating acceptance or nonacceptance of a broader message about reducing consumption of saturated fat. Importantly, no involvement of a health professional is required to assess these behaviors and many are potentially amenable to mass interventions. These behaviors are within the grasp of most individuals with adequate resources and supportive environments. In addition, once adopted, many can become permanent, even automatic parts of an individual's lifestyle. They become habits that are truly healthy and for which only very modest ongoing mental effort is required for their maintenance. For example, it is not a matter of permanently being on a diet, but one of having adopted a pattern of eating and drinking that is enjoyable but also consistent with best available medical knowledge and not conducive to gaining weight.

Several of the behaviors in **Table 4** are determinants of medically defined risk factors such as hypertension or hypercholesterolemia. A focus on the prudent lifestyle therefore addresses primary prevention and obviates the need for screening that is inherent in the high-risk approach (Rose, 1981). This distinction is in keeping with Rose's description of mass strategies as being radical, in the sense of preventing the development of risk, while

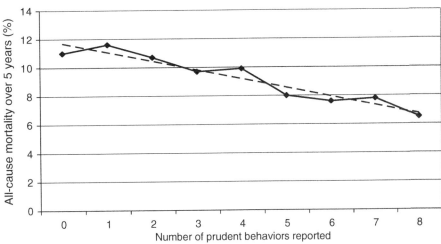

Figure 1   Five-year mortality (%) by Prudence Score in 12 203 men screened for abdominal aortic aneurysm. Reproduced with permission from Spencer CA, Jamrozik K, Norman PE, and Lawrence-Brown MM (2005) A simple lifestyle score predicts survival in healthy elderly men. *Preventive Medicine* 40: 712–717.

high-risk strategies are palliative, because they address risk that has become established (Rose, 1981).

While the components of a prudent lifestyle may be largely amenable to individual choice, many are also strongly affected by cultural norms (such as the Mediterranean diet), legislative controls (for example, on smoking), and environmental factors (for example, promoting opportunities for physical activity).

Prevalence of a Prudent Lifestyle

As part of the baseline assessment undertaken in the course of a population-based trial of screening for abdominal aortic aneurysm (AAA), Spencer *et al.* ascertained the adherence of 12 203 men aged 65–83 years to eight of the behaviors listed in **Table 4** (Spencer *et al.*, 2005). The resulting lifestyle scores, calculated as the simple sum of eight dichotomous answers, showed a bell-shaped distribution, indicating that the majority of these individuals already exhibited some health consciousness. By the same token, however, the majority also has scope to adopt additional elements of the prudent lifestyle. Combining these two interpretations suggests that most individuals have a base of health-related self-efficacy upon which they could draw when attempting to make changes to their lifestyle.

Prospective follow-up over 5 years of these men showed that, among those with no history of major cardiovascular events or angina, cumulative all-cause mortality decreased in an almost linear fashion from 12% among those with a lifestyle score of 0 to 6% among those with the maximum prudence score of 8 (see **Figure 1**) (Spencer *et al.*, 2005). When the data were divided at the median lifestyle score of 4, the lower half had a hazard ratio for all-cause mortality of 1.3 (95% CI, 1.1–1.5) relative to the

upper half. The findings in men with clinically evident vascular disease were similar. Thus the Prudence Score is not only simple to calculate, it also has considerable prognostic significance.

Conclusion

Atherosclerotic cardiovascular disease is the leading cause of death of humans. Our knowledge of factors contributing to the risk of CVD is both extensive and very detailed. We now understand that, for many of the important causal factors, risk rises progressively with the degree of exposure rather than exhibiting some sort of threshold. Thus, while easy to apply, clinical dichotomies between 'normal' and 'at risk' are simplistic and misleading. Further, there is abundant evidence from both observational studies and randomized trials that reducing levels of major modifiable factors is quickly followed by decreases in the incidence of major cardiovascular events. It follows that advice regarding prudent lifestyle and behavior in relation to risk of CVD is almost universally relevant and should not be delivered only to a selected subgroup of the population bearing a particularly adverse profile of risk factors. The pressing challenge is to broaden the understanding and application of this principle among both health professionals and policy makers; it is to apply better what we already know to control CVD in population, not to search for new risk factors.

> We have left undone those things which we ought to have done; and we have done those things which we ought not to have done; and there is no health in us.
>
> (Church of England, 1992)

Citations

Asia Pacific Cohort Studies Collaboration (Writing Committee: Patel A, Barzi F, Jamrozik K, Lam TH, Lawes C, Ueshima H, Whitlock G, Woodward M) (2004) Serum triglycerides as a risk factor for cardiovascular disease in the Asia Pacific region. *Circulation* 110: 2678–2686.

Baigent C, Keech A, Kearney PM, *et al.* (2005) Efficacy and safety of cholesterol-lowering treatment: Prospective meta-analysis of data from 90,056 participants in 14 randomised trials of statins. *Lancet* 366: 1267–1278.

Beaglehole R and Magnus P (2002) The search for new risk factors for coronary heart disease: Occupational therapy for epidemiologists? *International Journal of Epidemiology* 31: 1117–1122.

Blair SN, Cheng Y, and Holder JS (2001) Is physical activity or physical fitness more important in defining health benefits? *Medicine and Science in Sports and Exercise* 33(supplement 6): S379–S399.

Boushey CJ, Beresford SA, Omenn GS, and Motulsky AG (1995) A quantitative assessment of plasma homocysteine as a risk factor for vascular disease. Probable benefits of increasing folic acid intakes. *Journal of the American Medical Association* 274: 1049–1057.

Braunwald E (1997) Cardiovascular medicine at the turn of the millennium: Triumphs, concerns and opportunities. *New England Journal of Medicine* 337: 1360–1369.

Bunker SJ, Colquhoun DM, Esler MD, *et al.* (2003) "Stress" and coronary heart disease: Psychosocial risk factors. *Medical Journal of Australia* 178: 272–276.

Church of England (1992) *Book of Common Prayer.* Ebury.

Doll R, Peto R, Boreham J, and Sutherland I (2004) Mortality in relation to smoking: 50 years' observations on male British doctors. *British Medical Journal* 328: 1519.

Hemingway H and Marmot M (1999) Evidence-based cardiology: Psychosocial factors in the aetiology and prognosis of coronary heart disease. Systematic review of prospective cohort studies. *British Medical Journal* 318: 1460–1467.

Jamrozik K, Norman P, Spencer CA, *et al.* (2000) Screening for abdominal aortic aneurysm: Lessons from a population-based study. *Medical Journal of Australia* 173: 345–350.

Leone A (2007) Smoking, haemostatic factors, and cardiovascular risk. *Current Pharmaceutical Design* 13: 1661–1667.

MacMahon S, Peto R, Cutler J, *et al.* (1990) Blood pressure, stroke, and coronary heart disease. Part 1. Prolonged differences in blood pressure: Prospective observational studies corrected for the regression dilution bias. *Lancet* 335: 765–774.

Marmot M and Elliott P (eds.) (2005) *Coronary Heart Disease Epidemiology: From Aetiology to Public Health,* 2nd edn. Oxford, UK: Oxford University Press.

McElduff P and Dobson AJ (1997) How much alcohol and how often? Population-based case-control study of alcohol consumption and risk of a major coronary event. *British Medical Journal* 314: 1159–1164.

Misra A, Wasir JS, and Vikram NK (2005) Waist circumference criteria for the diagnosis of abdominal obesity are not applicable uniformly to all populations and ethnic groups. *Nutrition* 21: 969–976.

National Center for Chronic Disease Prevention and Health Promotion (1996) Physical activity and health: A report of the Surgeon General. Atlanta, GA: Centers for Disease Control and Prevention.

Paffenbarger RS, Hyde RT, Wing AL, and Steinmetz CH (1984) A natural history of athleticism and cardiovascular health. *Journal of the American Medical Association* 252: 491–495.

Rose G (1981) Strategy of prevention: Lessons from cardiovascular disease. *British Medical Journal* 282: 1847–1851.

Schmidt FB, Arnesen H, Christensen JH, Rasmussen LH, Kristensen SD, and De Caterina R (2005) Marine n-3 polyunsaturated fatty acids and coronary heart disease: Part II. Clinical trials and recommendations. *Thrombosis Research* 115: 257–262.

Smith SC, Jackson R, Pearson TA, *et al.* (2004) Principles for national and regional guidelines on cardiovascular disease prevention: A scientific statement from the World Heart and Stroke Forum. *Circulation* 109: 3112–3121.

Spencer CA, Jamrozik K, Norman PE, and Lawrence-Brown MM (2005) A simple lifestyle score predicts survival in healthy elderly men. *Preventive Medicine* 40: 712–717.

Stamler J, Wentworth D, and Neaton JD (1986) Is relationship between serum cholesterol and risk of premature death from coronary heart disease continuous and graded? Findings in 356,222 primary screenees of the Multiple Risk Factor Intervention Trial (MRFIT). *Journal of the American Medical Association* 256: 2823–2828.

Tunstall-Pedoe H (ed.) (2003) *MONICA Monograph and Multimedia Sourcebook.* Geneva, Switzerland: World Health Organization.

UK Prospective Diabetes Study (UKPDS) Group (1998) Intensive blood-glucose control with sulphonylureas or insulin compared with conventional treatment and risk of complications in patients with type 2 diabetes (UKPDS 33). *Lancet* 352: 837–853.

Vickers MR, MacLennan AH, Lawton B, *et al.* (2007) Main morbidities recorded in the women's international study of long duration oestrogen after menopause (WISDOM): A randomised controlled trial of hormone replacement therapy in postmenopausal women. *British Medical Journal* 335: 239–252.

Writing Group for the Women's Health Initiative Investigators (2002) Risks and benefits of estrogen plus progestin in healthy postmenopausal women: Principal results from the Women's Health Initiative randomized controlled trial. *Journal of the American Medical Association* 288: 321–333.

World Health Organization (2002) *The World Health Report 2002 – Reducing Risks and Promoting Healthy Life.* Geneva, Switzerland: World Health Organization.

Epidemic Investigation

E Mathieu, Centers for Disease Control and Prevention, Atlanta, GA, USA
Y Sodahlon, Mectizan Donation Program, Decatur, GA, USA

Published by Elsevier Inc.

Introduction

One of the key roles of public health is to manage outbreaks that endanger the public's health. The nature of an outbreak can range from infectious, zoonotic, or chronic diseases to injury, exposure to toxic substances, or health-damaging behavior. The cause can be incidental, accidental, or intentional, as in the case of a bioterrorism attack. Outbreaks require public health investigators to respond quickly and to make reasonable judgments from a dynamically unfolding set of information. Speed, coordination, and informed judgment are critical in these situations, as problems that at first appear limited may actually be significant outbreaks. A variety of approaches to outbreak detection and identification are possible, but the main points to keep in mind are described in the following section.

Outbreak Detection

An outbreak is traditionally characterized by an increasing number of persons who are showing a specific clinical pattern unusual for that particular situation or location. Public health concerns can range from two cases of Chagas' disease in a nonendemic area after organ transplantation to hundreds of cases of diarrhea due to a drinking water-related *Cryptosporidium* outbreak (MacKenzie *et al.*, 1994; Centers for Disease Control and Prevention [CDC], 2006).

Outbreaks can be detected in different ways. Thorough surveillance of diseases of public health importance forms the basis of public health investigations and research (**Figure 1**). Health departments can also be contacted by health professionals or members of communities (e.g., school, day care) where an unusual number of cases of a certain disease are noticed. One of the functions of a surveillance system is to monitor trends in a disease or other event. If there is an indication of a possible increase

in cases, rapid assessment is required and immediate action is recommended.

Measles surveillance is an example of intensive surveillance and rapid assessment of cases in the United States. Measles are currently very rare in the Western hemisphere: The number of reported cases between 1997 and 2004 was less than 200 per year (Atkinson *et al.*, 2007). This highly contagious disease is currently most common in the United States among persons that refuse vaccination for personal or religious reasons. Outbreaks are often related to the importation of a case from abroad that acts as a source case for an outbreak (Atkinson, 2007). In the United States, suspected measles cases have to be promptly reported to the CDC and to the National Notifiable Diseases Surveillance System (NNDSS), after which an investigation is launched (CDC, 2008).

To detect outbreaks in this way, the surveillance system has to be sensitive and the data have to be collected in a timely manner and regularly analyzed. To ensure that the surveillance system is able to detect cases in a timely fashion, the system itself has to be monitored. One indicator to follow in the measles surveillance system for example is the median interval between onset of rash and notification to the public health authority. This indicator measures the time lost to contain the spread of the infection. This is shown by a measles outbreak that occurred in the United States after a 34-year-old minister with an undocumented history of vaccination became infected while traveling abroad (Rooney *et al.*, 2004). The first symptoms were noticed in 1999 on September 2; the case was diagnosed on September 5 and the health department was informed on September 7. An epidemiologic and laboratory investigation identified 15 cases linked with the source case (**Figure 3**).

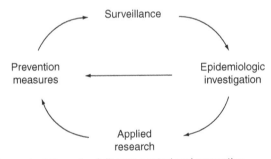

Figure 1   Life cycle of disease control and prevention.

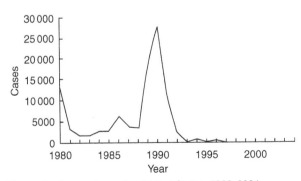

Figure 2   Cases of measles, United States, 1980–2004. Data from CDC Summary of Notifiable Diseases, available at http://www.cdc.gov/mmwr/PDF/wk/mm5653.pdf

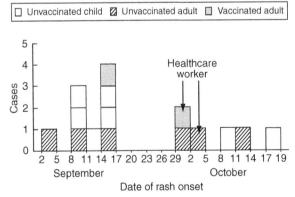

Figure 3   Epidemic curve depicting date of rash onset and vaccination status for case patients in measles outbreak, United States, September–October 1999. Reproduced from Rooney JA, Milton DJ, *et al.* (2004) The largest outbreak of measles in the United States during 1999: Imported measles and pockets of susceptibility. *Journal of Infectious Diseases* 189(supplement 1): S78–S80.

Another method of outbreak detection is through syndromic surveillance, which monitors nonspecific clinical syndromes. Once a possible outbreak is detected, a specific diagnosis is required to assess whether an outbreak has occurred. Since 1999, the New York City Department of Health has been monitoring and evaluating emergency medical service calls on a daily basis to identify an increase in respiratory illnesses that might represent an infectious disease outbreak (Mostashari *et al.*, 2003). This is also the recommended method to detect possible intentional outbreaks due to bioterrorism (CDC, 2003). Data sources used often already exist but have not been designed specifically for public health surveillance purposes. An example is the *International Classification of Diseases* (ICD-10), which contains coded health information from physician visit records. Data abstracted from emergency department logs or 911 calls can also be used through analysis of text or other developed coding systems (Pavlin *et al.*, 2003). In the case of a chemical agent, unexplained deaths among young or healthy persons or emission of unexplained odors by patients could indicate an outbreak.

Laboratory tests also play an important role. Cases are not always geographically clustered and for that reason are not always easily linked to an outbreak. The CDC and several state health departments established PulseNet, a molecular subtyping network for foodborne disease surveillance to facilitate the detection and investigation of foodborne outbreaks (Swaminathan *et al.*, 2001). Pulsed-field gel electrophoresis (PFGE) patterns of DNA from bacterial isolates are submitted to the national database and can help link apparently unrelated cases that are geographically dispersed. Though PulseNet can detect clusters of potentially related organisms, epidemiologic assessment is required to determine if the cluster contributes to an outbreak. PulseNet laboratories operate in public health departments in all 50 U.S. states and several national health and agriculture agencies. Most foodborne outbreaks are related to a local contamination such as in a restaurant, but a significant number are due to wide distribution of food contaminated at various points of production. An example is an *E. coli* O157 outbreak in 1992 linked with contaminated hamburgers that made more than 500 persons sick in 4 days and caused the deaths of four children (CDC, 1993). It took 39 days for the public health system to recognize it as an outbreak and another 10 days to investigate and institute a recall of the contaminated meat. PulseNet can now increase the sensitivity of outbreak detection in many instances. For example, in September 2006, state and CDC officials were able to detect and link multiple small clusters of *E. coli* O157:H7 infections across the United States within days using PulseNet information. This allowed investigators to rapidly identify fresh spinach as the source of infection (CDC, 2007). More than 200 cases were detected in 26 states and Canada (**Figure 4**).

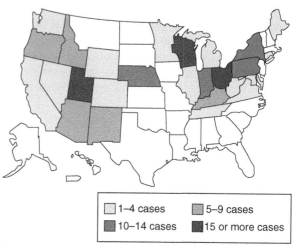

☐ 1–4 cases	▨ 5–9 cases
▩ 10–14 cases	■ 15 or more cases

Figure 4   Number of confirmed cases of *E. coli* O157:H7 by state, United States, October 2006. Reproduced from Centers for Disease Control and Prevention (2007b) Ongoing multistate outbreak of Escherichia coli serotype O157:H7 infections associated with consumption of fresh spinach – United States, September 2006. *MMWR Morbidity and Mortality Weekly Report* 55.

Organizing an Outbreak Investigation

Once an outbreak is identified, epidemiologic assessment assistance is started by a local public health authority, such as the health department. Depending on the context, other hierarchies or special jurisdictions are involved such as the World Health Organization (WHO) for an international investigation (Gregg, 1996). In the case of an international investigation, the World Health Organization (WHO) is often involved. The WHO coordinates the Global Outbreak Alert and Response Network (GOARN). This is a technical collaboration of existing institutions and networks that pool human and technical resources for rapid identification, confirmation, and response to outbreaks of international importance.

As soon as a response is initiated, it is important to inform public health authorities at appropriate government levels about the ongoing outbreak. Local and reference laboratories must be informed so that they can prepare for processing specimens (see the section 'Laboratory preparations'). A core team should be assembled made up of persons with epidemiologic, laboratory, communications, and possibly other expertise, such as statistical expertise. This core team should establish a hierarchy for decision and information sharing. They should then create objectives for the investigation and develop plans for reevaluating the objectives as the investigation evolves. It is important to delineate roles and responsibilities for the relevant agencies and to agree on a timeline for reevaluating those roles. A lead agency and principal investigator should be identified. In the case of a large, complex outbreak, the need for additional human resources also has to be discussed. A list of types of expertise (e.g., epidemiologic, laboratory, statistical, communications) is required and availability of experts should be made known so that any gaps in expertise can be filled.

Laboratory Preparations

An important aspect of preparing an outbreak investigation is the logistics involved in conducting laboratory or environmental testing. This includes not only collecting and testing the specimens, but also tracking and monitoring the shipments of specimens. Some of this responsibility falls within the laboratory domain, but field investigators may also have to undertake some of these functions. The first step is to develop specimen collection and shipping protocols. This includes information about the samples that have to be included, such as type, quantity, and timing vis-à-vis disease onset and treatment, but also the type of containers, transport media, and preservatives needed. The protocol must address information to be included on the labels, pre-shipping requirements, and instructions for shipping.

The next step is to develop specimen processing and testing protocols for the receiving laboratories. These include not only the tests each laboratory will conduct but also how the results will be determined and interpreted and how and to whom the results will be released. If indicated, obtain the materials and supplies such as collection kits, testing reagents, control specimens, labels, and shipping supplies and ship it to the outbreak location. Once the specimens are collected, it is important to label them well and track them. In October 2001, a bioterrorism-related anthrax outbreak in New York City occurred. For weeks the New York Bioterrorism Response Laboratory (BTRL) was overwhelmed by the increasing number of environmental samples. To deal with the situation, a laboratory bioterrorism command center was established and protocols for sample intake, processing, reporting, security, testing, staffing, and quality control were developed (Heller et al., 2002). The specimen load increased from 1 every 2 to 3 months to 2700 nasal swabs in 2 weeks and 3200 environmental specimens in 2 months. Staff increased from 2 to 75 persons and 6 tons of laboratory supplies were flown in from the CDC. **Figure 5** shows the data flowchart adopted soon after the surge of isolates after the bioterrorism attack.

Objectives for an Investigation

In most cases, an investigation is initiated to limit the spread of a particular illness. Through identification of the cause, source, and mode of transmission, public health measures can be taken to stop the expansion of the outbreak. On October 8, 2000 the Acting District Director of Health Services in Gulu District, Uganda, received two reports concerning unusual illness and deaths (Lamunu et al., 2004). One day later, an outbreak investigation was launched and 2 days later the first interventions to contain the outbreak were instituted: An isolation unit was set up in the local health-care facility, protective material for health staff was dispatched, and the public was alerted of the risk of infection during funerals. On October 14, the National Ebola Task Force was constituted to coordinate and mobilize resources for the outbreak, which lasted for more than four months. A total of 425 confirmed cases of Ebola were recorded, with 224 deaths among them.

Identification of the origin or source of the disease by a trace back environmental investigation to prevent further illness is another important aspect of an outbreak investigation. This was done during a multicluster outbreak in Massachusetts. Between February 2003 and May 2004, ten outbreaks of gastrointestinal illness among schoolchildren at nine different schools were reported to the Department of Public Health (CDC, 2006). All the children ate lunch provided by the schools and the disease was characterized by short incubation periods and short durations of illness. Based on prior investigations, a biotoxin or chemical agent was suspected. An environmental investigation identified three distributors who provided the schools with tortillas of different sizes and under various brand names but from one manufacturer. Several deficiencies at the plant were noted such as improper storage, use, and labeling of chemicals, food ingredients and additives, and food contact surfaces were not protected from environmental contamination. Samples were collected and analyzed. After the manufacturer was informed about the suspected cause of the outbreak, the recipe was changed and the amount of calcium propionate and potassium bromate used was lowered (CDC, 2006).

Outbreak investigations can also lead to national policy and regulatory changes. In the fall of 1996, 70 cases of E. coli O157:H7 infections were epidemiologically linked to a particular brand of unpasteurized apple juice in Canada; four persons developed hemolytic uremic syndrome, and one person died (Cody et al., 1999). Recalled apple juice grew E. coli O157:H7 with the same PFGE pattern as those from the case isolates. The magnitude and severity of this outbreak led the Food and Drug Administration (FDA) to propose two new regulations (Troxell, 2005). First, all unpasteurized fruit and vegetable juices would have to carry a label stating, "Warning: this product has not been pasteurized and therefore may contain harmful bacteria that can cause serious illness in children, elderly, and persons with weakened immune systems." The second regulation is the application of Hazard Analysis and Critical Control Point (HACCP) principles

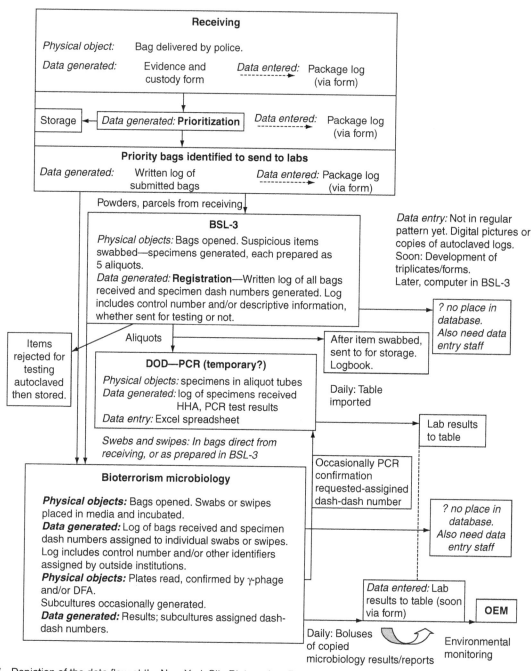

Figure 5 Depiction of the data flow at the New York City Bioterrorism Response Laboratory adopted soon after a surge of isolates after a bioterrorism attack, New York City, 2001. BSL: Biosafety Level; DOD: Department of Defense; OEM: Office of Emergency Management. Reproduced from Heller MB, Bunning ML, France ME, et al. (2002) Laboratory response to anthrax bioterrorism, New York City, 2001. *Emerging Infectious Diseases* 8(10): 1096–1102.

to fruit and vegetable juice processing (see the section 'Relevant Websites'). A HACCP program is a systematic method of identifying key production steps in which contamination may occur and instituting specific monitoring and interventions, such as pasteurization, at those steps.

Outbreaks also provide a natural, observational laboratory for evaluating and identifying defects in public health and regulatory programs.

Confirmation of an Outbreak

The first step in an investigation is to confirm the outbreak. The total number of cases is less relevant than analysis of the whole situation. The critical question is: Are there really more cases of a certain disease than normally expected in that time and location? In 1999, two cases of *Plasmodium vivax* in the United States among children without travel exposure to an endemic area were the cause of an epidemiologic, entomologic, and environmental outbreak investigation in Suffolk County, New York (CDC, 2000).

Surveillance data can indicate if there is an outbreak, but an increase in the number of reports of a certain disease can be due to several factors, including a random increase in the number of cases, a higher awareness of the disease, a new diagnostic tool, a misdiagnosis, or a change in reporting requirements or forms. For this reason it is important to collect preliminary demographic, geographic, and epidemiologic information to link the cases. When in doubt, one should treat the cases as an outbreak but avoid labeling them before possessing appropriate scientific evidence.

Although incubation periods and clinical syndromes are important as an indication of the source, it is recommended that the diagnosis be confirmed by laboratory tests. While it is often not necessary to confirm the diagnosis for all cases, in the initial phase of an outbreak, the diagnosis of a substantial proportion of the cases should be confirmed. The CDC published a table with possible etiologies of foodborne disease outbreaks and defined an outbreak as an incident in which two or more persons experience a similar illness resulting from the ingestion of a common food (CDC, 2007a). The table includes not only information about incubation periods and clinical syndromes, but also describes the laboratory tests needed to confirm the outbreak etiology.

Confirming an outbreak or its extent may also require active case finding. For example, in a recent outbreak of *Acanthamoeba* keratitis (AK), the Illinois Department of Public Health investigated a possible increase in AK at one ophthalmology center during the previous 3 years. As a result, the CDC initiated a retrospective survey of 22 ophthalmology centers nationwide to assess whether cases were increasing throughout the United States. Data received from 13 centers demonstrated an increase in culture-confirmed cases of AK across the United States. This triggered a large, multistate investigation at the national level (CDC, 2007).

Case Definition

One of the most important steps in an outbreak investigation is to develop the case definition. The definition has to be broad enough to capture most if not all cases but should not be so vague that every possible sick person in the targeted location is included. This balance is not always easy to achieve. One solution is to start with a very sensitive but less specific case definition based on preliminary information, which is then adapted after more information is collected and the etiology of the outbreak is clearer.

A case definition always includes information about three factors: person, time, and place. Person-related information includes symptoms, but also demographic information such as gender, age, or profession. There are several possible ways to approach defining symptoms. A case can be defined as having a few symptoms present for each case, or one can give a list and specify a minimum number of symptoms for a case to be included, or a combination of both can be used. If the symptoms are very common, such as cough or diarrhea, or very vague, such as fatigue, many unrelated background cases can be unintentionally included. As a result, the case definition tends to become more stringent in the later stages of an outbreak and includes a specific etiologic diagnosis if possible.

The time and place definition is used to ensure that only cases related with this outbreak are included. In the case of an outbreak, one is not interested in cases throughout the whole country or during the whole year. An example is the case definition used in the previously mentioned *Cryptosporidium* outbreak: "a person who lived in or visited central Ohio between June 17 and August 18, 2000 and who had three or more loose stools in a 24-hour period" (Mathieu *et al.*, 2004: 582). In the same investigation, a laboratory-confirmed case patient was defined as "a person who lived in or visited central Ohio between June 17 and August 18, 2000, who had a positive stool test result for *C. parvum,* along with either diarrhea (three or more loose stools during a 24-hour period), vomiting or abdominal cramps" (Mathieu *et al.*, 2004: 583).

Case Ascertainment

There should be an active search for cases that fall within the case definition as soon as there is suspicion of an outbreak. If the case definition includes laboratory confirmation, all the labs in the area should be contacted and probed for information. If the case is associated with a school or a certain community, messages can be passed through school authorities or the media to ask persons with certain symptoms to inform their local health department. In the case of an outbreak linked to a particular venue, a list of persons who attended a particular event can be obtained. By way of a short questionnaire, crucial information, including contact information, date of onset, and some questions related to the possible source of the outbreak should be collected from each person who could be considered a potential case. This information can be used to create a line listing, which is a table that includes key variables on each ill person (**Table 1**) (CDC, 2004). This makes it easy to visualize and summarize important information and to establish a hypothesis for the outbreak by identifying commonalities among the cases.

Table 1   A line listing for a possible hepatitis outbreak (CDC, 2004)

Case#	Initials	Date of report	Date of onset	Physician diagnosis	N	V	A	F	DU	J	HAIgM	Other	Age	Sex
												Lab		
							Signs and symptoms							
1	JG	10/12	12/6	Hep A	+	+	+	+	+	+	+	SGOT ↓	37	M
2	BC	10/12	10/5	Hep A	+	−	+	+	+	+	+	Alt ↓	62	F
3	HP	10/13	10/4	Hep A	±	−	+	+	+	S*	+	SGOT ↓	30	F
4	MC	10/15	10/4	Hep A	−	−	+	+	?	−	+	Hbs/Ag−	17	F

S*, Sclera; N, Nausea; V, Vomiting; A, Anorexia; F, Fever; DU, Dark urine; J, Jaundice; HAIgm, Hepatitis AIgM antibody test.
Centers for Disease Control and Prevention (2004) *Epidemiology in the Classroom: How to Investigate an Outbreak: Steps of an Outbreak Investigation.* http://www.cdc.gov/excite/classrom/outbreak/.

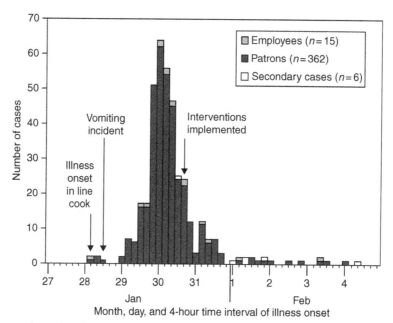

Figure 6   Number of cases of norovirus illness by 4-hour intervals of illness onset, among patrons and employees of a restaurant, Eaton County, Michigan, January 28–February 4, 2006. Reproduced from Centers for Disease Control and Prevention (2007) Norovirus outbreak associated with ill food-service workers – Michigan, January–February 2006. *MMWR Morbidity and Mortality Weekly Report* 56(46): 1212–1216.

Descriptive Epidemiology

An important part of the descriptive epidemiology of an outbreak is the epicurve, which will not only indicate when the outbreak started but may also provide clues to the source of the exposure. Traditionally, the number of cases is depicted on the y-axis and time on the x-axis. The time interval chosen can be months, weeks, days, or hours, depending on the estimated incubation period. Traditionally, the time intervals are one-fourth to one-third of the probable incubation period. An epicurve allows visualization of the epidemic's magnitude and the trend over time, and can predict the end of an epidemic.

The curve also helps to estimate the incubation time, which can assist in defining the causative agent. An outbreak with a point source in time and place will give a tight temporal clustering of cases. An example is a norovirus outbreak in the United States linked with a specific restaurant in Eaton County, Michigan, in February 2007. The epicurve shown in **Figure 6** reveals a peak in onset of disease around January 30 and a median incubation time of 32 hours. Investigation showed that more than 360 restaurant patrons became ill after eating in the restaurant on 2 consecutive days (CDC, 2007c). If there is person-to-person transmission, each case can cause more cases, shown on the curve as a series of successive peaks.

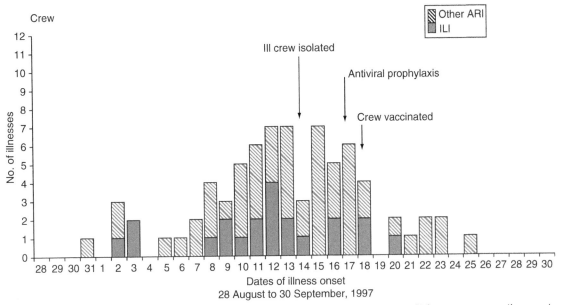

Figure 7 Number of medically attended respiratory illnesses (ARI) and influenza-like illnesses (ILI) among crew on three cruises of one ship during August and September 1997, by date of onset. Reproduced from Miller JM, Tam TWS, *et al.* (2000) Cruise ships: High-risk passengers and the global spread of new influenza viruses. *Clinical Infectious Diseases* 31(2): 433–438.

In 1997, passengers and crew members on a cruise ship developed acute respiratory illnesses possibly due to influenza (Miller *et al.*, 2000). The epicurve of the outbreak among the crew members is shown in **Figure 7**. If the source is intermittent or continues over a long period of time, the curve will show a mix of individual and clustered cases during a relatively protracted time frame.

Description of the geographic distribution of an outbreak provides information about the extent of the problem and can show any clustering or patterns that might provide more information on the source. Depending on the situation, cases can be mapped according to residence, place of occupation, and school or childcare settings, or related to possible relevant activities such as swimming or grocery shopping. A classic example is the map John Snow made to trace the source of a cholera outbreak in Soho, England, in 1854 (**Figure 8**) (Snow, 1855).

Another aspect of the descriptive epidemiology of an outbreak is the characterization of cases. Depending on the outbreak etiology and source, variables used to characterize the cases can include age, sex, race, occupation, leisure activities, health status, and drug use. The purpose is to identify common potential risk factors among cases.

Hypothesis

Based on the potential etiologic agents and vehicles, potential mode of transmission, types of exposure, population exposed, and timing and extent of exposure, hypotheses

can be developed. This information is collected through the descriptive epidemiology and line listing as mentioned previously; however, in some cases, in-depth interviews with a limited number of suspect cases may also be indicated.

Testing of the Hypothesis

The next step is to design the appropriate study to test the hypothesis. The purpose is to assess and quantify the relationship between an exposure and the outbreak-related event. Even if the hypothesis seems easy to accept, a study must be considered (Reingold, 1998). In case there are several possible exposures linked with the outbreak, all exposures must be tested. The general idea is to compare observed outbreak data with data collected from a comparison group that provides baseline or 'expected' data (Gregg, 1996). If the outbreak occurred in a well-defined population, a cohort study is recommended; otherwise, a case-control study is conducted.

In a cohort study, the occurrence of an event is compared among persons who were and were not exposed to a certain risk factor. The advantage of a cohort study is that attack rates and relative risk can be directly calculated. This design better suits outbreaks in which a limited and identifiable number of people were exposed to the risk factor or where one risk factor can have different outcomes. A typical example is a food-related outbreak at an event with a known guest list such as a wedding. People attending the event are asked if they became ill (thus meeting the case definition)

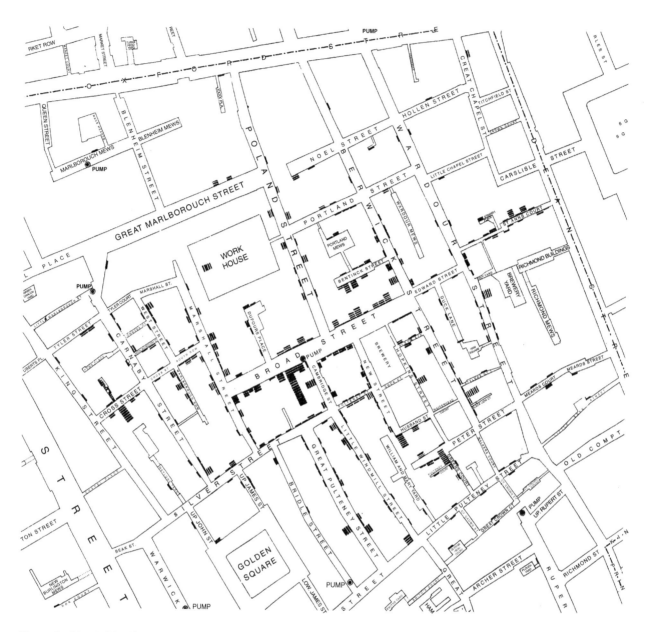

Figure 8   Map to identify cause of cholera outbreak, Soho, England, 1854. Reproduced from Snow J (1855) *On the Mode of Communication of Cholera.* London: John Churchill (available at http://www.ph.ucla.edu.epi/snow/snowmap1_1854_lge.htm).

but also which dishes they ate. This enables the investigators to calculate attack rates of disease among people who ate from certain dishes. The attack rate is the incidence of disease in a defined group.

$$\text{Attack rate}_{\text{exposed}} = \frac{\text{\# of people exposed to a factor who became ill}}{\text{\# of people exposed to a risk factor}}$$

$$\text{Attack rate}_{\text{unexposed}} = \frac{\text{\# of people unexposed to a factor who became ill}}{\text{\# of people unexposed to a risk factor}}$$

The relative risk qualifies the relationship between the risk factor and the outbreak-related disease. It indicates how much more likely a person who is exposed to a certain risk factor is to develop the outbreak-related illness compared with a person who was not exposed. **Table 2** shows the data of a classic outbreak investigation related to a salmonellosis outbreak at a church dinner in Oswego, New York, in 1940 (CDC, 2004). The relative risk related to ice cream was much higher than those of other food items, indicating that the outbreak was related to the ice cream.

Table 2 Number of ill and healthy people who ate certain food items, attack rates, and relative risk for each food item – outbreak of salmonellosis, Oswego, New York, 1940

	Number of persons who ate item			Number of persons who did not eat item			
	Ill	Total	Attack rate%	Ill	Total	Attack rate	Relative risk
Baked ham	29	46	63	17	29	59	1.07
Spinach	26	43	60	20	32	62	0.97
Potatoes	23	37	62	23	37	62	1.00
Jells	16	23	70	30	52	58	1.21
Rolls	21	37	57	25	38	66	0.86
Coffee	19	31	61	27	44	61	1.00
Cake	27	40	68	19	35	54	1.26
Ice cream	43	54	80	3	21	14	5.71[a]

[a]$p < 0.001$.

Centers for Disease Control and Prevention, steps of an outbreak investigation, (available at: http://www.cdc.gov/excite/classroom/outbreak/steps.htm (accessed June, 2008)).

The relative risk is calculated by the ratio of the attack rates:

$$\text{Relative risk} = \frac{\text{attack rate among the people exposed to the risk factor}}{\text{attack rate among the people not exposed to the risk factor}}$$

$$\text{Relative risk} = (a/H_1)/(c/H_0)$$

	Ill	Well	
Exposed	a	b	H_1
Unexposed	c	d	H_0
Total	V_1	V_0	T

A relative risk of 1 means that the risk of illness is the same among exposed and nonexposed persons and that the exposure is not associated with the event. A relative risk greater than 1 means that the risk of illness is greater among exposed than among nonexposed persons and that the exposure could be associated with the event. A relative risk smaller than 1 means that the risk of illness is smaller among exposed than among nonexposed persons and that the exposure could be protective.

A case-control study design compares past exposures among people who have ('cases') and do not have ('controls') the outbreak-related illness. Continuing with the wedding example, in the case of a foodborne outbreak, sick and healthy attendees are questioned about the dishes they consumed. Exposures to the factor of interest are compared for the cases and controls. If the exposure to the factor is the same in the two groups, it is unlikely that that factor caused the outbreak-related event. A case-control study requires fewer financial and human resources. This design is also better if multiple exposures are related to the outbreak. The measure of association between exposure and disease is quantified by an odds ratio that is the ratio of the odds of a certain outcome. It is often used as an approximation for the relative risk. Using the data layout and notation mentioned above:

$$\text{Odds ratio} = ad/bc$$

An important activity in designing a case-control study is the selection of controls. Controls provide information about the estimated exposure that is expected in the studied population if the exposure was not related to the illness in question. Controls must be selected independently from their exposure status, representative of the population in question, and should have the potential to be exposed to the risk factor without having the disease in question. An example is a large hepatitis A outbreak that occurred among patrons in a Pennsylvania restaurant (Wheeler *et al.*, 2005). For the case-control study, 240 cases, as many as could be interviewed in a 2-week time period, were included. The 130 controls included meal companions of patients or persons who were identified through credit card receipts as having dined in the restaurant during a certain time period. Controls were excluded if they reported having symptoms or a history of acute hepatitis A or were vaccinated for hepatitis A. In March 2003, a nosocomial outbreak of severe acute respiratory syndrome (SARS) occurred in a hospital in Singapore (Teleman *et al.*, 2004). To investigate factors associated with the transmission of SARS, a case-control study was conducted with 36 cases and 50 controls. The controls were selected among health-care workers working in the same ward as the cases, but who did not develop the disease although they had a history of exposure (exposure defined as being within close physical proximity [1m] of a patient subsequently confirmed with SARS).

As the previous examples show, controls can be selected among different population groups, depending on the outbreak. In a community outbreak, a random sample of the healthy population may, in theory, be the best control group. In practice, however, persons in a random sample may be difficult to contact and enroll. Often random digit dialing is used, though this method has a potential for selection bias (Bunin *et al.*, 2007).

The number of controls depends on the required precision and the number of cases. If there are more than 50 cases, one control can be selected for each case. If there are fewer cases, two or three controls per case may be needed to obtain sufficient statistical power to identify significant association.

Results from case-control and cohort studies have to be interpreted with caution as much will depend on the sample size and the related precision of the outcome. Tests of statistical significance must be used to determine the probability that an observed relative risk could have been found due to chance alone. This probability is called the *p*-value. A very small *p*-value means that the chances of finding relative risk due to chance alone are very small. If the *p*-value is smaller than a predetermined cutoff, often 0.05, the relative risk is considered statistically significant. The most used statistical test is the X^2:

$$X^2 = \frac{T(|ad - bc| - (T/2))^2}{V_1 \times V_0 \times H_1 \times H_0}$$

(The corresponding *p*-value for the chi-square can be found in a chi-square distribution table.)

Communication

From the time a possible outbreak is detected until it is under control, communication is very important. The amount of information to be shared is crucial, as well as the method of communication to the right persons and groups at the right time. During the investigation, the epidemiologist should maintain regular briefings with local health officials. However, communication with the public is just as crucial. Often one person will be designated to communicate with the press and public. The content, frequency, and form of communication (e.g., internal meetings, email, press releases, or press conferences) have to be adapted to the target audience. The need to protect the public's health as well as innocent stakeholders who may or may not be responsible for the outbreak must be carefully balanced. As much specific information as is possible and appropriate about etiologic agents, mode of transmission, source and mode of contamination, and interventions and prevention measures should be provided.

Although the need for communication with the public is important, communication with other agencies implicated in the investigation must not be overlooked. There exist several ways to inform public health professionals about ongoing outbreaks. An example is Epi-X, a web-based system that enables state and local health departments, poison control centers, and other public health professionals to access and share preliminary health surveillance information. Health Alert Network provides health information and

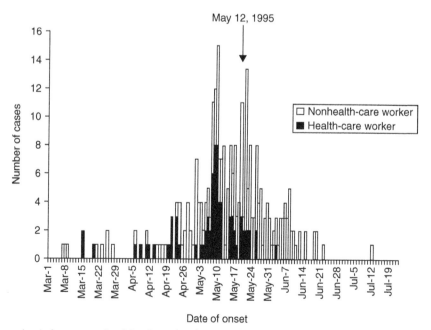

Figure 9 Ebola hemorrhagic fever cases by date of onset and occupation, Bandundu region, Democratic Republic of the Congo, March 1 to July 21, 1995. The arrow indicates date of initiation of upgraded infection control practices. Reproduced from Khan *et al.*, for the Commission de Lutte contre les Epidémies à Kikwit (1999) The reemergence of Ebola hemorrhagic fever, Democratic Republic of the Congo, 1995. *Journal of Infectious Diseases* 179(supplement 1): S76–S86.

Table 3 Distribution scheme for protective equipment initially used in care of patients with Ebola hemorrhagic fever, Bandundu region, Democratic Republic of the Congo, 1995

Individuals involved with	Isolation ward			Burial	Emergency ward	Health center	Home visitor	Home health-care giver
	Isolation	Cleaning	'Garde malade'[a]					
Protective equipment								
Plastic goggles	X	X	X	X				
Surgical mask with HEPA filter	X	X	X	X				
Disposable surgical mask					X	X	X	
Disposable gloves	X	X	X	X	X	X		
Surgical cap	X	X		X				
Long-sleeved surgical blouse (cotton)	X	X	X	X	X	X		
Surgical trousers (cotton)	X	X		X				
Long plastic aprons (multiple use)	X	X	X	X	X			
Rubber boots		X		X				
Rubber kitchen gloves		X		X				X
Burial								
Body bags				X		X		
Disinfectant and other material								
Hypochlorite		X		X	X	X		
Chloramine tablets			X			X		X
Jerrycan, 20 L						X		X
Plastic basin						X		X
Soap		X		X	X	X		X
Plastic container (100 L) with tap		X				X		
Sprayer		X		X				

[a]Relative taking care of patient.
Reproduced from Kerstiëns B and Matthys F (1999) Interventions to control virus transmission during an outbreak of Ebola hemorrhagic fever: Experience from Kikwit, Democratic Republic of the Congo, 1995. *Journal of Infectious Diseases* 179(supplement 1): S263–S267.

has the infrastructure to support the dissemination of that information at the state and local levels in the United States.

Completion of an Investigation

At the end of the investigation, investigators should present findings to local health authorities responsible for implementing control and prevention measures. In addition to an oral briefing, a scientific written report documenting the investigation should be presented. This report can also serve as reference for similar situations in the future and should include all details of the investigation, conclusions, and recommendations.

It is important to discuss at the beginning of the investigation what must occur following the outbreak investigation. One of the most important steps is to conduct a 'lessons learned' meeting and to communicate this information to all partners. These findings should be written in a report and if appropriate, published. In this way, the international scientific community can be aware of lessons learned.

Related Issue: Protection of Investigators

In the case of investigation of lethal and easily transmitted disease, the necessary precaution measures must be undertaken to protect health staff and outbreak investigators, because they are vulnerable to contracting the disease in question. During the Ebola outbreak in Kikwit, Democratic Republic of Congo, in 1995, 80 of the 315 laboratory-confirmed cases were in health-care workers (Khan *et al.*, 1999). Only one health-care worker developed the disease after the implementation of personal preventive measures (**Figure 9**). Among the protective equipment were disposable gloves, different types of surgical masks, long-sleeved blouses, and boots (**Table 3**) (Kerstiens and Matthys, 1999).

See also: Clinical Epidemiology; Demography, Epidemiology and Public Health; Disease Classification; Surveillance of Disease.

Citations

Atkinson WHJ, McIntyre L, and Wolfe S (eds.) (2007) *Epidemiology and Prevention of Vaccine-Preventable Diseases.* Washington, DC: Public Health Foundation.

Bunin GR, Spector LG, *et al.* (2007) Secular trends in response rates for controls selected by random digit dialing in childhood cancer studies: A report from the Children's Oncology Group. *American Journal of Epidemiology* 166(1): 109–116.

Centers for Disease Control and Prevention (1993) Update: Multistate outbreak of *Escherichia coli* O157:H7 infections from hamburgers – Western United States, 1992–1993. *MMWR Morbidity and Mortality Weekly Report* 42(14): 258–263.

Centers for Disease Control and Prevention (2000) Probable locally acquired mosquito-transmitted plasmodium vivax infection – Suffolk County, New York, 1999. *MMWR Morbidity and Mortality Weekly Report* 49(22): 495–498.

Centers for Disease Control and Prevention (2003) Syndrome definitions for diseases associated with critical bioterrorism-associated agents. http://www.bt.cdc.gov/surveillance/syndromedef/index.asp (accessed January 2008).

Centers for Disease Control and Prevention (2006) Chagas' disease after organ transplantation – Los Angeles, California, 2006. *MMWR Morbidity and Mortality Weekly Report* 55(29): 798–800.

Centers for Disease Control and Prevention (2006) Multiple outbreaks of gastrointestinal illness among school children associated with consumption of flour tortillas – Massachusetts, 2003–2004. *MMWR Morbidity and Mortality Weekly Report* 55(1): 8–11.

Centers for Disease Control and Prevention (2007a) Guide to confirming a diagnosis in foodborne disease. http://www.cdc.gov/foodborneoutbreaks/guide_fd.htm (accessed January 2008).

Centers for Disease Control and Prevention (2007c) Norovirus outbreak associated with ill food-service workers – Michigan, January–February 2006. *MMWR Morbidity and Mortality Weekly Report* 56(46): 1212–1216.

Centers for Disease Control and Prevention (2008) Measles, mumps, and rubella – vaccine use and strategies for elimination of measles, rubella, and congenital rubella syndrome and control of mumps: Recommendations of the Advisory Committee on Immunization Practices (ACIP). *MMWR Morbidity and Mortality Weekly Report* May 22, 1998/47(RR-8): 1–57.

Cody SH, Glynn MK, *et al.* (1999) An outbreak of Escherichia coli O157:H7 infection from unpasteurized commercial apple juice. *Annals of Internal Medicine* 130(3): 202–209.

Gregg M (1996) *Field Epidemiology.* New York: Oxford, Oxford University Press.

Heller MB, Bunning ML, France ME, *et al.* (2002) Laboratory response to anthrax bioterrorism, New York City, 2001. *Emerging Infectious Diseases* 8(10): 1096–1102.

Khan AS, Tshioko FK, Heymann DL, *et al.* (1999) The reemergence of Ebola hemorrhagic fever, Democratic Republic of the Congo, 1995. *Journal of Infectious Diseases* 179(supplement 1): S76–S86.

Kerstiëns B and Matthys F (1999) Interventions to control virus transmission during an outbreak of Ebola hemorrhagic fever: Experience from Kikwit, Democratic Republic of the Congo, 1995. *Journal of Infectious Diseases* 179(supplement 1): S263–S267.

Lamunu M, Lutwama JJ, *et al.* (2004) Containing a haemorrhagic fever epidemic: The Ebola experience in Uganda (October 2000–January 2001). *International Journal of Infectious Diseases* 8(1): 27–37.

MacKenzie WJ, Hoxie NJ, *et al.* (1994) A massive outbreak in Milwaukee of cryptosporidium infection transmitted through the public water supply. *New England Journal of Medicine* 331(3): 161–167.

Mathieu E, Levy DA, *et al.* (2004) Epidemiologic and environmental investigation of a recreational water outbreak caused by two genotypes of Cryptosporidium parvum in Ohio in 2000. *American Journal of Tropical Medicine and Hygiene* 71(5): 582–589.

Miller JM, Tam TWS, *et al.* (2000) Cruise ships: High-risk passengers and the global spread of new influenza viruses. *Clinical Infectious Diseases* 31(2): 433–438.

Mostashari F, Fine A, Das D, Adams J, and Layton M (2003) Use of ambulance dispatch data as an early warning system for community-wide influenza-like illness, New York City. *Journal of Urban Health* 80(supplement 1): i43–i49.

Pavlin JA, Mostashari F, *et al.* (2003) Innovative surveillance methods for rapid detection of disease outbreaks and bioterrorism: Results of an interagency workshop on health indicator surveillance. *American Journal of Public Health* 93(8): 1230–1235.

Reingold AAL (1998) Outbreak investigations – a perspective. *Emerging Infectious Diseases* 4(1): 21–27.

Rooney JA, Milton DJ, *et al.* (2004) The largest outbreak of measles in the United States during 1999: Imported measles and pockets of susceptibility. *Journal of Infectious Diseases* 189(supplement 1): S78–S80.

Snow J (1855) *On the Mode of Communication of Cholera.* London: John Churchill.

Swaminathan B, Barrett TJ, *et al.* (2001) PulseNet: The molecular subtyping network for foodborne bacterial disease surveillance, United States. *Emerging Infectious Diseases* 7(3): 382–389.

Teleman MD, Boudville IC, *et al.* (2004) Factors associated with transmission of severe acute respiratory syndrome among health-care workers in Singapore. *Epidemiology and Infection* 132(5): 797–803.

Troxell T (2005) Letter to state regulatory agencies and firms that produce treated (but not pasteurized) and untreated juice and cider. U.S. Department of Health and Human Services Food and Drug Administration, and Center for Food Safety and Applied Nutrition. http://www.cfsan.fda.gov/mdms/juicgul4.html.

Wheeler C, Vogt TM, *et al.* (2005) An outbreak of hepatitis A associated with green onions. *New England Journal of Medicine* 353(9): 890–897.

Further Reading

Gregg M (1996) *Field Epidemiology.* New York: Oxford, Oxford University Press.

Reingold AAL (1998) Outbreak investigations – A perspective. *Emerging Infectious Diseases* 4(1): 21–27.

Centers for Disease Control and Prevention *Principles of Epidemiology.*

Relevant Websites

http://www.cdc.gov/epix – Epi-X: The Epidemic Information Exchange (CDC).

http://www.who.int/csr/outbreaknetwork/en – Global Outbreak Alert and Response Network (WHO).

http://www.cfsan.fda.gov/~lrd/haccp.html – Hazard Analysis and Critical Control Point (HACCP).

http://www2a.cdc.gov/HAN – Health Alert Network (CDC).

http://www.cdc.gov/mmwr – Morbidity and Mortality Weekly Report (MMWR).

http://www.bt.cdc.gov/surveillance/syndromedef/index.asp – Syndrome Definitions for Diseases Associated with Critical Bioterrorism-associated Agents (CDC).

Governance of Epidemics: Trust and Health Consensus Building*

Stella R Quah, Duke-NUS Graduate Medical School, Singapore

In a free society organized along democratic principles, *governance* refers to the management of the affairs of the collective to ensure safety, fairness, and equality of opportunity for all its individual members. Social science and medical research indicate that epidemics test a society's governance effectiveness by endangering the lives of individuals, families, and entire communities (Whitman, 2000: 6–10; Taylor, 2002: 976–77; Blumenthal and Hsiao, 2005; Patterson and London, 2002; Haines *et al.*, 2004; Fidler, 2004a). HIV/AIDS and SARS are two of the major infectious disease epidemics we face today. The contrast between these two epidemics offers a singular lesson in public health governance for nations around the world. If the current avian influenza outbreak becomes a human epidemic, we will be preparing for a third major health crisis. It is timely, then, to learn as much as we can from the successes and failures in the governance of HIV/AIDS and SARS.

The governance of epidemics must be carefully scrutinized from both macro-(community) and micro-level (individual) perspectives. Examining micro-level data, I have discussed elsewhere (Quah, 2007) how the individual's perception of disease severity and of his/her own susceptibility to the disease help to shape the public image of HIV/AIDS and SARS. These two elements in turn help to explain the differing prevention effectiveness of the two diseases. In this chapter, I follow a macro-level perspective to address another major factor in the governance of epidemics: the need to nurture public consensus or "collective informed consent" on the nature of the problem and the range of solutions available. I would argue that the presence of collective informed consent is a crucial prerequisite for the successful governance of epidemics. Here, I propose and explore four major factors that influence the presence of collective informed consent. The first and most immediate factor is the level of community's trust in the health authorities' expertise and integrity to solve health crises fairly and successfully. The level of trust, in turn, is influenced by three other factors: the transparency of state's actions and decision-making; the state's implementation of consensus-building by disseminating objective information on the nature of the problem, the available and recommended solutions, and incentives to facilitate preventive

action; and the facilitation of community involvement in decision-making and crisis management.

These four factors must be present if the health authorities are to obtain collective informed consent and gain the corresponding cooperation from the community to address the epidemic promptly and effectively. These factors are dynamic and do not necessarily constitute a chain of events but, rather, a set of prerequisites to achieve collective informed consent. After considering the notion of collective informed consent, I discuss each of the four background factors separately, and then explain their impact on the successful governance of epidemics.

Collective Informed Consent

In the world of clinical trials and biomedical care, the concept of informed consent as applied to individuals is essential and well understood. The human subject or patient must be respected as a rational, autonomous person who is entitled to make decisions and weigh the benefits and risks of alternative solutions to his/her health problem or a health threat. Autonomy is a value that connotes "self-government and freedom of choice" and consequently, "consent given by the patient is the only legitimate ground for almost any interference in their lives or any intrusion upon their person" (Engelhard, 1986, cited in Harrington, 2002: 1426). Following regulations agreed upon by the international community represented in the membership of the World Health Organization (WHO), informed consent must be implemented daily and routinely in biomedical interventions and clinical trials (USFDA, 1998; USFDA, 2006). According to informed consent guidelines, clear, complete, and unambiguous explanation of a given procedure—including its justification, benefits, and all known risks—must be given to the patient or human subject. Questions are encouraged, and answered. Once the patient/subject is satisfied with the information, then he/she is invited to participate and, if he/she accepts, to sign a consent form to proceed with the intervention or clinical trial, as the case may be.

In some instances, the clinical context of individual informed consent intersects with public health practice. For example, medical practitioners offer immunization and/or screening tests for an infectious disease, or bring these options to the attention of their patients. Prenatal HIV testing for pregnant women (Lo, Wolf, and Sengupta, 2000)

---

* This chapter is reprinted from S.R. Quah, ed. (2007) *Crisis Preparedness — Asian and the Global Governance of Epidemics.* Stanford, CA: Walter H. Shorenstein Asia-Pacific Research Centre, Stanford University, 113–133.

and routine HIV testing for other individuals also provide relevant illustrations of this intersection. Both situations tend to occur as practitioner-patient interactions in a private context, but it is widely acknowledged that patients' private decisions have significant public consequences for the management of the HIV/AIDS epidemic (Baldwin, 2005: 287; D'Amelio *et al.*, 2001: 7–11; United Nations, 1985). Unfortunately, the concept of informed consent remains anchored in the doctor-patient encounter. If informed public choices are mentioned in the realm of public health, their discussion regularly focuses on the needs of decision-makers (Haines *et al.*, 2004). It is thus necessary to consider the scope of informed consent at the wider, community level.

What is collective or community informed consent? The concept of community informed consent differs from individual informed consent in two ways. First, in community informed consent the subject is a collective entity: the community affected by the disease or disease threat. Let us understand community to mean the total population, involving persons affected by the disease (e.g., persons living with HIV/AIDS, SARS patients), their immediate families and networks, and the rest of the population residing in the same political jurisdiction (city, municipality, county, state, province, or nation state) and enjoying autonomy in health policy decisions. So defined, the community should be treated as a collectivity of rational and autonomous individuals, entitled to make decisions and weigh the benefits and risks of alternative solutions to their health problems or a health threat. The same requirements of informed consent mentioned earlier apply: clear, complete, and unambiguous explanations of the nature of the problem or health threat should be distributed, including suggested solutions, their justification, benefits, and all known risks; and questions should be encouraged and answered. Second, community informed consent differs from individual informed consent in the manner in which the consent is taken. With community informed consent, the process should include an assessment of the community's level of information on the problem and on what is needed to solve it, and the community's level of agreement or consensus on what is needed to implement the solution. Halperin and colleagues (2004) offer a good illustration of this process in their discussion of the distribution of information on all possible preventive measures against HIV/AIDS infection.

To deal successfully with an infectious disease epidemic, health authorities need an informed and committed community as an active partner. Health authorities cannot deal with a crisis without the community's cooperation, regardless of the expertise and number of healthcare personnel and the level of medical technology available. We know of severe difficulties that public health practitioners and lay community members have faced in battling disease outbreaks or epidemics (e.g., Singer, 1994;

Rollins, 2004; Baldwin, 2005; Barry, 2004). The seriousness of the crisis is compounded when health authorities fail to mobilize the indispensable cooperation from a community of uninformed, indifferent or, at worst, misinformed and hostile individuals or groups. In other words, the most immediate factor influencing the successful governance of an epidemic is the presence of community informed consent. Because the containment and preventive measures vary in each epidemic and the socioeconomic, cultural, and political contexts are constantly changing, collective informed consent must be obtained for each public health crisis.

The Challenge of Building Trust

The history of epidemics around the world (e.g., Harrison, 2004; Baldwin, 2005) is rich with instances of reasons people have for trusting—or distrusting—the state in general, or government officials, or health authorities. Research findings have stressed the importance of patients' trust for the successful management of the HIV/AIDS epidemic (Burris, 2000; Valdiserri *et al.*, 2000; Klosinski, 2000; Lo, Wolf, and Sengupta, 2000), but we need to analyze trust in the context of public health more specifically.

I propose that trust is a precondition to informed consent, and that in the context of public health, the level of trust the community places in the health authorities influences the likelihood of granting informed consent. Put differently, it is reasonable to assume that you would consent to undergo a medical procedure, intervention, or action provided that you understood the problem (threat or danger) and the solution intellectually and trusted the people who informed you and who would work on the solution.

The discussion of trust has occupied philosophers and social scientists for a long time. Summarizing the definitions provided by seven scholars from 1958 to 1993, Deborah Welch Larson concludes that trust is understood as "a judgment that one can rely on another party's word or promise at the risk of a bad outcome should the other cheat or renege" (2004: 35). In the context of family relations, trust may mean "the willingness to accept risk based upon stable, positive expectations of a partner's intentions" (Brown, 2004: 168). On the other hand, trust in formal interactions among "anonymous actors", is defined as "the belief that other agents will act in a predictable way without special sanctions" (Radaev, 2004: 233). More generally, trust is "placing valued outcomes at risk to others' malfeasance, mistakes, or failures" (Tilly, 2005: 12). At an even higher level of abstraction, trust is found at both the socio-emotional and the rational spheres of social life. In the socio-emotional sphere, trust is embedded in the everyday life norms, roles, and expectations that hold a community together. That is, trust "may be regarded as an expectation that relevant others will behave according to certain norms that make their behavior dependable, predictable, or, as we say, trustworthy" (Wuthnow, 2004: 146). The rational sphere of trust involves exchange interactions and the calculation of risk (however subjective). In other words, trust "is part of a rational actor's effort to calculate the cost and benefits of entering into a specified relationship with another person" (Wuthnow, 2004: 148).

Both the socio-emotional sphere and the rational sphere of trust are relevant in the analysis of what influences the presence of informed consent required to manage epidemics successfully. These two spheres point to the importance of the social context in which trust may exist or be impeded. Wuthnow (2004: 154) identifies ten reasons—or "warrants"—for why A may trust B:

- *Sincerity*, whereby "A is persuaded" of the sincerity of B
- *Empathy*, whereby A believes "B cares about A";
- *Affinity*, when "A senses that A and B have a shared identity, common values, or mutual understanding";
- *Altruism*, when "A expects B to exercise restrain over B's self-interest and to behave in a way that takes account of A's interests and needs";
- *Accessibility*, whereby "A anticipates that B will be available" when needed and "that A has a valid claim to B's time and resources";
- *Effectiveness*, when "A regards B as efficacious, as able to get the job done or to achieve the desired results" and that B has the required "resources" and is able to mobilize them;
- *Competence*, when "A perceives B as having appropriate training, information, skills, and talents for performing the role in question";
- *Congeniality*, whereby "A regards B as capable of engaging" in the task with ease, politeness, and friendliness;
- *Fairness*, whereby "A expects B to follow prescribed procedures and abide by formal rules pertaining to B's roles, thus treating A similarly to people who are in similar situations and not rendering arbitrary judgments";
- *Reliability*, whereby "A regards B as being dependable or stable by virtue of expecting B to behave in similar ways under similar circumstances over time."

Applying Wuthnow's trust "warrants" to the matter of epidemics, we may ask: Why should members of a community trust their health authorities? Research findings based on direct data (Quah and Lee, 2004; Quah, 2007) and indirect and historical data (Barry, 2004: 448–61; Rollins, 2004; Kleinman and Watson, 2006; Lee and Yun, 2006; Zhang, 2006) suggest that of the ten warrants outlined by Wuthnow, nine are directly relevant to the presence of community consensus and cooperation (informed

consent) in a public health crises. People in the target community tend to trust (or distrust) the government and/or health authorities based on their perception of the government's sincerity, empathy, affinity, altruism, accessibility, effectiveness, competence, fairness, and reliability.

Citizens' perception of these attributes on the part of the government (or government agencies, or officials) are shaped primarily by citizens' inferences from their observations of and experience with government's past behavior and actions (Hardin, 2002:153-156).[1] Sociological research demonstrates that trust is embedded in the community's values and norms (Hardin, 2004; Wuthnow, 2005; Tilly, 2005). But time is crucial. Psychological and sociological studies show that building trust is a slow process: the bricks of the trust edifice are the accumulated positive interactions among the individuals concerned over a period of time (Murnighan, Malhotra and Weber, 2004: 294). The level of trust may increase with time, "as each additional positive interaction becomes more valuable in establishing mutual trust" (2004: 294), but this general trend may not apply to intimate relations (2004: 320). The history of the interaction or relationship is also important, even as we acknowledge that "the trust development process is neither neat nor strictly rational" (Murnighan, Malhotra and Weber, 2004: 315; Taylor-Gooley and Zinn, 2006: 399). Consequently, the community's warrants for trust in their government and health authorities need to be nurtured and strengthened over time—well before a health crisis strikes. The HIV/AIDS and SARS epidemics have brought to light this simple but important principle. Indeed, M.H. Merson's views on trust and the early detection of HIV infection underscore it:

> There is a wide consensus that early detection of HIV infection to increase access to care and to decrease risky behavior in order to prevent infection is a laudable goal that should be vigorously pursued and researched. But enthusiasm for testing must always be tempered by the need for acceptance and trust of individuals and communities. This can only come through dialogue and partnership; it can never be legislated" (Merson, 2000: S159).

In the case of SARS, the initial reaction to the outbreak, both among health authorities and the public, differed markedly from country to country: there are

---

[1] Some readers may like to know that Russell Hardin (2002: 155–56) labels this citizens-government situation "quasi trust." In Hardin's opinion, "quasi trust" differs from individual-to-individual trust relations, in which each individual has some knowledge of the other that helps him/her to estimate the other's trustworthiness. Hardin suggests that "quasi trust" occurs in all situations involving institutions and other collective entities because "it is grounded in inductive extrapolation from past behavior or reputation" (2002: 156). Hardin correctly points to extrapolations, but it is commonly recognized in the literature that such an extrapolation is present in most situations involving trust. I therefore continue to use the term "trust" in this discussion.

indications that governance effectiveness in controlling the outbreak differed across countries in tandem with a given country's governance style and a given community's level of trust in their health authorities (Zhao, 2003; Quah and Lee, 2004; Fidler, 2004b; Chiu and Galbraith, 2004; Kleinman and Lee, 2006).

Building Warrants for Trust

The discussion of trust raises three factors that contribute to the building of warrants for trust: transparency in state's actions and decision-making, implementation of consensus-building mechanisms, and facilitation of community's involvement in crisis resolution.

Transparency in State Actions and Decision-making

In a democratic system, it is expected that government actions and decisions will be accessible to the citizenry and open to scrutiny. Openness or transparency makes it easier for citizens to know how their government operates and why decisions are made, thus providing information that can nurture trust. Therefore, the building of warrants for trust depends, among other things, on transparency in the state's actions and decision-making. Transparency is important in normal times, but it becomes crucial in times of crisis. In the case of an infectious disease epidemic, distribution of information on the disease and rapid response are vital for the effective prevention and containment of the disease. With the current speed of transmission of infectious diseases such as HIV/AIDS and SARS, and the heavy toll that epidemics inflict on individuals and communities, timely and effective distribution of information on infectious disease outbreaks is needed to improve the global disease monitoring capabilities recommended by the United Nations (UN) (United Nations, 2004: 29–31; Fidler, 2004a: 801; Gostin, 2004).

The need for transparency and, specifically, for global reporting guidelines is well understood and generally accepted by most UN member nations (Sim and Mackie, 2006; Olowokure and Roth, 2006; Shaw, 2006). But the implementation of collaborative guidelines is less than ideal, even among modern industrialized countries. The European Community, for example, is still fine-tuning a system of collaboration in global case reporting and there is hope that the European Centre for Communicable Diseases will provide the answer. Along the same line of thought, experts in England are studying the role played by the Health Protection Agency during the SARS outbreak (Goddard *et al.*, 2006).

The slow pace of implementing transparency measures is problematic but not as serious as the problem of complete secrecy. Regrettably, historical and current events suggest that until the problem is verified, until a solution or way of controlling the danger is found, or until it becomes politically appropriate to reveal it, secrecy or concealment tend to be the most common impulse of officials who discover a potential danger. Indeed, concealing a threat or danger has been justified in many ways. For example, it has been cited as an effort to protect the community, to avoid panic, to keep the bad news from enemies or competitors, or to maintain for as long as possible the normal pace of work of those affected (Barry, 2004: 169–75; Garrett, 2005). In some countries, concealing disease outbreaks may be actually mandated. A vivid illustration of this problem is China's silence in 2002–2003, during the crucial first months of the SARS epidemic.[2] One expert in international affairs writes that in Chinese law "epidemics fall under the classification of state secrets" and local officials "do not have the incentive" or "the power to make public comments about disease outbreaks before this has been announced by the authorities at the national level." Not surprisingly, this situation "encourages optimistic reporting and the suppression of bad news." In the case of SARS, this feature of Chinese governance caused "the delay in timely reporting and exacerbated the impact of the disease, causing precisely the kind of domestic and international crisis that the system is designed to prevent" (Saich, 2006: 73).

In addition, at the micro-level, state secrecy confounds and interrupts the lives of individual members of the community facing a health crisis. State secrecy in a health crisis not only impedes a rapid and effective response to epidemics but also breeds, at best, misinformation, and at worst, panic among individuals and families. Without accurate information on what is happening and why, people activate their informal networks in whatever way possible—face-to-face, by telephone, through mobile phone text messages, and through email. People who can avoid or overcome panic resort to their traditional ways of thinking and of doing things, including traditional healing practices. During the SARS outbreak in Guangzhou, Hong Kong, and Taiwan, for example, rumors of disaster circulated, fast creating panic buying of traditional remedies like herbal medicines to increase body strength, and white vinegar. Residents believed that boiling white vinegar in a room would prevent the disease by killing germs

---

[2] The first SARS cases were seen in Foshan, a city in the southern Chinese province of Guangzhou, in November 2002. Clinicians originally mistook these cases as possible avian flu but later labeled them "atypical pneumonia." However, no reports or surveillance followed because "pneumonia, atypical or otherwise" is not on China's list of communicable infectious diseases. As a result, the outbreak "was kept from the public in Guangdong until February 11", when the epidemic was reported to the World Health Organization (WHO) after the Guangdong Provincial Health Bureau "initiated an inquiry based upon reports received from Hong Kong's Global Outbreak Alert and Response Network (GOARN)", a network set up by WHO" after September 11, 2001 (Kaufman, 2006: 53–68).

(SARS Expert Committee, 2003: 13; Kaufman, 2006: 65). Unfortunately, families used charcoal stoves to boil pots of vinegar inside closed rooms and this method led to cases of carbon monoxide poisoning (Abdullah *et al.*, 2003: 1043). However, some traditional procedures people used in the absence of other guidelines may turn out to be useful. The traditional Chinese belief in the sterilizing properties of white vinegar has been confirmed by scientific research: white vinegar has sterilizing properties not when it is boiled but when added to diluted household bleach (Miner *et al.*, 2006).

The personal experience of one 23-year old medical student as a SARS patient in Guangzhou during the time of official concealment (Ho, 2006), offers a compelling example of the danger, unnecessary anxiety, and suffering that state secrecy inflicts upon individuals. The medical student fell ill after treating a patient with severe pneumonia during a 20-minute ride in an ambulance on January 31, 2003. His own knowledge of medicine made him realize his symptoms were more serious than those of the common flu. The ambulance driver fell sick the next day. Both the patient and the driver died some days later. For the first week of his illness the medical student dealt with his symptoms alone. At first he remained in his dormitory alone by choice. But when he sought medial attention later, the Emergency Room staff simply gave him "some acetaminophen and sent me back to the dorm." Although the hospital had been dealing with at least two patients with "severe pneumonia", when the student became sicker and returned to the ER, they gave him "some antibiotics". He added: "And [they] sent me home again . . . I stayed in my bed for another two days with fever. I did not contact anyone and no one contacted me." As the disease progressed the student was finally warded. He went through a very critical period and survived SARS. His perspective on the silence of the medical professionals with whom he worked and interacted is informative, since it suggests the state's preference for secrecy had spilled over into the healthcare system: "We all knew that the one [patient] transferred from a rural district north of Guangzhou had infected nine hospital staff before his transfer to our hospital, but we hardly talked about it." There was also the plight of "nursing aids", one of the lowest ranks of temporary workers who are hired by relatives to look after patients at the hospital "for a small fee". The medical student observed that during the SARS outbreak nursing aids "were infected just like many doctors and nurses. They disappeared from the hospital site as soon as they got sick, for they could no longer work, nor could they afford the enormous medical fees." M.S. Ho, the author who interviewed the student, noted that nursing aids who fell ill "would return to their hometowns and blend in with the 800 million farmers in the vast rural areas of China, carrying with them the SARS virus from Guangdong" (Ho, 2006: 7). This is yet one more example of the tragedy of secrecy: when the state remains silent and abstains from urgently needed action, it leaves citizens to cope with the crisis on their own, and inflicts most pain on the weakest, least educated, and poorest members of the community.

Consensus-building and Community Involvement

I indicated earlier that three factors are associated with the creation of warrants for trust: transparency in state's actions and decision-making, implementation of consensus-building mechanisms, and facilitation of the community's involvement in crisis resolution. I turn now to the second and third factors.

The consensus-building mechanisms I discuss here are most likely to be devised in democratic systems of government, because these mechanisms presuppose respect for citizenry and a commitment to share rather than to conceal information. State authorities need to concern themselves with consensus-building to bring all the different sectors of the community together as partners in the collective endeavor of conquering a common problem or threat, whether it is poverty, crime, addiction, or an infectious disease epidemic, or other shared problem. For public health, three consensus-building mechanisms are necessary. First is the distribution of objective—that is, empirically verifiable—information on the problem, its nature, etiology, diagnosis, and prognosis. Second is the distribution of objective—again, empirically verifiable—information on the range of available solutions, and on the known benefits and risks of the recommended solutions. The key feature of these two types of information is that they *must* be empirically verifiable, which makes them the exact opposite of propaganda. Propaganda is the exercise in "mass suggestion or influence through . . . the dexterous use of images, slogans and symbols that play on our prejudices and emotions" (Pratkanis and Aronson, 2001: 11). History shows that opportunistic politicians and interest groups do not hesitate to use propaganda to take advantage of people's vulnerability during a health crisis (Barry, 2004; Baldwin, 2005). In contrast, in the battle against an epidemic, the goal is to educate the population on all known relevant aspects of the problem at hand, all possible solutions available, and the current limits of that knowledge.

These two first steps toward consensus-building provide the community with complete and useful information on the problem and on what the community can do, collectively and individually, to solve the problem. As discussed earlier, information sharing in a transparent and verifiable manner is conducive to creating and strengthening trust.

However, research findings indicate that information on a disease threat and possible preventive action does not necessarily lead the target population to put into practice the recommended actions. In other words, information alone is insufficient to motivate preventive behavior (Gochman, 1997; Quah, 1985, 1988; Quah and Lee, 2004). Thus, a third step is necessary: to identify and introduce incentives to practice preventive action. This third consensus-building mechanism is indispensable, because in the prevention of infectious disease epidemics it is crucial to ensure that all members of the affected community follow the recommended preventive actions. Like all infectious disease epidemics, SARS showed us clearly that one individual's actions may be enough to spread the disease to unsuspecting communities.

When the problem or crisis is sufficiently serious—to the point of threatening life and limb—the desire for safety becomes the built-in incentive to follow a recommended course of action that is believed to be effective. This desire for safety works as an incentive if two of the warrants for trust (Wuthnow, 2004) are present: effectiveness and competence. Effectiveness occurs when the community regards health authorities as capable of getting the job done or achieving the desired results, and believes that the government has the required resources to deal with the crisis and is able to mobilize them. Competence applies when the community perceives the health authorities as having appropriate training, information, skills, and talents to control the crisis and protect the population.

To facilitate community's cooperation and involvement, the state must not only share information but also create diverse channels of communication. But effective communication must be a two-way system, rather than a top-down transmission of directives. Community feedback and queries from individuals, groups, associations and other sectors of civil society are crucial elements in the health authorities' search for solutions to the crisis and in its effective implementation of those solutions.

Toward Successful Governance of Epidemics

Legislation is integral part of the traditional management of epidemics, both in the national and international arenas (Gostin, 2004; Patterson and London, 2002; Taylor, 2002; Whitman, 2000; James *et al.*, 2006; Quah and Lee, 2004). In this discussion, however, I take legislation as a given and focus instead on this wider principle: The *sine qua non* of successful crisis governance is the groundwork that is laid before the crisis. This principle has been recognized in different fields. In his assessment of leadership moments in organizations, management expert Michael Useem (1998) explains that the required groundwork includes "a strong culture with good lines of interior

communication, mutual understanding, and shared obligation", all of which "are essential ingredients to ensure that your team, your organization, or your company will perform to its utmost when it is most needed" (1998: 64). Sociologist Amitai Etzioni (1993) stresses the same point with respect to government and the citizenry in nation states. My research indicates that the same requirement applies to the successful management of health crises (for example infectious disease epidemics) by the state and its citizens. I propose in this chapter that community involvement, transparency, consensus-building, and efforts at strengthening trust constitute the groundwork needed to create prompt and effective responses to a crisis (**Figure 1**). These features take time to build. Crises are likely to cause more harm and take longer to resolve in countries where the spectrum of factors needed for successful governance (collective informed consent, transparency, procedures for consensus-building mechanisms, and the warrants for trust) is weak or not present when the crisis strikes.

The governance of SARS in some Asian countries illustrates the importance of preliminary groundwork. For example, community involvement and the three consensus-building mechanisms were already present in Singapore before SARS struck (Quah and Lee, 2004). Whatever medical experts knew at the outset about the disease's etiology, diagnosis, and prognosis was passed to the population through all mass media channels. New channels were created to reach more people, including a dedicated television channel, several public websites, and other website pages that many organizations set up in order to provide SARS prevention guidelines to their members and employees. Technical and scientific information on the SARS coronavirus were publicized in various ways—from cartoons to pamphlets and from TV to radio programs—to facilitate understanding among people from all walks of life. Basic preventive actions that every person was to follow during the outbreak included taking and recording one's body temperature twice a day with one's personal thermometer;[3] washing hands thoroughly as often as necessary; modifying the daily practice of sharing meals by using separate serving utensils even when eating at home with one's family members (a traditional Asian practice is to serve dishes in common plates or large bowls from which each person around the table partakes); and strictly limiting outside-home activities (Quah and Lee, 2004; Chua, 2004; James *et al.*, 2006). Those preventive actions impinged upon everyone's daily lives but the major incentive of following the

---

[3] The Singapore government distributed free thermometers to all educational institutions' students and teachers, as well as to the armed forces, civil service, any other organizations that requested them, and to individuals through clinics and hospitals and other healthcare institutions (Chua, 2004; James *et al.*, 2006).

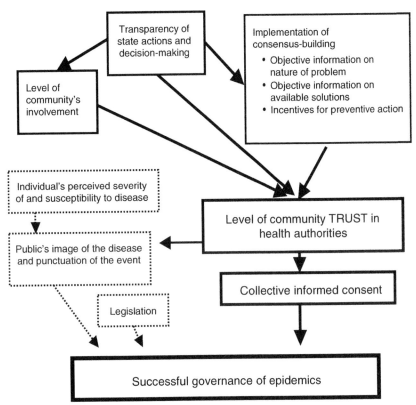

Figure 1 Main Factors Influencing the Governance of Epidemics.
Note: The solid line boxes indicate the factors discussed in this chapter. Factors in the dotted line boxes are discussed in Quah (2007).

recommended precautions was that those precautions were effective in preventing the spread of the disease.

It should be noted that at the start of the epidemic there was considerable uncertainty in medical circles about the nature of the infection and how to prevent it. This situation was conveyed to the population and information was updated continuously as more knowledge on the disease was acquired. Meanwhile, scientific research was accelerated through active networking on both the international and the local levels. One outcome of local research was the cooperation between two agencies, the Defense Science and Technology Agency and Singapore Technologies Engineering, to develop thermal imaging scanners which were installed at all Singapore's ports of entry to detect fever among passengers leaving and arriving. The scanners became "hot items sought by Asian governments battling SARS" including Hong Kong, the Philippines, China, Taiwan, and Thailand (Deutsche Press-Agentur, 2003).

Battling the SARS outbreak in Singapore was an exercise in collective learning, but the goal of collective action was safety: to control and stop the disease outbreak. This goal served as the best incentive for the community to follow the recommended preventive actions. Subsequently, as added incentives, arrangements were put in

place to minimize the financial cost of quarantine and other preventive measures for individuals and organizations (James *et al.*, 2006).

Many countries affected by the SARS outbreak could not respond in the same systematic manner. Within the health care system, hospitals were at the forefront of the epidemic, but as a study of hospitals in Laos, Taiwan, and Thailand reveals, there was discordance between the hospital epidemic control guidelines and the implementation of those guidelines (Lee *et al.*, 2004). Requests for preventive action by health authorities in several countries were originally greeted with noncooperation (Foreman, 2003). China's extremely inadequate governance of epidemics such as HIV/AIDS and SARS is well documented (Saich, 2006; Ho, 2006; Baldwin, 2005).

Other countries, too, have faltered. In the absence of the governance groundwork just discussed, Taiwan faced serious setbacks trying to manage the SARS outbreak at the beginning of the epidemic. One of the major management problems was the reluctance of the Taiwanese population and even healthcare personnel, to follow the health authorities' recommendations, particularly concerning quarantine. The first SARS case in Taiwan was diagnosed "in early March 2003" (Deng *et al.*, 2006: 16). On April 21, 2003, Taipei's health authorities declared the Hoping Hospital in quarantine for two weeks, as the hospital had ten probable SARS cases and some staff members had been infected. The public health experts had determined correctly that quarantine was the safest course of action. Even so, some 30 nurses and other health-care workers protested raucously. Some tossed "bottles and paper out of windows and displayed banners saying "Wrong Policy", and "Long, Long 14 days" (Foreman, 2003; Wu, 2003). Explaining to a reporter why people did not follow quarantine regulations, one Taiwanese public health expert said, "Taiwan is too democratic to execute quarantine with an iron fist like Singapore. But, more importantly, quarantining is disruptive of people's lives. The government needs . . . to find a way to accommodate their needs" (Shu, 2003). His comments reveal the absence of the necessary groundwork to face the epidemic, particularly the lack of accurate information on the nature of the disease, the low level of trust that the community placed in their health authorities, and consequently, the absence of collective informed consent.

By its very nature, informed consent cannot be forced upon a community. Baldwin explains this point well in his historical analysis of disease and democracy: "Modern democratic societies could not control citizens' behavior through prescribing conduct . . . . Instead, they sought to rear, educate and persuade inhabitants to act as members of a civilized polity" (2005: 263). As the SARS epidemic developed and spread to other countries, a process of learning by doing began to take place.

Conclusion

I have argued in this chapter that without the crucial factors of effective channels for community participation in decision-making, transparency, effective democratic mechanisms of consensus-building, warrants for citizens' trust in the health authorities, and collective informed consent, the prospect of successful governance of health crises remains uncertain.

Hopefully, today we are wiser from the SARS experience, but future epidemics may find some countries still unprepared. The governance of epidemics is a serious concern because in the realm of infectious disease epidemics, we live in a borderless world. A vivid reminder of this is the avian influenza threat, which comes from organized smuggling of poultry (either live birds or raw meat) across Asia and Europe (Rosenthal, 2006), and very likely in other world regions. In addition to natural bird migration, illegal trade fuels the spread of the A(H5N1) virus that causes avian influenza, and must be counteracted with "tough" legislation (Bradsher, 2006). But human air travel is potentially a more rapid mode for

transmitting the virus (compared to the usual "natural" spread through bird migration), and requires the urgent attention and cooperation of governments everywhere (Lim, 2006; Omi, 2006: viii).

Some of the actions taking place in countries currently battling the avian influenza outbreak among fowl give cause for optimism. One of the actions, for example, is to provide public announcements on what authorities are doing about the disease (Chou, 2005), such as setting up emergency surveillance arrangements. Such regular publicity keeps the topic in the media and ensures that people remain alert to the problem. Nevertheless, as one experienced epidemiologist declared, surveillance systems "can be set up very quickly" but "this is not a mode of operation we should come to depend on" (Foege, 2000: 214).

There are also indications that the groundwork for successful governance of future epidemics has not begun in some countries and that very few have learned from the SARS outbreak. International experts express concern about China's level of preparedness for a new epidemic, because of its inadequate monitoring mechanisms for infectious diseases at the county and village levels (Blumenthal and Hsiao, 2005: 1169); its persistent tendency toward secrecy (Agence France-Presse, 2005; Osnos, 2005; McCord, 2005); and the danger of corruption in handling a massive inoculation of poultry in the country (Bezlova, 2005). The manner in which culling of birds and poultry is being planned and implemented to avoid an Avian flu epidemic also indicates that the lessons from SARS on the importance of collective informed consent have not been learned. The task is multiple and challenging: to reach farmers (usually poorly educated) in remote rural areas, to communicate to them the seriousness of the disease and the necessity of bird culling—which typically terminates their main source of income—and to provide real incentives for their cooperation. However, in many affected countries, including Iran, Turkey, Romania, Ukraine, Moldova, and Nigeria, the health authorities apparently have concentrated their energies on the logistics of bird slaughtering (transport of slaughtering equipment, personnel, paraphernalia, and the like) but have neglected or paid less attention to informing the farmers of the etiology, diagnosis, and prognosis of the epidemic affecting their flocks and, particularly, to explaining the nature, justification, and effectiveness of culling as preventive action. Not surprisingly, farmers have protested and failed to cooperate. Some have even tried to salvage their source of livelihood by hiding their ducks and chickens from inspectors (Farmani, 2006; Cheviron, 2006; Ingham, 2006; Rompress, 2005; Chiriac, 2005; Akhaine *et al.*, 2006). The affected farmers are naturally anxious and wary of health inspectors, unwilling to trust government officials from faraway cities. In the farmers' eyes, most officials know nothing about farming and do not care about what happens to farmers.

Finally, then, in addition to the factors needed to create informed consent, the governance of a health crisis or epidemic must include effective international and national coordination. The international or global governance of infectious diseases has received considerable attention (Fidler, 2004a and 2004b; Whitman, 2000; Taylor, 2002; Gostin, 2005). Equally important are national governments' arrangements to adapt internal procedures and personnel and shift their civil service and health care systems into a crisis management mode. Such internal arrangements will vary across countries, given differences in political system, political ideology, geographical constraints, and socio-economic context. Still, irrespective of these differences, three arrangements are likely to bear fruit in most countries. The first is the active coordination of ministries and other state agencies to share information, to deal with the problem in a synchronized fashion, and to respond to the crisis promptly and consistently. The second is to design a multi-pronged approach to the solution of the health crisis. No single solution is likely to be sufficient in combating an epidemic. A multi-pronged approach means rallying of significant sectors of society to cooperate—including, among others, scientists, professionals, security experts, university students, schools, the armed forces, religious groups, retired people, businesses, and nongovernmental organizations. This collaborative effort may be formalized by establishing one or more task forces entrusted with specific responsibilities. The third arrangement begins by using existing legislation. Then, because each crisis or epidemic brings its own demands, health authorities must be prepared to introduce specifically designed regulations to deal with each crisis within the framework of collective informed consent. These three additional arrangements require, of course, constant fine-tuning, both in light of advances in technological and scientific knowledge, the nature of the disease, and changes in the demographic, socioeconomic, and cultural features of a given population.

References

Abdullah ASM, Tomlinson B, Cockram CS, and Thomas GN (2003) Lessons from the Severe Acute Respiratory Syndrome Outbreak in Hong Kong. *Emerging Infectious Diseases* 9: 1042–1045.

Agence France-Presse (2005) China Dismally Unprepared for Bird Flu Crisis: Expert. Paris: May 25.

Akhaine S, Obinor F, Adeyemi B, and Oluwole F (2006) Authorities Kill 45,000 Chickens in Northern Nigeria over Flu Fears. *The Guardian on Saturday.* Lagos: February 11.

Baldwin P (2005) *Disease and Democracy: The Industrialized World Faces AIDS.* Berkeley, California: University of California Press.

Barry JM (2004) *The Great Influenza: The Epic Story of the Deadliest Plague in History.* New York: Penguin Books.

Bezlova A (2005) Corruption May Stymie Fowl Inoculation Drive. *Inter Press Service.* Beijing: November 25.

Blumenthal D and Hsiao W (2005) Privatization and Its Discontents—The Evolving Chinese Health Care System. *New England Journal of Medicine* 11: 1165–1170.

Bradsher K (2006) Health Officials Call for Long-term Spending on Bird Flu. *New York Times,* January 17. www.nytimes.com/2006/01/17/health. Accessed: 17 Jan 2006.

Brown ML (2004) Compensating for Distrust among Kin. In: Hardin R (ed.) *Distrust,* pp. 167–191. New York: Russell Sage Foundation.

Burris S (2000) Surveillance, Social Risk, and Symbolism: Framing the Analysis of Research and Policy. *Journal of Acquired Immune Deficiency Syndromes* 25: 120–127.

Cheviron N (2006) Pigeon Culling in Turkey Ruffles Feathers. *Agence France-Presse.* Istanbul: January 19.

Chiriac L (2005) Poultry Slaughter Leaves Romanian Villagers Worried about Livelihood. *Agence France-Presse.* Ceamurlia de Jos, Romania: October 16.

Chiu W and Galbraith V (2004) Calendar of Events. In: Loh C and Civic Exchange (eds.) *At the Epicentre. Hong Kong and the SARS Outbreak,* pp. xv–xxviii. Hong Kong: Hong Kong University Press.

Chou J (2005) Bird Flu Measures Made Public. *Taipei Times,* October 22.

Chua MH (2004) *A Defining Moment: How Singapore Beat SARS.* Singapore: Institute of Policy Studies.

D'Amelio R, Tuerlings E, Perito O, Biselli R, Natalicchio S, and Kingma S (2001) Global Review of Legislation on HIV/AIDS: The Issue of HIV Testing. *Journal of Acquired Immune Deficiency Syndromes* 28: 173–179.

Deng JF, Olowokure B, Kaydos-Daniels CS, Chang HJ, Barwick RS, Lee ML, Deng CY, Factor SH, Chiang CE, and Maloney SA (The SARS International Field Team) (2006) Severe Acute Respiratory Syndrome (SARS): Knowledge, Attitudes, Practices, and Sources of Information among Physicians Answering a SARS Fever Hotline Service. *Public Health* 120: 15–19.

Deutsche Press-Agentur (2003) Singapore's Scanners to Detect Fevers are Hot Item in Asia. April 29. http://infoweb.newsbank.com. Accessed: 30 May 2003.

Engelhardt HT (1986) *The Foundations of Bioethics.* New York: Oxford University Press.

Etzioni A (1993) *The Spirit of Community: Rights, Responsibilities, and the Communitarian Agenda.* New York: Crown.

Farmani H (2006) Iran Villagers Part with Precious Poultry. *Agence France-Presse.* Barasb, Iran: January 18.

Fidler DP (2004a) Germs, Governance, and Global Public Health in the Wake of SARS. *The Journal of Clinical Investigation* 113(6): 799–804.

Fidler DP (2004b) *SARS, Governance and the Globalization of Disease.* New York: Palgrave.

Foege W (2000) Surveillance, Eradication and Control: Successes and Failures. In: Whitman J (ed.) *The Politics of Emerging and Resurgent Infectious Diseases,* pp. 203–219. London: Macmillan Press.

Foreman W (2003) *4,000 Told to Stay Home Due to SARS.* Associated Press News Service, Beijing. April 25. http://infoweb.newsbank.com. Accessed: 30 May 2003.

Garrett L (2005) The Lessons of HIV/AIDS. *Foreign Affairs* 84(4): 51–64.

Gochman DS (ed.) (1997) *Handbook of Health Behavior Research. Vol 1. Personal and Social Determinants.* New York: Plenum.

Goddard NL, Delpech VC, Watson JM, Regan M, and Nicoll A (2006) Lessons Learned from SARS: The Experience of the Health Protection Agency, England. *Public Health* 120: 27–32.

Gostin LO (2004) International Infectious Disease Law. Revision of the World Health Organization's International Health Regulations. *Journal of the American Medical Association* 291(21): 2623–2627.

Haines A, Becerra-Posada F, Berwick D, *et al.* (2004) Informed Choices for Attaining the Millennium Development Goals: Towards an International Cooperative Agenda for Health-Systems Research. *The Lancet.* November 27(364): 1913–1915.

Halperin DT, Steiner MJ, Cassell MM, *et al.* (2004) The Time Has Come for Common Ground on Preventing Sexual Transmission of HIV. *The Lancet,* November 27(364): 1913–1915.

Hardin R (2002) *Trust & Trustworthiness.* New York: Russell Sage Foundation.

Hardin R (ed.) (2004) *Distrust.* New York: Russell Sage Foundation.

Harrington JA (2002) The Instrumental Uses of Autonomy: A Review of AIDS Law and Policy in Europe. *Social Science & Medicine* 55: 1425–1434.

Harrison M (2004) *Disease and the Modern World: 1500 to the Present Day.* Cambridge, UK: Polity Press.

Ho MS (2006) I Think I Got 'That Disease': An Interview with a Medical Student Who Had Recovered from SARS in Guangzhou, China. *Public Health* 120: 6–7.

Ingham R (2006) Local Farming Practices, Monitoring Problems Helped Drive Bird Flu in Turkey. *Agence France-Presse.* Paris: January 9.

James L, Shindo N, Cutter J, Ma S, and Chew SK (2006) Public Health Measures Implemented during the SARS Outbreak in Singapore, 2003. *Public Health* 120: 20–26.

Kaufman J (2006) SARS and China's Health-care Response. Better to be Both Red and Expert! In: Kleinman A and Watson JL (eds.) *SARS in China. Prelude to Pandemic?* pp. 53–68. Stanford: Stanford University Press.

Kleinman A and Watson JL (eds.) (2006) *SARS in China. Prelude to Pandemic?* Stanford: Stanford University Press.

Kleinman A and Lee S (2006) SARS and the Problem of Social Stigma. In: Kleinman A and Watson JL (eds.) *SARS in China. Prelude to Pandemic?* pp. 173–195. Stanford: Stanford University Press.

Klosinski LE (2000) HIV Testing from a Community Perspective. *Journal of Acquired Immune Deficiency Syndromes* 25: S94–S96.

Lee DTS and Kwok WY (2006) Psychological Responses to SARS in Hong Kong—Report from the Front Line. In: Kleinman A and Watson JL (eds.) *SARS in China. Prelude to Pandemic?* pp. 133–147. Stanford: Stanford University Press.

Lee NE, Potjaman S, Tappero J, *et al.* (2004) Infection Control Practices for SARS in Lao People's Democratic Republic, Taiwan, and Thailand: Experience from Mobile SARS Containment Teams 2003. *American Journal of Infection Control* 32(7): 377–383.

Lim MK (2006) Bird Flu: Pandemic Flu Preparation: An Unheeded Lesson from SARS. *British Medical Journal,* April, 332: 913.

Lo B, Wolf L, and Sengupta S (2000) Ethical Issues in Early Detection of HIV Infection to Reduce Vertical Transmission. *Journal of Acquired Immune Deficiency Syndromes* 25: S136–S143.

McCord M (2005) Once Secretive Countries Opening Up about Bird Flu. *Agence France-Presse.* Hong Kong: October 25.

Merson MH (2000) Early Detection: The Next Steps. *Journal of Acquired Immune Deficiency Syndromes* 25: S157–S159.

Miner NJ, Dunham, Musgrove B, and Harris V (2006) A Commonly Available Household Sterilant. Paper presented at the American Society for Microbiology 2006 Biodefense Research Meeting, February 17, 2006. Washington DC: ASM.

Murnighan JK, Malhotra D, and Weber JM (2004) Paradoxes of Trust: Empirical and Theoretical Departures from a Traditional Model. In: Kramer RM and Cook KS (eds.) *Trust and Distrust in Organizations: Dilemmas and Approaches,* pp. 293–326. New York: Russell Sage Foundation.

Olowokure B and Roth C (2006) Mini-Symposium Severe Acute Respiratory Syndrome (SARS): Reshaping Global Public Health. *Public Health* 120: 3–5.

Omi S (2006) Overview. In: World Health Organization (ed.) *How a Global Epidemic Was Stopped,* pp. vii–x. Geneva: WHO.

Osnos E (2005) China's Past Stirs Fears of Future. Avian Flu Experts Are Wary of Nation's History of Secrecy and Delay in Handling Medical Crisis. *Chicago Tribune.* November 2, p. 1.

Patterson D and London L (2002) International Law, Human Rights, and HIV/AIDS. *Bulletin of the World Health Organization* 80(12): 964–969.

Pratkanis A and Aronson E (2001) *Age of Propaganda. The Everyday Use and Abuse of Persuasion,* Revised Edition. New York: Henry Holt & Company.

Quah SR (1985) The Health Belief Model and Preventive Health Behaviour in Singapore. *Social Science & Medicine* 21(3): 351–363.

Quah SR (1988) Private Choices and Public Health: A Case of Policy Intervention in Singapore. *Asian Journal of Public Administration* 10(2): 207–224.

Quah SR (2007) Public Image and Governance of Epidemics: Comparing HIV/AIDS and SARS. *Health Policy* 80: 253–272.

Quah SR and Lee HP (2004) Crisis Prevention and Management during SARS Outbreak, Singapore. *Emerging Infectious Diseases* 10(2): 364–368.

Radaev V (2004) Coping with Distrust in Emerging Russian Markets. In: Hardin R (ed.) *Distrust,* pp. 233–248. New York: Russell Sage Foundation.

Rollins J (2004) *AIDS and the Sexuality of Law: Ironic Jurisprudence.* New York: Palgrave.

Rompress (2005) Romania, Ukraine, Moldova Set Up Task Force to Combat Bird Flu. Bucharest: October 18.

Rosenthal E (2006) Bird Flu Virus May Spread by Smuggling. *New York Times.* April 15. www.nytimes.com/2006/04/15/world/europe/15bird.html. Accessed: 15 April 2006.

Saich T (2006) Is SARS China's Chernobyl or Much Ado about Nothing? In: Kleinman A and Watson JL (eds.) *SARS in China: Prelude to Pandemic?* Stanford: Stanford University Press.

SARS Expert Committee (2003) *SARS in Hong Kong: From Experience to Action.* Hong Kong: Report of the SEC, Hong Kong SAR Government.

Shaw K (2006) The 2003 SARS Outbreak and Its Impact on Infection Control Practices. *Public Health* 120: 8–14.

Shu SL (2003) SARS Epidemic Worsens in Taiwan. Home Quarantines Are Often Violated. *The Washington Post,* May 15, p. A16.

Sim F and Mackie P (2006) The Angel of Death: Reshaping Global Public Health. *Public Health* 120: 1–2.

Singer M (1994) The Politics of AIDS. *Social Science & Medicine* 38(10): 1321–1342.

Taylor AL (2002) Global Governance, International Health Law and WHO: Looking towards the Future. *Bulletin of the World Health Organization* 80(12): 975–980.

Taylor-Gooby P and Zinn JO (2006) Current Directions in Risk Research: New Developments in Psychology and Sociology. *Risk Analysis* 26(2): 397–411.

Tilly C (2005) *Trust and Rule.* Cambridge: Cambridge University Press.

United Nations (1985) *The Siracusa Principles: International Covenant on Civil and Political Rights.* Annex to UN Document E/CN.4/1985/4, September 28, 1984. New York: United Nations.

United Nations (2004) *A More Secure World: Our Shared Responsibility. Report of the Secretary-General's High-Level Panel on Threats, Challenges and Change.* New York: United Nations Department of Public Information.

Useem M (1998) *The Leadership Moment: Nine True Stories of Triumph and Disaster and Their Lessons for Us All.* New York: Three Rivers Press.

U.S. Food and Drug Administration (1998) *The Belmont Report: Ethical Principles and Guidelines for the Protection of Human Subjects of Research.* Washington, DC: USFDA. http://www.fda.gov/oc/ohrt/irbs/belmont.html. Accessed: 30 May 2006.

U.S. Food and Drug Administration (2006) *Guidance for Institutional Review Boards, Clinical Investigator Sponsors.* Washington, DC: USFDA. http://www.fda.gov/oc/ohrt/irbs/. Accessed: 30 May 2006.

Valdiserri RO, Janssen RS, Buehler JW, and Fleming PL (2000) The Context of HIV/AIDS Surveillance. *Journal of Acquired Immune Deficiency Syndromes* 25: S97–S104.

Welch Larson D (2004) Distrust: Prudent, If Not Always Wise. In: Hardin R (ed.) *Distrust,* pp. 34–59. New York: Russell Sage Foundation.

Whitman J (2000) *The Politics of Emerging and Resurgent Infectious Diseases.* London: Macmillan Press.

Wu S (2003) SARS Cases Rise at Sealed-off Taiwan Hospital; Patients Inside Protest. *BBC Monitoring International Reports.* Taipei: April, 26. http://infoweb.newsbank.com. Accessed: 10 Feb 2006.

Wuthnow R (2004) Trust as an Aspect of Social Structure. In: Alexander JC, Marx GT and Williams CL (eds.) *Self, Social Structure and Beliefs. Explorations in Sociology,* pp. 145–167. Berkeley: University of California Press.

Zhang H (2006) Making Light of the Dark Side: SARS Jokes and Humor in China. In: Kleinman A and Watson JL (eds.) *SARS in China. Prelude to Pandemic?* pp. 148–170. Stanford: Stanford University Press.

Zhao J (2003) The SARS Epidemic under China's Media Policy. *Media Asia* 30(4): 191–196.

Infectious Disease Modeling

M Kretzschmar, Julius Center for Health Sciences and Primary Care, University Medical Center Utrecht, Utrecht, The Netherlands

What Is Infectious Disease Modeling?

In recent years, mathematical models have been used increasingly to support public health policy making in the field of infectious disease control. Especially in developing public health response plans for a future pandemic outbreak of a new strain of influenza A, mathematical and computer modeling has been applied to investigate various intervention scenarios ranging from ring prophylactic treatment with antivirals to increasing social distance by school closure. There are several reasons to use mathematical modeling as a tool for an analysis of policy options. One is the complexity of infectious disease dynamics: Since transmission of infections involves contact between infectious and susceptible persons, the spread of an infectious disease depends on contact behavior and patterns in the population in combination with biological characteristics of the host–pathogen interaction. Second, it is not possible by pure reasoning to decide between a variety of different intervention strategies or possibly combinations of these strategies, because their effectiveness depends on many interrelated factors. Third, to conduct a sound cost-effectiveness analysis, the impact of intervention on the prevalence and incidence of an infectious disease should be taken into account, which requires quantitative estimates of the impact of different intervention options.

The central idea of transmission models as opposed to statistical models is a mechanistic description of the transmission of infection between two individuals. This mechanistic description makes it possible to describe the time evolution of an epidemic in mathematical terms and in this way connect the individual-level process of transmission with a population-level description of incidence and prevalence on an infectious disease. The rigorous mathematical way of formulating these dependencies requires analyzing in great detail all the dynamic processes that contribute to disease transmission. Therefore, developing a mathematical model helps to focus thoughts on the essential processes involved in shaping the epidemiology of an infectious disease and to reveal the parameters that are most influential and amenable for control. Mathematical modeling is therefore also integrative in combining knowledge from very different disciplines such as microbiology, social sciences, and clinical sciences.

The first roots of mathematical modeling date back to the eighteenth century, when Daniel Bernoulli used mathematical methods to estimate the impact of smallpox vaccination on life expectancy (Dietz and Heesterbeek, 2000). Later, Hamer (Hamer, 1906) used mathematical reasoning to argue that an epidemic can come to an end before all susceptible persons in the population have been infected, even without a decrease in the virulence of the pathogen. A rigorous mathematical framework was first worked out by Kermack and Mckendrick in 1927 (Kermack and McKendrick, 1991a, 1991b, 1991c). Their model has been the basis of all further modeling and is nowadays best known as the SIR model, although the theory developed by Kermack and McKendrick is much richer than what is usually meant by the SIR model. In their work, the central insight of the threshold value that determines whether a disease spreads or becomes extinct is first introduced. This threshold value is now better known as the basic reproduction number and will be explained in more detail in the section titled 'The SIR model and the basic reproduction number R_0' below. Research in mathematical modeling of infectious diseases increased and expanded out of the pure applied mathematics community into the public health community in the 1980s with the advent and problems of the spread of HIV/AIDS. But only in recent years has mathematical modeling been recognized as a valuable tool for public health policy makers and has the interaction between modelers and policy makers become direct and intense. Examples such as the outbreak of SARS in 2003, the need to design response plans for renewed smallpox outbreaks, and the need to prepare for the event of an outbreak with a pandemic strain of influenza A have shown public health policy makers the power of using models to test intervention strategies in the face of infectious disease threats that are newly emerging or yet to come.

The SIR Model and the Basic Reproduction Number R_0

The SIR model contains all the essential elements of a mathematical model for the transmission of an infectious disease. Its basic assumption is that the human population is subdivided into three groups or compartments: The group of susceptible persons (denoted by S), the group of infected persons (denoted by I) and the group of removed persons (removed from the process of transmission by immunity) (denoted by R). The mathematical

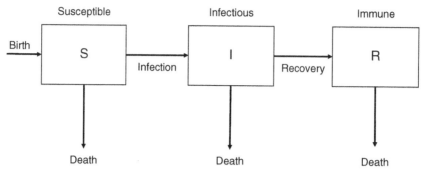

Figure 1 Flow chart of the SIR model.

model provides a precise description of the movements in and out of the three compartments. Those movements are birth (flow into the compartment of susceptibles), death (flow out of all compartments), transmission of infection (flow from S into I) and recovery (flow from I into R) (**Figure 1**).

Transitions between compartments are governed by rates, which in the simplest version of the model are assumed to be constant in time. The birth rate ν describes the recruitment of new susceptibles into the population, the death rate μ the loss of individuals due to a disease-unrelated background mortality, and γ denotes the recovery rate of infected individuals into immunity. The key element of the model is the term describing transmission of infection according to a rate β using a mass action term. The idea behind using a mass action term to describe transmission is that individuals of the population meet each other at random and each individual has the same probability per unit time to meet each other individual. Therefore, for a susceptible person the rate of meeting infected persons depends on their density or prevalence in the population, or in mathematical terms $\lambda = \beta\,I$, where λ is the force of infection. The force of infection is a measure for the risk of a susceptible person to become infected per unit of time. It depends on prevalence, either in an absolute sense on the number of infected people in the population or in a relative sense on the fraction of infected people in the population. In the latter case, we would obtain $\lambda = \beta I/N$, with N denoting the total population size. The parameter β is a composite parameter measuring the contact rate κ and the probability of transmission upon contact q, so $\beta = \kappa q$. The flow chart in **Figure 1** can be translated into a system of ordinary differential equations as follows:

$$\frac{dS}{dt} = \nu - \beta S \frac{I}{N} - \mu S$$

$$\frac{dI}{dt} = \beta S \frac{I}{N} - \gamma I - \mu I$$

$$\frac{dR}{dt} = \gamma I - \mu R$$

with $N = S + I + R$. For a full definition of the model, the initial state of the system has to be specified, i.e., the

numbers or fractions of the population in the states S, I, and R at time $t = 0$ have to be prescribed. Values for the parameters ν, μ, γ, and β have to be chosen either based on estimates from data or based on assumptions. Then standard numerical methods can be used to compute the time evolution of the system starting from the initial state.

So far, the model describes disease transmission without any possible intervention. We will show how to incorporate vaccination of newborns into this simple system and how to obtain some important insights into the effect of universal newborn vaccination. We denote the fraction of newborns that are vaccinated immediately after birth by p. Then instead of having a recruitment rate of ν, the recruitment is now $(1-p)\nu$ into the susceptible compartment, while $p\nu$ is recruited directly into the immune compartment. In terms of model equations this leads to:

$$\frac{dS}{dt} = \nu(1 - p) - \beta S \frac{1}{N} - \mu S$$

$$\frac{dI}{dt} = \beta S \frac{I}{N} - \gamma I - \mu I$$

$$\frac{dR}{dt} = \nu p + \gamma I - \mu R$$

with $0 \le p \le 1$. We will now derive some basic principles using this model as an example.

Basic Concepts: Reproduction Number, Endemic Steady State, and Critical Vaccination Coverage

The most important concepts of epidemic models can be demonstrated using the SIR model. Let us first consider an infectious disease that spreads on a much faster time scale than the demographic process. On the scale of disease transmission, the birth rate ν and the death rate μ can be considered to be close to zero. When can the prevalence in the population increase? An increase in prevalence is equivalent with $dI/dt > 0$, which means that $\beta SI/N > \gamma I$. This leads to $\beta S/N > \gamma$ or equivalently to

$\beta S/(\gamma N) > 1$. In the situation where all individuals of the population are susceptible, we have $S = N$; this means that an infectious disease can spread in a completely susceptible population if $\beta/\gamma > 1$. The quantity $R_0 = \beta/\gamma$ is also known as the basic reproduction number and can in principle be determined for every infectious disease model and can be estimated for every infectious disease. In biological terms, the basic reproduction number describes the number of secondary infections produced by one index case in a completely susceptible population during his entire infectious period (Diekmann *et al.*, 1990; Diekmann and Heesterbeek, 2000).

If $R_0 > 1$ the infection can spread in the population, because on average every infected individual replaces himself by more than one new infected person. However, this process can only continue as long as there is a sufficient number of susceptible individuals available. Once a larger fraction of the population has gone through the infection and has become immune, the probability of an infected person to meet a susceptible person decreases and with it the average number of secondary cases produced. If – as we assumed above – there is no birth into the population, no new susceptible individuals are coming in and the epidemic outbreak will invariably end (**Figure 2(a)**). Analysis of the model shows, however, that the final size of the outbreak will never encompass the entire population, but there will always be a fraction of susceptible individuals left over

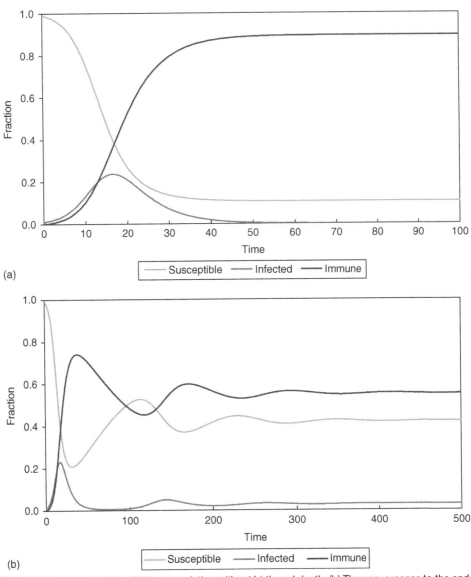

(a)

(b)

Figure 2 (a) The epidemic curve for $R_0 = 2.5$ in a population without birth and death. (b) The convergence to the endemic equilibrium for a population with birth and death. Adapted from Krämer A and Reintjes R (eds.) (2003) *Infectious Disease Epidemiology: Methods, Surveillance, Mathematical Models, Global Public Health* (in German). Heidelberg: Springer Verlag, with kind permission of Springer Science and Business Media.

after the outbreak has subsided. It can be shown that the final size A_∞ (attack rate in epidemiological terms) is related to the basic reproduction number by the implicit formula $A_\infty = 1 - \exp(-R_0 A_\infty)$. In other words, if the basic reproduction number of an infectious disease is known, the attack rate in a completely susceptible population can be derived.

The situation changes when we consider the system on a demographic time scale where births and deaths play a role (**Figure 2(b)**). Assuming now that ν and μ are positive, with the same arguments as above, we obtain that $R_0 = \beta/(\gamma + \mu)$. Now if $R_0 > 1$ the system can develop into an equilibrium state where the supply of new susceptible persons by birth is balanced by the transmission process and on average every infected person produces one new infection. This endemic equilibrium can be computed from the model equations by setting the left-hand sides to zero and solving for the variables S, I, and R in terms of the model parameters. First one obtains the steady state population size as $N^* = \nu/\mu$ (the superscript * denotes the steady state value). The steady state values for the infection-related variables are then given by:

$$S^* = \frac{(\gamma + \mu)\nu}{\beta\mu} = \frac{\nu}{\mu R_0}$$

$$I^* = \left(\frac{\nu}{\mu}\right)\left(\frac{\mu}{\gamma + \mu}\right)\left(1 - \frac{1}{R_0} - p\right)$$

$$R^* = \frac{\nu}{\mu} - S^* - I^*$$

Hence the fractions of the population that are susceptible, infected, and recovered in an endemic steady state are given by:

$$\frac{S^*}{N^*} = \frac{\gamma + \mu}{\beta} = \frac{1}{R_0}$$

$$\frac{I^*}{N^*} = \left(\frac{\mu}{\gamma + \mu}\right)\left(1 - \frac{1}{R_0} - p\right)$$

$$\frac{R^*}{N^*} = 1 - \frac{S^*}{N^*} - \frac{I^*}{N^*}$$

Note that the fraction of susceptible individuals S^*/N^* in the endemic steady state is independent of the vaccination coverage p. On the other hand, the prevalence of infection I^*/N^* depends on p: The prevalence decreases linearly with increasing vaccination coverage until the point of elimination is reached. This means we can compute the critical vaccination coverage p_c, i.e., the threshold coverage needed for elimination from $0 = 1 - 1/R_0 - p_c$ as $p_c = 1 - 1/R_0$. In other words, the larger the basic reproduction number, the higher the fraction of the population that has to be vaccinated in order to eliminate an infection from the population. For an infection such as smallpox with an estimated basic reproduction number of around 5, a coverage of 80% is needed for elimination, while for measles with a reproduction number of around 20 the coverage has to be at least 96%. This gives one explanation for the fact that it was possible to eradicate smallpox in the 1970s whereas we are still a long way from measles eradication. There are some countries, however, that have been successful in eliminating measles based on a consistently high vaccination coverage (Peltola *et al.*, 1997). A graphical representation of the relationship between the basic reproduction number and the critical vaccination coverage is given in **Figure 3**.

Advanced Models

Building on the basic ideas of the SIR framework, numerous types of mathematical models have been developed, all incorporating more structure and details of the transmission process and infectious disease dynamics.

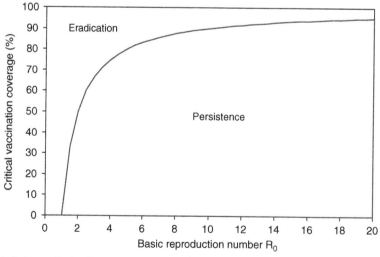

Figure 3   The relationship between the basic reproduction number R_0 and the critical vaccination coverage p_c. Adapted from Krämer A and Reintjes R (eds.) (2003) *Infectious Disease Epidemiology: Methods, Surveillance, Mathematical Models, Global Public Health* (in German). Heidelberg: Springer Verlag, with kind permission of Springer Science and Business Media.

More Complex Compartmental Models

A first obvious extension is the inclusion of more disease-specific details into the model. Compartments describing a latent period, the vaccinated population, chronic and acute stages of infection, and many more have been described in the literature (Anderson and May, 1991). Another important refinement of compartmental models is to incorporate heterogeneity of the population into the model, for example by distinguishing between population subgroups with different behaviors or population subgroups with differences in susceptibility, or geographically distinct populations. Heterogeneity in behavior was first introduced into models describing the spread of sexually transmitted infections by Hethcote and Yorke (Hethcote and Yorke, 1984). Later, during the first decade of the HIV/AIDS pandemic, efforts were made to describe models with sexual activity levels and mixing patterns between subgroups of various activity levels (Koopman et al., 1988). These models are still used frequently for assessing the effects of intervention in the spread of STI. Age structure has also been modeled as a series of compartments, with individuals passing from one compartment to the next according to an aging rate, but this requires a large number of additional compartments to be added to the model structure. This point also shows the limitation of compartmental models: With increasing structuring of the population, the number of compartments increases rapidly and with it the necessity to define and parametrize the mixing between all the population subgroups in the model. The theory of how to define and compute the basic reproduction number in heterogeneous populations was developed by Diekmann et al. (Diekmann et al., 1990). Geographically distinct but interacting population groups have been investigated using the framework of metapopulations for analyzing the dynamics of childhood infections.

Models with a Continuous Age Structure

Age structure can best be described as a continuous variable, where age progresses with time. Mathematically, this leads to models in the form of partial differential equations, where all variables of the model depend on time and age (Diekmann and Heesterbeek, 2000). Analytically, partial differential equations are more difficult to handle than ordinary differential equations, but numerically solving an age-structured system of model equations is straightforward.

Stochastic Transmission Models

In a deterministic model based on a system of differential equations, it is implicitly assumed that the numbers in the various compartments are sufficiently large that stochastic effects can be neglected. In reality, this is not always the case. For example, when analyzing epidemic outbreaks in small populations such as a school or a small village, typical stochastic events can occur such as extinction of the infection from the population or large stochastic fluctuations in the final size of the epidemic. Questions of stochastic influences on infectious disease dynamics have been studied in various ways, starting with the Reed-Frost model for a discrete time transmission of infection up to a stochastic version of the SIR model introduced above (Bailey, 1975; Becker, 1989). Finally, stochastic models have been investigated using simulation techniques also known as Monte-Carlo simulation. An important theoretical result from the analysis of stochastic models is the distinction between minor and major outbreaks for infectious diseases with $R_0 > 1$. While in a deterministic model a R_0 larger than unity always leads to an outbreak if the infection is introduced into an entirely susceptible population, in a stochastic model a certain fraction of introductions remain minor outbreaks with only a few secondary infections. This leads to a bimodal probability distribution of the final epidemic size following the introduction of one infectious index case (**Figure 4**). The peak for small outbreak sizes describes the situation where the infection dies out after only a few secondary infections; the peak for large outbreak sizes describes those outbreaks that take off and affect a large part of the population. The larger the basic reproduction number, the larger is the fraction of major outbreaks in the susceptible population (Andersson and Britton, 2000).

Network Models

Some aspects of contact between individuals cannot easily be modeled in compartmental models. In the context of the spread of sexually transmitted diseases, models were developed that take the duration of partnerships into account, called pair formation models. Extending those models to include also simultaneous long-term partnerships leads to the class of network models, where the network of contacts is described by a graph with nodes representing individuals and links representing their contacts. Different network structural properties have been related to the speed of spread of an epidemic through the population. In the small world networks, most contacts between individuals are local, but some long-distance contacts ensure a rapid global spread of an epidemic. Long-distance spread of infectious disease is becoming increasingly important in a globalizing world with increasing mobility, as demonstrated by the SARS epidemic in 2003. Recently, the concept of scale-free networks where the number of links per node follows a power law distribution was discussed in relation to the spread of epidemics. With respect to the spread of sexually transmitted diseases, a network structure where some individuals have very many partners while the majority of people have only a few might lead to great difficulties

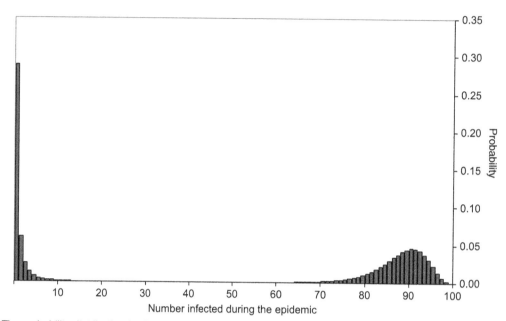

Figure 4 The probability distribution for the occurrence of minor and major outbreaks after the introduction of one infectious index case into a population of 100 susceptible individuals for an infection with basic reproduction number $R_0 = 2.5$. Adapted from Krämer A and Reintjes R (eds.) (2003) *Infectious Disease Epidemiology: Methods, Surveillance, Mathematical Models, Global Public Health* (in German). Heidelberg: Springer Verlag, with kind permission of Springer Science and Business Media.

in controlling the disease by intervention. Network concepts have also been applied to study the spread of respiratory diseases.

Use of Modeling for Public Health Policy

Mathematical models have been widely used to assess the effectiveness of vaccination strategies, to determine the best vaccination ages and target groups and to estimate the effort needed to eliminate an infection from the population. More recently, mathematical modeling has supported contingency planning in preparation for a possible attack with smallpox virus and in planning the public health response to an outbreak with a pandemic strain of influenza A. Other types of intervention measures have also been evaluated such as screening for asymptomatic infection with *Chlamydia trachomatis*, contact tracing, and antiviral treatment in the case of HIV. In the field of nosocomial infections and transmission of antibiotic-resistant pathogens, modeling has been used to compare hospital-specific interventions such as cohorting of health-care workers, increased hygiene, and isolation of colonized patients. In health economic evaluations, it has been recognized that dynamic transmission models are a necessary requisite for conducting good cost-effectiveness analyses for infectious disease control.

It is a large step from developing mathematical theory for the dynamics of infectious diseases to application in a concrete public health-relevant situation. The latter requires an intensive focusing on relevant data sources, as well as clinical and microbiological knowledge to make a decision on how to design an appropriate model. Appropriate here means that the model uses the knowledge available, is able to answer the questions that are asked by the policy makers, and is sufficiently simple so that its dynamics can be understood and interpreted. In the future it will be important to strengthen the link between advanced statistical methodology and mathematical modeling in order to further improve the performance of modeling as a public health tool.

See also: Biostatistics; Measurement and Modeling of Health-Related Quality of Life.

Citations

Anderson RM and May RM (1991) *Infectious Disease of Humans: Dynamics and Control.* Oxford, UK: Oxford University Press.

Andersson H and Britton T (2000) *Stochastic Epidemic Models and Their Statistical Analysis.* New York: Springer.

Bailey NTG (1975) *The Mathematical Theory of Infectious Diseases and Its Applications.* London: Griffin.

Becker NG (1989) *Analysis of Infectious Disease Data.* London: Chapman and Hall.

Diekmann O and Heesterbeek JAP (2000) *Mathematical Epidemiology of Infectious Diseases.* Chichester, UK: Wiley.

Diekmann O, Heesterbeek JA, and Metz JA (1990) On the definition and the computation of the basic reproduction ratio R0 in models for infectious diseases in heterogeneous populations. *Journal of Mathematical Biology* 28(4): 365–382.

Dietz K and Heesterbeek JA (2000) Bernoulli was ahead of modern epidemiology. *Nature* 408(6812): 513–514.

Hamer WH (1906) Epidemic disease in England – The evidence of variability and persistency of type. *Lancet* 1: 733–739.

Hethcote HW and Yorke JA (1984) *Gonorrhea Transmission Dynamics and Control*. New York: Springer Verlag.

Kermack WO and McKendrick AG (1991a) Contributions to the mathematical theory of epidemics – I. 1927. *Bulletin of Mathematical Biology* 53(1–2): 33–55.

Kermack WO and McKendrick AG (1991b) Contributions to the mathematical theory of epidemics – II. The problem of endemicity. 1932. *Bulletin of Mathematical Biology* 53(1–2): 57–87.

Kermack WO and McKendrick AG (1991c) Contributions to the mathematical theory of epidemics – III. Further studies of the problem of endemicity. 1933. *Bulletin of Mathematical Biology* 53(1–2): 89–118.

Koopman J, Simon C, Jacquez J, Joseph J, Sattenspiel L, and Park T (1988) Sexual partner selectiveness effects on homosexual HIV transmission dynamics. *Journal of Acquired Immune Deficiency Syndrome* 1(5): 486–504.

Krämer A and Reintjes R (eds.) (2003) *Infectious Disease Epidemiology: Methods, Surveillance, Mathematical Models, Global Public Health* (in German). Heidelberg, Germany: Springer Verlag.

Peltola H, Davidkin I, Valle M, *et al.* (1997) No measles in Finland. *Lancet* 350(9088): 1364–1365.

Further Reading

Ancel Meyers L, Newman ME, Martin M, and Schrag S (2003) Applying network theory to epidemics: Control measures for *Mycoplasma pneumoniae* outbreaks. *Emerging Infectious Diseases* 9(2): 204–210.

Baggaley RF, Ferguson NM, and Garnett GP (2005) The epidemiological impact of antiretroviral use predicted by mathematical models: A review. *Emerging Themes in Epidemiology* 2: 9.

Barnabas RV, Laukkanen P, Koskela P, Kontula O, Lehtinen M, and Garnett GP (2006) Epidemiology of HPV 16 and cervical cancer in Finland and the potential impact of vaccination: Mathematical modelling analyses. *PLo S Medicine* 3(5): e138.

Bootsma MC, Diekmann O, and Bonten MJ (2006) Controlling methicillin-resistant *Staphylococcus aureus*: Quantifying the effects of interventions and rapid diagnostic testing. *Proceedings of the National Academy of Sciences USA* 103(14): 5620–5625.

Coffee M, Lurie MN, and Garnett GP (2007) Modelling the impact of migration on the HIV epidemic in South Africa. *AIDS* 21(3): 343–350.

Eames KT and Keeling MJ (2003) Contact tracing and disease control. *Proceedings of the Royal Society B: Biological Sciences* 270(1533): 2565–2571.

Edmunds WJ, Medley GF, and Nokes DJ (1999) Evaluating the cost-effectiveness of vaccination programmes: A dynamic perspective. *Statistics in Medicine* 18(23): 3263–3282.

Ferguson NM, Keeling MJ, Edmunds WJ, *et al.* (2003) Planning for smallpox outbreaks. *Nature* 425(6959): 681–685.

Ferguson NM, Cummings DA, Fraser C, Cajka JC, Cooley PC, and Burke DS (2006) Strategies for mitigating an influenza pandemic. *Nature* 442(7101): 448–452.

Gay NJ, Hesketh LM, Morgan-Capner P, and Miller E (1995) Interpretation of serological surveillance data for measles using mathematical models: Implications for vaccine strategy. *Epidemiology and Infection* 115(1): 139–156.

Grundmann H and Hellriegel B (2006) Mathematical modelling: A tool for hospital infection control. *Lancet Infectious Diseases* 6(1): 39–45.

Hadeler KP, Waldstatter R, and Worz-Busekros A (1988) Models for pair formation in bisexual populations. *Journal of Mathematical Biology* 26(6): 635–649.

Hethcote HW (1997) An age-structured model for pertussis transmission. *Mathematical Biosciences* 145(2): 89–136.

Hufnagel L, Brockmann D, and Geisel T (2004) Forecast and control of epidemics in a globalized world. *Proceedings of the National Academy of Sciences USA* 101(42): 15124–15129.

Keeling MJ and Eames KT (2005) Networks and epidemic models. *Journal of the Royal Society Interface* 2(4): 295–307.

Kretzschmar M, Welte R, van den Hoek A, and Postma MJ (2001) Comparative model-based analysis of screening programs for *Chlamydia trachomatis* infections. *American Journal of Epidemiology* 153(1): 90–101.

Kretzschmar M, de Wit GA, Smits LJ, and van de Laar MJ (2002) Vaccination against hepatitis B in low endemic countries. *Epidemiology and Infection* 128(2): 229–244.

Liljeros F, Edling CR, Amaral LA, Stanley HE, and Aberg Y (2001) The web of human sexual contacts. *Nature* 411(6840): 907–908.

Longini IM Jr., Halloran ME, Nizam A, and Yang Y (2004) Containing pandemic influenza with antiviral agents. *American Journal of Epidemiology* 159(7): 623–633.

Roberts MG and Tobias MI (2000) Predicting and preventing measles epidemics in New Zealand: Application of a mathematical model. *Epidemiology and Infection* 124(2): 279–287.

Roberts T, Robinson S, Barton P, *et al.* (2004) The correct approach to modelling and evaluating chlamydia screening. *Sexually Transmitted Infections* 80(4): 324–325.

Rohani P, Earn DJ, and Grenfell BT (1999) Opposite patterns of synchrony in sympatric disease metapopulations. *Science* 286 (5441): 968–971.

Van Rie A and Hethcote HW (2004) Adolescent and adult pertussis vaccination: Computer simulations of five new strategies. *Vaccine* 22(23–24): 3154–3165.

Watts DJ and Strogatz SH (1998) Collective dynamics of 'small-world' networks. *Nature* 393(6684): 440–442.

Welte R, Postma M, Leidl R, and Kretzschmar M (2005) Costs and effects of chlamydial screening: Dynamic versus static modeling. *Sexually Transmitted Diseases* 32(8): 474–483.

Chronic Disease Modeling

J D F Habbema and R Boer, Erasmus MC, University Medical Center, Rotterdam, The Netherlands
J J Barendregt, School of Population Health, University of Queensland, Brisbane, Australia

Why and When to Use Modeling

Modeling of chronic diseases is undertaken to answer research questions on these diseases and their health impact. General background knowledge, data from research and disease registries, expert knowledge, and judgment are all crucial in modeling. Models are applied to explain observations and make predictions, similar to scientific theory in general. Modeling, which can be defined as reasoning and theorizing in the language of mathematics, is required when natural language becomes too ambiguous or too complex to address the questions at hand. Modeling is virtually mandatory when research questions involve changes over time. Consider, for example, the future prevalence of a chronic disease. A survey can give an estimate of the current prevalence, yet to assess future prevalence, more information is needed. The present prevalence is a result of past incidence and survival rates, and trends in these rates are important for estimating future prevalence. Incidence is – with delays – influenced by trends in risk factors. Finally, population dynamics will have to be taken into account. Thus, answering the seemingly simple question on future prevalence can require complex modeling.

Chronic Disease

A chronic disease is a disease of long duration. This definition is necessarily ambiguous, because every disease has a particular duration, and thus it is a matter of judgment whether a disease is considered of 'long' duration; it cannot be approximated by a specific endpoint in time.

A chronic disease is a dynamic entity whose consequences may change dramatically as medical interventions evolve. As knowledge of a disease and the array of available interventions for prevention, diagnosis, and treatment expands, modeling of the disease process may move accordingly. An impressive example is cervical cancer. Without treatment, as is often the case in resource-poor countries, it is a 100% lethal disease. With surgical and other treatment possibilities, stage distribution at diagnosis, and stage-specific survival become relevant. With the possibility of early detection by a Pap smear, models might expand to include preclinical stages and even preinvasive stages. With the discovery of the human papilloma virus (HPV) as a cause of cervical cancer, it is useful to further extend models to capture HPV-infection stages and HPV screening tests. And the recent development of HPV vaccination will make the next generation of cervical cancer models a combination of infectious disease and chronic disease modeling (Kim *et al.*, 2007).

Public Health Impact of Chronic Diseases

The significance of chronic diseases for public health includes concern for both mortality and morbidity. Mortality affects life expectancy, while morbidity causes loss in health-related quality of life. The quantity and quality aspects of disease burden can be combined in the overall measure of quality-adjusted life years (QALYs), disability-adjusted life years (DALYs), or other summary measures for population health (see Murray *et al.*, 2002). Models for chronic diseases require embedding in a population perspective to calculate public health impact.

A Basic Model

In what is a basic model for assessing the burden of a chronic disease (**Figure 1(a)**), a disease-specific, yearly mortality l acts on a stationary, homogeneous population (i.e., unstratified by age, sex, or other individual characteristics) and competes with a mortality rate m from other causes. These rates enable us to calculate life-years lost. The loss in life expectancy caused by the disease equals $1/m - 1/(l+m)$. For example, when death statistics indicate that m equals 0.012 and l equals 0.001, the life expectancy in the population equals 76.9 years, and with elimination of the disease the life expectancy would increase by 6.4 years to 83.3 years. When health-related quality of life, on a scale of 0 to 1, is measured to be 0.9 without the disease and 0.7 with the disease, the loss in QALYs because of the lower life expectancy equals 5.76, calculated as 6.4 years times the 0.9 quality-of-life value. When a health survey gives a disease prevalence of 0.01, we can calculate that persons live on average $0.01 \times 76.9 = 0.8$ years with the disease, and the QALY-loss during life because of the disease therefore equals $0.8 \times 0.2 = 0.16$ QALY. The total QALY-loss from this disease is 5.92 QALYs per person on average, being the sum of 5.76 and 0.16.

With this basic model we can not only calculate the impact on population health of total elimination of the disease, but also the impact of interventions that reduce mortality rate, incidence, and the loss in quality of life. Because the model describes its components in their mutual coherence, it allows us to calculate also the unobserved duration and incidence of the disease. The approximate disease duration is 10 years, obtained by dividing the prevalence of 0.01 by the cause-specific mortality rate of 0.001 (it will be somewhat shorter because of mortality from other causes). And, to keep prevalence at 0.01, the yearly incidence has to equal the loss in prevalence due to mortality.

Other models for chronic diseases can be considered as extensions of this basic model, by adding age and sex, risk factors, time trends, multiple disease states, unobserved heterogeneity between persons, population dynamics, and appropriate dependencies and stochasticities.

Research Question and Model Structure

Research question and model structure are intimately connected. **Figure 1** gives model structures that correspond to different research questions. **Figure 1(a)** describes the basic model discussed in the previous section. **Figure 1(b)** is an appropriate structure for modeling treatment improvements. It includes a cure rate, which can be influenced by treatment. **Figure 1(c)** distinguishes early disease from late disease. This is appropriate for exploring implications of shorter patient and doctor

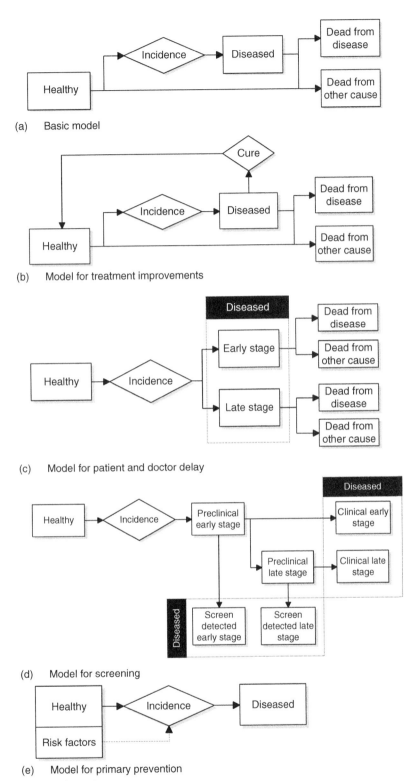

(a)   Basic model

(b)   Model for treatment improvements

(c)   Model for patient and doctor delay

(d)   Model for screening

(e)   Model for primary prevention

Figure 1   Chronic disease model structures.

delays, which lead to an earlier diagnosis, and for assessing new diagnostic techniques, which can lead to more accurate disease staging and better treatment choice. **Figure 1(d)** includes preclinical (screen-detectable) disease stages to model screening. **Figure 1(e)** gives a structure for primary prevention in which changes in risk-factor distribution lead to changes in incidence. More complex model structures are obtained by combining features of **Figures 1(a)–1(e)**.

Extension to several diseases can lead to great complexity and to demanding data requirements, and simplifications are needed to maintain tractability.

Time

Disease models will usually have 'age,' 'time,' and 'sex' as dimensions. Time and age are continuous phenomena, but many models use discrete time steps of, for example, 1 year. This is easy to implement but it also introduces a problem. Since we do not know where during the time step an event took place, we cannot tell by how much it changes the risk of other events. With continuous time modeling this problem does not exist. Therefore, continuous time modeling is preferred, but it is more difficult to implement. Two theories dealing with time underlie much of the modeling of transition rates. Life-table methods are almost exclusively in discrete time (Manton and Stallard, 1988). The continuous time theory of multistate models is firmly embedded in event-history analysis, survival analysis, and competing risk theory (Andersen and Keiding, 2002). Multistate models usually use Markov assumptions, which means that transition probabilities only depend on the current state and not on the duration *in* the state or on previous states. Markov models are much used in decision analytical modeling of chronic diseases (Beck and Pauker, 1983). A number of extensions have been developed by Manton and Stallard (1988) to account for age-dependence, individual differences, preclinical disease phases, disease dependency, and unobserved heterogeneity; they also propose a nonparametric modeling approach for situations in which there is insufficient background knowledge for building a more traditional multistate model.

Model Implementation: Macrosimulation and Microsimulation

For simple models with convenient assumptions, analytical and numerical solutions are possible. Otherwise, there are two main types of implementation of chronic disease models: macrosimulation and microsimulation (Law and Kelton, 1991).

In macrosimulation, the unit of simulation is a group. Applying the model equations to a group as a whole implies an assumption of homogeneity. When this assumption is not met, the group can be divided into more homogeneous subgroups. For example, there are usually separate life tables for men and women, and within each there is always a subdivision by age. Further subdivisions – for example, by health state – lead to a multistate life table. Subdivision works up to a point. With comorbidity, exposure to various risk factors (with possibly several exposure levels), and subdivision by time (since exposure, incidence, etc.), the

number of cells quickly gets unmanageable. Currently, most simulation models in public health and health care are macrosimulation models.

With microsimulation, a life history is simulated for each individual using an algorithm that describes the events that make up that life history. Random draws decide if and when specific events occur. Microsimulation population-level outcomes are obtained by aggregating over individual life histories. Microsimulation has the advantage in that there is no limit to what heterogeneity can be modeled. It produces individual-level artificial data that can be analyzed using standard statistical techniques. But microsimulation tends to be computationally intensive. Large runs are required because outcomes are stochastic. Additional assumptions are needed because the model is defined by distributions instead of single parameters. And the implications of the combined algorithmic assumptions defining the model can be so complex that they are discovered only through the simulation process itself. On the other hand, microsimulation can make exhaustive use of longitudinal, individual-level data in quantifying and fitting the model.

Population Models

For addressing public health questions, the chronic disease model has to be embedded in a population context. We will look at three types of population model: single cohort, multiple cohort, and dynamic population models.

A single cohort model is basically a period life table. A group of usually 100 000 people of an exact age (often 0) is subjected to cross-sectional ('period') mortality probabilities by age and followed until the cohort is extinct. In the multistate version, cross-sectional incidence and case fatality by age make it possible to calculate disease prevalence and mortality. The single cohort model is easy to implement, in particular when the discrete time/age option is chosen: a spreadsheet will suffice. The model has two mutually exclusive interpretations. One is the 'stationary population' interpretation: the life table is interpreted as a population of people of all ages at a single point in time. The second is the 'cohort' interpretation: the interpretation is of a cohort of people that is followed over time into the future while they age. Dynamic effects, defined as the time-delayed effects of a change, cannot be captured. Despite its strong limitations, the ease of use makes the single cohort model the natural starting point of almost any modeling exercise.

The multiple cohort model can be thought of as separate, single cohort models for each age group in the start population. All of these initial cohorts are followed over time until all are extinct. The sizes of these initial cohorts can be those of the real population. The model has both time and age, so trends and dynamic effects can be modeled, and the economic evaluation of costs and benefits at different points in time causes no problems. However, all evaluations apply to the current population only, so the population becomes increasingly incomplete with longer follow-up. When implemented as discrete time macrosimulation, it is still possible to use a spreadsheet for the multiple cohort model, although it tends to become rather big. Size can be reduced by taking, for example, 5-year instead of 1-year cohorts.

The dynamic population model adds births to the multiple cohort model. The population can be a life-table population ('dynamic life-table population') or the observed one ('dynamic real population'). Because the dynamic population model describes complete populations at every point in time, it can handle interventions for future populations, and is easily the most realistic of all population models, at the price of more complexity (especially when migration is also included). Implementation of a discrete time, macrosimulation, dynamic population model in a spreadsheet is a challenge, especially with long time horizons. It can be done, but using custom-made software for the task is a better option.

Validation

Validation refers to the process of increasing confidence that the model is producing the correct results. Face validity exists when a plain explanation of the model structure and assumptions appears reasonable to a critical audience. At the next level, the model assumptions can be justified by reference to an evidence base of results of good empirical research, and, when necessary, complemented by expert opinion. It is even better when model parameters are estimated by optimizing the fit between simulated and observed data, using, for example, least-squares, minimum chi-square, or maximum-likelihood methods. Fitting to data is well defined when a model is built for a particular intervention, and there are one or more randomized trials in which the effects of the intervention are reported in terms of end results and intermediate outcomes, which can be compared with model predictions. Often, the data to be fitted come from diverse studies and disease registries. In this case, expert judgment is required for assessing data quality and prioritizing data for their importance in fitting.

Internal validation of the model can subsequently be undertaken by assessing the quality of model predictions for data that were not used in the estimation process. Even more convincing is external validation in which the model is applied to prediction of future observations or prediction of outcomes in studies that were not used at all in the model quantification. A quite different type of validity is formal validity in which the modeler makes sure that the model indeed performs the calculations that it is supposed to do. This kind of validity is often taken for granted; to establish formal validity, extensive testing and analysis, in particular for complex models, may be required. For further discussion on model quality, including the role of sensitivity and uncertainty analysis, see Weinstein *et al.* (2003).

Actual Models

Until now we have discussed the different characteristics of models. In practice modelers will have to make many choices on how to proceed, and chronic disease models in public health can be seen as a cocktail of statistical, demographic, epidemiological, disease-course, and intervention modeling. We will briefly describe what choices have been made in some of the models developed over the last decades.

The model Prevent is a population-level model to evaluate the effect of changes in exposure to risk factors (Gunning-Schepers, 1989). It allows for multiple risk factors and multiple diseases, using independence assumptions and simple disease models to minimize complexity. Prevent uses macrosimulation, and the risk factors and diseases are embedded in a discrete time, dynamic population model. Applications include projections of future disease incidence, scenarios, and what-if questions (Brønnum-Hansen, 2002).

The DisMod model was developed for the Global Burden of Disease (GBD) project. The purpose of the model was to supplement incomplete data, and ensure that the disease data used in the GBD calculations were internally consistent (Barendregt and Ott, 2005). DisMod II (the current version of this model) allows input of three different disease variables, but usually only three suffice to calculate all seven. DisMod II is a macrosimulation, continous time, single cohort model, but switches to a multiple cohort model when time trends are incorporated in the input variables (Barendregt *et al.*, 2003). DisMod II is in the public domain, and can be downloaded at the World Health Organization's (WHO) website.

Popmod was developed for the WHO cost-effectiveness program, WHO-CHOICE. It models two diseases, in addition to a 'healthy' and a comorbid state, where the two diseases can interact. It evaluates the population-level effects of health-care interventions over time and age. Popmod is a continuous time, dynamic population model (Lauer *et al.*, 2003) and is available from the WHO on request (see Murray *et al.*, 2003 for an application to cardiovascular risk reduction).

The MISCAN model was developed to evaluate mass screening for cancer, including breast, cervical, prostate, and colorectal cancer. It is a microsimulation model with continuous time and discrete events that simulates a dynamic population (Habbema *et al.*, 1985).

The simulated life histories include date of birth and age at death from other causes than the disease, a preclinical, screen-detectable disease process and survival from diagnosis, and how the moment of death is affected by different possible screening programs. The MISCAN model has been used to design and monitor several cancer-screening programs and for surveillance of population trends (see, e.g., Koning *et al.*, 1991; for a review of screening models, see Stevenson, 2000).

The POHEM model of Statistics Canada is a micro-simulation model of a comprehensive series of chronic diseases intended to track health effects and costs resulting from the diseases and from interventions (Wolfson, 1994). It includes risk factors, disease onset, and progression, health-care resource utilization, direct medical care costs, and survival from a disease (see Evans *et al.*, 1995 for an application to lung cancer diagnosis and treatment).

The Coronary Heart Disease Policy Model has been developed to project the future mortality, morbidity, and cost of coronary heart disease (CHD) in the United States (Weinstein *et al.*, 1987). The model simulates the distribution of coronary risk factors and the incidence of CHD in a dynamic population; subsequent events in persons with a previous CHD event; and the effects of preventive and therapeutic interventions on mortality, morbidity, and costs. It is a discrete time, dynamic macrosimulation model. (For an application to risk factor modifications, see Tsevat *et al.*, 1991; for a review of heart disease models, see Cooper *et al.*, 2006.)

The Archimedes model is continuous in time and represents biological variables continuously by differential equations (Schlessinger and Eddy, 2002). It consists of components that represent the physiology of several organ systems and medical care processes. It comprises a general framework that is intended to represent a comprehensive set of diseases and care processes, and has so far been applied to diabetes (Eddy and Schlessinger, 2003). The extraordinary level of detail is intended to eventually represent complete, textbook-level details of medical practice.

In the CISNET cancer intervention and surveillance modeling network, many models have been developed for different cancer sites. For example, seven breast cancer models were developed and extensively discussed (Feuer *et al.*, 2006). All CISNET models are described using a newly developed 'model profiler' that facilitates description and comparison of models (CISNET, 2007).

See also: Infectious Disease Modeling.

Citations

Andersen PK and Keiding N (2002) Multi-state models for event history analysis. *Statistical Methods in Medical Research* 11: 91–115.

Barendregt JJ, van Oortmarssen GJ, Vos Th, and Murray CJL (2003) A generic model for the assessment of disease epidemiology: The computational basis of DisMod II. *Population Health Metrics, BioMed Central* 1: 4.

Barendregt JJ and Ott A (2005) Consistency of epidemiologic estimates. *European Journal of Epidemiology* 20: 827–832.

Beck JR and Pauker SG (1983) The Markov process in medical prognosis. *Medical Decision Making* 3: 419–458.

Brφnnum-Hansen H (2002) Predicting the effect of prevention of ischaemic heart disease. *Scandanavian Journal of Public Health* 30: 5–11.

CISNET (2007) Model profiles. Bethesda, MD: National Cancer Institute. http://cisnet.cancer.gov/resources (accessed February 2008).

Cooper K, Brailsford SC, Davies R, and Raftery J (2006) A review of health care models for coronary heart disease interventions. *Health Care and Management Sciences* 9: 311–324.

De Koning HJ, van Ineveld BM, van Oortmarssen GJ, et al. (1991) Breast cancer screening and cost-effectiveness; policy alternatives, quality of life considerations and the possible impact of uncertain factors. *International Journal of Cancer* 49: 531–537.

Eddy DM and Schlessinger L (2003) Archimedes: A trial-validated model of diabetes. *Diabetes Care* 26: 3093–3101.

Evans WK, Will BP, Berthelot JM, and Wolfson MC (1995) Estimating the cost of lung cancer diagnosis and treatment in Canada: The POHEM model. *Canadian Journal of Oncology* 5: 408–419.

Feuer EJ, Plevritis SK, Berry DA, and Cronin KA (eds.) (2006) The impact of mammography and adjuvant therapy on U.S. breast cancer mortality (1975–2000): Collective results from the Cancer Intervention and Surveillance Modelling Network. *Journal of the National Cancer Institute Monographs* 36: 1–126.

Gunning-Schepers LJ (1989) The health benefits of prevention: A simulation approach. *Health Policy* 12: 1–255.

Habbema JDF, van Oortmarssen GJ, Lubbe JT, and van der Maas PJ (1985) The MISCAN simulation program for the evaluation of screening for disease. *Computer Methods and Programs in Biomedicine* 20(1): 79–93.

Kim JJ, Kuntz KM, Stout NK, et al. (2007) Multiparameter calibration of a natural history model of cervical cancer. *American Journal of Epidemiology* 166: 137–150.

Lauer JA, Röhrich K, Wirth H, Charette C, Gribble S, and Murray CJL (2003) PoPMod: a longitudinal population model with two interacting disease states. *Cost Effectiveness and Resource Allocation, BioMed Central* 1: 6.

Law LM and Kelton WD (2000) *Simulation Modeling and Analysis*, 3rd edn. New York: McGraw-Hill.

Manton KG and Stallard E (1988) *Chronic Disease Modelling: Measurement and Evaluation of the Risks of Chronic Disease Processes*. New York: Oxford University Press.

Murray CJL, Salomon JA, Mathers CD, and Lopez AD (eds.) (2002) *Summary Measures of Population Health: Concepts, Ethics, Measurement and Applications*. Geneva, Switzerland: World Health Organization.

Murray CJ, Lauer JA, Hutubessy RC, et al. (2003) Effectiveness and costs of interventions to lower systolic blood pressure and cholesterol: A global and regional analysis on reduction of cardiovascular-disease risk. *The Lancet* 361: 717–725.

Schlessinger L and Eddy DM (2002) Archimedes: A new model for simulating health care systems – the mathematical formulation. *Journal of Biomedical Informatics* 35: 37–50.

Stevenson C (2000) Screening, models of. In: Armitage P and Colton T (eds.) *Encyclopedia of Biostatistics*, pp. 3999–4022. New York: Wiley

Tsevat J, Weinstein MC, Williams LW, Tosteson AN, and Goldman L (1991) Expected gains in life expectancy from various coronary heart disease risk factor modifications. *Circulation* 83: 1194–1201.

Weinstein MC, Coxson PG, Williams LW, Pass TM, Stason WB, and Goldman L (1987) Forecasting coronary heart disease incidence, mortality, and cost: The Coronary Heart Disease Policy Model. *American Journal of Public Health* 77: 1417–1426.

Weinstein MC, O'Brien B, Hornberger J, *et al.* (2003) Principles of good
practice for decision analytic modeling in health-care evaluation:
Report of the ISPOR Task Force on good research practices –
modeling studies. *Value in Health* 6: 9–17.
Wolfson MC (1994) POHEM – a framework for understanding and
modelling the health of human populations. *World Health Statistics
Quarterly* 47: 157–176.

Relevant Websites

http://cisnet.cancer.gov/resources – National Cancer Institute, Model
  Resources.
http://www.who.int – World Health Organization.

Cancer Screening

M Hakama and A Auvinen, University of Tampere School of Public Health, Tampere, Finland

Theory of Screening

The primary purpose of screening for cancer is to
reduce mortality. Besides the effect on the length of
life, screening also has other important consequences,
including a burden on economic resources and implications for the quality of life. Screening usually implies
an increase in health expenditure. The effects on the
quality of life of screened subjects can be both positive
and negative.

Cancers Suitable for Screening

Cancer is characterized both by an insidious onset and by
an improved outcome when it is detected early. For a
cancer to be suitable for screening, therefore, the natural
history of the disease should include a phase without
symptoms during which the cancer can be detected by a
screening test earlier than by ordinary clinical diagnosis
after the subject has experienced symptoms. The outcome
of treatment following diagnosis during this detectable,
preclinical phase (DPCP) (Cole and Morrison, 1978)
should also be better than following clinical detection.
Sometimes the screening program may reduce morbidity
or improve the quality of life. For example, a mammography program may increase the number of women undergoing surgery because of overdiagnosis; early diagnosis
increases the duration of sickness, but mammography
enables breast-conserving operations, which improves
the quality of life and produces less morbidity than the
treatment of more advanced disease.

The objective of screening is to reduce the burden of
disease. The impact of disease covers both death and
morbidity, that is, detriment of the disease for the patient
while alive, including reduced well-being and loss of
functional capacity. The prognosis should be better following early treatment of screen-detected disease than of
clinically detected disease. If a disease can be successfully
treated after it manifests clinically, there is no need for
screening. Screening should not be applied for untreatable diseases. Cancer is always a potentially lethal disease
and the primary goal of treatment is saving the patient's
life. Thus, a reduction of mortality is the most important
indicator of the effectiveness of screening.

The disease should be common enough to justify the
efforts involved in mounting a screening program. Disease
in the preclinical phase is the target of detection. The
frequency of preclinical disease in the population to be
screened depends on the incidence of clinical disease and
on the length of the detectable preclinical phase. Screening for disease is a continuous process. The prevalence of
disease at initial screening may be substantially different
from the prevalence at subsequent screens. This variation
in yield is not due to the length of the preclinical phase,
that is, the basic biological properties of the disease only,
but is simply a consequence of the length of intervals
between screening rounds, or the screening regimen.

The screening test must be capable of identifying
disease in the preclinical phase. For cancer, the earliest
stages of the preclinical phase are thought to occur in a
single cell, and they remain beyond identification. The
detectable preclinical phase starts when the disease
becomes detectable by the test and ends when the cancer
would surface clinically. The length of the DPCP is called
the sojourn time (Day and Walter, 1984). The sojourn time
is not constant, but varies from case to case. It can be
described with a theoretical distribution. Factors influencing the sojourn time include (1) the biological characteristics of the disease (growth and progression rate)
influencing the time from start of detectability to diagnosis at symptomatic stage, (2) the screening test and the
cut-off value or criteria for positivity, used for identifying
early disease (detectability threshold), and (3) behavioral
factors and health care affecting the end of DPCP, or the
time of diagnostic confirmation of the disease.

The occurrence of disease in a population is measured in terms of incidence or mortality rates. Stomach cancer is still common in middle-aged populations in many countries, but the risk is rapidly decreasing, which contrasts with a substantial increase for cancer of the breast, another disease occurring at a relatively early age in many countries. In contrast, the incidence of prostate cancer has been very low under 65 years of age, and the increase in incidence is mainly attributable to diagnostic activity. Therefore, the number of life-years that can potentially be saved by a (successful) screening program is small.

If screening postpones death, screening increases the prevalence of disease, that is, the number of people living who have been diagnosed with it at some time in the past. Prevalence may also increase as a consequence of earlier diagnosis or overtreatment, so the prevalence of disease and the survival of cancer patients are not appropriate indicators of the effect of screening.

Effects of screening on the quality of life and cost are in principle considered in decisions on whether or not to screen. In practice, however, public health policies related to cancer screening are invariably initiated, run, and evaluated by their effect on mortality. In fact, there is no agreement on how to apply criteria other than mortality to policy decisions about screening. Such a decision would require evidence on the magnitude of effect on these criteria, and agreement on how to weigh the benefits and harms in different dimensions of death, quality of life, and cost.

Benefits and Harms of Screening

Independently of effectiveness, screening has adverse effects. The effectiveness of screening is related to the degree to which the objectives are met. As indicated above, the purpose of screening is to reduce disease burden and the main goal is the reduction of deaths from the disease. If the treatment of screen-detected disease has fewer or less serious adverse effects than the treatment of clinical disease, then the iatrogenic morbidity for the patient is decreased. If late-stage disease is avoided, highly debilitating effects can be reduced. Costs can be saved if treatment and follow-up of early disease requires fewer resources than clinically detected cancer. A correct negative test also has a beneficial effect in terms of reassurance for those without disease.

Because screening requires preclinical diagnosis of disease, the period of morbidity is prolonged by the interval between diagnosis at screening and the hypothetical time when clinical diagnosis would have occurred if the patient had not been screened. This interval is called the lead time.

Screen-positive cases are confirmed by the standard clinical diagnostic methods. Many screen-detected cases are borderline abnormalities, some of which would progress to clinical disease, while some would not progress even if untreated. Cervical cancer screening results in detection of early intraepithelial neoplasia (premalignant lesions or *in situ* carcinomas), not all of which would progress to (fatal) cancer, even without treatment (IARC, 2005). Occult intraductal carcinomas of the breast (IARC, 2002), occult papillary carcinomas of the thyroid gland (Furihata and Maruchi, 1969), or occult prostatic cancer (Hugosson *et al.*, 2000) may fulfill the histological criteria for malignancy, but would remain indolent clinically. Any screening program will disclose such abnormalities, which are indistinguishable from a case that would progress into clinical disease during the person's lifetime, if not subjected to early treatment. Therefore, one of the adverse effects of screening is overdiagnosis, that is, detection of indolent disease and its unnecessary treatment (overtreatment), which results in anxiety and morbidity that would be avoided without screening and which is unnecessary for achieving the goals of screening.

A false-negative screening test (a person with disease that is not detected by the test) provides undue reassurance and may result in delayed diagnosis and worse outcome of treatment. In such cases, the effect of screening is disadvantageous.

Screening tests are applied to a population without recognized disease. In addition to the abnormal or borderline diagnoses, therefore, there will be false-positive screening results (a person without disease has a positive test), and these can cause anxiety and morbidity. The test itself may carry a risk. For example, screening for breast cancer is based on mammography, which involves a small radiation dose. The small risk of breast cancer induced by irradiating a large population should be compared with the benefits of mammography.

Validity of Screening

The validity of screening indicates the process or performance of screening and consists of two components: sensitivity and specificity. Sensitivity is an indicator of the extent to which preclinical disease is identified and specificity describes the extent to which healthy individuals are so identified. Predictive values are derived from those indicators and they describe the performance from the point of view of the person screened (the screenee).

The purpose of the screening test is to distinguish a subset of the population with a high probability of having unrecognized disease from the rest of the population, with average or low risk. Sensitivity is the proportion of persons who have a positive test among those with the disease in the DPCP (**Table 1**). Sensitivity is a basic performance measure because it indicates the proportion of early disease that is identified by screening. Specificity is the

Table 1 Validity of screening test

| Screening test | Disease in DPCP[a] | |
	Present	Absent
Positive	a	b
Negative	c	d

Sensitivity = a/(a+c)
Specificity = d/(b+d)
[a]DPCP, detectable preclinical phase.

proportion of persons with a negative test among all those screened who are disease-free. Specificity is a basic measure of the disadvantages of a test, since poor specificity results in high financial costs and adverse effects due to false-positive tests. Both the sensitivity and the specificity of a screening test are process indicators. A screening program based on a valid test may nevertheless fail in its objective of reducing mortality in the screened population.

As with clinical diagnostic procedures, the screening test is not always unambiguously positive or negative, and classification depends on the subjective judgment of the individual who is interpreting the test. The test result is often quantitative or semi-quantitative rather than dichotomous (positive or negative). Serum prostate-specific antigen (PSA) concentration is measured on a continuous scale and the results of Pap smear for cervical cancer were originally given on a 5-point scale of increasing degree of suspected malignancy (I, normal; II, benign infection; III, suspicious lesion; IV, probably malignant; V, malignant). The repeatability and validity of any classification are imperfect, because of both subjective interpretation and other sources of variation in the screening test. Because of this ambiguity, the cut-off point on the scale classifying the population in terms of screening positives and negatives can be selected at varying levels. The selection of the cut-off point crucially affects the test performance. Definition of a cut-off level influences both sensitivity and specificity in an opposite, counterbalancing fashion: a gain in sensitivity is inevitably accompanied by a loss in specificity.

Selection of a particular cut-off point will fix a particular combination of specificity and sensitivity. Several approaches have been proposed to select the cut-off point to distinguish best the high-risk group from the average-risk population. The simplest approach is to accept that cut-off which minimizes the total proportion of misclassification, which is equivalent to maximizing the sum of sensitivity and specificity. However, these two components of validity have different implications, which cannot be directly compared. Sensitivity is mainly related to the objective of screening and specificity to the adverse effects. When the total number of misclassified cases is minimized, sensitivity and specificity are considered of equal importance. This may be problematic, because it

implies that false negatives and false positives have a similar impact. The importance of sensitivity relative to specificity implies a weighted sum of misclassification as the basis to find a correct cut-off point. However, there are no objective weightings for sensitivity and specificity. Selection of a particular combination for validity components, that is, sensitivity and specificity, always involves value judgment.

This does not mean that any combination of specificity and sensitivity is acceptable. It depends on the test and the disease to be screened: for Pap smear some false positives are regarded as acceptable. This is because the yield is of primary importance and confirmation of the diagnosis is regarded, not necessarily correctly, as relatively reliable, noninvasive, and inexpensive. False-positive diagnoses pose a problem in breast cancer screening, because some degree of abnormality is common in the breast, but confirmation of a positive test is rather expensive. Low specificity is problematic because of the potentially high cost of diagnostic confirmation and exceeding the capacity of clinical diagnostic services with screen-positive cases.

Episode validity describes the ability of the screening episode to detect disease in the DPCP and to identify those who are healthy. Attempts to confirm the diagnosis after a positive screening test may fail to identify the disease and a (true-positive) case may thus be labeled as a false-positive screening test. For example, the PSA test has a high sensitivity (Stenman et al., 1994), but biopsy may fail to identify the malignant lesion. Therefore, many cases that are in the DPCP will not be diagnosed during the screening episode. The difference between test sensitivity and episode sensitivity is obvious for a screening test that is independent of the biopsy-based confirmation process. Screening for cervical cancer is based on exfoliated cells and the lesion where the malignant cells originated may not be detected at colposcopic biopsy. Even a biopsy for a breast cancer seen on screening mammography may fail to contain the malignant tissue.

Program validity is a public health indicator. Program sensitivity is related to the yield of the screening program, the detection of disease in DPCP in the target population. The program specificity indicates the correct identification of subjects free of the disease in the target population. Program validity depends on the screening test, confirmation of the test, attendance, the screening interval, and the success of referral for diagnostic confirmation of screen-positive cases.

Predictive Values of a Screening Test

Estimates of sensitivity are derived from the screening program itself. The most immediate indication of sensitivity is the yield, or cases detected at screen. The rate of detection is insufficient because it does not as such consider the total burden that stems from the cancers detected both at screen and clinically in between the screens if repeated. The relationship between these interval cancers and screen-detected cancers is not recommended as a measure of sensitivity because the cases that would not surface clinically if the population were not screened (overdiagnosis) cause a bias. Cancers diagnosed in nonattenders (those invited but not attended) at screening and in an independent control population contribute in estimating and understanding the screening validity. Methods are available that allow unbiased and comparable estimation of test, episode, and program sensitivity (IARC, 2005; Hakama *et al.*, 2007).

For the screenee, it is important to know the consequences of the result of a screening test and episode (including also the subsequent examinations). These can be described by the predictive values of a test and episode (**Table 2**). The positive predictive value (PPV) is the proportion of persons who do have unrecognized (preclinical) disease among those who have a positive test or episode. The negative predictive value (NPV) is the proportion of those who are free from the target condition among those with a negative episode. The predictive values depend on the validity of the test and the episode and on the prevalence of the disease in the DPCP (**Table 3**). High predictive values require valid screening and diagnostic tests. Particularly for a rare disease, PPV is usually low and the majority of positive screening tests will then occur among those who do not have the disease. In contrast, if the prevalence is low, the NPV is high, that is, a negative test gives a very high probability of absence of the disease. Many of those who attend a screening program are seeking reassurance that they do not have the disease. In practice, this is the most frequent benefit of screening for rare diseases, and it emphasizes the importance of high specificity.

Table 2   Predictive values of a screening test

	Disease	
Screening	Present	Absent
Positive	a	b
Negative	c	d

Positive predictive value = a/(a+b)
Negative predictive value = d/(c+d)

Table 3   The effect of preclinical prevalence on the predictive value assuming specificity = sensitivity = 95%

	Predictive value (%)	
Prevalence in DPCP[a] (%)	Positive	Negative
10	68	99.4
1	16	99.9
0.1	2	99.99

[a]DPCP, detectable preclinical phase.

Evaluating the Effect of Screening

An effective program shows an impact in the process indicators, that is, intermediate end points in screening. Such proxy measures reflect the performance of the program, but are only indirect indicators of the ultimate goal, which is mortality reduction. To be effective, mammographic screening for breast cancer must provide sufficient coverage of the target population, identify preclinical breast cancer reliably, and lead to the detection of early cancers that are more curable than those diagnosed without screening. An evaluation of the effect of a screening program based on process indicators alone is inadequate: these are necessary but not sufficient requirements for effectiveness, because an ineffective program may still produce favorable changes in process indicators.

The screening test detects disease in the DPCP and the yield depends on the prevalence of unrecognized disease. Prevalence depends on the length of DPCP. For many cancers, the length of DPCP correlates with the prognosis: fast-growing cancers with a short DPCP have a poor prognosis. Screening detects a disproportionate number of slow-growing cancers compared with normal clinical practice, especially when pursuing a high sensitivity. Therefore, screen-detected disease tends to have a more favorable survival than clinically detected disease, because the cancers are selected to be more slow-growing than clinically detected ones. The bias introduced by this selection is called length bias (Feinleib and Zelen, 1969). Length bias cannot be directly estimated and adjustment for it is cumbersome. Therefore, study designs and measures of effect that are free from length bias should be used to assess the effectiveness of screening. They are based on the total target population. Randomized screening trials evaluating mortality outcome are free from bias caused by overdiagnosis, length bias, and lead time.

Lead time (Hutchison and Shapiro, 1968) is the amount of time by which the diagnosis of disease is brought forward compared with the absence of screening. By definition, an effective screening program gives some lead time, since earlier diagnosis is a requirement for achieving the goals of screening. The maximum lead time is equivalent to the length of the DPCP, or sojourn time. Therefore, even if screening does not postpone death, survival from the time of diagnosis is longer for a screen-detected case than for a clinically detected case. Comparison of survival between screen-detected and symptom-detected patients is therefore biased unless it can be corrected for lead time. Such corrections remain crude at best, and survival is not a valid indicator of the effectiveness of screening.

Length bias and lead time are theoretical concepts of key importance in screening. Empirical assessment of length bias and lead time can provide valuable information on the natural history of the disease and the effects of screening (Day *et al.*, 1984). These sources of bias, in addition to overdiagnosis, make indicators such as survival unsuitable for the evaluating the effectiveness of screening programs.

Evaluation of the effectiveness of screening should therefore be made in terms of the outcome, which for cancer is mortality. However, screening programs also affect morbidity and, more broadly, quality of life. Such effects should also be taken into account in screening decisions although they should not be mixed with process indicators of the program. For example, fertility may be maintained after treatment for a screen-detected precursor lesion of cervical cancer, and breast-conserving surgery with less cosmetic and functional impairment may be used for screen-detected breast cancer compared with clinically detected cancer. Such procedures may reduce physical invalidity and adverse mental effects, and thereby improve the quality of life. However, the process measures, for example, the number of conisations of the cervix or breast-conserving surgery or their proportion of all surgical procedures, are invalid indicators of effect, because of potential overdiagnosis. Overdiagnosis increases the proportion of cases with favorable features because healthy individuals are misclassified as cases of disease.

A randomized preventive trial with mortality as the end point is the optimal and often the only valid means of evaluating the effectiveness of a screening program. Cohort and case-control studies are often used as a substitute for trials. Most evidence on the effectiveness of screening programs stems from comparisons of time trends and geographical differences between populations subjected to screening of different intensity. These nonexperimental approaches remain crude and insensitive, however, and do not provide a solid basis for decision making.

Several biases may distort comparability between attenders and nonattenders at screening. The most obvious is the 'healthy screenee' effect: an individual must be well enough to attend if he or she is to participate. Furthermore, a patient with, for example, a previous diagnosis or who is already under close medical surveillance due to a related disorder has no reason to attend a program aimed at detection of that disease. Elimination of bias in a nonexperimental design is likely to remain incomplete. In randomized trials, previously diagnosed cancer is an exclusion criterion, that is, prevalent cases are excluded and randomization with analysis based on the intention-to-screen principle guarantees comparability.

The randomized screening effectiveness trials with mortality as end point provide a solid basis for a routine screening program that is run as a public health policy. Such mass screening programs should be evaluated and monitored. Intervention studies without a control group (also called demonstration projects or single-arm trials) and other nonexperimental designs (cohort and case-control studies) have been proposed for this type of evaluation, but each approach has inherent biases.

A randomized approach with controls must be considered the gold standard, to be adopted if possible.

All routine screening programs are introduced gradually. Extension from the initial stage requires time and planning and involves more facilities. In several countries, use of Pap smears developed from very infrequent to become part of normal gynecological practice or public health service within about 10 years. It follows that a screening program can be introduced as a public health policy in an experimental design, with comparison of screened and unscreened groups formed by random allocation. Under such circumstances, provision of screening can be limited to a randomly allocated sample of the population, instead of a self-selected or haphazardly selected fraction of the population. As long as the resources for the program are only adequate for a proportion of the population, it is ethically acceptable to randomize, because screening is not withheld from anybody. There is, *a priori*, an equal chance for everybody in the target population to receive the potential benefit of the program and to avoid any adverse effects of the program. In this context, the equipoise (lack of firm evidence for or against an intervention), which is an ethical requirement for conducting a randomized trial, gradually disappears as evidence is accrued within the program. For those planning public health services, this will provide the most reliable basis for accepting or withholding new activities within the services.

Organizing a Screening Program

Screening is a chain of activities that starts from defining the target population and extends to the treatment and follow-up of screen-detected patients. A screening program consists of several elements that are linked together.

Different cancer screening programs consist of different components. In general, they can be outlined as eight distinct steps, divided into four components.

Population component:

1. Definition of target population.
2. Identification of individuals.
3. Measures to achieve sufficient coverage and attendance, such as personal letter of invitation.

Test execution component:

4. Test facilities for collection and analysis of the screen material.
5. Organized quality control program for both obtaining screen material and its analysis.

Clinical component:

6. Adequate facilities for diagnosis, treatment, and follow-up of patients with screen-detected disease.

Coordination component:

7. A referral system linking the screenee, laboratory (providing information about normal screening tests), and clinical facility (responsible for diagnostic examinations following an abnormal screening test and management of screen-detected abnormalities).
8. Monitoring, quality control, and evaluation of the program: availability of incidence and mortality rates for the entire target population, and separately for both attenders and non-attenders.

Routine screening can be divided into opportunistic (spontaneous, unorganized) and organized screening (mass screening, screening program). The major differences are related to the level of organization and planning, systematic nature, and scope of activity. The components described previously are characteristics of an organized screening program. Most of them are not found in opportunistic screening.

Spontaneous screening frequently focuses on high sensitivity at the cost of low specificity. This is due to several factors including economic incentives (fee-for-service) and risk-averse behavioral models (avoiding neglect, fear of litigation). However, more emphasis on specificity would be consistent with the primary ethical responsibilities of the physician under the Hippocratic oath: First, do no harm. For a high-technology screening program, such as mammography for breast cancer, low specificity results in high cost and frequent adverse effects. Furthermore, in countries with limited resources for the follow-up of screen-positive cases, screening competes for scarce resources that could be used for the treatment of overt disease with worse outcomes.

Major organizational considerations of any screening program are the age range to be covered and screening interval. For example, in Western populations with similar risk of disease and available resources, cervical cancer screening policies range from annual testing from the start of sexual activity to a smear every 5 years from age 30 to age 55. Hence, the difference in the cumulative number of tests over a lifetime varies from 6 to more than 60, that is, 10-fold.

In general, only organized screening programs can be evaluated. An organized program with individual invitations can prevent excessively frequent screening and overuse of the service, and is therefore less expensive. If screening appears ineffective, an organized screening program is also easier to close than a spontaneous activity. Therefore, organized screening programs should be recommended over opportunistic screening.

Cancer Screening by Primary Site

The following sections on cervical, breast, and colorectal cancer screening describe cancer screening with proven effectiveness.

Cervical Cancer Screening

Cervical cancer is the second most common cancer among women worldwide, with 493 000 new cases in 2002 and 273 000 deaths. The great majority of the burden is in developing countries, with highest incidence rates in Africa and Latin America.

Natural history

Cervical cancer is thought to develop gradually, through a progression of a series of precursor lesions from mild abnormality (atypia) into more aberrant lesions (dysplasia) and eventually malignant changes (initially *in situ*, then microinvasive and finally invasive carcinoma). Human papillomavirus (HPV) infection is a common early event. Most infections are cleared spontaneously within 6–12 months or less. Early precursor lesions seem to be a rare consequence of persistent infection with oncogenic HPV types. High-grade neoplasia occurs rarely without persistent HPV infection and viral load also predicts the probability of progression. Regression of lesions occurs commonly at early stages and the rate of progression is likely to increase during the process, with accumulation of abnormalities. The duration of the detectable, preclinical phase has been estimated at as long as 12–16 years.

Screening with cervical smears

Screening for cervical cancer is based on detecting and treating unrecognized disease, primarily premalignant lesions to prevent their progression into invasive carcinoma. Traditional techniques are based on cytological sampling of cells from the cervix. The classical smear is based on cytological assessment of exfoliated cervical cells from the transformation zone, where the squamous epithelium changes into columnar epithelium. The sample is collected from the vaginal part of the cervix using a spatula and from the endocervix with a brush or swab. Sampled cells are fixed on a glass slide for evaluation with microscope.

There are several classifications for cytological and histopathological abnormalities of the cervix. The present Bethesda 2001 system consists of two classes of benign atypical findings (atypia thought to occur as reactive change related to infection; atypical squamous cells of unknown significance [ASCUS], or a result that cannot exclude higher grade lesion, ASC-H) and two classes of more aberrant changes (low- and high-grade squamous intraepithelial lesion, LSIL and HSIL, respectively). The diagnostic classification of preinvasive changes is based on cervical intraepithelial neoplasia (originally CIN1–3, corresponding to mild, moderate, and severe dysplasia [including carcinoma *in situ*], modified by combining mild, moderate, and *in situ* into high-grade CIN).

Diagnostic assessment requires colposcopic examination (microscopic visualization with 6- to 40-fold magnification) for assessment of morphological features of the cervix. Histologic assessment is based on colposcopy-directed punch or cone biopsy.

The incidence of cervical cancer is very low in the first year following a negative smear and increases gradually, returning to baseline at about 10 years. The risk has still been 50% lower at 5 years, compared with unscreened women. The risk of cancer decreases further with the number of consecutive negative tests.

Effectiveness of screening

The objective of cervical cancer screening is to reduce both cervical cancer incidence and mortality. A successful screening program detects early, preinvasive lesions during the preclinical detectable phase and is able to reduce deaths by preventing the occurrence of invasive cancer.

No randomized trials were conducted to evaluate the mortality effects of cervical cancer screening at the time when it was introduced. There is, however, evidence for substantial incidence and mortality reduction from non-randomized studies conducted in several countries when screening was introduced. In such studies, a screened population is identified at the individual level. The screened and unscreened women may however not be comparable in terms of disease risk, which can induce selection bias. Several such studies have been summarized by IARC (2005). In British Columbia, Canada, a screening program was introduced in 1949. During 1958–1966, the incidence of cervical cancer among 310 000 women screened at least once was well below the rates preceding the screening project (standardized incidence ratio (SIR) 0.16, 13 cases), while 230 000 unscreened women showed no decrease (SIR 1.08, 67 cases). In Finland, a population-based cervical cancer screening program was started in 1963 and evaluation of more than 400 000 women covered showed effectiveness of 60% at 10 years in terms of incidence reduction. A Norwegian study with 46 000 women invited for screening showed approximately 20% lower cervical cancer incidence and mortality among participants than among the reference population.

Several case-control studies have been carried out in Denmark, Latin America, Canada, South Africa, and other countries to evaluate the efficacy of cervical cancer screening. Most have shown odds ratios in the range of 0.3–0.4 for invasive cervical cancer associated with ever versus never having had a screening test, but the results are prone to selection bias (IARC, 2005).

In ecological analyses without individual data, introduction of screening has been associated with a reduction in cervical cancer incidence and mortality. Major differences in the timing of introduction and the extent of cervical cancer screening between Nordic countries with similar baseline risk has allowed assessment of the effect of screening on cervical cancer incidence and mortality. Adoption of screening as a public health policy has been followed by a sharp reduction in cervical cancer occurrence. Comparison between counties in Denmark with and without cervical cancer screening showed that both incidence of and mortality from the disease were lower by a third in the areas with organized mass screening. Conversely, in an area where organized screening had been discontinued, increased incidence of invasive cancer was found. An analysis of 15 European countries was also consistent with a 30–50% reduction in cervical cancer incidence related to organized cervical cancer screening. Similar reductions in cancer incidence and/or mortality have been reported after launching screening programs in England and Wales, the United States, and Australia.

Screening programs

The recommended interval between screens has ranged from 1 to 5 years. Most screening programs start from 18–30 years of age and are discontinued after age 60–70 years. The most intensive screening protocols with an early start and frequent testing involve 10 times as many tests over a woman's lifetime as the most conservative approaches. Organized programs with large, population-based target groups tend to be least intensive, but nevertheless able to produce better results than less organized efforts, with ambitious screening regimens but very incomplete coverage of the target population and a weaker link among the program components (testing, diagnosis, and treatment). In some programs, the frequency of screening has been modified according to the screening result, either starting at annual screening, for example, and increasing the interval after negative results, or conversely, offering initially a longer, 3–5-year interval that is shortened if there is any abnormality.

Adverse effects of screening

Overdiagnosis of preinvasive lesions (i.e., detection and treatment of changes that would not have progressed into malignancy) appears common in cervical cancer screening, as only a small proportion of preinvasive lesions would develop into a cancer, even if left untreated. The cumulative risk of an abnormal screening test is relatively high compared with lifetime risk of cancer in the absence of screening (10–15% or higher versus approximately 3%). Treatment has several adverse effects. Excisional treatments are associated with pregnancy complications, including preterm delivery and low birth weight. Hysterectomy, quite obviously, leads to loss of fertility.

Other screening tests

Direct visualization of the cervix has been evaluated as a screening method that does not require sophisticated technology or highly trained personnel. Unaided visual inspection (also known as downstaging) can identify bleeding, erosion, and hypertrophy. Low-level magnification ($\times$ 2–4) has not been shown to improve performance of visual inspection. Use of acetic acid in visual inspection results in white staining of possible neoplastic changes and improves test sensitivity. Lugol's solution (or Schiller's iodine test) stains neoplastic epithelium yellow and it appears to have similar or better performance than acetic acid. Visual inspection with iodine solution or acetic acid offers an effective and affordable screening approach. With trained personnel and quality control a 25% reduction in cervical cancer mortality can be achieved (Sankaranarayanan et al., 2007).

Commercially available HPV tests are based on nucleic acid hybridization and are able to identify more than 10 different HPV types. No trials have been completed that have compared effectiveness of HPV testing with cytological smears. Yet, preliminary findings indicate that HPV screening is likely to be at least as effective as screening based on smears, but is also likely to have more adverse effects including lower specificity. Etiology-based screening may label cervical cancer as a sexually transmitted disease, despite common nonsexual transmission of the virus. This may reduce the acceptability of screening and reduce participation. One hazard is the stigmatization of the woman carrying the virus, regardless of the route of transmission (e.g., infidelity of the woman's partner), especially in cultures where the norms guard female sexuality more strictly than that of men.

In summary, the effectiveness of cytological smears in cervical cancer screening has never been established with current, methodologically stringent criteria. However, there is extensive and consistent evidence showing that a well-organized screening program will reduce both the incidence of and mortality from invasive carcinoma.

In the future, HPV vaccination has the potential to influence profoundly the conditions in which screening operates, and possibly to reduce the demand for cervical cancer screening by lowering the risk of the disease. This may take at least one generation to achieve.

Breast Cancer Screening

Breast cancer is the most common cancer among women and it accounts for a fifth of all cancers among women worldwide. Approximately 1 150 000 new cases occurred in the world in 2002. The number of breast cancer deaths in 2002 was estimated at 410 000. Increasing incidence rates have been reported in most populations. The highest incidence rates have been reported in high-income countries, in North America, Europe, as well as in Australia and New Zealand. Yet, in terms of numbers of cases, the burden of breast cancer is comparable in rich and poor countries of the world.

Natural history

In a synthesis of seven reports on breast cancer as an autopsy finding, the median prevalence of invasive breast cancer at autopsy was 1.3%. The mean sojourn time has been estimated at 2–8 years. Sojourn times tend to be longer for older ages and may depend on the histological type of breast cancer.

Mammography screening

In screening, the primary target lesion is early invasive cancer, but ductal carcinoma *in situ* is also detected with a frequency about 10–20% that of invasive cancer.

Mammography is X-ray imaging of the breast with a single or two views read by one or two radiologists. The screen-positive finding is a lesion suspicious for breast cancer, appearing typically as an irregular, starlike lesion or clustered microcalcifications. Two views are likely to increase detection rates by approximately 20%, with most benefit for detection of small cancers among women with radiologically dense breasts. In some screening programs, two views are used only at first screening, with only one view (mediolateral oblique) subsequently. Similarly, double reading appears to increase both the recall rate and detection of breast cancer by some 10%. Currently, digital mammography is replacing film technology.

Screen-positive findings result in the recall of 2–15% of women for additional mammographic examinations, with biopsy in approximately half of these women. Detection rates vary between populations of 3–11 per 1000, corresponding to PPVs of 30–70% for biopsied women. Sensitivity has been estimated at 60–70% in most randomized trials and close to that also in service screening. Specificity (the proportion of true negatives among all negative screens) has been reported at 95–98% in most studies, with lower figures in the initial (prevalence) screen than in subsequent screens.

Effectiveness of screening

Twelve randomized trials have evaluated mortality reduction in mammography screening (**Table 4**). In the age range 50–69, the trials have shown relatively consistent mortality reduction in the range of 20–35%. Excluding the Canadian trial with women 50–59 years, which showed no benefit, estimates of the number of women needing to be screened (NNS) to prevent one death from cervical cancer has ranged from 1000 to 10 000 women at 10 years.

The Health Insurance Plan trial in New York was the first randomized screening trial. It had approximately 60 000 women randomized pair-wise. The subjects were aged 40–64 years at entry. Four screening rounds with 1-year intervals were performed using two-view mammography and clinical breast examination (CBE). CBE was also used in the intervention arm. Causes of death were evaluated by a committee unaware of the allocation. Breast cancer mortality was reduced in the

Table 4   Randomized trials evaluating mortality effects of mammography screening

Reference	Setting	Sample size	Age range	Follow-up (years)	Mortality[a] (10^{-5})
Shapiro, 1988	Greater NY	60 995	40–64	18	23/29
Andersson and Janzon, 1997	Malmö	42 283	45–70	19	45/55
	Malmö	17 793	43–49	9	26/38
Tabár, 2000b	Kopparberg	56 448	40–74	20	27/33
Nyström et al., 2002	Östergotland	76 617	40–74	17	30/33
Alexander et al., 1999	Edinburgh	52 654	45–64	13	34/42
Miller et al., 2002	Canada	50 430	40–49	13	37/38
Miller et al., 2000	Canada	39 405	50–59	13	50/49
Moss et al., 2006	UK	160 921	39–41	11	18/22
Nyström 2002	Stockholm	60 117	40–64	15	15/17
Bjurstam et al., 2003	Gothenburg	51 611	39–59	13	23/30
Hakama et al., 1997	Finland	158 755	50–64	4	16/21

[a]Screening/control.

screening arm by 20% (5.5 vs. 6.9 per 100 000). In the analysis with the longest follow-up, the mortality difference persisted after 18 years of follow-up.

Several cluster-randomized screening trials have been carried out in Sweden. In the Kopparberg trial with three screening rounds, an 18% reduction in breast cancer mortality was reported after 20 years of follow-up. The Östergötland study showed 13% lower breast cancer mortality in the screening arm after four screening rounds and 17 years of follow-up. The Malmö trial with 22 000 women aged 45–69 years reported an 18% reduction in breast cancer mortality for the screening group after 19 years. In the Stockholm trial, nearly 40 000 women aged 40–64 years were enrolled and breast cancer mortality was 12% lower in the screening group after 15 years of observation.

Two mammography screening trials have been conducted in Canada. Both were started simultaneously, one enrolling volunteers aged 40–49 (Canadian National Breast Screening Study (CNBBS1) 50 000 women) and the other 50–59 years (NBBS2 40 000 women). Intervention was annual two-view mammography and CBE for 5 years in both trials, with no intervention for the control arm in the younger group and CBE only in the older cohort. No reduction in breast cancer mortality was found in either age group in analyses covering 13 years of follow-up.

The Edinburgh trial used cluster randomization based on general practices, with more than 44 000 women aged 45–64 years at entry. The screening interval was 12 or 24 months and covered four screening rounds. After 13 years of follow-up, breast cancer mortality was 19% lower in the screening arm.

The randomized trials have been criticized for methodological weaknesses (Olsen and Gøtzsche, 2001), especially for incorrect randomization and postrandomization exclusions leading to lack of comparability between the trial arms. In a systematic review excluding studies with possible shortcomings, only two trials were finally evaluated and no benefit was demonstrated (Olsen and

Gotzsche, 2001). It was also argued that breast cancer mortality is not a valid end point for screening trials. However, the validity of these criticisms has been rebutted by several investigators and international working groups. The dismissal of studies based on mechanistic evaluation of technical criteria of questionable relevance has been considered inappropriate.

Service screening

National breast cancer screening programs are ongoing in several European countries. They are organized either regionally or nationally and use guidelines and quality assurance systems for both radiology and pathology. Common features are target groups at ages 50–69 and 2-year intervals. In several Northern European countries, participation around 80% has been achieved with recall rates of 1–8%. PPVs have been in the range of 5–10% and detection rate of invasive cancer generally has been at 4–10 per 1000 in the initial screen and 2–5 per 1000 in subsequent rounds (IARC, 2002). In the evaluation of effectiveness, nonrandomized approaches have been used (with the exception of Finland where screening was introduced using a randomized design). In such studies, definition of controls and estimation of expected risk of death is problematic. Extrapolations of time trends and comparisons between geographical areas have been used as in evaluation of effectiveness. Yet, comparability between screened and nonscreened groups in such studies is questionable. Also, exclusion criteria are not as strict as in randomized trials and exclusion of prevalent cancers at baseline has not always been possible.

In Finland, the female population was divided into a screening group and a control group based on birth year. The women were aged 50–59 at entry and 89 000 women born on even years were invited to mammography screening every second year, while 68 000 born on odd years were not invited but served as a reference group. Participation was 85%. Refined mortality was used, that is, breast cancers diagnosed before the start of the screening program were excluded. Overall, a 24% reduction in breast cancer mortality was reported at 5 years, which did not reach statistical significance.

In the Netherlands, a statistically significant reduction in breast cancer mortality was reported following introduction of mammography screening. The target age group was 50–69 years and participation reached 80%. Compared to rates before screening, the reduction in mortality was 19% at 11 years of follow-up (85.3 vs. 105.2 per 100 000). No similar decrease was found for women in older age groups, suggesting that the reduction was attributable to screening and not to improvement in treatment.

In an evaluation of mammography screening in Sweden, mortality from breast cancers diagnosed during the screening period was evaluated in seven counties between 1978 and 1990. A statistically significant 32% reduction in refined breast cancer mortality was observed following introduction of screening in counties with 10 years of screening and an 18% reduction in areas with shorter screening periods. A more recent assessment showed a 26% mortality reduction after 11 years among 109 000 women with early screening, compared with areas with later introduction of screening.

In England and Wales, breast cancer mortality decreased by 21% after introduction of mammography screening for women aged 50–69 years compared to that expected in the absence of screening (predicted from underlying trend). The estimated reduction in breast cancer mortality gained by screening was 6%, while the rest was attributed to improvements in treatment.

A Danish study showed a significant 25% reduction in nonrefined breast cancer mortality within 10 years after introduction of screening in Copenhagen for the age group 50–69 years compared with earlier rates and control areas.

No substantial effect on breast cancer mortality at population level was shown in an early analysis of a screening program in Florence, Italy. During the first 9 years of the program, breast cancer mortality declined by merely 3%, which was attributed to the relatively low coverage of the program (60%).

In a comparison of Swedish counties that introduced mass screening with mammography in 1986–87 with those starting after 1992, only a nonsignificant 10% mortality reduction from breast cancer was found at 10 years among women aged 50–69 at entry. Among women aged 70–74 years, the mortality reduction was even less (6%).

The results from nonrandomized evaluation are consistent with a mortality reduction obtained in screening trials and suggest that mortality reduction is achievable when mammography screening is applied as public health policy, though it may be somewhat less than the average effect of approximately 25% seen in randomized trials. Further, improvement in quality of life can be gained by early diagnosis, allowing a wider range of treatment options, with the possibility of avoiding radical surgery (and possibly adjuvant chemotherapy).

Adverse effects

The extent of overdiagnosis and subsequent unnecessary treatment of lesions that would not have progressed may not be as large for breast cancer screening as for several other cancer types. The estimates of overdiagnosis have been in the range of 3–5%.

Preinvasive cancer (*in situ* carcinoma) is detected at screening with a frequency of approximately 1 per 1000 screens and is commonly treated surgically, even if all cases would not progress to cancer. Mammography causes a small radiation dose (1–2 mGy) to the breast, which can be expected to increase breast cancer risk. The excess risk is, however, likely to remain very small (in the range of 1–3% or less increase in the relative risk).

Other screening tests

Digital mammography has been adopted recently. It appears to yield a higher detection rate than conventional film mammography, but correspondingly, specificity seems lower. It remains unclear if the higher detection rate also increases overdiagnosis. No studies have evaluated the effect of digital mammography on breast cancer mortality.

Studies of magnetic resonance imaging among high-risk groups have suggested higher sensitivity compared with mammography, but no randomized trials have compared its effect on mortality with mammography. An advantage is avoidance of exposure to ionizing radiation. Yet, it is also more expensive and time-consuming.

CBE consists of inspection and palpation of the breasts by a health professional to identify lumps or other lesions suspicious for cancer. No randomized trials have evaluated the effectiveness of CBE alone, but it was included in the intervention arm of the Health Insurance Plan (HIP), Canadian, and Edinburgh trials. It may increase the sensitivity of screening if combined as an ancillary test in a mammography screening program.

Breast self-examination (BSE) has been evaluated as a resource-sparing option for early detection of breast cancer. A randomized trial in Shanghai showed no reduction in breast cancer mortality following instruction in BSE. A similar conclusion was reached also in a trial carried out in the former Soviet Union.

Several randomized trials have shown that mammography screening can reduce mortality from breast cancer and evidence from studies evaluating service screening indicates a similar or slightly smaller effect at population level. The age group with most benefit is 50–69 years. The methodological limitations of the studies are not severe enough to justify ignoring their results.

Colorectal Cancer Screening

Colorectal cancer ranks as the second most common cause of cancer death. There were more than 1 million new cases in 2002, with more than 500 000 deaths.

Natural history

The majority of colorectal carcinomas are thought to arise from benign precursor lesions (adenoma). Adenoma (particularly those with a diameter of up to 1 cm, or dysplasia) and early carcinoma make up the principal target of screening. The duration of the detectable preclinical phase has been estimated at 2–6 years.

Screening tests

Several screening methods are available for colorectal cancer screening, including fecal occult blood testing (FOBT) and endoscopic examination (sigmoidoscopy or colonoscopy) as well as radiographic examination (double-contrast barium enema).

FOBT is based on detection of hemoglobin in stools using guaiac-impregnated patches, where an oxidative reaction (pseudoperoxidase activity) results in color change, which is detectable on inspection. The most commonly used test, Hemoccult II, is not specific to human blood. Other tests are also available that immunologically detect human hemoglobin, but they are also more expensive. Rehydration (adding water to the specimen) can be used to increase the detection rate, but this also leads to more false-positive results. For screening, two specimens are usually obtained on 3 consecutive days. Dietary restrictions (avoiding red meat, vitamin C, and nonsteroidal anti-inflammatory drugs) and combination of tests may increase specificity, but can also reduce acceptability.

The detection rate of carcinoma with FOBT has been 0.2–0.5% for biennial screening. Sensitivity is considerably lower for detection of polyps, which do not bleed as frequently as cancers. The PPV has been 10% for cancer and 25–50% for adenoma.

Effectiveness of FOBT

Two-year screening intervals have been most widely used and most studies have targeted the age groups 45–75 years. Three randomized trials evaluating incidence and mortality have been reported (**Table 5**).

They show a consistent 6–18% reduction in mortality with biennial screening. A systematic review showed a 16% (95% confidence interval [CI] 7–23%) reduction in mortality. The NNS to prevent one colorectal cancer death was estimated as less than 1200 at 10 years, given two-thirds participation.

In the Nottingham (UK) trial, more than 150 000 subjects aged 45–74 years were recruited between 1981 and 1991 and randomized by household. No reduction in colorectal cancer incidence was shown, but mortality was 19% lower in the screening arm after a median 12 years of follow-up.

In the Danish Funen study, approximately 62 000 subjects aged 45–75 were enrolled in 1985. Randomization was performed in blocks of 14 persons (with spouses always in the same arm). The mortality reduction was 11% after a mean follow-up of 14 years. No decrease in colorectal cancer incidence was observed.

In the Minnesota (United States) trial, 46 551 volunteers aged 50–80 years were recruited between 1975 and 1977. After a mean follow-up of 15 years, a mortality reduction of 33% was shown in the annual screening group and 21% in the biennial screening group, compared with the control arm. The incidence of colorectal cancer was also approximately 20% lower in the screened groups.

Service screening

Provision of colorectal cancer screening for the population has been tested in several countries. In France, a 16% mortality reduction was reported in a population of 90 000 offered screening, compared with control districts in the same administrative area. The incidence of colorectal cancer was similar in both populations during 11 years of follow-up.

Finland was the first country to launch a population-based FOBT screening program, in 2004. It was introduced using individual randomization, but the effects on colorectal cancer incidence and mortality have not been evaluated yet.

Adverse effects of screening

FOBT is safe, but a positive result requires further diagnostic examinations such as endoscopy, which cause inconvenience, rare complications (e.g., perforation), and

Table 5 Randomized trials evaluating mortality effects of colorectal cancer screening based on fecal occult blood testing (FOBT)

Reference (setting)	Sample size	Age range	Follow-up (years)	Mortality (RR)[a]
Mandel et al., 1999 (Minnesota, U.S.)	46 551[b]	50–80	15	0.67 (0.51–0.87)
Scholefield et al., 2002 (Nottingham, UK)	152 850	45–74	11	0.87 (0.78–0.97)
Kronborg et al., 2004 (Fynen, Denmark)	61 933	45–75	11	0.89 (0.78–1.01)
			14	0.82 (0.69–0.97)

[a]RR, ratio of mortality rates in screening arm and no-screening arm.
[b]Three arms, annual and biennial screening with control.

costs. Some overdiagnosis is likely, because not all precursor lesions would advance to cancer. Yet, the morbidity related to the removal of polyps is very moderate.

Other screening tests

Flexible sigmoidoscopy covers approximately 60 cm of the distal colon, where roughly half of all colorectal cancers occur. Any adenomas detected can be removed during the procedure. Compliance with sigmoidoscopy as a screening investigation has only been 50% or less. The detection rate is higher than with FOBT, suggesting higher sensitivity. Three case-control studies and a cohort study have suggested lower mortality from colorectal carcinoma following sigmoidoscopy, as well as lower incidence. These studies do not provide evidence as strong as that from randomized intervention trials, because selection bias and other systematic errors may affect the results. Therefore, the mortality reduction achievable with sigmoidoscopy remains unclear. A population-based randomized trial is ongoing in Norway with 20 000 subjects aged 50–64, comparing one sigmoidoscopy with no intervention. It is expected to provide important new information.

Screening colonoscopy has the advantage of covering the entire colon, but the procedure is expensive, bears substantial discomfort and has the potential for complications such as perforation (reported in 1–2 patients per 10 000). No trials have evaluated the effectiveness of screening colonoscopy.

Recently, fecal DNA analysis has been introduced as a new option for colorectal cancer screening, but no studies assessing its effectiveness have been conducted.

In summary, FOBT has been shown to decrease mortality from colorectal cancer in several randomized trials. It appears to be an underutilized opportunity for cancer control. Other screening modalities are also available, but there is currently no solid evidence for their effectiveness.

Screening for other cancers

Some evidence for effectiveness is available for oral cancer and liver cancer screening, but it is not as well established as for cervical, breast, and colorectal cancers.

Oral cancer is among the most common cancers in some areas of the world, largely due to the habit of tobacco chewing. Globally, more than 270 000 cases are detected annually, primarily in developing countries. A recent cluster-randomized trial of visual inspection for oral cancer demonstrated a 20% reduction in mortality among more than 190 000 subjects (Sankaranarayanan et al., 2005).

Liver cancer is the sixth most common cancer in the world, with more than 600 000 new cases in 2002. In terms of cancer deaths it ranks third, with nearly 600 000 deaths annually. Serum alpha-fetoprotein (AFP) and ultrasound have been used as a screening test for

hepatocellular cancer. Two randomized trials have been carried out in China, both among chronic carriers of hepatitis B virus, who are at high risk of liver cancer. The smaller study found a nonsignificant 20% reduction associated with 6-monthly AFP tests among 5500 men in Qidong county (Zhang et al., 2004). Another trial involved 18 000 people and showed a one-third mortality reduction at 5 years with 6-monthly AFP and ultrasonography (Chen et al., 2003).

The following section, 'Lung Cancer Screening,' describes cancer screening with evidence against effectiveness.

Lung Cancer Screening

Lung cancer is the most common cancer in many countries. Mortality rates are very similar to incidence due to its very poor prognosis. In 2002, the global number of cases was 1.35 million and there were 1.18 million deaths.

Natural history, diagnosis, and treatment

The target lesion for lung cancer screening is early, resectable (stage 1) carcinoma. Diagnostic examinations may include high-resolution computerized tomography (CT), positron-emission tomography (PET), transthoracic needle biopsy, and thoracotomy. A conclusive diagnosis of early lung cancer is based on biopsy.

Screening with chest X-rays, with or without sputum cytology

The plain chest X-ray was evaluated as a screening test in several randomized screening trials in the 1960s and 1970s. Commonly, it was combined with cytological assessment of exfoliative cells that are most commonly detected in squamous cell carcinoma.

Small nodules are easily missed in chest X-rays and sensitivity is low, with specificity above 90%. Detection rates have been 0.1–0.8% and positive predictive value 40–60%. False-negative results in sputum cytology are common among patients with lung cancer; its sensitivity is also regarded as inferior to that of chest X-rays.

Effectiveness of screening

Four randomized trials of lung cancer screening with chest X-rays have been conducted, but only one compared chest X-ray screening against no intervention (until the end of the 3-year study period, **Table 6**). One compared chest X-ray and sputum examination offered within the trial against a recommendation to have such tests. The other two trials assessed the impact of chest X-ray alone with chest X-ray and sputum cytology. The interval between rounds ranged between 4 months and 1 year. The detection rate of lung cancer at baseline examination has been 0.1–0.8%. In a meta-analysis, lung

Table 6 Randomized trials assessing mortality effect of lung cancer screening based on chest X-ray with or without sputum cytology

Reference (setting)	Study subjects[a]	Follow-up (years)	Mortality rate per 1000 (no. of deaths)[a]
Studies comparing chest X-ray during vs. after study period			
Kubik, 1990 (Czechoslovakia)	3172+3174	6 (15)	6.0 vs. 4.5 (247 vs. 216)
Studies comparing chest X-ray with sputum cytology vs. chest X-ray alone			
Melamed 1984 (Sloane-Kettering U.S.)	4968+5072	8	2.7 vs. 2.7
Levin, 1982 (Johns Hopkins U.S.)	5161+5225	8	3.4 vs. 3.8
Marcus *et al.*, 2000 (Mayo Clinic, U.S.)	4618+4593	20	4.4 vs. 3.9 (337 vs. 303)

[a]Intervention vs. control.

cancer mortality was increased by 11% with the more intensive screening.

Adverse effects of screening

A false-positive test leads to invasive diagnostic procedures. Overdiagnosis has been estimated as 15% based on long-term follow-up in one of the trials.

Other screening methods

In spiral low-dose CT, the screen-positive finding is a noncalcified nodule, usually at least 1 cm in diameter. For smaller lesions, follow-up examinations may be needed to define whether the nodule is growing.

No randomized trials have been done, so the effect on mortality has not been established. Adverse effects due to false-positive results appear common but the extent of overdiagnosis has not been established. In the United States, the National Lung Screening Trial is comparing annual chest radiography with annual low-dose CT among 50 000 smokers.

To conclude, chest X-rays have been shown *not* to reduce mortality from lung cancer. Opportunities provided by novel radiological technology have been eagerly advocated for screening, but currently there is no evidence on the effectiveness of screening based on spiral CT.

Screening for other cancers

Neuroblastoma is a tumor of the sympathetic nervous system in children, with an overall annual incidence rate of approximately 1 per 100 000 under the age of 15 years. Peak incidence is during the first year of life, and occurrence decreases after that. The natural course is highly variable. Early-stage disease, occurring mainly in young children, has a very favorable prognosis, while diagnosis at an advanced stage (and usually above 1 year of age) is associated with poorer survival. There is a subgroup of tumors with the potential to disappear spontaneously or mature into a benign tumor (ganglioneuroma), even in the presence of metastasis. Hence there is obvious potential for overdiagnosis. Screening is possible using urine tests for metabolites of the neuronal transmitters, catecholamines (homovanillic acid and vanillylmandelic acid),

which are secreted by most (60–80%) tumors. Studies in Germany, Canada, and Japan have compared screened and unscreened cohorts to evaluate the effects of screening. Screening has led to a two- to sixfold *increase* in the recorded incidence of neuroblastoma, and an increase at young ages has not been counterbalanced by a reduction at older ages. No reduction in mortality or in the occurrence of advanced disease has been demonstrated. Screening for neuroblastoma is therefore not recommended, even if no randomized trials have been conducted. Screening was recently discontinued in Japan.

The follow section, 'Prostate Cancer Screening,' including other cancers, describes cancer screening without sufficient evidence for or against effectiveness.

Prostate Cancer Screening

The recorded incidence of prostate cancer has increased rapidly in the past 10–15 years in most industrialized countries and it is currently the most common cancer among men in several countries. Globally, 679 000 prostate cancers were diagnosed in 2002, with 221 000 deaths from it.

Natural history

The target lesion in prostate cancer screening is early invasive prostate cancer. The natural course of prostate cancer is highly variable, ranging from indolent to highly aggressive. Premalignant lesions such as prostatic intra-epithelial neoplasia (PIN) exist, but are not strongly predictive of prostate cancer and are not considered as an indication for treatment. Latent prostate cancer is a common autopsy finding. It has been detected in more than 10% of men dying before the age of 50 years, and much more frequently in older men. The common occurrence of indolent prostate cancer is a clear indication for potential overdiagnosis. The mean lead time in prostate cancer has been estimated as 6–12 years.

Prostate cancer screening based on PSA

PSA is a serine protease secreted by the prostate and it is usually found in low concentrations in serum, with levels increased by prostate diseases such as benign prostatic hyperplasia, prostatitis, or prostate cancer.

The specificity of PSA has been estimated as approximately 90%. Detection rates have ranged from less than 2% to above 5%, depending on the cut-off and population. In serum bank studies, where no screening has been offered, but baseline PSA levels have been used to predict subsequent incidence of prostate cancer, sensitivity has been estimated as 67–86% at 4–6 years.

Effectiveness of PSA screening

Mortality analysis has been published from only one, relatively small, randomized trial. A study carried out in Quebec, Canada, randomized 46 500 men aged 45–80 years in 1988 with two-thirds allocated into the screening arm (Labrie *et al.*, 2004). Compliance with screening was only 24%. Screening interval was 1 year, with PSA cut-off 3 ng/ml. By the end of 1999, the mean length of follow-up was 10 years among unscreened men and 7 years in the screened group. When analyzed by trial arm (intention to screen analysis), no reduction in prostate cancer mortality was seen.

Two large randomized trials are being carried out, one in Europe and the other in the United States. The European Randomized trial of Screening for Prostate Cancer (ERSPC) has eight centers in the Netherlands, Finland, Sweden, Italy, Belgium, Spain, Switzerland, and France. It has recruited a total of more than 200 000 men aged 50–74 years. The first mortality analysis is planned in 2010.

In the United States, the Prostate, Lung, Colorectal and Ovary screening trial (PLCO) recruited 76 705 men aged 55–74 years in the prostate screening component between 1993 and 2001. Both serum PSA and digital rectal examination are used as screening tests. No mortality results are available yet.

Four case-control studies have evaluated prostate cancer screening, but they have not given consistent results. At any rate, the evidence from such nonrandomized studies should be seen as tentative.

Several ecological studies and time series analyses have been published, correlating the frequency of PSA testing (or the incidence of prostate cancer as a surrogate for PSA testing) with prostate cancer mortality. The results have been inconsistent. Given the shortcomings inherent in these approaches, the findings do not have the potential to provide valid conclusions.

Adverse effects of screening

Overdiagnosis is potentially a major problem in prostate cancer screening. It has been estimated that 30–45% of the cancers detected by screening would not have been diagnosed in the absence of screening during the man's expected lifetime. Overdiagnosis leads to unnecessary treatment of prostate cancer, which has several major adverse effects, including high rates of erectile dysfunction and urinary incontinence with surgery, as well as urinary incontinence and irritation of the rectum or bladder (chronic radiation cystitis and proctitis) with radiotherapy.

Other screening tests

The effect of digital rectal examination (DRE) as a screening test on death from prostate cancer has not been evaluated in randomized studies. Five case-control studies have yielded inconsistent results, which is thought to be due to the low sensitivity of DRE for the detection of early disease.

In summary, no effect on mortality from prostate cancer with screening by serum PSA or other means has been established. Screening should be limited to randomized trials. Randomized trials are on-going and should provide important evidence.

Screening for other cancers

Ovarian cancer is among the 10 most common cancers among women. In 2002, 204 000 new cases were diagnosed globally and there were 124 000 deaths from ovarian cancer.

The natural history of ovarian carcinoma is not well understood. It is unclear how commonly cancers develop from benign or borderline lesions to malignant disease, relative to carcinoma arising *de novo*. Similarly, the duration of the detectable preclinical phase remains unknown. Screening tests include transvaginal or transabdominal ultrasound for imaging and serum CA-125 as a biochemical marker. There is no evidence on the effectiveness of ovarian cancer screening in terms of mortality reduction. Preliminary results obtained from nonrandomized studies are not encouraging: the sensitivity is low and false-positive findings are common.

Cutaneous melanoma incidence has been increasing rapidly in most industrialized countries and it now ranks among the 10 most common cancers in several European countries. There are approximately 160 000 new cases diagnosed annually in the world. Some of the increase may be due to more active case finding and changes in diagnostic criteria. Mortality has not shown a similar increase. Survival is favorable in the early stages. A substantial proportion of melanomas (approximately a fifth) arise from atypical moles (naevi). Visual inspection can be used to identify early melanomas (or premalignant lesions). Diagnostic assessment requires a skin biopsy. No randomized trials have been conducted to evaluate the effect of screening on melanoma mortality.

Gastric carcinoma is the third most common cancer in the world with 930 000 cases in 2002. With 700 000 deaths annually, it is the second most common cause of cancer death globally. Fluoroscopic imaging (photofluorography) and endoscopy have been used in screening for stomach cancer. As no randomized trials have been reported, there is not sufficient evidence to allow sound evaluation of effectiveness or to make recommendations concerning screening.

Cancer Screening Guidelines

Several international and national organizations have given recommendations for cancer screening as public health policy (**Table 7**). They have been based on a variety of approaches from expert opinion and consensus development conferences to more objective methods of evidence synthesis. There is some degree of consistency between the guidelines, but also differences. For some organizations, the rationale for evaluation has been strictly based on evidence for effectiveness, with the goal of assessing whether there is sufficient high-quality research to justify screening. Other organizations, notably the American Cancer Society, have adopted a more ideological approach, with a bias in favor of screening (a low threshold for advocating screening). Similarly, medical

Table 7 Cancer screening recommendations by various organizations

Organization	Cervical cancer	Breast cancer	Colorectal cancer	Prostate cancer
WHO	Recommended without details	Every 2–3 years at ages 50–69 years	Mortality can be reduced; no clear recommendation	Not recommended
UICC	Pap smear every 3–5 years from age 20–30 until 60 years or later	Mammography every 2 years at ages 50–69	FOBT every 2 years at ages above 50 years	No evidence
EU	Start at ages 20–30, screening interval 3–5 years, discontinue at age 60 or later	Mammography every 2–3 years at ages 50–69 years	FOBT every 1–2 years at ages 50–74 years	Not recommended
Canadian Taskforce on Preventive Health Care	Pap test every year from age 18 or start of intercourse; frequency every 3 years after two negative smears; discontinue at age 69	Mammography every 1–2 years at ages 50–59 years	Insufficient evidence	Not recommended
U.S. Preventive Services Taskforce	Pap smear at least every 3 years among sexually active women until age 65 years	Mammography every 1–2 years at ages 50–69 years	Yearly FOBT after age 50 years; sigmoidoscopy as alternative	Not recommended
American Cancer Society	Pap test annually since age 18 or start of intercourse; less frequently after 2–3 negative smears	Mammography annually from age 40 years	Annual FOBT and sigmoidoscopy after age 50 years; alternatively colonoscopy every 10 years or barium enema every 5–10 years	Annual DRE and PSA from age 50 years

Table 8 Summary of evidence for cancer screening

Primary site	Screening method	Efficacy		Effectiveness	
		Nonrandomized	Randomized	Randomized trial	Service screening
Cervical cancer	Pap smear		NA[a]	NA	0–80%
	Visual inspection			NA	NA
	HPV testing		NA	NA	NA
Breast cancer	Mammography		35%	15–25%	6–20
Colorectal cancer	Fecal occult blood		24	15	NA
	Sigmoidoscopy		NA	NA	NA
	Colonoscopy		NA	NA	NA
Lung cancer	Chest X-ray ± sputum cytology		None		NA
	Low-dose CT		NA	NA	NA
Prostate cancer	Serum PSA		NA	NA	NA
	Digital rectal exam	None	NA	NA	NA
Oral cancer	Visual inspection		20%		NA
Liver cancer	Serum AFP ± ultrasound		20–33%		NA
Ovarian cancer	Ultrasound with CA-125		NA	NA	NA

[a]NA, not available.

specialty societies tend to adopt screening recommendations relatively eagerly (not included in the table).

The role of the organization or the task of the working group also affects the outcome, so that groups with more responsibility for planning health-care services tend to apply more stringent evaluation criteria than those without such responsibility. Countries with publicly financed health-care systems tend to be more conservative than countries with systems based on fee-for-service health-care systems.

Conclusion

In summary, establishing the benefits of screening usually requires evidence of a significant reduction in mortality from large randomized trials. Such a knowledge base exists for cervical, breast, and colorectal cancer (**Table 8**). The evidence is more limited for oral and liver cancer. Screening tests exist for numerous primary sites of cancer, but either their effectiveness has not been adequately evaluated, or a lack of effectiveness has been demonstrated. Even after randomized trials have shown efficacy (typically in specialist centers with volunteer subjects), the introduction of mass screening requires that pilot studies should first be done to demonstrate feasibility. After an organized screening program has been implemented, continuous evaluation is required to ensure that the benefits are maintained. Ideally, this is achieved by introducing a mass screening program with a randomized design, that is, comparing subjects randomly allocated to early entry with those covered only later. This approach is particularly important when the effect demonstrated in trials of efficacy is small. It is also highly recommended when an established technique is being replaced with a new one.

Citations

Alexander FE, Anderson TJ, Brown HK, *et al.* (1999) Fourteen years of follow-up from the Edinburgh randomised trial of breast-cancer screening. *The Lancet* 353: 1903–1908.

Andersson I and Janzon L (1997) Reduced breast cancer mortality in women under age 50: updated results from the Malmo mammographic screening program. *Journal of the National Cancer Institute Monograph* 22: 63–67.

Bjurstam N, Björneld L, Warwick J, *et al.* (2003) The Gothenburg breast screening trial. *Cancer* 97: 2387–2396.

Chen JG, Parkin DM, Chen QG, *et al.* (2003) Screening for liver cancer: Results of a randomised controlled trial in Qidong, China. *Journal of Medical Screening* 10: 204–209.

Cole P and Morrison AS (1978) Basic issues in cancer screening. In: Miller AB (ed.) *Screening in Cancer* vol. 40, pp. 7–39. Geneva, Switzerland: UICC UICC Technical Report Series.

Day NE and Walter SD (1984) Simplified models for screening: Estimation procedures from mass screening programmes. *Biometrics* 40: 1–14.

Day NE, Walter SD, and Collette B (1984) Statistical models of disease natural history: Their use in the evaluation of screening programmes. In: Prorok PC and Miller AB (eds.) *Screening for Cancer I – General*

Principles on Evaluation of Screening for Cancer and Screening for Lung, Bladder and Oral Cancer, UICC Technical Report Series. vol. 78, pp. 55–70. Geneva, Switzerland: UICC.

Feinleib M and Zelen M (1969) Some pitfalls in the evaluation of screening programs. *Archives of Environmental Health* 19: 412–415.

Furihata R and Maruchi N (1969) Epidemiological studies on thyroid cancer in Nagano prefecture, Japan. In: Hedinger CE (ed.) *Thyroid Cancer,* UICC Monograph Series. vol. 12, p. 79. Berlin: Springer-Verlag.

Hakama M, Auvinen A, Day NE, and Miller AB (2007) Sensitivity in cancer screening. *Journal of Medical Screening* 14: 174–177.

Hugosson J, Aus G, Becker C, *et al.* (2000) Would prostate cancer detected by screening with prostate specific antigen develop into clinical cancer if left undiagnosed. *British Journal of Urology* 85: 1978–1984.

Hutchison GB and Shapiro S (1968) Lead time gained by diagnostic screening for breast cancer. *Journal of the National Cancer Institute* 41: 665–681.

IARC (2002) *Breast Cancer Screening. IARC Handbooks of Cancer Prevention* vol. 7. Lyon, France: IARC Press.

IARC (2005) *Cervix Cancer Screening. IARC Handbooks of Cancer Prevention* vol. 10. Lyon, France: IARC Press.

Kronborg O, Jorgensen OD, Fenger C, and Rasmussen M (2004) Randomized study of biennial screening with a faecal occult blood test: results after nine screening rounds. *Scandinavian Journal of Gastroenterology* 39: 846–851.

Kubik A, Parkin DM, Khlat M, Erban J, Polak J, and Adamec M (1990) Lack of benefit from semi-annual screening for cancer of the lung: follow-up report of a randomized controlled trial on a population of high-risk males in Czechoslovakia. *International Journal of Cancer* 45: 26–33.

Labrie F, Candas B, Cusan L, *et al.* (2004) Screening decreases prostate cancer mortality: 11-year follow-up of the 1988 Quebec prospective randomized controlled trial. *Prostate* 59: 311–318.

Levin ML, Tockman MS, Frost JK, and Ball WC (1982) Lung cancer mortality in males screened by chest X-ray and cytologic sputum examination: a preliminary report. *Recent Results in Cancer Research* 82: 138–146.

Mandel JS, Church TR, Ederer F, and Bond JH (1999) Colorectal cancer mortality: effectiveness of biennial screening for fecal occult blood. *Journal of the National Cancer Institute* 91: 434–437.

Marcus PM, Bergstralh EJ, Fagerstrom RM, *et al.* (2000) Lung cancer mortality in the Mayo Lung Project: impact of extended follow-up. *Journal of the National Cancer Institute* 92: 1308–1316.

Melamed MR, Flehinger BJ, Zaman MB, *et al.* (1984) Screening for early lung cancer. Results of the Memorial Sloan-Kettering study in New York. *Chest* 86: 44–53.

Miller AB, To T, Baines CJ, and Wall C (2000) Canadian National Breast Screening Study-2: 13-year results of a randomized trial in women aged 50–59 years. *Journal of the National Cancer Institute* 92: 1490–1499.

Miller AB, To T, Baines CJ, and Wall C (2002) The Canadian National Breast Screening Study-1: breast cancer mortality after 11 to 16 years of follow-up. A randomized screening trial of mammography in women age 40 to 49 years. *Annals of Internal Medicine* 137: 305–312.

Moss S, Cuckle H, Evans A, Johns L, Waller M, and Bobrow L (2006) Effect of mammographic screening from age 40 years on breast cancer mortality at 10 years' follow-up: a randomised controlled trial. *Lancet* 368: 2053–2060.

Nyström L, Andersson I, Bjurstam N, Frisell J, Nordenskjöld B, and Rutqvist LE (2002) Long-term effects of mammography screening: updated overview of the Swedish randomised trials. *Lancet* 359: 909–919.

Olsen O and Gøtzsche PC (2001) Cochrane review on screening for breast cancer with mammography. *Lancet* 358: 1340–1342.

Sankaranarayanan R, Esmy PO, Rajkumar R, *et al.* (2007) Effect of visual screening on cervical cancer incidence and mortality in Tamil Nadu, India: a cluster-randomised trial. *Lancet* 370: 398–406.

Sankaranarayanan R, Ramadas K, Thamas G, *et al.* (2005) Effect of screening on oral cancer mortality in Kerala, India: a cluster-randomised controlled trial. *Lancet* 365: 1927–1933.

Scholefield JH, Moss S, Sufi F, Mangham CM, and Hardcastle JD (2002) Effect of faecal occult blood screening on mortality from colorectal cancer: results from a randomised controlled trial. *Gut* 50: 840–844.

Shapiro S, Venet W, Strax P, and Venet L (1988) Current results of the breast cancer screening randomized trial: The Health Insurance Plan (HIP) of Greater New York Study. In: Day NE and Miller AB (eds.) *Screening for Breast Cancer*, pp. 3–15. Geneva, Switzerland: International Union Against Cancer.

Stenman UH, Hakama M, Knekt P, Aromaa A, Teppo L, and Leinonen J (1994) Serum concentrations of prostate specific antigen and its

complex with α1-ACT 0–12 years before diagnosis of prostate cancer. *Lancet* 344: 1594–1598.

Tabár L, Vitak B, Chen HH, *et al.* (2000) The Swedish Two-County Trial twenty years later. Updated mortality results and new insights from long-term follow-up. *Radiologic Clinics of North America* 38: 625–651.

Zhang BH, Yang BH, and Tang ZY (2004) Randomized controlled trial of screening for hepatocellular carcinoma. *Journal of Cancer Research and Clinical Oncology* 131: 417–422.

Measurement and Modeling of Health-Related Quality of Life

R D Hays, University of California at Los Angeles, Los Angeles, CA, USA
B B Reeve, National Cancer Institute, Bethesda, MD, USA

Introduction

Health-related quality of life (HRQOL) refers to how well a person functions in their life and his or her perceived well-being in physical, mental, and social domains of health. HRQOL includes whether the person can carry out a range of activities of daily living such as bathing or dressing him- or herself (physical functioning). It also includes whether the person can climb stairs, walk, or run. Other relevant aspects of functioning include the extent to which one is able to interact with family, friends, and others (social functioning). The functional part of HRQOL consists of behaviors that can be observed by other people.

The well-being part of HRQOL refers to internal, subjective perceptions such as vitality, pain, anxiety, depressive symptoms, and general health perceptions. These perceptions are not directly observable by others. A person who is anxious might look nervous to an external observer or someone in pain might grimace, but these external signs can be hidden, difficult to detect, and provide at best an indirect indicator of the way the person feels.

Methods of Assessing Health-Related Quality of Life

The target person is considered the best source of information about his or her functioning and well-being. Hence, the usual mode of assessing HRQOL is through self-reports. HRQOL data are typically gathered using either self-administered surveys (e.g., mail) or interviewer-administration (e.g., telephone).

When it is not possible to obtain HRQOL data from the target respondent, HRQOL data can be collected using a proxy (e.g., family member or clinician). Proxy responses are more often used in studies of children or adults who are severely ill or cognitively impaired. Agreement between proxy and self-reports tends to be better for more observable aspects of HRQOL, such as physical functioning, than for internal perceptions such as emotional well-being (Hays *et al.*, 1995; Magaziner *et al.*, 1997).

Generic versus Targeted HRQOL Profile Measures

Generic HRQOL measures are analogous to intelligence tests in that they are designed to be relevant to anyone and allow different people to be compared to one another because they have taken the same test. Generic profile measures yield scores on multiple aspects of HRQOL.

The SF-36 is the most well-recognized generic HRQOL profile measure in the world today. It comprises 36 items selected from a larger pool of items used in the RAND Corporation's Medical Outcomes Study (MOS). Twenty of the items are administered using a 'past four weeks' reporting interval. The SF-36 assesses eight health concepts using multi-item scales (35 items): physical functioning (10 items), role limitations caused by physical health problems (4 items), role limitations caused by emotional problems (3 items), social functioning (2 items), emotional well-being (5 items), vitality (4 items), pain (2 items), and general health perceptions (5 items). An additional item assesses change in perceived health during the last twelve months.

Generic HRQOL profile measures such as the SF-36 are often used to compare the relative burden of disease for different groups of patients. For example, SF-36 physical functioning and emotional well-being scores for 2864 HIV-infected individuals in a probability sample of adults with HIV receiving health care in the United States were compared to patients with other chronic diseases and to the general U.S. population (Hays *et al.*, 2000). SF-36 physical functioning scores were about the same for adults with asymptomatic HIV disease as compared with the U.S. general population but were much worse for those with symptomatic HIV disease (by one standard deviation [SD]), and worse still (by another standard deviation) for those who met criteria for AIDS. Patients with AIDS had worse physical functioning than those with some of the other chronic diseases (epilepsy, gastroesophageal reflux disease, clinically localized prostate cancer, clinical depression, diabetes). SF-36 emotional well-being was comparable among patients with various stages of HIV disease, but was significantly worse than the general U.S. population and patients with other chronic diseases with the exception of depression. In a separate analysis from the same dataset, HRQOL for HIV patients coinfected with chronic viral hepatitis was shown to be similar to those with HIV monoinfection (Kanwal *et al.*, 2005).

HRQOL Targeted Profile Measures

Targeted measures are constructed to fill the gaps in generic instruments by tapping aspects of HRQOL that have particular relevance to people with the characteristic of interest (e.g., age, gender, disease). A common target for these measures is a particular disease or condition. Patrick and Deyo (1989) recommended use of both a generic measure and disease-targeted items. For instance, the Kidney Disease Quality of Life (KDQOL) instrument (Hays *et al.*, 1994) includes the SF-36 as the generic core plus items that assess symptoms and problems associated with kidney disease such as the effects of the disease on daily activities, burden of kidney disease, work, quality of social interaction, sexual function, and sleep.

Disease-targeted measures have the potential to be more sensitive to smaller differences and smaller change over time than generic measures because they are selected to be relevant to a given condition. In a study of HRQOL in men treated for localized prostate cancer, there were no differences on the SF-36 between those treated with surgery, radiation, watchful waiting, or an age- and zip-coded matched control group (Litwin *et al.*, 1995). However, disease-targeted measures of sexual, urinary and bowel function, and distress revealed worse HRQOL among the treatment groups (e.g., radiation, surgery).

A fundamental consideration for including disease-targeted measures in tandem with generic cores is the unique information they capture. The National Eye Institute Refractive Error Quality of Life (NEI-RQL) multi-item scales were found to account for 29% of the variance in satisfaction with vision correction item beyond that explained by the SF-36 and the National Eye Institute

Visual Functioning Questionnaire (NEI-VFQ) (Hays *et al.*, 2003). In a study of 598 persons with chronic eye diseases, the NEI-VFQ scales were found to have low correlations with the SF-36 (Mangione *et al.*, 1998). While the SF-36 was not associated with self-rated severity of gastrointestinal tract involvement, disease-targeted scales in the Scleroderma Gastrointestinal Tract 1.0 survey were sensitive to differences in disease severity (Khanna *et al.*, 2007).

Summary Scores for HRQOL Profile Measures

Profile measures provide multiple scores (one for each domain assessed) and more comprehensive information about a person on a range of HRQOL indicators (e.g., the eight SF-36 scales). However, there are times when summary scores are preferred. Summary scores provide parsimony, but provide less information. Factor analyses are employed to examine how higher-order factors or summary measures can be constructed over a range of HRQOL indicators. Factor analyses of the SF-36 in the United States provide strong support for two underlying factors with physical health defined primarily by measures of physical functioning, pain, and role limitations due to physical health problems, and by mental health reflected primarily by measures of emotional well-being and role limitations caused by emotional problems (Hays *et al.*, 1994). General health perceptions, vitality, and social functioning represent both physical and mental health about equally.

The SF-36 Physical Component Summary (PCS) and Mental Component Summary (MCS) scores were derived using an orthogonal (i.e., uncorrelated) factor model (Ware *et al.*, 1995). Inconsistent results have been found between scale scores and the PCS and MCS because 'mental health' scales receive negative weightings in creating the PCS whereas 'physical health' scales receive negative weightings in constructing the MCS. Thus, better mental health tends to lower the PCS and better physical health tends to lower the MCS. For example, a study of 536 primary care patients who initiated antidepressant treatment found that the SF-36 physical functioning, role limitations due to physical health, pain, and general health perceptions scales improved significantly by 0.3 to 0.5 standard deviations over time, but the PCS did not change significantly (Simon *et al.*, 1998). Inconsistency can arise whenever the physical and mental scales change in a consistent direction.

Hays and colleagues (1998) derived physical and mental health summary scores using a correlated factor model in a sample of 255 female and 245 males stratified by age, race/ethnicity, and educational level to reflect the U.S. population. Farivar *et al.* (2007) derived alternative summary scores for the SF-36 based on a correlated factor model. The difference in factor scoring coefficients for the PCS were as follows (standard scoring vs. alternative): physical functioning (0.42 vs. 0.20), role limitations due to physical health problems (0.35 vs. 0.31), bodily pain (0.32 vs. 0.23), general health perceptions (0.25 vs. 0.20), vitality (0.03 vs. 0.13), social functioning (−0.01 vs. 0.11), role limitations due to emotional problems (−0.19 vs. 0.03) and emotional well-being (−0.22 vs. −0.03). For the MCS the differences in factor scoring coefficients was as follows: physical functioning (−0.23 vs. −0.02), role limitations due to physical health problems (−0.12 vs. 0.03), bodily pain (−0.10 vs. 0.04), general health perceptions (−0.02 vs. 0.10), vitality (0.24 vs. 0.29), social functioning (0.27 vs. 0.14), role limitations due to emotional problems (0.43 vs. 0.20) and emotional well-being (0.48 vs. 0.35). The alternative scoring reduces the number and size of negative weights that produce inconsistencies between scale and summary scores.

Preference-Based HRQOL Measures

While profile measures provide a wealth of information over multiple HRQOL domains, if an intervention shows improvements in some HRQOL scales and decrements in others, it may be difficult to make an overall conclusion. In addition, attrition due to mortality poses a unique problem for profile measures. If those who die are dropped from the analysis, results can be biased. Some proposals for imputing HRQOL scores for the dead have been made (e.g., Diehr *et al.*, 1995), but no one approach is entirely satisfactory.

Preference-based measures are designed to integrate across domains of health to produce a single summary score for each health state anchored relative to 'dead' (score of 0) and 'perfect health' (score of 1). The preference-based measure SF-6D is derived using a six-dimensional health classification scheme (physical functioning, role functioning, emotional well-being, pain, social functioning, and vitality) and a subset of items and categories from the SF-36. Preference weights for 9000 health states defined by combinations of responses to the SF-36 health survey were derived. Visual analogue and standard gamble estimating equations were developed to predict preference scores for each possible health state. The 166 participants in the valuation study consisted of health professionals, health service managers and administrators, staff at the University of Sheffield medical school, undergraduates, and patients at hospital outpatient clinics (Brazier *et al.*, 1998). A larger study of 611 people from the UK general population was used to finalize the scoring function (Brazier *et al.*, 2002).

O'Brien *et al.* (2003) compared the SF-6D with the Health Utilities Index, Mark 3 (HUI3) in a sample of 246 patients at increased risk of sudden cardiac death who were participating in a randomized trial of implantable defibrillator therapy. Mean scores differed significantly ($p < 0.05$) for the SF-6D (0.58) and HUI3 (0.61). Product-moment and intraclass correlations between the two measures were only 0.58 and 0.42. Hence, future work is needed to document and explain the variation in scores produced by different preference-based measures.

Attributes of Good Measures

The ability of HRQOL data to enhance decision making in health care, research, practice, and policy depends on the quality of the instrument used. As reviewed in the following subsections, key characteristics of a good HRQOL measure include the conceptual and measurement model, reliability, validity, minimally importance differences and interpretation of scores, respondent and administrative burden, alternative assessment modalities, and language translations.

Conceptual/Measurement Model

The U.S. Food and Drug Administration (2006) guidance on patient-reported outcomes (PROs) for labeling and promotional claims emphasizes the importance of identifying concepts and domains that are important to patients (**Figure 1**). In addition, the document argues for a clear conceptual framework or specification of how items are grouped into domains. The mapping of items to the concepts they represent is a fundamental step in the development and evaluation of HRQOL measures.

Focus groups and cognitive interviews can be very helpful in developing and evaluating the conceptual framework. Focus groups typically consist of a moderator interacting with six to twelve people representing the target population, significant others (e.g., family), or health-care providers of the target population. Focus groups may be used during all stages of instrument development and evaluation. In early stages, focus groups may respond to open-ended questions that elicit information about important issues and concerns about the HRQOL construct. This may uncover cultural differences in the experiences of the HRQOL domain. Further, it is possible to use focus groups to obtain feedback on item formulation and how items are perceived. For lengthy instruments, focus group members typically complete the instrument in advance and the moderator may ask individuals to discuss complex terms and identify unclear items. Focus groups may also help in generating hypotheses or explanations for interpreting data that have been collected (Aday, 1996).

Cognitive interviewing is a powerful tool for gaining a better understanding of the underlying or covert process

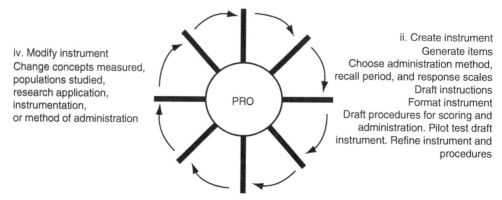

i. Identify concepts and develop conceptual framework
Identify concepts and domains that are important to patients
Determine intended population and research application
Hypothesize expected relationships among concepts

ii. Create instrument
Generate items
Choose administration method,
recall period, and response scales
Draft instructions
Format instrument
Draft procedures for scoring and
administration. Pilot test draft
instrument. Refine instrument and
procedures

iv. Modify instrument
Change concepts measured,
populations studied,
research application,
instrumentation,
or method of administration

PRO

iii. Assess measurement properties
Assess score reliability, validity, and ability to detect change
Evaluate administrative and respondent burden. Add, delete, or revise items
Identify meaningful differences in scores. Finalize instrument formats,
scoring, procedures, and training materials

Figure 1 How are PROs developed?: The FDA perspective.

involved in responding to survey items through the use of verbal probing techniques (Willis, 2005). It is used to evaluate the quality of each item in terms of a person's understanding of the item, ability to retrieve the appropriate information, decision making on reporting retrieved information, and selection of the response. Further, cognitive interviews can be used to examine relationships between participant characteristics, such as ethnicity, and responses to HRQOL items.

The cognitive interview process includes both the administration of an instrument and the collection of additional verbal information about the survey responses (Beatty, 2004). Cognitive interviewing encompasses the more specific practice of cognitive debriefing. The term cognitive debriefing is typically associated with following up with a respondent through the use of retrospective probes, after he or she has completed an instrument with a line of questions aimed at uncovering any difficulties the person may have experienced with either the item content or instructions. For cognitive interviews that involve concurrent probing, the interviewer follows each question with a series of probes to capture participant understanding. In contrast to the retrospective cognitive debriefing, concurrent probing can yield information about the cognitive processing of the item at a point close in time to when it is first presented. It is recommended that five to twelve persons are used for cognitive interviews with a second, iterative round of testing to evaluate items revised from the first round (Willis, 2005).

Cognitive interviews can include both scripted probes to ensure that particular information is collected in every interview and then could be compared across all interviews and emergent, nonscripted probes that help interviewers make sense of gaps or contradictions in participants' responses and provide contextual information needed to precisely define item problems. If sufficient numbers of cognitive interviews are conducted, a coding mechanism allows researchers to use quantitative methods (e.g., logistic regression) to determine if problems encountered during the interviews are due to a number of factors including cultural effects. Cognitive interviewing has been employed as an instrument evaluation tool in several HRQOL studies.

Reliability

The first attribute evaluated and reported typically is reliability, the extent to which a measure yields the same number or score each time when the construct being measured has not changed. Internal consistency reliability, the primary method of estimating reliability for multi-item scales, provides information about the associations among different items in the scale. Internal consistency is typically indexed by coefficient alpha, which is estimated using a two-way fixed-effect analysis of variance (ANOVA) that partitions the 'signal' (i.e., between person variance) from the 'noise' (i.e., interaction between people and responses to different items). Alpha can also be expressed as: $\alpha = (K \times Rii)/(1 + (K - 1) \times Rii)$. This alternative expression illustrates how reliability increases with the number of items (K) in a scale and the intraclass correlation (estimated reliability for a single item), which is based on the correlations among items (*Rii*). A multi-item scale is typically more reliable than a single-item measure.

Test-retest reliability is the only option available for single item scales, but can be used for multi-item scales as well. Picking the optimal time interval for test-retest reliability may be difficult. It should not be too soon such that responses at the second assessment are simply memories of the first assessment, yet not so long that true change in the construct has occurred during the time interval between the initial and subsequent HRQOL assessment.

Reliability coefficients range in theory between 0 and 1, with 0.70 the standard threshold for adequate reliability for use of measures for group comparisons. For individual applications, a more stringent minimum threshold of 0.90 reliability has been suggested (Nunnally, 1978). The higher standard is needed because the error around an individual's score is larger than the error around a group mean score. For example, even with a reliability of 0.90, the individual's standard error of measurement – SD × square root of $(1 - \text{reliability coefficient}) = 0.30 \times$ SD. If the SD of a measure is 10 as it is with the SF-36v2 scales, then the width of the 95% confidence interval around an individual's score is 12 points (greater than a SD) as it extends from 6 points below to 6 points above the estimated true score. Using the same instrument in a group, a sample size of 25 people would result in the width of the 95% confidence interval around the group mean to be 2.4 points (approximately one-quarter of a SD).

Reliability and standard error of measurement (SEM) are inversely related; the more reliable the instrument, the smaller the SEM. This association has important implications for the sample size needed to detect group differences in HRQOL measures. For example, adjusting for the SEM, the required sample size per group to detect a difference between baseline and follow-up of about one-third of a SD is about 297 versus 227 per group if the reliability is 0.69 versus 0.84, respectively (Zimmerman and Williams, 1986).

The limitation of the traditional measures of reliability is that they assume that the reliability of a scale is fixed for all score levels. For example, a pain instrument with a reliability of 0.82 would be considered acceptable for measuring a group's average state of pain no matter if the group experiences mild, average, or severe levels of pain. In contrast, item response theory (IRT) provides an alternative assessment of reliability in terms of item and scale information curves. The IRT information curve indicates the precision (reciprocal of the error variance) of an item or scale for measuring different levels along its underlying HRQOL trait continuum. Thus, the reliability of an item or scale varies depending on the trait level one is assessing. Items are most useful when they are appropriate or matched to the individual completing it. For instance, asking a person who is generally happy and content with life about thoughts of suicide in the last week is not likely to be informative for measuring his/her emotional distress level. Items are most informative when the answer that someone will give is less certain probabilistically (e.g., just as likely to say 'yes' as 'no' to a dichotomous question). Because of the emphasis on assessing dysfunction, information curves for measures often reflect higher precision for measuring worse HRQOL than for measuring better HRQOL. This is appropriate for determining if an intervention has an effect on the population if dysfunction is the range of the continuum targeted by the measure.

Validity

Validity is the extent to which an instrument measures that which it was intended to measure and not something else. There are three main subtypes of validity: content, criterion, and construct. Content validity is the extent to which a measure represents the appropriate content and the variety of attributes that make up the measured construct. Another way of expressing content validity is the adequacy of sampling of the material in the measure. Adequate sampling is best ensured by a plan for content and item construction before the measure is developed. Focus groups and other qualitative methods (e.g., cognitive testing) are sources for appropriate content. A group of experts can examine items and can either endorse the content validity or identify any important gaps in content. Face validity is considered a form of content validity in which the content of a scale is evaluated in terms of the extent to which it is perceived to be measuring what it is supposed to measure by patients or experts.

Criterion-related validity refers to the extent to which the measure agrees with an external standard, typically a 'gold standard' measure. An example would be the development of an observational measure of how well an individual is breathing and comparing it to the gold standard of a pulse oximeter that measures oxygen saturation. Because there is typically no gold standard for HRQOL measures, criterion-related validity is usually not applicable. For situations in which it is appropriate, evaluation of criterion-related validity would involve determining the extent to which the new measure is consistent or captures the essence of the gold standard measure. For example, one might employ contingency table analyses of sensitivity and specificity or area under the curve analyses to assess the level of agreement of the new measure with the standard.

Construct validity is the extent to which the measure 'behaves' in a way consistent with theoretical hypotheses and represents how well scores on the instrument are indicative of the theoretical construct. Construct validity evaluation includes the degree to which a measure correlates with other measures to which it is similar and does not correlate with (diverges from) measures that are dissimilar. A surplus of terminology exists in the literature that falls into the general class of construct validity. For example, the multitrait, multimethod approach to validity assessment refers to convergent and discriminant validity as aspects of construct validity. Although responsiveness (i.e., an instrument's ability to capture sensitivity to change) is often described as a separate psychometric property of HRQOL instruments, in actuality it is one aspect of the construct validity of a measure because a valid measure should change in accordance with true underlying change (Hays and Hadorn, 1992).

Construct validity is typically examined using bivariate correlations, factor analysis, and multivariate regression models. For example, one could hypothesize that a breast cancer patient's self-esteem was positively associated with breast-conserving surgery. One could regress self-esteem on type of surgery (e.g., lumpectomy, partial mastectomy, radical mastectomy) and background variables such as age, marital status, and educational level. A statistically significant finding for type of surgery would support the hypothesis and construct validity of the measure of self-esteem. A more complicated example is as follows. Suppose one hypothesized that larger breast size was associated with lower self-esteem in men but higher self-esteem in women. One could then compute rank order correlations separately by gender between a category measure of size (A, B, C, D, DD) and a self-esteem measure. In addition, one could regress self-esteem on a gender dummy variable (female = 1; male = 0), breast size, the interaction of female gender with size, and some background variables such as age and educational attainment. The presence of a positive significant interaction term would support the hypothesis and construct validity of the measure of self-esteem. One might also imagine more refined hypotheses, such as a quadratic effect among females such that intermediate cup size (e.g., B or C), are associated with the highest level of self-esteem.

Minimally Important Difference and the Interpretation of Scores

The minimally important difference (MID) is the smallest change in HRQOL that is perceived by patients as beneficial or that would result in a change in treatment (Guyatt *et al.*, 2002). Evaluating the MID is a special case of examining responsiveness to change that focuses on the people who are deemed to have had 'minimal' change. Hence, a fundamental aspect of estimating the MID is identifying the subgroup of people who have changed by a minimal amount. The essential step is to use external information or anchors (retrospective measures of change, knowledge about the course of health over time, clinical parameters) to identify those who have changed.

The best anchors are ones that identify those who have changed but not too much. In other words, it is important to identify the subset of people who have experienced minimal, but detectable, change. **Figure 2**, for example, shows a hypothetical plot of the impact on physical function of four life interventions. The change from preintervention to postintervention is displayed on the y-axis. Changes in physical function for getting hit by a feather, rock, bike, and car are 0, 2.5, 12.5, and 20, respectively. Assuming the physical function scale has a standard deviation of 10, the getting hit by a car intervention results in a substantial impact on physical function (two standard deviations). At the other extreme, the feather has no detectable impact on physical function. The bike impacts physical function by 1.25 standard deviations and the rock impacts it by about a quarter of a standard deviation. If one had the highest possible physical functioning at baseline, a decline of 1.25 standard deviations on the SF-36 physical functioning scale would occur at follow-up by a report of being limited 'a lot' in vigorous activities, limited 'a little' in moderate activities, and limited a lot in climbing several flights of stairs. A decrease by one quarter of a standard deviation would occur if one reported being limited a little in vigorous activities.

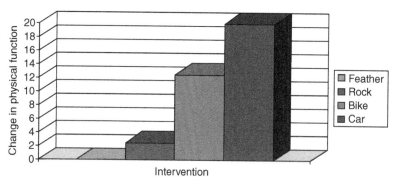

Figure 2 Hypothetical change in physical function (T-score units) by magnitude of intervention.

The car, bike, and feather interventions would not be good anchors for estimating the MID because they would be expected to produce changes in physical function that are either nonexistent (feather) or too large (bike or car). One might argue, however, that getting hit by a rock could be an anchor that might be useful for estimating the MID in physical function.

One type of anchor that has been used in the past is asking study participants at follow-up to report how much they changed since baseline of a study using a multiple categorical response scale such as 'got a lot better,' 'got a little better,' 'stayed the same,' 'got a little worse,' 'got a lot worse.' People who reported either getting a little better or a little worse constitute the minimal change subgroup. The change in HRQOL reported by this subgroup of people would then be the estimate of the MID as perceived by the patient. One should look at change for those getting worse versus getting better separately first and if the results are consistent pool them together after accounting for the difference in the direction of change (e.g., multiplying the change for those who got a little worse by negative one to account for the direction difference). It may also be informative to evaluate whether the MID estimate is invariant to location of the scale (low or high on the construct).

Retrospective self-reports are known to be subject to recall bias (Schwartz and Sudman, 1994). When retrospective change items are used as anchors, it is useful to determine if they reflect the baseline (pretest) and present (posttest) status equally. In theory, retrospective change items should correlate positively with the posttest and have a negative correlation of equal magnitude with the pretest as illustrated in the following formulas: $r(x, y - x) = r(x, y)$ and $r(y, y - x) = r(y, -x) = -r(x, y)$, where r is the correlation, x is the pretest, and y is the posttest. In reality, retrospective self-reports tend to correlate more strongly with the posttest than they do with the pretest because current status unduly influences the retrospective perception of change.

As with any anchor, use of clinical anchors requires establishing the amount of change that is a reasonable indicator of 'minimal.' Kosinski et al. (2000) defined minimal improvement on their clinical measures as 1–20% improvement in the number of swollen and tender joints in a study of 693 patients with rheumatoid arthritis. Although this may be a reasonable threshold, other investigators might argue for something different.

The variety of possible anchors and uncertainty in the anchor cut point that defines a minimal difference makes a single estimate of MID problematic. Using the retrospective report anchor as an example, the recall item might refer globally to change in 'health,' 'health-related quality of life,' or 'quality of life.' Moreover, the anchor might be worded more specifically such as 'physical functioning,' 'pain,' 'getting along with family,' etc. The choice of words could lead to variability in the performance of the anchor. Any specific anchor may be more or less appropriate for different HRQOL domains. For example, a vitality scale might be expected to change more than a pain scale in response to change in hematocrit. Interpreting change in response to a particular anchor should take into consideration that not all domains should change or change equally in tandem with the anchor. Other factors that can lead to variation in the estimation of the MID include whether the people being evaluated are high or low on the measure at baseline, whether they improve or decline in HRQOL over time, and whether they have similar demographic, clinical, and other characteristics (Hays and Woolley, 2000).

Respondent and Administrative Burden

Respondent burden is the time, effort, and other demands imposed on respondents to a survey. Administrative burden is the demand on those who administer the survey. A measure that has adequate reliability and validity will not be used in practice if the burden on the respondent or those who administer it is excessive.

A rule of thumb is that about 3–5 survey items can be administered per minute. Of course, these rules of thumb are general and do not take into account the nature of the items. Survey items with fewer response options are more quickly administered. For example, Hays et al. (1995) found that 832 clients enrolled in treatment programs for impaired (drinking) drivers completed about 4.5 items per minute for an alcohol screening scale with polytomous response options but they were able to complete about 8 items per minute for scales with dichotomous response options.

There is no absolute time threshold for survey administration, but surveys that can be administered in 15–30 minutes are preferred over longer surveys. Applying the 3–5 items per minute rule of thumb, 45–65 items can be administered in 15 minutes while 90–150 items can be administered in 30 minutes. Because the survey needs to be accessible to slower respondents, the lower end of the range should be used in planning survey length.

Availability in Alternate Forms

Alternative forms refer to the ability of the HRQOL instrument to be administered in different modes (e.g., mail self-administration, telephone interviews, web self-administration). The equivalence of alternative modes of administration is especially important in vulnerable and hard-to-reach populations given the advantages of mixed mode data collection for enhancing study participation rates (Brown et al., 1999).

There is consistent evidence that interviewer-administration yields more socially desirable (better HRQOL) responses than self-administration (Dillman *et al.*, 1996). Indeed, there is consistent evidence that interviewer administration results in more positive HRQOL reports than does self-administration (McHorney *et al.*, 1994; Weinberger *et al.*, 1996; Jones *et al.*, 2001). For example, persons randomized to telephone interviews had more positive SF-36 scores than those randomized to mail self-administration, leading McHorney *et al.* (1994: 565) to recommend mode-specific norms.

Translations

Establishing the conceptual and linguistic equivalence of translated and original versions of HRQOL survey instruments is necessary. The international adaptation and evaluation of the SF-36 health survey has been one of the most systematic and coordinated efforts to date (Ware and Gandek, 1998). Efforts such as this suggest a series of important steps in translation of instruments.

If one is trying to translate an instrument developed by someone else, it is a good idea to contact the developer to obtain approval for translation and to work out an acceptable mechanism for proceeding (Acquadro *et al.*, 1996). Working closely with the developers can be mutually beneficial and synergistic. The primary goal of the effort is to produce a translation that is linguistically and conceptually equivalent to the original version. Equivalence can only be obtained if the original and translated versions have the same meaning. Translators should be instructed to produce colloquial translations that will be understood by the general public (Acquadro *et al.*, 1996).

The instructions, items, and response choices should be translated independently by at least two trained bilingual translators. Ideally, these translations should be carried out by local teams and both translators should be native speakers of the language into which the measure is being translated. Translators can rate the difficulty of translating each item and response scale using a 0 (not at all difficult) to 100 (most difficult) scale (Ware *et al.*, 1996). To help select equivalent response options, the Thurstone and Chave (1929) method of equal-appearing intervals can be employed. In this method, a sample of raters ($n = 25$ or so) is asked to rate the position of intermediate response choices using a 10-cm line anchored by the extreme (lowest and highest) response choices (Ware *et al.*, 1996). The translators should compare their translations and reconcile discrepancies.

Two different translators should then rate the quality of the reconciled forward translation. Each item and response scale is rated for its conceptual equivalence to the original version using a 0 (not at all equivalent) to 100 (exactly equivalent) scale. Items and response scales that are rated less than 75 on the 0 to 100 scale are retranslated by the original translators until an acceptable independent rating of equivalence is obtained.

The resulting translation should then be cognitively tested in a small sample (about 10) of patients. This testing should take the form of concurrent or think-aloud interviews as well as self-administration followed by retrospective interviews (Jobe and Mingay, 1990). Following cognitive testing, the item and response options should be rewritten as necessary and a new version of the translation produced. Ideally, the next step is to convene a panel that includes the forward translators, a survey design expert, a patient, and a clinician. The panel's job is to evaluate the conceptual equivalence of the translation and the original survey instrument. The forward translation is then finalized based on the panel's feedback.

After approval of the process by the developers, the final forward translation should be back-translated by two other translators. Both of these translators should be native speakers of the original language of the survey. These two translators should compare their backward translations and come to agreement about discrepancies. The reconciled back translation will then be compared against the original and each item and response scale rated for equivalence to the original version using a 0 (not at all equivalent) to 100 (exactly equivalent) rating scale. Items and response scales should be rated highly (e.g., 75 or higher on the 0–100 scale) for the translation to be approved.

The next step is field testing the translated survey instrument. At a minimum, the translation should be administered to a sample of 75 people who are native speakers of the target language. Scale equivalence should be assessed by performing standard reliability and validity testing and comparing these results to those obtained for the original sample (Hays *et al.*, 1995). Ideally, the translated and the original versions of the instrument should be administered to a bilingual sample in counterbalanced order to allow for direct comparisons of responses for the same respondent (c.f. Coons *et al.*, 1998).

Meaningful and valid comparisons of different groups assume that the generic measure is equivalent in the different groups. This means that the HRQOL scales should have the same level of acceptability, reliability, and validity in different segments of the population. In HRQOL studies, some attention has been paid to evaluating cross-group equivalence involving different language or race/ethnic subgroups. For example, Yu *et al.* (2003) compared the reliability and mean scores of the English and Chinese versions of the SF-36 in a sample of 309 Chinese nationals bilingual in Chinese and English living in the United States. Similarly, the International Quality of Life Assessment Project evaluated the equivalence between the U.S. English and translations versions of the SF-36 into multiple languages including Dutch, Spanish, German, Japanese, and Italian (Gandek *et al.*, 1998).

Item Banking

An item bank is a collection of items that measure a single HRQOL domain that have undergone rigorous qualitative, cognitive, and psychometric review (including cross-cultural group validations), and that have been IRT-calibrated with a set of properties allowing instrument developers to select an item set matched to the characteristics of the study population (Reeve and Fayers, 2005). The bank can be used to develop short-form instruments selecting the best set of items, or used for computerized-adaptive testing (CAT). Instruments built from item banks can yield reliable and valid measurement with reduced response burden.

Another advantage of item banks is the ability in a comparison trial to tailor the item severity (not content) to the target group. For one reason or another, one group may have more depression or pain than another. The item bank can provide different sets of items (but all measuring the same construct) to the different groups, yet because the items come from the same item bank, scores can be compared. Further, item banks can offer the ability to administer repeated HRQOL assessment in a short time frame and not have to worry about issues related to memory effects for responses given on previous assessments. A well-populated item bank can provide alternative HRQOL scales all linked on the same metric.

The strength of a bank to deliver precise, valid, and efficient measurement depends, like any other HRQOL instrument, on the developmental process. An item bank should start with a conceptual framework that leads to identifying existing items that measure that domain and/or developing new items. Once the item pool has been built of old and new items, a thorough qualitative review phase must begin evaluating the items using the techniques described above including focus groups and cognitive interviewing. Next, response data with a large sample representative of the target population must be collected and used to quantitatively review the item performance and make IRT-calibrations.

Use of Measures in Research, Population Surveillance, and Clinical Practice

HRQOL measures can be used for a range of potential applications. The most common application to date has been for group-level comparisons in research. For example, Lorenz et al. (2006) found that each additional symptom at follow-up was associated with worsened overall health and overall quality of life ratings in a nationally representative cohort of 2267 patients in care for HIV who were surveyed in 1996 and again in 1998.

HRQOL measures are also used for population surveillance. For example, one study of U.S. Medicare managed-care beneficiaries found that age- and gender-adjusted annual expenditures in the year after a self-rating of health varied from \$8743 for those who rated their health as poor to \$1656 for those rating their health as excellent (Bierman et al., 1999). The SF-36 has been administered to Medicare beneficiaries enrolled in managed care as part of a project to monitor performance and stimulate quality improvement in managed care plans (Haffer and Bowen, 2004; Jones et al., 2004). The HUI was administered in the Joint Canada/United States Survey of Health, a binationally representative random-digit-dial telephone survey administered in both the United States and Canada to compare the health of those 18 and older in the two countries (Sanmartin et al., 2006). The Medical Expenditure Panel Survey is a nationally representative survey of health-care utilization and expenditures for the U.S. noninstitutionalized civilian population (Cohen et al., 1996) that included the SF-12 version 1 and the EQ-5D in some administrations.

Investigators with the Dartmouth Cooperative Information Project (COOP) were pioneers in the use of HRQOL measures in clinical practice. The COOP chart system was developed by a network of community medical practices that cooperate on primary care research activities. The COOP charts were developed for the purpose of making a brief, practical, and valid method to assess the functional status of adults and adolescents.

The charts are similar to Snellen charts, which are used medically to measure visual acuity quickly in busy clinical practices. Each chart consists of a title, a question referring to the status of the patient over the past 2–4 weeks, and five response choices. Each response is illustrated by a drawing that depicts a level of functioning or well-being along a 5-point ordinal scale (Nelson et al., 1990). The illustration makes the charts appear friendly without seeming to bias their responses (Larson et al., 1992).

In one study of 29 intervention and 27 control group physicians, the Dartmouth COOP Charts were used to assess HRQOL of adult patients during a single clinical encounter (Wasson et al., 1992). The ordering of tests and procedures for women was increased by exposure to the COOP Charts (52% vs. 35%; $p < 0.01$); the effect in men was not as significant (37% vs. 23%; $p = 0.06$). Although women reported no change in satisfaction with care, men claimed that the clinician helped in the management of pain ($p = 0.02$).

A prospective randomized study of 28 oncologists and 286 cancer patients documented more frequent discussion of chronic nonspecific symptoms ($p = 0.03$) in the intervention group. HRQOL improvement was associated with use of HRQOL data ($p = 0.016$) and discussion of pain and role function ($p = 0.046$).

Despite some encouraging results in the use of HRQOL measures in clinical practice, Greenhalgh *et al.* (2005) argued that more attention needs to be given to the mechanism linking HRQOL assessment to better outcomes to maximize its impact on clinical decisions.

Wasson and James (2001) discussed how HRQOL assessment and feedback could be used at multiple levels including clinic, school, workplace, and community. They note that in the clinic patients and providers are encouraged to discuss the patient's HRQOL. In the school system, aggregated information can be used to target programs to meet student needs. Health assessment and personal feedback at school (Wasson *et al.*, 1995) or in the workplace can be offered to improve health and reduce health-care costs. Finally, the Internet provides a means by which health assessment and feedback can be used to improve the health of the community.

Acknowledgments

Ron Hays was supported by the National Institutes of Health through the NIH Roadmap for Medical Research Grant (AG015815), PROMIS Project, a P01 grant (AG20679-01) from the National Institutes of Aging, UCLA/DREW Project EXPORT, National Institutes of Health, National Center on Minority Health and Health Disparities, (P20-MD00148-01), a UCLA Center for Health Improvement in Minority Elders/Resource Centers for Minority Aging Research, National Institutes of Health, National Institute of Aging, (AG-02-004), and a cooperative agreement (2 U18 HS09204) from the Agency for Healthcare Research and Quality.

See also: Clinical Trials; Health Surveys; Methods of Measuring and Valuing Health; Measuring the Quality of Life of Children and Adolescents.

Citations

Acquadro C, Jambon B, Ellis D, and Marquis P (1996) Language and translation issues. In: Spilker B (ed.) *Quality of Life and Pharmacoeconomics in Clinical Trials*, 2nd edn., pp. 575–585. Philadelphia, PA: Lippincott-Raven

Bierman AS, Bubolz TA, Fisher ES, and Wasson JH (1999) How well does a single question about health predict the financial health of Medicare managed care plans? *Effective Clinical Practice* 2: 56–62.

Brazier J, Usherwood T, Harper R, and Thomas K (1998) Deriving a preference-based single index from the U.K. SF-36 Health Survey. *Journal of Clinical Epidemiology* 51: 1115–1128.

Brazier J, Roberts J, and Deverill M (2002) The estimation of a preference-based measure of health from the SF-36. *Journal of Health Economics* 21: 271–292.

Brown JA, Nederend SE, Hays RD, Short PF, and Farley DO (1999) Special issues in assessing care of Medicaid recipients. *Medical Care* 37: MS79–MS88.

Cohen JW, Monheit AC, Beauregard KM, *et al.* (1996) The Medical Expenditure Panel Survey: A national health information resource. *Inquiry* 33: 373–389.

Coons SJ, Alabdulmohsin SA, Draugalis JR, and Hays D (1998) Reliability of an Arabic version of the RAND 36-Item Health Survey 1.0 (a.k.a. SF-36) and its equivalence to the U.S.-English version. *Medical Care* 36: 428–432.

Diehr P, Patrick D, Hedrick S, *et al.* (1995) Including deaths when measuring health status over time. *Medical Care* 33: AS164–A172.

Dillman DA, Sangster RL, Tarnai J, and Rockwood TH (1996) Understanding differences in people's answers to telephone and mail surveys. In: Braverman MT and Slater JK (eds.) *Advances in Survey Research: New Directions for Evaluation* vol. 70, pp. 45–62. San Francisco, CA: Jossey-Bass.

Farivar SS, Cunningham WE, and Hays RD (2007) Correlated physical and mental health summary scores for the SF-36 and SF-12 health survey, vol. 1. *Health and Quality of Life Outcomes* 5: 54.

Gandek B, Ware JE, Aarons NK, *et al.* (1998) Tests of data quality, scaling assumptions, and reliability of the SF-36 in eleven countries: Results from the IQOLA Project. *Journal of Clinical Epidemiology* 51: 1149–1158.

Greenhalgh J, Long AF, and Flynn R (2005) The use of patient reported outcome measures in routine clinical practice: Lack of impact or lack of theory? *Social Science and Medicine* 60: 833–843.

Guyatt GH, Osoba D, Wu AW, *et al.* (2002) Methods to explain the clinical significance of health status measures. *Mayo Clinic Proceedings* 77: 371–383.

Haffer SC and Bowen SE (2004) Measuring and improving health outcomes in Medicare: The Medicare HOS program. *Health Care Financing Review* 25: 1–3.

Hays RD and Hadorn D (1992) Responsiveness to change: An aspect of validity, not a separate dimension. *Quality of Life Research* 1: 73–75.

Hays RD, Marshall GN, Wang EYI, and Sherbourne CD (1994) Four-year cross-lagged associations between physical and mental health in the Medical Outcomes Study. *Journal of Consulting and Clinical Psychology* 62: 441–449.

Hays RD, Kallich JD, Mapes DL, Coons SJ, and Carter WB (1994b) Development of the Kidney Disease Quality of Life (KDQOL) Instrument. *Quality of Life Research* 3: 329–338.

Hays RD, Anderson R, and Revicki DA (1995) Psychometric evaluation and interpretation of health-related quality of life data. In: Shumaker S and Berzon R (eds.) *The International Assessment of Health-Related Quality of Life: Theory, Translation, Measurement and Analysis*, pp. 103–114. Oxford, UK: Rapid Communications.

Hays RD, Merz JF, and Nicholas R (1995b) Response burden, reliability, and validity of the CAGE, Short-MAST, and AUDIT alcohol screening measures. *Behavior Research Methods, Instruments, and Computers* 27: 277–280.

Hays RD, Vickrey B, Hermann B, *et al.* (1995c) Agreement between self reports and proxy reports of quality of life in epilepsy patients. *Quality of Life Research* 4: 159–168.

Hays RD, Mangione CM, Ellwein L, *et al.* (2003) Psychometric properties of the National Eye Institute – Refractive Error Quality of Life Instrument. *Ophthalmology* 110: 2292–2301.

Hays RD, Prince-Embury S, and Chen H (1998) *RAND-36 Health Status Inventory*. San Antonio, TX: Psychological Corporation.

Hays RD, Cunningham WE, Sherbourne CD, *et al.* (2000) Health-related quality of life in patients with human immunodeficiency virus infection in the United States: Results from the HIV Cost and Services Utilization Study. *American Journal of Medicine* 108: 714–722.

Jobe JB and Mingay DJ (1990) Cognitive laboratory approach to designing questionnaires for surveys of the elderly. *Public Health Reports* 105: 518–524.

Jones D, Kazis L, Lee A, *et al.* (2001) Health status assessments using the Veterans SF-12 and SF-36: Methods for evaluating outcomes in the Veterans health administration. *Journal of Ambulatory Care Management* 24: 68–86.

Jones N, Jones SL, and Millar NA (2004) The Medicare Health Outcomes Survey program: Overview, context, and near-term prospects. *Health and Quality of Life Outcomes* 2: 33.

Kanwal F, Gralnek IM, Hays RD, *et al.* (2005) Impact of chronic viral Hepatitis on health-related quality of life in HIV: Results from a nationally representative sample. *American Journal of Gastroenterology* 100: 1984–1994.

Khanna D, Hays RD, Park GS, *et al.* (2007) Development of a preliminary scleroderma gastrointenstinal tract 1.0 (SSC-GIT 1.0) quality of life instrument. *Arthritis Care and Research* 57: 1280–1286.

Kosinski M, Zhao SZ, Dedhiya S, Osterhaus JT, and Ware JE (2000) Determining the minimally important changes in generic and disease-specific health-related quality of life questionnaires in clinical trials of rheumatoid arthritis. *Arthritis and Rheumatolgy* 43: 1478–1487.

Larson CO, Hays RD, and Nelson EC (1992) Do the pictures influence scores on the Dartmouth COOP charts? *Quality of Life Research* 1: 247–249.

Litwin M, Hays RD, Fink A, *et al.* (1995) Quality of life outcomes in men treated for localized prostate cancer. *Journal of the American Medical Association* 273: 129–135.

Lorenz KA, Cunningham WE, Spritzer KL, and Hays RD (2006) Changes in symptoms and health-related quality of life in a nationally representative sample of adults in treatment for HIV. *Quality of Life Research* 15: 951–958.

Magaziner J, Zimmerman SI, Gruber-Baldini AL, Hebel R, and Fox KM (1997) Proxy reporting in five areas of functional status: Comparison with self-reports and observations of performance. *Amercian Journal of Epidemiology* 146: 418–428.

Mangione CM, Lee PP, Pitts J, Gutierrez P, Berry S, and Hays RD (1998) Psychometric properties of the National Eye Institute Visual Function Questionnaire, the NEI-VFQ. *Archives of Ophthalmology* 116: 1496–1504.

McHorney CA, Kosinski M, and Ware JE (1994) Comparisons of costs and quality of norms for the SF-36 health survey collected by mail versus telephone interview: Results from a national survey. *Medical Care* 32: 551–567.

Nelson EC, Landgraf JM, Hays RD, Wasson JH, and Kirk JW (1990) The functional status of patients: How can it be measured in physicians' offices? *Medical Care* 28: 1111–1126.

Nunnally J (1978) *Psychometric Theory,* 2nd edn. New York: McGraw-Hill.

O'Brien BJ, Spath M, Blackhouse G, Severens JL, Dorian P, and Brazier J (2003) A view from the bridge: Agreement between the SF-6D utility algorithm and the Health Utilities Index. *Health Economics* 12: 975–981.

Patrick DL and Deyo RA (1989) Generic and disease-specific measures in assessing health status and quality of life. *Medical Care* 27: S217–S232.

Reeve BB and Fayers P (2005) Applying item response theory modeling for evaluating questionnaire items and scale properties. In: Fayers P and Hays R (eds.) *Assessing Quality of Life in Clinical Trials: Methods and Practice*, pp. 55–73. Oxford, UK: Oxford University Press.

Sanmartin C, Berthelot JM, Ng E, *et al.* (2006) Comparing health and health care use in Canada and the United States. *Health Affairs* 25: 1133–1142.

Schwartz N and Sudman S (1994) *Autobiographical Memory and the Validity of Retrospective Reports.* New York: Springer-Verlag.

Simon GE, Revicki DA, Grothaus L, *et al.* (1998) SF-36 summary scores: Are physical and mental health truly distinct? *Medical Care* 36: 567–572.

Thurstone LL and Chave EJ (1929) *The Measurement of Attitude.* Chicago, IL: University of Chicago Press.

U.S. Food and Drug Administration (2006) Draft guidance for industry on patient-reported outcome measures: Use in medicinal product development to support labeling claims. *Federal Register* 71: 5862–5863.

Velikova G, Booth L, Smith AB, *et al.* (2005) Measuring quality of life in routine oncology practice improves communication and patient well-being: A randomized controlled trial. *Journal of Clinical Oncology* 22: 714–724.

Ware JE and Gandek B (1998) Overview of the SF-36 health survey and the international quality of life assessment (IQOOLA) project. *Journal of Clinical Epidemiology* 51: 903–912.

Ware JE, Kosinski M, Bayliss MS, *et al.* (1995) Comparison of methods for the scoring and statistical analysis of SF-36 health profile and summary measures: Summary of results from the Medical Outcomes Study. *Medical Care* 33: AS264–279.

Ware JE, Gandek BL, and Keller SD and the IQOLA Project Group (1996) Evaluating instruments used cross-nationally: Methods from the IQOLA project. In: Spilker B (ed.) *Quality of Life and Pharmacoeconomics in Clinical Trials*, pp. 681–692. Philadelphia, PA: Lippincott-Raven.

Wasson J, Hays R, Rubenstein L, *et al.* (1992) The short-term effect of patient health status assessment in a health maintenance organization. *Quality of Life Research* 1: 99–106.

Wasson JH, Kairys SW, Nelson EC, *et al.* (1995) Adolescent health and social problems: A method for detection and early management. The Dartmouth Primary Care Cooperative Information Project (COOP). *Archives of Family Medicine* 4: 51–56.

Wasson JH and James C (2001) Implementation of web-based interaction technology to improve the quality of a city's health care. *Journal of Ambulatory Care Management* 24: 1–9.

Weinberger M, Oddone EZ, Samsa GP, and Landsman PB (1996) Are health-related quality-of-life measures affected by the mode of administration? *Journal of Clinical Epidemiology* 49: 135–140.

Yu J, Coons SJ, Draugalis JR, Ren XS, and Hays RD (2003) Equivalence of the Chinese version and the U.S.-English version of the SF-36 Health Survey. *Quality of Life Research* 12: 449–457.

Zimmerman DW and Williams RH (1986) Note on the reliability of experimental measures and the power of significance tests. *Psychological Bulletin* 100: 123–124.

Further Reading

Hahn EA, Cella D, Chassany O, Fairclough DL, Wong GY, and Hays RD (2007) A comparison of the precision of health-related quality of life data relative to other clinical measures. *Mayo Clinic Proceedings* 82(10): 1244–1254.

Hays RD, Brodsky M, Johnston MF, Spritzer KL, and Hui K (2005) Evaluating the statistical significance of health-related quality of life change in individual patients. *Evaluation and the Health Professions* 28: 160–171.

Reeve BB, Hays RD, Bjorner JB, *et al.* (2007) Psychometric evaluation and calibration of health-related quality of life item banks: Plans for the Patient-Reported Outcome Measurement Information System (PROMIS). *Medical Care* 45: S22–S31.

Revicki DA, Cella D, Hays RD, Sloan JA, Lenderking WR, and Aaronson NK (2006) Responsiveness and minimal important differences for patient reported outcomes. *Health and Quality of LifeOutcomes* 4: 70.

Methods of Measuring and Valuing Health*

J Brazier, Sheffield University, Sheffield, UK
J Ratcliffe, University of South Australia, Adelaide, Australia

Introduction

The quality-adjusted life year (QALY) combines length of life and health-related quality of life (HRQOL) into a single measure. To put the 'Q' into a QALY requires an index for valuing health states. The increasing application of economic evaluation, and specifically the use of the incremental cost per QALY to assess cost effectiveness, has resulted in an enormous growth in the demand for health states values for use in decision-analytic models and clinical trials comparing alternative health-care interventions.

The range of tools for valuing health states has expanded considerably from the early notion of a health index in the United States (Fanshel and Bush, 1970) to the emergence of the EQ-5D in Europe (Brooks *et al.*, 2003) and the Health Utilities Index (HUI) in Canada (Feeny *et al.*, 2002). At the same time there have been important debates in the literature concerning the core issues of what to value (or how to define health), how to value it, and who should do the valuing. This article aims to provide the reader with an overview of these issues and then focuses on methods for valuing health (see Brazier *et al.*, 2007).

The article begins by outlining these core issues. It then describes the main techniques for the direct valuation of health states, including the conventional cardinal techniques (like standard gamble) and their advantages and disadvantages, and ordinal methods (like ranking and pairwise choices) that are starting to be used to value health states. The article then addresses the question of whose values to use and whether values should be based on preferences (as is usually the case in economics) or experiences. Finally, there is a brief review of the most widely used generic preference-based measures of health (such as EQ-5D, SF-6D, and HUI3).

The Core Questions to Address When Valuing Health States

To calculate QALYs it is necessary to represent health on a scale in which death and full health are assigned values of 0 and 1, respectively. Therefore, states rated as better than dead have values between 0 and 1 and states rated as worse than dead have negative scores that in principle are bounded by negative infinity. One of the most commonly used instruments for estimating the value of the 'Q' in the QALY is a generic preference-based measure of health called the EQ-5D (Brooks *et al.*, 2003). This instrument has a structured health state descriptive system with five dimensions of mobility, self-care, usual activities, pain/discomfort, and anxiety/depression (**Table 1**). Each dimension has three levels: no problem (level 1), moderate or some problem (level 2), and severe problem (level 3). Together these five dimensions define a total of 243 health states formed by different combinations of the levels (i.e., 3^5), and each state is described in the form of a five-digit code using the three levels (e.g., state 12321 means no problems in mobility, moderate problems in self-care, etc.). It can be administered to patients or their proxy using a short one-page questionnaire with five questions.

The EQ-5D can be scored in a number of ways depending on the method of valuation and source country, but the most widely used to date is the UK York TTO Tariff shown in **Table 2**. This population value set was obtained using the time trade-off (TTO) method with a sample of about 3000 members of the UK general population; similar tariffs have been estimated for other countries, including the United States. Different valuation methods and the appropriateness of obtaining values from the general population are reviewed later in the article.

The EQ-5D provides a useful starting point for the rest of this article, because it demonstrates the key features of any method for measuring and valuing health. Underpinning the EQ-5D and similar instruments are a number of core methodological questions: How should health be described, how should it be valued, and who should provide the values? The first part of the question concerns the aspects of health (and/or quality of life) that should be covered by the measure. The next part concerns the valuation technique that should be used. The EQ-5D has been valued using TTO and visual analogue scale (EQ VAS). Other generic preference-based measures such as the HUI3 and SF-6D used the standard gamble (SG) method, which some have argued should be the gold standard method of valuation in this field. The last part of the question concerns the source of values, and whether they should be obtained from patients themselves, their carers and medical professionals, or members of the general population. The remainder of this article addresses

---

* This chapter is reprinted from Measurement and Valuation of Health for Economic Evaluation, International Encyclopedia of Public Health, 2008, 4, 252–261.

these three questions. (For discussion on whether the QALY is an appropriate measure and how QALYs should be aggregated and used to inform health policy, see Brazier *et al.*, 2007.)

How Should Health Be Described?

There are two broad approaches to describing health for deriving health state values. One is to construct a custom-made description of the condition and/or its treatment and the other is to use a standardized descriptive system (such as the EQ-5D). A bespoke description, sometimes referred to as a vignettes in the literature, can take the form of a text narrative or a more structured description using a bullet point format. More recently

researchers have begun to explore alternative narrative formats, such as the use of videos or simulators. The use of custom-made vignettes was more common in the early days of obtaining health state values, however, in recent years the standardized descriptive systems have tended to dominate.

The other approach has been to use generic preference-based measures of health such as the EQ-5D. These have two components, the first a system for describing health or its impact on quality of life using a standardized descriptive system, and the second an algorithm for assigning values to each state described by the system. A health state descriptive system is composed of a number of multilevel dimensions that together describe a universe of health states (such as the EQ-5D described earlier). Generic instruments have been developed for use across all groups by focusing on core aspects of health.

Generic preference-based measures have become the most widely used and this stems from their ease of use, their alleged generic properties (i.e., validity across different patient groups), and their ability to meet a number of requirements of agencies such as the National Institute for Health and Clinical Excellence (NICE). Furthermore, they come 'off the shelf,' with a questionnaire and a set of weights for each health state defined by the classification already provided. The questionnaires for collecting the descriptive data can be readily incorporated into most clinical trials and routine data collection systems with little additional burden for respondents, and the valuation of their responses can be done easily using the scoring algorithms provided by the developers.

However, there are concerns about the sensitivity of the generics and their relevance for some conditions. As a result, there has been work to develop condition-specific descriptive systems (Brazier *et al.*, 2007) and there continues to be an interest in using custom-made vignettes. This raises the question as to whether health state utilities derived from specific descriptive systems are generalizable.

Table 1   EQ-5D classification

Dimension	Level	Description
Mobility	1	No problems walking about
	2	Some problems walking about
	3	Confined to bed
Self-care	1	No problems with self-care
	2	Some problems washing or dressing self
	3	Unable to wash or dress self
Usual activities	1	No problems with performing usual activities (e.g., work, study, housework, family, or leisure activities)
	2	Some problems with performing usual activities
	3	Unable to perform usual activities
Pain/discomfort	1	No pain or discomfort
	2	Moderate pain or discomfort
	3	Extreme pain or discomfort
Anxiety/ depression	1	Not anxious or depressed
	2	Moderately anxious or depressed
	3	Extremely anxious or depressed

Table 2   Descriptive systems of generic preference-based measures

Instrument	Dimension	Levels	Health states
QW	Mobility, physical activity, social functioning	3	945
B	27 symptoms/problems	2	
HUI-2	Sensory, mobility, emotion, cognitive, self-care, pain	4–5	24 000
	Fertility	3	
HUI-3	Vision, hearing, speech, ambulation, dexterity, emotion, cognition, pain	5–6	972 000
EQ-5D	Mobility, self-care, usual activities, pain/discomfort, anxiety/depression	3	243
15D	Mobility, vision, hearing, breathing, sleeping, eating, speech, elimination, usual activities, mental function, discomfort/symptoms, depression, distress, vitality, sexual activity	4–5	31 billion
SF-6D	Physical functioning, role limitation, social functioning, pain, energy, mental health	4–6	18 000 (SF-36 version) 7500 (SF-12 version)
AQoL	Independent living (self-care, household tasks, mobility), social relationships (intimacy, friendships, family role), physical senses (seeing, hearing, communication), psychological well-being (sleep, anxiety and depression, pain)	4	16.8 million

Source: Brazier J, Ratcliffe J, Salomon J, and Tsuchiya A (2007) *Measuring and Valuing Health Benefits for Economic Evaluation.* Oxford, UK: Oxford University Press.

This is important for economic evaluations in which the purpose is often to inform resource allocation decisions across patient groups. Even if values are obtained using the same techniques and from similar populations, differences may persist due to preference interactions between dimensions in the descriptions and those outside the system. The impact of asthma on health state utility values, for example, may be altered by the presence of pain from a comorbid condition. Of course, this problem exists for generic descriptive systems; it is just more likely to be a problem with specific systems. Ultimately it is a trade-off between the greater relevance and sensitivity of some specific systems and the limitations on generalizability.

There are also important issues about the appropriate conceptual basis for a descriptive system; some instruments cover quite narrowly defined aspects of impairment and symptomology associated with medical conditions, while others consider a higher level and broader conception of quality of life.

Valuation Techniques

To be used in economic evaluation, health state valuations need to be placed on a scale ranging from 0 to 1, where 0 is for states regarded as equivalent to dead and 1 is for a state of full health. Within the health state valuation process it is also necessary to allow for states that could be valued as worse than being dead. The three main techniques for valuing health states are the SG, the TTO, and the EQ VAS. This section describes how each technique can be used to value chronic health states.

The Visual Analogue Scale (EQ VAS)

The EuroQol Visual Analogue Scale (EQ VAS) is usually represented as a line with well-defined endpoints, on which respondents are able to indicate their judgments, values, or feelings (thus it is sometimes called a 'feeling' thermometer). The distances between intervals on a EQ VAS should reflect an individual's understanding of the relative differences between the concepts being measured. EQ VAS is intended to have interval properties, so that the difference between 3 and 5 on a 10-point scale, for example, should equal the difference between 5 and 7.

In the health context, EQ VAS has been widely used as a measure of symptoms and various domains of health including the direct measurement of a patient's own health or as a means of valuing generic health state classifications including the Quality of Well-Being scale (QWB) (Kaplan and Anderson, 1988), the HUI (Feeny *et al.*, 2002) and the EQ-5D (Brooks *et al.*, 2003). **Figure 1** presents an example of the EQ VAS developed by the Euroqol group. EQ VAS can also be used to elicit the value attached to temporary health states (e.g., those lasting for a specified period of time after which

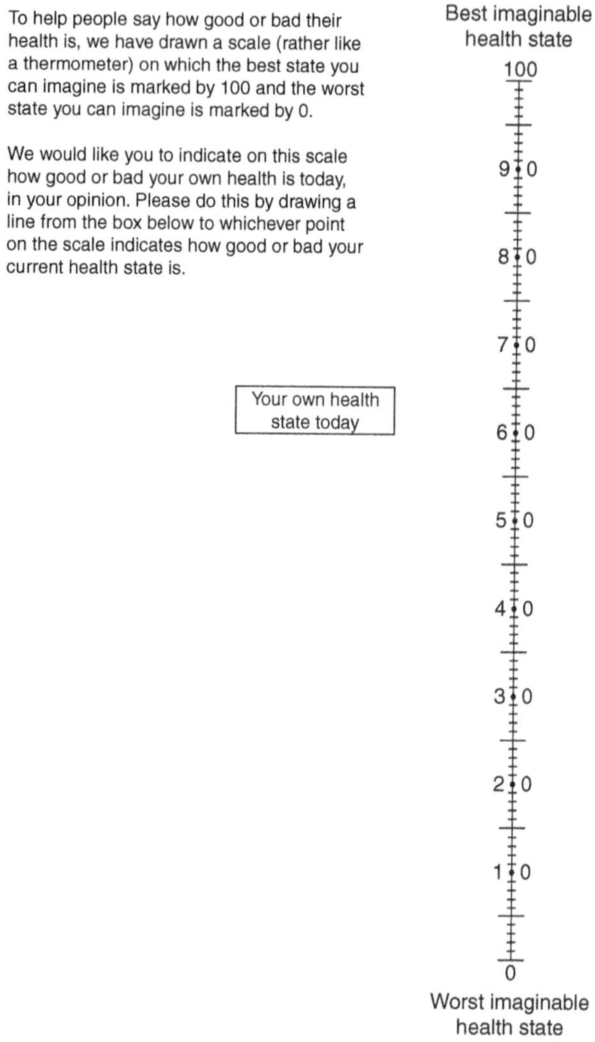

To help people say how good or bad their health is, we have drawn a scale (rather like a thermometer) on which the best state you can imagine is marked by 100 and the worst state you can imagine is marked by 0.

We would like you to indicate on this scale how good or bad your own health is today, in your opinion. Please do this by drawing a line from the box below to whichever point on the scale indicates how good or bad your current health state is.

Your own health state today

Best imaginable health state

100
9 0
8 0
7 0
6 0
5 0
4 0
3 0
2 0
1 0
0

Worst imaginable health state

Figure 1 Example of a visual analogue scale for own health representing the EQ VAS portion of the EQ-5D. EQ-5D™ is a trademark of the EuroQol Group. Figure is reproduced with permission from the 1990 EuroQol Group.

there is a return to good health in contrast to chronic health states which are assumed to last for the rest of a person's life) and states considered worse than death.

The Standard Gamble (SG)

The SG comes from expected utility theory, which postulates that individuals choose between prospects – for example, different ways of managing a medical condition – in such a way as to maximize their 'expected' utility. The SG method gives the respondent a choice between a certain intermediate outcome and the uncertainty of a gamble with two possible outcomes, one of which is better than the certain intermediate outcome and one of which is worse. The SG task for eliciting the value attached to health states considered better than dead is displayed in **Figure 2**. The respondent is offered two alternatives. Alternative 1 is

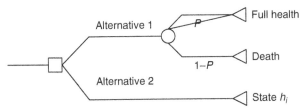

Figure 2 Standard gamble for a chronic health state preferred to death.

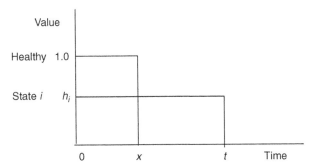

Figure 3 Time trade-off for a chronic health state preferred to death.

a treatment with two possible outcomes: either the patient is returned to normal health and lives for an additional t years (probability $= P$), or the patient dies immediately (probability $= 1 - P$). Alternative 2 has the certain outcome of chronic state h_i for life (t years). The probability P of the best outcome is varied until the individual is indifferent between the certain intermediate outcome and the gamble. This probability P is the utility for the certain outcome, state h_i. This technique is then repeated for all intermediate outcomes. The SG can also be modified to elicit the value attached to health states considered worse than death and temporary health states.

The SG technique has been widely applied in the decision-making literature and has also been extensively applied to medical decision making, including the valuation of health states, in which it has been used (indirectly via a transformation of EQ VAS) to value the HUI2 and HUI3 (Torrance et al., 1996; Feeney et al., 2002) and to directly value SF-6D (Brazier et al., 2002) and a number of condition-specific health state scenarios or vignettes (Brazier et al., 2007). There are many variants of the SG technique that differ in terms of the procedure used to identify the point of indifference, the use of props, and the method of administration (e.g., by interviewer, computer, or self-administered paper questionnaire).

The Time Trade-Off (TTO)

The TTO technique was developed specifically for use in health care in an effort to overcome the problems associated with SG in explaining probabilities to respondents. TTO asks respondents to choose between two alternatives of certainty rather than between a certain outcome and a gamble with two possible outcomes. The application of TTO to a chronic state considered better than dead is illustrated in **Figure 3**.

The approach involves presenting individuals with a paired comparison. For a chronic health state preferred to death, alternative 1 involves living for period t in a specified but less than full health state (state h_i). Alternative 2 involves full health for time period x where $x < t$. Time x is varied until the respondent is indifferent between the two alternatives. The score given to the less than full health state is then x/t. The TTO task can be modified to con-

sider chronic health states considered worse than death and temporary health states. In common with SG, there are numerous variants of TTO using different elicitation procedures, props (if any), and modes of administration.

Pros and Cons of Valuation Techniques

Visual Analogue Scales (EQ VAS)

EQ VAS achieves high response rates and high levels of completion. EQ VAS methods tend to be less expensive to administer than TTO or SG methods due to their relative simplicity and ease of completeness. There is also a significant amount of empirical evidence to demonstrate the reliability of EQ VAS methods in terms of inter-rater reliability and test–retest reliability. However, the lack of choice and direct nature of the EQ VAS tasks have given rise to concerns over the ability of this technique to reflect preferences on an interval scale.

There is also a concern that EQ VAS methods are susceptible to response spreading, whereby respondents use all areas on the valuation scale when responding, especially where multiple health states are valued on the same scale. Response spreading can lead to health states that are very much alike, being placed at some distance from one another on a valuation scale, and health states that are essentially vastly different being placed very close to one another, as the respondent seeks to place responses across the whole (or a specific portion) of the available scale. If response spreading does occur, then this implies that EQ VAS techniques do not generate an interval scale and the numbers obtained may not be meaningful in cardinal terms.

More generally, EQ VAS is prone to context effects in which the average rating for items is influenced by the level of other items being valued and by endpoint bias whereby health states at the top and bottom of the scale are placed further apart on the scale than would be suggested by a direct comparison of differences.

In summary, EQ VAS techniques appear to measure aspects of health status changes rather than the satisfaction or benefit conveyed by such changes. Qualitative evidence of respondents seeing EQ VAS methods as an expression of numbers in terms of 'percentages of the best imaginable state,' or a 'percentage of functioning scale' rather than eliciting information about their preferences for health states provides support for this hypothesis. There is a large body of evidence to suggest that unadjusted EQ VAS scores do not provide a valid measure of the strength of preference that can be used in economic evaluation.

Given the evidence that EQ VAS may not produce health state utilities that can be used directly in the calculation of QALYs, there has been interest in mapping EQ VAS values to SG or TTO utility values. This has the advantage of retaining the ease of use of EQ VAS with the theoretical advantages of a choice-based measure of health. However, the extent to which a stable mapping function can be found between EQ VAS and SG or TTO has been disputed (Stevens *et al.*, 2006).

Standard Gamble

Many SG studies, across different respondent groups, have reported completion rates in excess of 80%, with some studies reporting completion rates as high as 95–100%, indicating that the SG appears to be acceptable in terms of its practicality. The SG has also been found to be feasible and acceptable among varied types of patient groups and clinical areas including cancer, transplantation, vascular surgery, and spinal problems.

SG is rooted in expected utility theory (EUT). EUT has been the dominant theory of decision making under uncertainty for over half a century. EUT theory postulates that individuals choose between prospects (such as different ways of managing a medical condition) in such a way as to maximize their 'expected' utility. According to this theory, for a given prospect such as having a surgical operation, a utility value is estimated for each possible outcome, good or bad. These values are multiplied by their probability of occurring and the result summed to calculate the expected utility of the prospect. This procedure is undertaken for each prospect being considered. The key assumption made by EUT over and above conventional consumer theory is independence, which means that the value of a given outcome is independent of how it was arrived at or its context. In decision tree analysis this is the equivalent of saying that the value of one branch of the tree is unaffected by the other branches.

Due to its theoretical basis, the SG is often portrayed as the classical method of decision making under uncertainty, and due to the uncertain nature of medical decision making the SG is often classified as the gold standard. As medical decisions usually involve uncertainty the use of the SG method would seem to have great appeal. However, the type of uncertain prospect embodied in the SG may bear little resemblance to the uncertainties

in various medical decisions, so this feature may be less relevant than others have suggested.

The status of SG as the gold standard has been criticized given the existence of ample evidence that the axioms of EUT are violated in practice. One response in health economics (as elsewhere) has been that EUT should be seen as a normative rather than a descriptive theory, that is, it suggests how decisions should be made under condition of uncertainty. However, this still does not alter the concern that the values generated by SG do not necessarily represent people's valuation of a given health state, but incorporate other factors, such as risk attitude, gambling affects, and loss aversion.

Time Trade-Off

The TTO technique is a practical, reliable, and acceptable method of health state valuation as evidenced by the wide variety of empirical studies that have applied this method (Brazier *et al.*, 2007). The TTO has been mainly interviewer-administered although it has also been used in a self-administered and computer-based applications.

The applicability of the TTO in medical decision making may be questioned because the technique asks respondents to make a choice between two certain outcomes, when health care is characterized by conditions of uncertainty. It is potentially possible to adjust TTO values to incorporate individuals' attitudes to risk and uncertainty, though this is rarely done. Furthermore, adjusting for risk attitude is difficult when there are strong theoretical and empirical grounds for arguing there is not a constant attitude to risk.

An underlying assumption of the TTO method is that individuals are prepared to trade off a constant proportion of their remaining life years to improve their health status, irrespective of the number of years that remain. This is a very strong assumption and it seems reasonable to expect that the valuation of a health state may be influenced by a duration effect relating to the time an individual spends in that state. There may be a 'maximal endurable time' for some severe health states beyond which they yield negative utility. Furthermore, for short survival periods, individuals may not be willing to trade survival time (measured in life years) for an improvement in quality of life, implying that individuals' preferences are lexicographic for short time durations. If individuals do not trade off a constant proportion of their remaining life expectancy in the valuation of health states, then values elicited using specific time durations (e.g., 10 years) cannot be assumed to hold for states lasting for different time periods.

The impact of 'time preference' on valuations is another issue that causes theoretical concerns with the TTO. If individuals have a positive rate of time preference they will give greater value to years of life in the near future than to those in the distant future. Alternatively respondents may prefer to experience an episode of ill health immediately to eliminate 'dread' and move on. For instance, this hypothesis may explain why some women with a family history of breast cancer opt for mastectomy before any breast cancer is detected. In practice, the majority of individuals exhibit positive time preferences for health, although empirically the validity of the traditional (constant) discounting model in health has been challenged in favor of a model that allows for decreasing time aversion (implying that the longer the period of delay for the onset of ill health, the lower the discount rate). TTO values are rarely corrected for time preference.

Which Valuation Technique Should Be Used?

Health economists have tended to favor the choice-based scaling methods of SG and TTO in the context of cost per QALY analysis and a choice-based method is also recommended by NICE. Each of the SG and TTO methods starts with the premise that health is an important argument in an individual's utility function. The welfare change associated with a change in health status can then be determined by the compensating change required in one of the remaining arguments in the individual's utility function that leaves overall utility unchanged. In the SG, the compensating change is valued in terms of the risk of immediate death. In the TTO, the compensating change is valued in terms of the amount of life expectancy an individual is prepared to sacrifice.

SG has the most rigorous foundation in theory in the form of EUT theory of decision making under uncertainty. However, there are theoretical arguments against the use of SG in health state valuation and there is little empirical support for EUT. There are also concerns about the empirical basis of the TTO technique. There is also concern that duration effects and time preference effects can have an impact on the elicitation of TTO values.

In summary, there are theoretical concerns with all three valuation techniques. We argue that unadjusted EQ VAS values do not provide a valid basis for estimating preferences over health states and satisfactory adjustments remain elusive. For trade-off-based valuations from an individual perspective, the current choice is between SG and TTO, but for the reasons outlined above the values they generate are distorted by factors apart from preferences over health states, and currently there is no compelling basis on which to select one or the other. This is one reason why researchers in the field have begun to examine the potential role of ordinal techniques such as ranking and discrete choice experiments (DCEs) in health state valuation.

The Use of Ordinal Techniques

Ordinal methods simply ask respondents to say whether they prefer one state to another but not by how much. Two well-known ordinal methods are ranking and pairwise comparisons. Typically, with ranking, respondents are asked to rank a set of health states from best to worst. The pairwise comparison limits the comparison to two states and has been used widely in DCEs in health economics, though not usually to value health *per se*. To use them to value health states it is necessary to include full health and death in the comparisons or to introduce valuations for these states from other sources (e.g., Ratcliffe *et al.*, 2006).

Until recently the use of ordinal data in health state valuation has largely been ignored. Ranking exercises have traditionally been included in health state valuation studies as a warm-up procedure prior to the main cardinal method to familiarize the respondent with the set of health states to be valued and with the task of preference elicitation between health states. Often these data may not be used at all in data analysis, or they may be used to check consistency between the ordinal ranking of health states and the ranking of health states according to their actual values obtained using a standard elicitation technique (e.g., TTO or SG). Thurstone's law of comparative judgment offers a potential theoretical basis for deriving cardinal values from rank preference data. Thurstone's method considers the proportion of times that one health state (A) is considered worse than another health state (B). The preferences over the health states represent a latent cardinal utility function and the likelihood of health state A being ranked above health state B when health state B is actually preferred to health state A is a function of how close to each other the states lie on this latent utility function.

Salomon (2003) used conditional logistic regression to model rank data from the UK measurement and valuation of health (MVH) valuation of the EQ-5D. He was able to estimate a model equivalent to the original TTO model by rescaling the worst state using the observed TTO value. Other methods of rescaling were also considered, including normalization to produce a utility of 0 for death, but these were found not to provide the best-fitting predictions.

DCEs have their theoretical basis in random utility theory. Although DCEs have become a very popular tool for eliciting preferences in health care, the vast majority of published studies using DCE methodology have tended to focus on the possibility that individuals derive benefit from nonhealth outcomes and process attributes in addition to health outcomes. A limited number of studies have used DCEs to estimate values for different health state profiles and few have linked these values to the full-health dead scale required for the calculation of QALYs. Ratcliffe *et al.*, (2006) used an external valuation of the worst state of health defined by the classification (i.e. PITS state by TTO to recalibrate the results of a DCE onto the conventional 0 to 1 scale. Brazier *et al.* (2007) have finally used DCE data on their own by setting death to 0 and including death in some of the comparisons. The use of DCE – and to a lesser extent ranking data for this purpose – is at an early stage of development, however, it offers promise as an alternative to cardinal methods.

The Impact of Different Variants of the Valuation Techniques

Although the academic literature has tended to focus on the most appropriate technique for valuation, it is important to remember that there are many variants of each technique and these too may have important implications. Techniques vary in terms of their mode of administration (e.g., interview or self-completion, computer or paper administration), search procedures (e.g., iteration, titration, or open-ended), the use of props and diagrams, time allowed for reflection, and individual versus group interviews. There have been few publications in the health economics literature comparing these alternatives, but what evidence there is suggests that health state values vary considerably between variants of the same technique (Brazier *et al.*, 2007).

There is evidence that the wording of questions affects the answers. This finding has a number of implications. To cite two examples, first, it demonstrates the importance of using a common variant to ensure comparability between studies. Second, there might be scope for correcting for some of these differences if they prove to be systematic. However, there has been little of this work to date.

More fundamentally, this evidence suggests that people do not have well-defined preferences over health prior to the interview, but rather their preferences are constructed during the interview. This would account for the apparent willingness of respondents to be influenced by the precise framing of the question. This may be a consequence of the cognitive complexity of the task. Evidence from the psychology literature suggests that respondents faced with such complex problems tend to adopt simple-decision heuristic strategies (Lloyd, 2003). Much of the interview work has been done using cold-calling techniques. There is a strong case for allowing respondents more time to learn the techniques, to ensure they understand them fully, and to allow them more time to reflect on their health state valuations. An implication may be to move away from the current large-scale surveys of members of the general public involving one-off interviews, to smaller-scale studies of panels of members of the general

public who are better trained and more experienced in the techniques and who are given time to fully reflect on their valuations (Stein *et al.*, 2006).

Who Should Value Health?

Values for health could be obtained from a number of different sources including patients, their carers, health professionals, and the community. Health state values are usually obtained from members of the general public trying to imagine what the state would be like, but in recent years the main criticism of this source has come from those who believe values should be obtained from patients.

The choice of whose values to elicit is important, as it may influence the resulting values. A number of empirical studies have been conducted that indicate that patients with firsthand experience tend to place higher values on dysfunctional health states than do members of the general population who do not have similar experience, and the extent of this discrepancy tends to be much stronger when patients value their own health state. There are a number of possible contributing factors for observed differences between patient and general population values including poor descriptions of health states (for the general population), use of different internal standards, or response shift and adaptation.

Why Use General Population Values?

The main argument for the use of general population values is that the general population pays for the service. However, while members of the general population want to be involved in health-care decision making, it is not clear that they want to be asked to value health states specifically. At the very least, it does not necessarily imply the current practice of using relatively uninformed general population values.

Why Use Patient Values?

A common argument for using patient values is that patients understand the impact of their health on their well-being better than someone trying to imagine it. However, this requires a value judgment that society wants to incorporate all the changes and adaptations that occur in patients who experience states of ill health over long periods of time. It can be argued that some adaptation may be regarded as laudable, such as skill enhancement and activity adjustment, whereas cognitive denial of functional health, suppressed recognition of full health, and lowered expectations may be seen as less commendable. Furthermore, there may be a concern that patient values are context based, reflecting their recent experiences of ill health and the health of their immediate peers. In addition, there are practical problems in asking patients to value their own health, many of whom will by definition be quite unwell.

Finally, to obtain values on the conventional 0 to 1 scale required for QALYs, valuation techniques require patients to compare their existing state to full health, which they may not have experienced for many years. For patients who have lived in a chronic health state like chronic obstructive pulmonary disease or osteoarthritis, for example, the task of imagining full health is as difficult as a healthy member of the general population trying to imagine a poor health state.

A Middle Way – Further Research

It has been argued that it seems difficult to justify the exclusive use of patient values or the current practice of using values from relatively uninformed members of the general population. Existing generic preference-based measures already take some account of adaptation and response shift in their descriptive systems, but whether this is sufficient is ultimately a normative judgment. If it is accepted that the values of the general population are required to inform resource allocation in a public system, it might be argued that respondents should be provided with more information on what the states are like for patients experiencing them.

Generic Preference-Based Measures of Health

Description of Instruments

Generic preference-based measures have become one of the most widely used set of instruments for deriving health state values. As already described, generic preference-based measures have two components: the first is their descriptive system that defines states of health and the second is an algorithm for scoring these states. The number of generic preference-based measures has proliferated over the last two decades. These include the QWB scale; Rosser Classification of illness states; HUI Marks 1, 2, and 3 (HUI1, HUI2, and HUI3); EQ-5D; 15D; SF-6D, a derivative of the SF-36 and SF-12; and AQOL (see Brazier *et al.*, 2007 for further details of each of these instruments and their developers). This list is not complete and does not account for some of the variants of these instruments, but it includes the vast majority of those that have been used.

While these measures all claim to be generic, they differ considerably in terms of the content and size of their descriptive system, the methods of valuation, and the populations used to value the health states (though most aim for a general population sample). A summary of the main characteristics of these seven generic preference-based measures of health is presented in **Table 2** and **Table 3**. Table 2 summarizes the descriptive content of these measures including their dimensions and dimension levels. Each instrument has a questionnaire for completion by the patient (or proxy), or administration by interview, that is used to assign them a health state from the instrument's descriptive system. These questions are mainly designed for adults, typically 16 or older, although the HUI2 is designed for children. **Table 3** summarizes the valuation methods used in terms of the valuation technique and the method of modeling the preference data.

Comparison of Measures

The agreement between measures was generally found to be poor to moderate (about 0.3–0.5 as measured by the intraclass correlation coefficient). Whereas differences in mean scores have often been found to be little more than 0.05 between SF-6D, EQ-5D, and HUI3, this mean statistic masks considerable differences in the distribution of scores.

Table 3   Valuation methods of generic preference-based measures

	Country[a]	Valuation technique[b]	Method of extrapolation
QWB	USA [San Diego]	EQ VAS	Statistical – additive, except for symptom/problem complexes
HUI2	Canada [Hamilton], UK	EQ VAS transformed into SG	MAUT – multiplicative
HUI3	Canada [Hamilton], France	EQ VAS transformed into SG	MAUT – multiplicative
EQ-5D	Belgium, Denmark, Finland, Germany, Japan, Netherlands, Slovenia, Spain, UK, USA, Zimbabwe	TTO, EQ VAS, ranking	Statistical – additive, with interaction term
15D	Finland	EQ VAS	MAUT – additive
SF-6D	Hong Kong, Japan, UK, Portugal, Brazil	SG, ranking	Statistical – additive with interaction term
AQoL	Australia	TTO	MAUT – multiplicative

[a]See 'Further reading' section in text or visit the instrument's website.
[b]EQ VAS, visual analogue scale; TTO, Time trade-off; SG, standard gamble; MAUT, multiattribute utility theory.

Given the differences in coverage of the dimensions and the different methods used to value the health states, it is not surprising the measures have been found to generate different values. The choice of generic measure has been a point of some contention, since the respective instrument developers have academic and in some cases commercial interests in promoting their own measure. The recommended approach to instrument selection has been to compare their practicality, reliability, and validity (Brazier *et al.*, 2007). Although all these instruments are practical to use and achieve good levels of reliability, the issue of validity has been more contentious and difficult to prove.

Validity can be broken down into the validity of the descriptive system of the instrument, the validity of the methods of valuation, and the empirical validity of the scores generated by the instrument. In terms of methods of valuation, the QWB and the 15D would be regarded by many health economists as inferior to the other preference-based measures due to their use of EQ VAS to value the health descriptions. HUI2 and HUI3 would be preferred to the EQ-5D by those who regard the SG as the gold standard, but this is not a universally held view in health economics. A further complication is that the SG utilities for the HUIs have been derived from EQ VAS values using a power transformation that has been criticized in the literature (Stevens *et al.*, 2006). There is evidence in terms of descriptive validity that some measures perform better for certain conditions than others (Brazier *et al.*, 2007); however, there are no measures that have been shown to be better across all conditions. The validity of the descriptive system relates to the condition and treatment outcomes associated with the treatment being evaluated.

Conclusions

This article has described the key features of the instruments available for estimating health state values for calculating QALYs. It has shown the large array of methods available for deriving health state values. This richness in methods comes at a price, because the analyst, and perhaps more importantly the policy maker, must decide on the methods to use for informing resource allocation decisions. Some of the issues raised can be resolved by technical means, using theory (such as the use of EQ VAS) or empirical evidence (such as the descriptive validity of different generic measures). Others require value judgments about the appropriateness of using general population instead of patient values.

For policy makers wishing to make cross-program decisions, the Washington, DC panel on Cost Effectiveness in Health and Medicine and some other public agencies (such as NICE) have introduced the notion of a reference case that has a default for one or other of the (usually generic) measures. Given that more than one measure is likely to be used for the foreseeable future, and perhaps for good reason, there is a need for further research to focus on mapping or 'cross walking' between measures.

See also: Biostatistics; Measurement and Modeling of Health-Related Quality of Life; Meta-Analysis; Systematic Reviews in Public Health.

Citations

Brazier J, Roberts J, and Deverill M (2002) The estimation of a preference-based single index measure for health from the SF-36. *Journal of Health Economics* 21(2): 271–292.

Brazier J, Ratcliffe J, Salomon J, and Tsuchiya A (2007) *Measuring and Valuing Health Benefits for Economic Evaluation.* Oxford, UK: Oxford University Press.

Brazier J, Murray C, Roberts J, Brown M, Symonds T, Kelleher C (in press) Estimation of a preference-based index from a condition specific measure: The King's Health Questionnaire. *Medical Decision Making.*

Brooks R, Rabin RE and de Charro FTH (eds.) (2003) *The Measurement and Valuation of Health Status Using EQ-5D: A European Perspective.* The Netherlands: Kluwer Academic Press.

Fanshel S and Bush J (1970) A health status index and its application to health service outcomes. *Operations Research* 18: 1021–1066.

Feeny D, Furlong W, Torrance G, et al. (2002) Multiattribute and single attribute utility functions for the Health Utilities Index Mark 3 system. *Medical Care* 40: 113–128.

Kaplan RM and Anderson JP (1988) A general health policy model: Update and applications. *Health Services Research* 23(2): 203–235.

Lloyd AJ (2003) Threats to the estimation of benefit: Are preference elicitation methods accurate? *Health Economics* 12(5): 393–402.

Ratcliffe J, Brazier JE, Tsuchiga A, Symonds T, and Brown M (2006) Estimation of a preference based single index from the sexual quality of life questionnaire (SQOL) using ordinal data. Health Economics and Decision Science Discussion Paper 06/06, ScHARR. University of Sheffield. http://www.sheffield.ac.uk/scharr/sections/heds/discussion.html (accessed September 2007).

Salomon JA (2003) Reconsidering the use of rankings in the valuation of health states: A model for estimating cardinal values from ordinal data. *Population Health Metrics* 1(1): 12.

Stein K, Ratcliffe J, Round A, Milne R, and Brazier J (2006) Impact of discussion on preferences elicited in a group setting. *Health and Quality of Life Outcomes* 4(1): 22.

Stevens K, McCabe C, and Brazier J (2006) Mapping between Visual Analogue Scale and Standard Gamble data: Results from the UK Health Utilities Index 2 valuation survey. *Health Economics* 15(5): 527–533.

Torrance G, Feeny D, Furlong W, Barr R, Zhang Y, and Wang Q (1996) Multiattribute utility function for a comprehensive health status classification system. Health Utilities Index Mark 2. *Medical Care* 34: 702–722.

Further Reading

Brazier J, Ratcliffe J, Salomon J, and Tsuchiya A (2007) *Measuring and Valuing Health Benefits for Economic Evaluation.* Oxford, UK: Oxford University Press.

Measuring the Quality of Life of Children and Adolescents

E Davis, E Waters, A Shelly, and L Gold, McCaughey Centre, VicHealth Centre for the Promotion of Mental Health and Community Wellbeing, School of Population Health, University of Melbourne, Carlton, VIC, Australia and School of Health and Social Development, Deakin University, Burwood, VIC, Australia

Introduction

Consistent with the World Health Organization's definition of health as "a state of complete physical, mental, and social well-being and not merely the absence of disease or infirmity" (WHO, 1948: 100) the concept of good health has moved from the absence of disease to a more positive concept that embraces subjective well-being and quality of life (QOL). In pediatrics and child health, as in other areas of health care, awareness is growing that traditional outcome measures such as survival or reduction of symptoms do not capture the whole range of ways in which a patient may be affected by illness or treatment. The inclusion of more holistic outcomes such as measures of QOL and health-related quality of life (HRQOL) is gaining increasing interest.

Emergence of QOL in Pediatrics and Child Health

There are now a range of potential interventions for children and adolescents with chronic illnesses and disabilities, as well as a spectrum of public health population-based interventions. Over the past 10 years, there have been increasing efforts to demonstrate empirically that interventions are effective in improving a child's life. A range of outcome measures is used depending on the disability or illness; however, they are often focused on outcomes at the level of body structure and function. These outcomes on their own are inadequate for evaluating medical and health interventions that not only impact on symptoms but on a child's whole life. For example, some interventions may result in discomfort, pain, inconvenience, or embarrassment for the child, as well as increased well-being, self-esteem, happiness, or improved sleeping. To examine the impact of an intervention on a child's whole life, researchers and clinicians increasingly refer to a child's QOL. The realization that measures of emotional and social health and well-being are equally as important as measuring the reduction of symptoms and improved survival to evaluate medical outcomes has brought about the measurement of QOL. QOL is now considered to be a key outcome variable to evaluate the effectiveness of interventions for children and adolescents.

Unfortunately, the field of QOL measurement of children and adolescents lags behind that of adults. Although there are now over 30 000 publications relevant to QOL in medicine, only 12% of these are related to children and adolescents, and most of these involve theoretical and conceptual work. There are unique measurement challenges in assessing the QOL of children and adolescents. The language, content, and setting all need to be pertinent to the activities and stages of children's experience and development.

Defining QOL and HRQOL for Children and Adolescents

Quality of Life

Due to differing opinions, theories, and professional perspectives, QOL is variously defined. For example, researchers often cite the World Health Organization's definition of QOL as "the individual's perception of their position in life, in the context of culture and value systems in which they live and in relation to their goals, expectations, standards and concerns" (WHOQOL, 1993). Other researchers develop their own definitions for children, such as "QOL includes, but is not limited to the social, physical and emotional functioning of the child, and when indicated, his or her family, and it must be sensitive to the changes that occur throughout development" (Bradlyn et al., 1996). Although there are many different definitions, one core theme is that QOL refers to well-being, or feelings about life, across multiple domains of life.

Objective and Subjective QOL

QOL can be measured by objective indicators and subjective indicators, although the latter are more common. Objective indicators of QOL can be observed by other people, such as family income, number of sick days from school, and number of medications a person takes. Subjective indicators, in theory, cannot be completed by another person as they refer to a person's feelings such as their feelings about their health, school, or family. Objective indicators of QOL generally have a poor relationship with subjective indicators. A child may take several medications but may still perceive their health to be good. This highlights the complexity in the subjective QOL construct, which may be influenced by personality, coping style, and attitudes. The remainder of this article, as with much of the empirical literature on QOL, concerns subjective QOL.

Is QOL the Same as Health-Related QOL?

Although, in the past, researchers and clinicians have used the terms QOL and HRQOL interchangeably, there is now recognition that these terms are not interchangeable, nor are the instruments used to assess them. Definitions of HRQOL tend to focus on the health domain, that is, symptoms and functioning. HRQOL is considered to be a subdomain of the more global construct of QOL. For example, HRQOL has been defined as "a multidimensional functional effect of an illness or a medical condition and its consequent therapy upon the child" (Schipper *et al.*, 1990).

Measuring QOL

Multidimensional versus Global Instruments

QOL is quantifiable and there are two major types of instruments. Multidimensional instruments focus on domains of life and assess well-being, or feelings about each domain (e.g., health, school, family, friends). Global instruments ask the person to rate his or her whole life, and include more general questions such as 'Overall, how do you feel about your life as a whole?' For children, the majority of instruments are multidimensional.

Condition-Specific and Generic Instruments

The QOL literature includes generic and condition-specific instruments, both of which have different purposes. Generic instruments are designed to be applicable to all population subgroups. They are useful for comparing outcomes between groups, such as the QOL of children with asthma compared to the QOL of children with diabetes. They are less useful to evaluate the effectiveness of an intervention for children with a specific illness or disability because they do not include domains that are specific to the illness or disability. Hence, if a child with asthma completed a generic QOL instrument, the scores may not completely capture their QOL, as some important domains that impact their life (i.e., medication) would not be assessed.

Condition-specific instruments are designed to be applicable to one group (i.e., individuals with asthma) and are useful to detect changes following an intervention. As they include domains that are specific to an illness, it is more likely that if a change occurs as the result of an intervention, it will be detected.

Increasingly, instrument developers are producing QOL instruments that have a generic core and additional condition-specific modules. This means that even for a specific condition, the core module can be compared to the general population. For example, KIDSCREEN is a generic cross-cultural QOL instrument that assesses the subjective health and well-being of children and adolescents aged 8–18 years. The KIDSCREEN instrument comes in 10-, 27-, and 52-item versions and has child/adolescent self-report and parent-proxy versions. The core QOL domains included in the KIDSCREEN-52 are physical well-being, psychological well-being, moods and emotions, self-perception, autonomy, parent relation and home life, financial resources, peers and social support, and school environment and bullying (Ravens-Sieberer *et al.*, 2005). KIDSCREEN also has condition-specific instruments referred to as DISABKIDS Disease Modules that include arthritis, asthma, atopic dermatitis, cerebral palsy, cystic fibrosis, diabetes, and epilepsy (Baars *et al.*, 2005).

Challenges in Measuring QOL/HRQOL for Children and Adolescents

One of the reasons that the child QOL literature lags behind that of the adult is the measurement challenges of childhood. There is consensus that the language and content of children's QOL instruments need to be appropriate to children's experience and development, and therefore researchers have been reluctant to simply apply the principles and definitions of adult QOL to child and adolescent QOL. One issue that has generated much discussion concerns the reporter of QOL.

Child Self-Report and Parent-Proxy

In the adult QOL literature, QOL refers to an individual's perceptions and self-report questionnaires are regarded as the primary method of assessing QOL. In the child QOL literature, it is proposed that because of children's cognitive immaturity, limited social experience, and continued dependency, parents may be more able to rate some aspects of their child's QOL than the child themselves. Increasingly, in an attempt to capture both parent and child opinions, instrument developers are now producing parent-proxy and child/adolescent self-report versions. The majority of child self-report instruments start at about 8 or 9 years of age. This is because, according to Piaget, children at age 7 are in their preoperational stage of development, which means that their understanding is limited by their inability to carry out a variety of logical operations (Piaget, 1929).

Parents are generally able to estimate their child's well-being, and daily monitoring of a child's well-being can alert parents to small behavioral changes or physical symptoms. However, parents may easily over- or under-estimate the importance their child attributes to certain aspects of his or her well-being at a specific point in time. For example, peer-related issues may be far more important to an adolescent than parents might think they are. Moreover, parental expectations and previous experiences with the child may influence their views of the child's current health state.

Researchers have commenced examining the degree of concordance between parent-proxy and child self-report scores. A systematic review of 14 studies assessing the relationship between parent-proxy and child self-reported QOL demonstrated that the level of agreement between parents and children appeared to depend on the domain (Eiser and Morse, 2001). Generally there was good agreement (correlations >0.5) between parents and children for domains reflecting physical activity, functioning, and symptoms and there was poor agreement (correlations <0.30) for domains that reflected more social or emotional areas.

The differences between parent-proxy reported QOL and child self-reported QOL become particularly problematic when only parent-proxy data can be collected, due to a variety of reasons such as the child's age, severity of illness, type of disease, cognitive ability, or communication ability. In these cases, where parent-proxy reported QOL is used to guide clinical decisions, it is important to understand how and why scores differ.

There are several reasons why parents and children may report different levels of QOL. Parents and children may think about different events that have happened, or interpret events differently. Additionally, parents and children may use different response styles (i.e., approach questions, items, response scales differently). Finally, parents and children may also differ in their understanding and interpretation of the items. We recently conducted a qualitative study with parents and children to examine possible reasons for discordance. The results suggest that the major reasons for discordance were that parents and children were providing different reasons for the answers and had different response styles (Davis et al., 2007).

Child Development

There are several developmental issues that researchers and clinicians need to be aware of when measuring a child's QOL using self-report methods. The child needs to understand the question, understand the response scale, and be able to formulate a response. There is some variation in the type of response scale that is used, such as Likert scale, happy–sad faces scale, and visual analogue scale. Although a happy–sad faces scale appears to be a suitable option for young children, the scale

is based on the assumption that pointing to faces to indicate relative levels of satisfaction or happiness is a simpler task than verbal responding; however, this assumption has not been tested. Furthermore, often questions require the child to think about the previous week or month. The child's ability to respond to a time frame will be influenced by their developmental status. Often, in order to address these developmental issues, instrument developers produce separate instruments for children based on their age. For example, the Pediatric QOL Inventory has several versions (2–4 years, 5–7 years, 8–12 years, 13–18 years) (Varni et al., 2003).

Domains of QOL

In designing a pediatric QOL instrument, one question that requires consideration is which domains constitute QOL for children. Although in the past domains of QOL were decided *a priori* by researchers and clinicians, there is increasing recognition that families and children need to be consulted in this process. Qualitative research is the most suitable design for researching the underpinning elements of QOL for children. For example, Ronen and colleagues identified domains of QOL for children with epilepsy by conducting focus groups with both parents and children to discuss how epilepsy impacted on their lives (Ronen et al., 1999).

QOL Instruments for Children and Adolescents

Condition-Specific and Generic Instruments

Many pediatric QOL instruments have been developed and several reviews have been published (see section titled 'Further reading'). We recently conducted a review of QOL instruments for children, identifying 14 generic and 25 condition-specific instruments (Davis et al., 2006). Condition-specific instruments were identified for a range of illnesses including asthma, cancer, and spina bifida.

Domains of QOL

Common domains of QOL included in pediatric QOL instruments are emotional well-being, social interactions, medical treatments, cognition, activities, school, family, independence/autonomy, pain, behavior, future, leisure, and body image. Common domains for adolescents include emotional well-being, social well-being, self-esteem, physical health, relationships, school, environment, participation, and leisure.

Some of the domains may be different in condition-specific instruments, as the factors that impact on QOL may vary by condition. For example, domains of QOL that children with cerebral palsy and their parents believe are important include social well-being and acceptance, functioning, participation and physical health, emotional well-being, access to services, pain and impact of disability, and family health.

QOL Items

Items measuring QOL are often framed in terms of problems or difficulties, intensity of feelings, frequency of feelings, or comparisons between current state and ideal self or other children. Instruments that examine problems include items such as 'How much of a problem have you had with … ?' 'Have you had any difficulty with … ?' and 'How much were you bothered by … ?' Instruments that assess intensity of feelings examine feelings of satisfaction and being upset such as 'How do you feel about … ?' Instruments that examine frequency of feelings include items such as 'Have you felt … ?' (never–always). Instruments that examine comparisons between actual self and ideal self or other children include items such as 'How much are you like … ?' and 'How much do you want to be like … ?'

Scoring and Interpretation of QOL Instruments

Each QOL instrument has specific scoring instructions; however, most QOL instruments provide domain scores and/or a total QOL score. To calculate domain scores, items within each domain are totaled or averaged. A total QOL score is the (weighted) average of all the domain scores. Scores must be calculated separately for parent-proxy reports and child/adolescent self-reports. Although the level of agreement between the two scores can be calculated, it is important to note that unlike the adult QOL literature, one score is not superior to the other. Neither parents nor children are right or wrong; they may simply have different views. It is recognized however that if parent and child scores are significantly different, it may be difficult to select an appropriate course of action. In a clinical context, if parent and child scores are very different, it may be useful to interview the parent and child together to understand why the discrepancy exists. In a research context, a follow-up qualitative study with a subsample of parents and children may be useful.

Example of a Generic Instrument: KIDSCREEN

KIDSCREEN is a generic HRQOL instrument for children and adolescents. KIDSCREEN was developed across seven European countries, and participants of the project include Austria, Czech Republic, France, Germany, Greece, Hungary, Ireland, Poland, Spain, Switzerland, The Netherlands, and the United Kingdom. KIDSCREEN consists of 10 dimensions: physical well-being, psychological well-being, mood and emotions, self-perceptions, autonomy, parent relations and home life, peers and social support, school environment, bullying, and financial resources. There are two versions of KIDSCREEN: one for child and adolescent self-report (8–18 years) and one for parent-proxy report (8–18 years). KIDSCREEN can be administered in hospitals, medical establishments, and schools by professionals in the fields of public health, epidemiology and medicine.

Example of a Condition-Specific Instrument: Cerebral Palsy QOL for Children

The cerebral palsy QOL questionnaire for children (CP QOL – Child) is a condition-specific QOL questionnaire for children with cerebral palsy aged 4–12 years. The CP QOL – Child was developed by an international team of researchers. The CP QOL – Child has seven domains: social well-being and acceptance, feelings about functioning, participation and physical health, emotional well-being, access to services, pain and feelings about disability, and family health (refer to **Figure 1** for sample items). There are two versions of the CP QOL – Child: a primary caregiver-proxy report for children aged 4–12 years (66 items) and a child self-report for children aged 9–12 years (52 items) (Waters *et al.*, 2007).

Economic Evaluation

Resources (both workforce and health budgets) are limited and treatment for children with chronic illnesses or disabilities can be expensive. Researchers, clinicians, and policy makers increasingly need to demonstrate that the effects of a treatment warrant the costs. Economic evaluation builds on the results of analyses of clinical effectiveness to explicitly compare the effectiveness of an intervention (over and above the best alternative care) to the additional costs of that intervention. Economic evaluation produces estimates of the cost-effectiveness of interventions in a variety of formats, most frequently in the form of 'additional cost per additional unit of effect' using clinical outcome measures in their natural measurement units (e.g., 'additional cost per unit increase in PEV'). Expressing cost-effectiveness in natural units of clinical outcome measures makes it hard to compare the cost-effectiveness of different interventions that are competing for the same limited health-care resources. Even when cost-effectiveness is expressed using QOL measures, the outcomes are not comparable if different QOL measures have been used to evaluate different interventions.

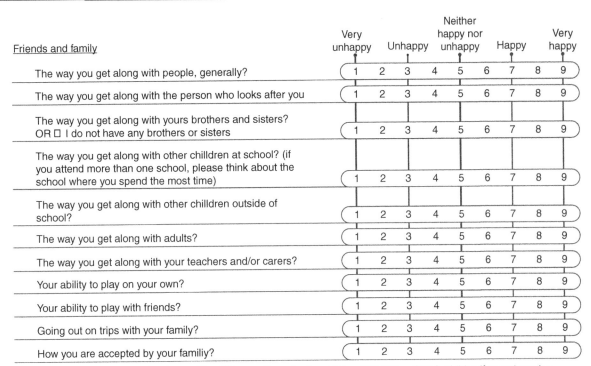

Figure 1 Example of the cerebral palsy quality of life questionnaire for children (CP QOL – Child), child self-report version.

Quality-Adjusted Life Years

The quality-adjusted life year (QALY) is a composite health outcome measure that combines a measure of QOL with a measure of survival. QALYs provide a common currency for measuring the extent of health gain that results from health-care interventions and, when combined with the costs associated with the interventions, can be used to assess their relative worth from an economic perspective. QALYs therefore offer the potential for all evaluations of child health interventions to be comparable in terms of the improvement to generic child health and, where economic evaluation has been included, in terms of the relative value-for-money of the intervention.

However, to combine QOL and survival, the QOL measure used to construct QALYs must have particular methodological properties. The QOL measure must be able to express any health state as a single numerical utility score, where a utility score of 0 equates to being dead (the absence of health status) and a score of 1 equates to perfect health. Negative scores can be used to represent health states considered worse than being dead. Current generic QOL measures of child and adolescent health, such as KIDSCREEN and PedsQL, do not hold these properties. There are generic adult QOL measures that can be used to construct QALYs (such as SF-36, Health Utility Index [HUI], and EQ-5D), although the only measure derived from a child or adolescent population is the HUI (Feeny *et al.*, 1998). As detailed above, there are additional domains that are particularly relevant to child health (including autonomy, body image, cognitive skills, and family relationships) that are not captured by these generic QOL measures.

In the absence of an existing suitable QOL measure for child and adolescent health, there are a number of ways to generate health utility scores to express the outcomes of an intervention in QALY terms. Three broad strategies include expert judgment, indices from relevant literature, and direct measurement of the preferences of an appropriate population (Dolan, 2000). The third strategy is the most common, given that experts may focus on different attributes than patients, and valuations in one study may be inappropriate for another study. There are several ways to obtain direct measures of preferences, including visual analogue scale (EQ VAS), standard gamble (SG), and the time trade-off (TTO). The EQ EQ VAS requires respondents to directly rate their health state on a scale from 0–1. The standard gamble asks the respondent to choose between the certainty of an intermediate health state and the uncertainty of a treatment with two possible outcomes, one of which is better than the certain outcome and one of which is worse. The time trade-off asks the respondent to choose between a defined length of life in an intermediate health state and a shorter length of life in full health. Use of these measures in pediatrics and child health has been vigorously debated. As children do not have the cognitive ability to comprehend and complete valuation or preferences, parent-proxy reports are required, which may be influenced by the parent's beliefs (Griebsch *et al.*, 2005).

Evaluating and Selecting QOL Instruments

There are an increasing number of QOL questionnaires for children and adolescents and it is becoming increasingly difficult for researchers and clinicians to choose the best instrument. A good QOL instrument is

- Appropriate for children's developmental status (i.e., number of items, wording of items, response scales, age groupings)
- Based on a clear, accepted definition of QOL
- Piloted with an appropriate sample to ensure the items are acceptable
- Structured using domains of QOL that are based on consultations with children/adolescents and parents
- Available in parent-proxy and child/adolescent self-report format
- Reliable and valid (for the particular country and sample)
- Sensitive to clinically significant change in condition.

(Further information is provided in the next section about the desired psychometrics properties.)

Reliability

A measure is judged to be reliable when it consistently produces the same results when applied to the same subjects, when there is no evidence of underlying change in the health state being assessed. Reliability of an instrument is most frequently evaluated by internal consistency and test–retest reliability. For internal consistency, Cronbach's alpha coefficient (α) measures the average correlation among the items in the scale. This measure has a range of 0–1 with higher values indicating a closer correlation, which suggests that the set of questions is assessing a single domain. A low alpha coefficient (e.g., <0.5) indicates that the item does not arise from the same conceptual domain. If the coefficient is too high, it is likely to indicate that some of the items are unnecessary and the scale may be too narrow in its scope to have much validity. Coefficients greater than 0.7 and probably less than 0.9 are recommended.

Test–retest reliability is assessed when the instrument is administered to the same population on two occasions and the results are compared by correlation. However,

repeating a QOL instrument to assess its stability or reliability over time is often not as simple as repeating a measurement in the physical sciences. The main problem is that the second response to a question is likely to be affected by the previous administration. A subjective report on QOL may change between administrations depending on what life experiences have occurred in the intervening time.

Agreement and association are measures of the discrepancies between pairs of ratings such as between a mother and her child. Agreement may be assessed by examining the distribution in the score given for a particular domain between a pair of reporters. Association refers to the relationship between two sets of scores, for example, parent scores with child scores, and is usually tested by a correlation coefficient.

Validity

Validity is defined as the extent to which the instrument measures what it is intended to measure. Face validity refers to the extent to which the scale appears to be a good test of the construct in question (i.e., whether the items and scales look reasonable at face value). Criterion validity establishes whether the variable or concept can be measured with accuracy by comparison with an existing gold standard, and whether the instrument can substitute for the gold standard or vice versa. Testing this involves application of the two measures simultaneously or randomly to alternate subjects, and is important when you are attempting to develop a scale that is simpler or less expensive to administer than an existing measure. Construct validity requires establishing theories and testing these theories and models against the relationships of the measure. Establishing construct validity is an ongoing process, as often there is no one single study that can satisfy the criteria. Discriminant validity assesses the 'success' of an item to correlate more strongly with its hypothesized scale than with any other scale within a questionnaire, and provides evidence of the conceptual logic for placing an item within a particular scale relative to other scales within the instrument.

Sensitivity to Change

When examining the effectiveness of interventions in increasing children's QOL, it can be difficult to interpret QOL scores. Researchers and clinicians may detect a statistically significant difference of 5 points, however, this then leads to the question about what those 5 points mean. Does it mean their QOL is improved? Are they noticing differences in their everyday life? These questions are referring to the detection of clinically important differences. There has been much research in the area of minimal clinically importance differences, which is "the smallest difference in score in the domain of interest which patients perceive as beneficial and which would mandate, in the absence of troublesome side-effects and excessive cost, a change in the patient's management" (Jaeschke *et al.*, 1989).

Conclusion and Recommendations for Future Research

The field of pediatric QOL, and in particular the measurement of child and adolescent QOL, has advanced significantly within the last decade. There are now several generic and condition-specific QOL instruments for children and adolescents. Many of these instruments now have both parent-proxy and child self-report versions and adequate reliability and validity. One concern, which requires urgent action, is the small number of instruments that have examined sensitivity to change. This is essential, particularly if the instrument is to be used to evaluate the effectiveness of interventions. We need to know whether, for example, a 5-point difference in QOL makes a meaningful difference to a child's QOL.

Another concern, also related to sensitivity to change, is the lack of understanding about the process by which children, adolescents, and parent-proxies determine QOL. If child QOL is greatly determined by personality, then it must be questioned whether an intervention can increase a child's QOL. More importantly, if we understood the determinants of children's QOL, interventions can be designed to ensure they increase a child's QOL.

See also: Health Surveys; Measurement and Modeling of Health-Related Quality of Life; Methods of Measuring and Valuing Health.

Citations

Baars RM, Atherton CI, Koopman HM, Bullinger M, and Power M (2005) The European DISABKIDS project: Development of seven condition-specific modules to measure health related quality of life in children and adolescents. *Health and Quality of Life Outcomes* 3: 70.

Bradlyn AS, Ritchey AC, Harris CV, *et al.* (1996) Quality of life research in pediatric oncology: Research methods and barriers. *Cancer* 78: 1333–1339.

Davis E, Waters E, Mackinnon A, *et al.* (2006) Paediatric quality of life instruments: A review of the impact of the conceptual framework on outcomes. *Developmental Medicine and Child Neurology* 48: 311–318.

Davis E, Nicolas C, Waters E, *et al.* (2007) Parent-proxy and child self-reported health-related quality of life: Using qualitative methods to explain the discordance. *Quality of Life Research* 16(5): 863–871.

Dolan P (2000) A note on QALYs versus HYEs. Health states versus health profiles. *International Journal of Technology Assessment in Health Care* 16(4): 1220–1224.

Eiser C and Morse R (2001) Can parents rate their child's health-related quality of life? Results of a systematic review. *Quality of Life Research* 10(4): 347–357.

Feeny D, Furlong W, and Barr RD (1998) Multiattribute approach to the assessment of health-related quality of life: Health utilities index. *Medical and Pediatric Oncology* 30: 54–59.

Griebsch I, Coast J, and Brown J (2005) Quality-adjusted life-years lack quality in pediatric care: A critical review of published cost-utility studies in child health. *Pediatrics* 115(5): e600–e614.

Jaeschke R, Singer J, and Guyatt GH (1989) Ascertaining the minimal clinically important difference. *Controlled Clinical Trials* 10: 407–415.

Piaget J (1929) *The Child's Conception of the World.* New York: Harcourt, Brace Jovanovich.

Ravens-Sieberer U, Gosch A, Rajmil L, *et al.* (2005) KIDSCREEN-52 quality-of-life measure for children and adolescents. *Expert Review of Pharmacoeconomics and Outcomes Research* 5(3): 353–356.

Ronen GM, Rosenbaum P, Law M, and Streiner DL (1999) Health-related quality of life in childhood epilepsy: The results of children's participation in identifying the components. *Developmental Medicine and Child Neurology* 41: 554–559.

Schipper H, Clinch J, and Powell V (1990) Definitions and conceptual issues. In: Spilker B (ed.) *Quality of Life Assessment in Clinical Trials,* pp. 11–24. New York: Raven Press.

Varni JW, Burwinkle TM, Seid M, and Skarr D (2003) The PedsQL 4.0 as a pediatric population health measure: Feasibility, reliability, and validity. *Ambulatory Pediatrics: The Official Journal of the Ambulatory Pediatric Association* 3(6): 329–341.

Waters E, Davis E, Mackinnon A, *et al.* (2007) Psychometric properties of the quality of life questionnaire for children with CP. *Developmental Medicine and Child Neurology* 49: 49–55.

World Health Organization (1948) Preamble to the Constitution of the World Health Organization as adoped by the International Health Conference, New York, 19–22 June 1946. *Official Records of the World Health Organization* 2: 100.

WHOQOL Group and World Health Organization (WHO) (1993) Study protocol for the World Health Organization project to develop a Quality of Life assessment instrument. *Quality of Life Research*. 2: 153–159.

Further Reading

Bullinger M and Ravens-Sieberer U (1995) Health-related QOL assessment in children: A review of the literature. *European Review of Applied Psychology* 45(4): 245–254.

Crosby RD, Kolotkin RL, and Williams GR (2003) Defining clinically meaningful change in health-related quality of life. *Journal of Clinical Epidemiology* 56: 395–407.

Eiser C and Morse R (2001) A review of measures of quality of life for children with chronic illness. *Archives of Disease in Childhood* 84(3): 205–211.

Harding L (2001) Children's quality of life assessments: A review of generic and health related quality of life measures completed by children and adolescents. *Clinical Psychology and Psychotherapy* 8: 79–96.

Levi R and Drotar D (1998) Critical issues and needs in health-related quality of life assessment of children and adolescents with chronic health conditions. In: Drotar D (ed.) *Measuring Health-Related Quality of Life in Children and Adolescents*, pp. 3–24. Mahwah, NJ: Lawrence Erlbaum.

Matza LS, *et al.* (2004) Assessment of health-related quality of life in children: A review of conceptual, methodological, and regulatory issues. *Value in Health* 7(1): 79–92.

Rajmil L, *et al.* (2004) Generic health-related quality of life instruments in children and adolescents: A qualitative analysis of content. *Society for Adolescent Medicine* 34: 37–45.

Schmidt LJ, Garratt AM, and Fitzpatrick R (2002) Child/parent-assessed population health outcome measures: A structured review. *Child: Care, Health and Development* 28(3): 227–237.

White-Koning M, *et al.* (2005) Subjective quality of life in children with intellectual impairment – how can it be assessed? *Developmental Medicine and Child Neurology* 47(4): 281–285.

Relevant Websites

http://acqol.deakin.edu.au – Australian Centre on Quality of Life (ACQOL).

http://disabkids.org – DISABKIDS.
http://www.healthutilities.com – Health Utilities Index.
http://www.isoqol.org – International Society of Quality of Life Research (ISOQOL).
http://www.isqols.org – International Society for Quality-of-Life Studies (ISQOLS).
http://kidscreen.org – KIDSCREEN.
http://www.mapi-research.fr – MAPI Research Institute.
http://www.pedsql.org – Pediatric Quality-of-Life Inventory (PedsQL).

Systematic Reviews in Public Health

R Armstrong, Cochrane HPPH Field, Victoria, Australia
E Waters, University of Melbourne, Carlton, VIC, Australia
H Roberts, Institute of Education, University of London, London, UK
L M Anderson, US Centers for Disease Control and Prevention, Atlanta, GA, USA
S Oliver, University of London, London, UK
M Petticrew, London School of Hygiene and Tropical Medicine, London, UK

Introduction to Evidence-Based Public Health

Public health decision making can concern questions regarding what programs might work; the impact of illness or disease; the causes of disease and health outcomes; barriers to better health; and views people have regarding health, illness, treatments or interventions, and government priorities. Thus, a wide range of evidence is required involving a wide range of methods and processes.

Systematic reviews are now being applied more frequently to questions of intervention effectiveness. The development of methods to assess interventions is closely related to the emergence of evidence-based practice (EBP). EBP has evolved as a process in which 'best available' research evidence is incorporated into practice to inform decision making. More recently there has been a focus on studying the process of implementation, establishing what works (or does not), for whom, and why.

Interest in evidence-based public health is prompted by several factors. As with other groups within the health sector and beyond, there has been an increasing public and political expectation to demonstrate outcomes and to prioritize the use of available resources. One of the options available is to synthesize previous research to identify what programs provide the most likely way forward. Thus, as a field of endeavor, researchers engage in the critical appraisal, synthesis, exchange, and translation of knowledge acquired through research investments to provide access to relevant, easily usable, and high-quality public health evidence for consumers, practitioners, researchers, and policymakers.

Systematic Reviews and Their Contribution to Evidence-Based Public Health

Over the past 20 years the generation of information has increased markedly, fueled by information technology advances. This has stimulated the need to develop efficient methods to review, synthesize, and summarize the interventions undertaken in a particular area. In public health, topics range from specific interventions (for instance, a review of school-based driver education) or a broader range of interventions addressing specific problems (such as the social exclusion associated with unintended teenage pregnancy).

A systematic review is defined as "a review of the evidence on a clearly formulated question that uses systematic and explicit methods to identify, select, and critically appraise relevant primary research, and to extract and analyze data from the studies that are included in the review" (NHS Centre for Reviews and Dissemination, 2001). This type of review provides a comprehensive summary of rigorous studies conducted to address a question of interest. This synthesis is important as single studies, which can generate a large amount of publicity, can be misleading. Systematic reviews are therefore a powerful tool in supporting both policy and practice. They differ from a traditional or narrative review that describes and appraises previous work, but tends to be less comprehensive and transparent in identifying included studies and thus is more prone to bias. They also differ from meta-analyses, which are simply a statistical combination of results from a number of studies. Where the process for identifying studies included in a meta-analysis is not systematic, meta-analysis may not be considered as a systematic review. Some systematic reviews may, however, include a meta-analysis in their results section.

Systematic review methods can be applied across research questions and methods. The majority of published systematic reviews have sought to address an intervention-related question: Does the intervention work (effectiveness)? More recent studies have addressed these questions as well: how and why the intervention works (or not), how acceptable the intervention is, whether there are any unanticipated harms associated with it, and what its costs are in relation to its effectiveness. Systematic reviews of complex health promotion and public health interventions can be extremely challenging methodologically (Jackson *et al.*, 2005). A systematic review is therefore ideally conducted by a team, in which some members bring knowledge about the topic and others bring skills in the methodology. Users, or stakeholders, increasingly play a role in identifying salient questions, advising on scope, and sometimes participating in other ways in the review process.

The majority of the methodological work regarding the effectiveness of interventions has been undertaken on questions for which the randomized controlled trial (RCT) is considered the strongest possible study design to minimize bias. In these contexts, good RCTs are more likely to provide answers about effectiveness than studies of lower quality (e.g., uncontrolled studies). However, depending on the question the review seeks to answer, the full spectrum of study designs related to public health questions may be included. Systematic reviews of effectiveness have included a range of other study designs, where appropriate, such as quasi-randomized trials, controlled before-and-after studies, and interrupted time-series studies. For questions of harm, well-conducted cohort or case-control studies may be recommended and included in meta-analyses of observational studies (Egger *et al.*, 1998). It is also becoming more common to see qualitative studies included in systematic reviews of effectiveness that seek to understand people's experiences (Evans and Fitzgerald, 2002) or views (Harden *et al.*, 2004).

Research findings are often only a small part of the policy debate. Other influences include judgment, resources, values and policy context, habits and traditions, lobbyists and pressure groups, pragmatics and contingencies, and experience and expertise (Davies, 2005). However, rigorously conducted research and high-quality systematic reviews may increase the impact of research evidence on decision making (Petticrew and Roberts, 2006). This impact can be further enhanced by an understanding of the broad processes that link research, knowledge synthesis, translation and distribution of knowledge, and evaluation of public health impacts. By enhancing the capacity for evidence-based practice through its summary of existing knowledge and identification of opportunities

for innovation/further research, systematic reviews enable practitioners to respond to the increasing pressure to use evidence to justify their approach and to contribute to the evidence base (Petticrew and Roberts, 2006).

Conducting Systematic Reviews of Public Health Interventions

This section is based on the *Guidelines for Conducting Reviews of Health Promotion and Public Health Interventions* developed by the Cochrane Health Promotion and Public Health Field in Victoria, Australia, with the involvement of 16 experienced international public health methodologists and practitioners.

Planning the Review

It may be useful to establish an advisory group to assist with framing the question, determining the scope of the review, and ensuring that the end product meets the needs of users. Defining the scope of the review requires the authors to consider the practical application of the review in question. They must make pragmatic decisions about time and resources available to carry out the review. At this point, they must decide which populations and interventions of interest to review and which outcomes to use to determine intervention effectiveness. The relevance of an outcome for decision making can vary according to one's point of view as a consumer, practitioner, policymaker, researcher, or member of the public.

Study Designs to Include

The review question will determine the types of study designs to be included. For example, a question about effectiveness is best answered by systematic reviews followed by RCTs, whereas a question about the acceptability of day care for families living in disadvantaged areas is more likely to benefit from a range of qualitative research methods (Petticrew and Roberts, 2006). A broad test search (often referred to as a scoping search) will assist in the identification of study designs used to address the question of interest in a particular topic area. The decisions about which type(s) of study designs to include will influence subsequent phases of the review, particularly searching the literature, quality assessment, and analysis (especially for meta-analyses). Although RCTs may be the 'gold standard' for questions of effectiveness, they may not always be appropriate for your question.

Searching the Public Health Literature

Searching for literature on public health interventions is difficult. Studies are often poorly indexed by medical databases, and the terminology used in studies may differ across journals and contexts. Research on interventions may be published in a range of multidisciplinary sources (Jackson *et al.*, 2005; Petticrew and Roberts, 2006). Many studies of public health interventions are never published in peer-review journals and are referred to as 'gray literature,' which may appear as reports to government agencies, books, or chapters in books. As part of the scope of a review, it is important to consider the pros and cons of including these types of studies before devising an appropriate search strategy.

Quality Assessment

Quality assessment of studies to be included in systematic reviews refers to assessing the degree to which the study is free from methodological biases (including selection bias, response bias, and observer bias). If studies of varying levels of quality are summarized together to estimate an effect size, the results of the review may be biased. Authors need to be explicit about the approach used to assess quality and draw conclusions about the strength of evidence. A range of tools have been developed and are appropriate for use in systematic reviews of public health interventions (Petticrew and Roberts, 2006). Currently, there is no single validated checklist to use for all types of qualitative studies. Where possible, authors using checklists should report on their usefulness to advance research methodologies.

Theoretical Framework

Although it is not known whether theoretical frameworks have an impact on the effectiveness of interventions, many interventions are based either explicitly or implicitly on a theory about what works. At the systematic review level, capturing, synthesizing, and interpreting information about the theoretical bases of included studies may provide the decision maker with insight into how the program designer thinks the intervention brings about change. This may be useful information when considering how applicable the intervention is to a particular context or population. When reporting systematic review results, it may be useful to tabulate the theoretical perspectives used in each intervention.

Integrity of Intervention

The integrity (or fidelity) of the intervention is the degree to which the intervention is implemented as planned. Dane and Schneider (1998) describe six aspects of integrity/fidelity: adherence (whether components were delivered as prescribed), exposure (the number and length of sessions within a program), quality of delivery (related to staff involved in program delivery), participant

responsiveness (including participation and enthusiasm), program differentiation (ensuring that participants only received planned interventions), and heterogeneity in public health reviews (the differences in included studies including populations, contexts, and outcomes measured).

Integrating Qualitative and Quantitative Studies

Combining a synthesis of qualitative studies with a synthesis of quantitative data from research trials can provide greater insights into developing, evaluating, and implementing interventions (Oliver *et al.*, 2005). When the synthesis of trials includes a meta-analysis, the method allows the integration of quantitative estimates of benefit and harm with qualitative understanding from people's lives. The insights gained from the synthesis of qualitative studies allows exploration of statistical heterogeneity in ways that it would be difficult to imagine in advance (Thomas *et al.*, 2004).

Ethics and Inequalities

Systematic review methods for addressing health-care inequalities are in their infancy, and as a result, with some admirable exceptions (Kristjansson *et al.*, 2007) few systematic reviews currently include this type of information. This is primarily because information on equity tends to be underreported in primary studies. Where possible, it may be useful to use PROGRESS (place of residence, race/ethnicity, occupation, gender, religion, education, socioeconomic position [SES] and social capital) to assess issues of equity. It is also important to consider the ethical implications of every decision made throughout the review process. Ethical issues may arise during many stages of the review, including when making these decisions: the topic of the review, who is involved throughout it, and which interventions and outcomes to include.

Sustainability

Users of reviews are often interested in knowing whether the health benefits (e.g., reductions in specific diseases or improvements in health) from an intervention are going to be sustained beyond the life of the intervention.

Shediac-Rizkallah and Bone (1998) present a useful framework for addressing sustainability. It defines key aspects of program sustainability as (1) maintenance of health benefits from the program, (2) institutionalization of a program within an organization, and (3) capacity building in the community. Key factors influencing sustainability are those in the broader environment, those within the organizational setting, and project design and implementation factors.

Context

The context (e.g., political, organizational, social, or economic) in which an intervention is conducted can affect its subsequent success or failure. It is therefore often difficult to make generalizations about whether an intervention included in a review may work in other contexts (Roberts *et al.*, 2006). Often this contextual information is not included in primary studies, and the review author may need to contact the original researchers to obtain it. Systematic reviews of public health interventions should highlight what context-specific information was included in the studies and identify further information required, such as features of the host organization, staff, and healthcare system and characteristics of the target population (e.g., socioeconomic, cultural, literacy levels, place of residence) (Hawe *et al.*, 2004).

Applicability

External validity is the extent to which the findings of a study or a systematic review are relevant to other populations and contexts. Sometimes referred to as generalizability, it allows decision makers to consider how the findings of a systematic review might be adopted or adapted for effective practice or policy within their setting (Wang *et al.*, 2006).

Infrastructure and Activity to Support Systematic Reviews of Public Health Interventions

Both the development and implementation of systematic reviews need to be supported by appropriate infrastructure. This section of the study describes programs/activities being undertaken to support review production and knowledge translation and exchange. It may include an acknowledgment of the work being conducted by the following groups:

- **Cochrane Collaboration,** established in 1993, is an international organization with the aim of preparing and maintaining systematic reviews of the effects of health interventions and making this information available to all practitioners, policymakers, and consumers. The Cochrane Health Promotion and Public Health Field, an organization of the Cochrane Collaboration, was established in 1996 and has been funded by the Victorian Health Promotion Foundation since 2000. The Collaboration and its entities have contributed to the development of methods for conducting reviews and the translation of findings of systematic reviews into policy and practice.
- **The Canadian Institutes of Health Research** (CIHR), established in 2000, is the government of Canada's health research funding agency. Knowledge translation is the cornerstone of CIHRs mandate and involves the exchange, synthesis, and application of knowledge to accelerate use of the best available evidence in the interest of improving the health of Canadians. Within CIHR, the Institute of Population and Public Health actively contributed to the establishment of the National Collaborating Centres for Public Health (NCCs), a Public Health Agency Canada initiative to make public health research more accessible for practice and policy decisions.
- **Health-evidence.ca** is a website that forms part of a randomized controlled trial to test the effectiveness of three knowledge translation strategies: website, targeted evidence messages, and a knowledge broker. The trial is funded by several sources including the Canadian Institutes of Health Research. Although there is a significant investment in knowledge translation strategies, very little is known about which strategies are most likely to result in the use of evidence to inform decision making. This project seeks to inform this debate.
- **National Institute for Health and Clinical Excellence** in the UK is an independent organization responsible for providing national guidance on promoting good health and preventing and treating ill health. It makes recommendations on interventions to promote a healthy lifestyle or reduce the risk of developing a disease or condition. This guidance may focus on a topic (such as smoking), particular population (such as young people), or a particular setting (such as the workplace).
- **U.S. Guide to Community Preventive Services** summarizes what is known about the effectiveness, economic efficiency, and feasibility of interventions to promote community health and prevent disease. Established in 1996, the Task Force on Community Preventive Services, a nongovernmental body whose work is supported by the U.S. Centers for Disease Control and Prevention, makes recommendations for the use of public health interventions based on evidence gathered in systematic reviews of published studies conducted by the review teams of the Community Guide.

Citations

Dane A and Schneider B (1998) Program integrity in primary and early secondary prevention: Are implementation effects out of control? *Clinical Psychology Review* 18(1): 23–45.

Davies P (2005) *Workforce Development to Support Evidence-informed Public Health*. Presentation at Cutting Edge Debates, Vic Health, Melbourne. Victoria, Australia: VicHealth.

Egger M, Schneider M, and Davey-Smith G (1998) Spurious precision? Meta-analysis of observational studies. *British Medical Journal* 316 (7125): 140–144.

Evans D and Fitzgerald M (2002) The experience of physical restraint: A systematic review of qualitative research. *Contemporary Nurse* 13 (2–3): 126–135.

Harden A, Garcia J, Oliver S, *et al.* (2004) Applying systematic review methods to studies of people's views: An example from public health research. *Journal of Epidemiology and Community Health* 58(9): 794–800.

Hawe P, Shiell A, Riley T, *et al.* (2004) Methods for exploring implementation variation and local context within a cluster randomised community intervention trial. *Journal of Epidemiology and Community Health* 58(9): 788–793.

Jackson N and Waters E and the Guidelines for Systematic Reviews in Health Promotion and Public Health Taskforce (2005) *Guidelines for Systematic Reviews in Health Promotion and Public Health.* Melbourne, Australia: Cochrane Health Promotion and Public Health Field.

Kristjansson E, Robinson V, Petticrew M, *et al.* (2007) School feeding for improving the physical and psychosocial health of disadvantaged elementary school children. *Cochrane Database of Systematic Reviews* 1: CD004676.

NHS Centre for Reviews and Dissemination (2001) Undertaking systematic reviews of research on effectiveness. CRD's guidance for those carrying out or commissioning reviews. *CRD Report Number 4 (2dn edn.).* New York, UK: NHS Centre for Reviews and Dissemination.

Oliver S, Harden A, Rees R, *et al.* (2005) An emerging framework for including different types of evidence in systematic reviews for public policy. *Evaluation: The International Journal of Theory, Research and Practice* 11(4): 428–446.

Petticrew M and Roberts H (2006) *Systematic Reviews in the Social Sciences: A Practical Guide.* Oxford, UK: Blackwell Publishing.

Roberts H, Arai L, Roen K, *et al.* (2006) It might work in a trial, but how do we make it work round here? In: Kelly M, Kanaris A Morgan A, *et al. Evidence at the Crossroads: New Directions in Changing the Health of the Public: A Manual.* Oxford, UK: Oxford University Press.

Shediac-Rizkallah MC and Bone LR (1998) Planning for the sustainability of community-based health programs: Conceptual frameworks and future directions for research, practice and policy. *Health Education Research* 13(1): 87–108.

Thomas J, Harden A, Oakley A, *et al.* (2004) Integrating qualitative research with trials in systematic reviews: An example from public health. *British Medical Journal* 328: 1010–1012.

Wang S, Moss JR, and Hiller J (2006) Applicability and transferability of interventions in evidence-based public health. *Health Promotion International* 21(1): 76–83.

Further Reading

EPPI-Centre (2006) EPPI-Centre methods for conducting systematic reviews. *Report of the EPPI-Centre.* London: University of London.

Harden A, Brunton G, Fletcher A, Oakley A, Burchett H, and Backhans M (2006) Young people, pregnancy and social exclusion: A systematic synthesis of research evidence to identify effective, appropriate and promising approaches for prevention and support. *Report of the EPPI-Centre.* London: University of London.

Higgins JPT and Green S (eds.) (2006) *Cochrane Handbook for Systematic Reviews of Interventions 4.2.6.* Chichester, UK: John Wiley & Sons.

Roberts I and Kwan R (2001) School based driver education for the prevention of traffic crashes. *Cochrane Database of Systematic Reviews* 1: CD003201.

Jackson N and Waters E (2004) The challenges of systematically reviewing public health interventions. *Journal of Public Health* 26(3): 303–307.

Relevant Websites

http://www.health-evidence.ca – Canadian Institutes of Health Research.

http://www.thecommunityguide.org – Centers for Disease Control and Prevention (CDC).

http://www.cochrane.org – Cochrane Collaboration.

http://www.vichealth.vic.gov.au – Cochrane Health Promotion and Public Health Field.

http://eppi.ioe.ac.uk – EPPI-Centre.

http://www.nice.org.au – National Institute for Health and Clinical Excellence (NICE).

SECTION 2
FIELDS OF EPIDEMIOLOGY

Clinical Epidemiology

D L Sackett, Kilgore S. Trout Research and Education Center at Irish Lake, Markdale, ON, Canada

Definitions of Clinical Epidemiology

Clinical epidemiology is the application of epidemiological and related methods from a clinical (rather than public health) perspective. Whereas classical epidemiology studies the distribution and determinants of disease at a population level, clinical epidemiology employed these methods to study the diagnosis, prognosis, and treatment of individual and groups of patients. In its inception in the mid-nineteenth century, clinical epidemiology employed methodological strategies and tactics mostly confined to epidemiology and biostatistics. Over the past six decades it has evolved in two ways. First, it has widened the research methods it employs, including health economics and the social and behavioral sciences. Second, it has expanded the uses to which these methods are put: the explosion in the generation of relevant evidence, the critical appraisal of that evidence for its validity and clinical applicability, the efficient storage and retrieval of that evidence, the development of evidence-based medicine and health care, and the systematic review and synthesis of evidence.

A Brief History of Clinical Epidemiology

The term 'clinical epidemiology' was introduced by John Paul (born 1893, died in 1971), an infectious disease internist who was appointed head of the Section of Preventive Medicine in Yale's Department of Medicine in 1940. In his president's address to the American Society for Clinical Investigation in 1938 (when it was still an organization with broad interests that included intact humans), he proposed clinical epidemiology as a "new basic science for *preventive* medicine" in which the exploration of relevant aspects of human ecology and public health began with the study of individual patients (Paul, 1938). Dr. Paul wrote the first book and offered the first course in clinical epidemiology for undergraduate medical students. However, his concept of clinical epidemiology had a population rather than individual patient orientation in which he described the role of the clinical epidemiologist as being "like that of a detective visiting the scene of the crime" who then "branches out into the setting in which that individual became ill." Thus the procedure in his course for third and fourth year Yale medical students was to "start the student at the bedside and lead him gradually away from it." This was in sharp contrast to the orientation

of other pioneers who, although they didn't refer to themselves as clinical epidemiologists, exemplified the application of epidemiology in bedside neonatology (where William Silverman showed that the traditional prophylactic antimicrobial therapy of babies with kernicterus did more harm than good) and gastroenterology (where Thomas Chalmers showed that the traditional regimen of prolonged bed rest for Type A hepatitis was unnecessary).

The shift in the focus of clinical epidemiology from community ecology to individual patients and groups of patients took place in the 1960s in the form of the first Clinical Epidemiology Research Unit in the Department of Medicine at the State University of New York at Buffalo, United States, in 1966, followed shortly by the Department of Clinical Epidemiology and Biostatistics at McMaster Medical School in Canada in 1967. In the prospectus for each of them clinical epidemiology was defined as

> the application, by a physician who provides direct patient care, of epidemiologic and biostatistical methods to the study of diagnostic and therapeutic processes in order to effect an improvement in health.   (Sackett, 1969)

Thus, at McMaster the external, public health orientation was set aside and replaced with a focus on individual patients and groups of patients in clinical, not community, settings.

In 1968 Alvan Feinstein published a series of papers on clinical epidemiology in the *Annals of Internal Medicine* (Feinstein, 1968). He defined the "territory" of clinical epidemiology as:

> the clinicostatistical study of diseased populations. The intellectual activities of this territory include the following: the occurrence rates and geographic distribution of disease; the patterns of natural and post-therapeutic events that constitute varying clinical courses in the diverse spectrum of disease; and the clinical appraisal of therapy. The contemplation and investigation of these or allied topics constitute a medical domain that can be called clinical epidemiology.

Thus, he cast a wider net, and included elements of classical epidemiology and public health. His inclusion of public health in his definition of clinical epidemiology was repeated 18 years later in his book of that name:

> clinical epidemiology represents the way in which classical epidemiology, traditionally oriented toward general

strategies in the public health of community groups, has been enlarged to include clinical decisions in personal-encounter care for individual patients.

Early clinical epidemiologists received important encouragement from Archie Cochrane, who provided a powerful rationale for the rigorous scientific evaluation of diagnosis, treatment, and preventive medicine (Cochrane, 1972). The first modern textbook in clinical epidemiology was written by Robert Fletcher, Suzanne Fletcher, and Edward Wagner at the University of North Carolina, published in 1982. Now in its fourth edition, it continues to be a favored introductory text. It was followed by ones from McMaster (now in its third edition) and Yale in 1985, from the University of Washington in 1986 (now in its third edition), and from McGill in 1988. Each has its own flavor and niche, and they are now available in several languages.

Typical Clinical Epidemiologic Investigations

Typical clinical epidemiological investigations include:

1. Comparing patients' symptoms and signs with the results of 'reference standard' diagnostic tests. High-quality studies of this sort sample patients in whom it is clinically sensible to suspect a specific diagnosis (e.g., patients suspected of chronic airflow limitation), carry out specific bits of the clinical examination (e.g., the position of the thyroid cartilage relative to the suprasternal notch), and then carry out an independent, reference standard test (e.g., spirometry) while 'blind' to the results of the clinical examination. The results of these studies, commonly expressed as likelihood ratios, improve both the accuracy and efficiency of the clinical examination. In doing so, they have confirmed the usefulness of some traditional signs and symptoms (e.g., the presence of an S3 gallop on cardiac auscultation of a patient with suspected heart failure), added new signs and symptoms (e.g., clinical prediction rules for deep vein thrombosis and the 'Ottawa ankle rule' for ruling out the need for ankle radiographs), and, equally important, shown that other signs and symptoms are useless (e.g., the tourniquet test for carpal tunnel syndrome).
2. Relating patients' later outcomes (prognoses) to the results of earlier (baseline) clinical and laboratory findings. High-quality studies of this sort sample patients at the very start of their illness (an inception cohort), perform baseline clinical and laboratory examinations on them, and then follow them to the conclusion of their disease. The results of these studies provide more accurate predictions and advice to patients at the start of an illness.
3. Randomized clinical trials in which consenting patients are assigned, by a system analogous to tossing a coin, to

receive or not receive a new (experimental) treatment and then closely followed for the occurrence or prevention of unfavorable outcomes. High-quality studies of this sort have now been applied not only to medications (e.g., caffeine for premature babies), but also to operations (e.g., carotid endarterectomy for threatened stroke), behavioral and educational interventions (e.g., behavioral maneuvers for improving compliance with medications and exercise), health professionals (e.g., the nurse practitioner), and the like. The results of these studies determine whether new treatments or other health-care interventions do more good than harm. For example, the preventive and therapeutic interventions for coronary heart disease that have been validated in randomized trials are credited with halving both the incidence and case-fatality of myocardial infarction in high-income countries.

Education Programs for Training Clinical Epidemiologists

Opportunities for clinicians to obtain education and training in clinical epidemiology gradually spread from Yale and McMaster to other North American health sciences centers and to centers in Europe and the Far East. Combined training in clinical medicine and clinical epidemiology greatly expanded in the United States in 1974 with the creation of the Robert Woods Johnson Clinical Scholars Program. The internationalization of clinical epidemiology began in 1980 when Kerr White and the Rockefeller Foundation initiated the International Clinical Epidemiology Network (INCLEN). In this program, young clinicians from low-income countries came for training in clinical epidemiology to 'training centers' at McMaster in Canada, Newcastle in Australia, and the University of Pennsylvania. A key element of their career development was linkage to a mentor who spent part of each year working with them back at their home institutions. The organization now includes 64 medical institutions in 26 countries. In the eyes of many, its most important accomplishments have been the repeated redefinition of clinical epidemiology to suit local needs and the taking over of the training of clinical epidemiologists by regional centers in Africa, China, India, Latin America, and South East Asia.

Clinical Epidemiology's Detractors

Clinical epidemiology has not been without its detractors, especially among more traditional epidemiology departments who perceived (often correctly) their loss of resources and bright young minds to this new discipline. For example, in 1983 Walter Holland urged the abandonment of the term 'clinical epidemiology' altogether (Holland, 1983). While acknowledging its usefulness over the previous 15 years, he now found it a divisive term that conferred "respectability" only on those epidemiologists who practiced medicine, created the impression that one form of teaching (using epidemiology for solving clinical problems) was more appropriate than another (mastering classical epidemiological methods), and fashioned students' perceptions of the priorities and needs of societies. In response to his criticism, it was suggested that the distinction between clinical and nonclinical epidemiologists was on a nominal, not ordinal, scale, but that his other criticisms were not only true, but to be applauded: clinical epidemiology was a better way to teach medical students, and clinical epidemiology was reshaping the perceptions of not only medical students (who began to see it as a relevant basic science) but also entire faculties (departments of clinical epidemiology were growing in number and size; clinical departments were carrying out more and better 'clinical-practice' research), and learned societies were acknowledging the relevance of clinical epidemiology to 'clinical research' in ways that classical epidemiology had been unable to achieve (Sackett, 1984).

The Current State of Clinical Epidemiology

Having established itself, gained formal recognition at universities, granting agencies, and learned societies, and populated academic departments and research groups around the world, the field of clinical epidemiology became increasingly able to emphasize its similarities to, rather than its differences from, classical public health epidemiology and the related sciences of economics, political science, psychology, and sociology. This is perhaps best seen in low- and middle-income countries, where clinical epidemiologists have begun to perform highly pragmatic cluster trials of public health interventions (such as insecticide-bearing mosquito nets) that have incorporated economic analyses and sociological inquiries. As predicted by Walter Spitzer, all of these disciplines carry out and collaborate in studies of "diagnostic and therapeutic processes in order to effect an improvement in health" (Spitzer, 1986).

Clinical Epidemiology and the Clinical Journals

Although a wide spectrum of clinical journals have published the concepts, methods and results of clinical epidemiological research, and the *Journal of Clinical Epidemiology* has been a natural home for the discipline, some general medical journals also fostered the field and its recent evolutions. In the 1970s the *Journal of Clinical*

Pharmacology and Therapeutics turned Donald Mainland's "Notes from a Laboratory of Medical Statistics" over to Alvan Feinstein for his landmark series in "Clinical Biostatistics." In the 1980s the *Canadian Medical Association Journal* hosted series on "How to Read Clinical Journals" and "How to Interpret Diagnostic Data" from the clinical epidemiology group at McMaster. In the 1990s, the *Journal of the American Medical Association* initiated the "Rational Clinical Examination" series that hosted reviews of the accuracy and precision of the clinical history and examination. It went on to host a series of "Users' Guides to the Medical Literature" that were collated into a major text. Throughout this era, the *Annals of Internal Medicine* published several fundamental papers and series, culminating in the *ACP Journal Club* and *Evidence-Based Medicine* series of journals of secondary publication. The *British Medical Journal* edited several 'evidence-based' journals and became a major international publisher of clinical epidemiological research.

Clinical Epidemiologic Contributions to Five Recent Evolutions

Clinical epidemiology has played a central or major role in five recent evolutions (some say revolutions) in health care: in evidence generation, its rapid critical appraisal, its efficient storage and retrieval, evidence-based medicine, and evidence synthesis.

Evolution 1: Evidence Generation

The evolution in evidence generation since 1970, although most easily documented in the growth in reports of and about the randomized trial (with more of them published in the single year 2000 than in the entire decade 1965–1975), is paralleled by similar, although less spectacular, increases in the numbers and sophistication of reports about diagnosis, prognosis, and the appropriateness and quality of clinical care. Clinical epidemiologists are providing leadership in both the generation and continuing methodological development of this burgeoning body of clinically relevant evidence.

Evolutions 2 and 3: The Critical Appraisal, Storage, and Retrieval of Evidence

The price to be paid for this vast increase in relevant evidence was an increasing difficulty in finding it, retrieving it, and keeping up-to-date with it. By 1972 there were about 4M articles published in the biomedical literature per year (in all languages). Restricting one's reading to just the journals that provided the content that is sound and relevant for internal medicine required clinicians to read 33 articles every day of the year. When the dramatic decline in general medical knowledge after certification was documented by a group of clinical epidemiologists, it became impossible to ignore this growing problem. A second problem became evident when this growing body of evidence was subjected to the critical appraisal of its validity: the majority of it was found wanting. These two situations combined to place clinicians at increasing risk of "drowning in doubtful data." The parallel evolutions in (1) the rapid critical appraisal of evidence (for its validity and potential clinical usefulness) and in (2) the efficient storage and rapid retrieval of evidence combined to rescue clinicians who were striving to track down the evidence than might help their patients. Several clinical epidemiologists, as well as library scientists, statisticians, and qualitative researchers, made contributions to these parallel evolutions, most notably Brian Haynes at McMaster University, who brought these evolutionary streams together in powerful and clinically relevant ways (Haynes *et al.*, 1994). The example he set by reducing the internal medicine literature to just the 2% that was both valid and clinically relevant in the *ACP Journal Club* introduced the revolution that today provides frontline clinicians in a number of clinical fields with manageable chunks of up-to-date, reliable evidence, right at the bedside (Wu and Straus, 2006).

Evolution 4: Evidence-Based Medicine

As more and more clinicians, armed with the strategies and tactics of clinical epidemiology, cared for more and more patients, they began to evolve the final, vital link between evidence and direct patient care. Building on the prior evolutions, and manifest in clinically useful measures such as Andreas Laupacis's NNT (the Number of patients a clinician would Need to Treat in order to prevent one more bad outcome) (Laupacis *et al.*, 1988), and often incorporating the patient's own values and expectations as in Sharon Straus's LHH (the Likelihood that a treatment would Help vs. Harm the patient's achievement of their health objectives) (Straus, 2002), the *Revolution of Evidence-Based Medicine* was introduced by Gordon Guyatt (Evidence-Based Medicine Working Group, 1992). Since its first mention in 1992, its ideas about the use (rather than just critical appraisal) of evidence in patient care and in health professional education have spread worldwide and have been adopted not only by a broad array of clinical disciplines but also by health-care planners and evaluators. In 2006, the *British Medical Journal* designated evidence-based medicine one of the 15 greatest medical breakthroughs since 1840.

Evolution 5: Evidence Synthesis and the Cochrane Collaboration

Simultaneous with these other evolutions and revolutions, and both supporting and building upon them, has been the evidence-synthesis evolution of strategies and tactics for assembling and systematically reviewing the totality of evidence about the effects of health care. This evolution is epitomized in the Cochrane Collaboration, a worldwide collaboration of patients, clinicians, and methodologists, who prepare, maintain, and promote the accessibility of systematic reviews of the effects of health-care interventions (Cochrane Collaboration, 2007). Conceived and initiated by Iain Chalmers in Oxford, this undertaking has been characterized as equal in importance to the human genome project. Many consider the contributions of clinical epidemiologists to evidence synthesis their greatest accomplishment since the term was introduced 65 years ago.

See also: Clinical Epidemiology; Environmental and Occupational Epidemiology; Epidemiology of Injuries; Observational Epidemiology; Psychiatric Epidemiology; Social Epidemiology.

Citations

Cochrane AL (1972) *Effectiveness and Efficiency: Random Reflections on Health Services*. London: Nuffield Provincial Hospitals Trust.

Cochrane Collaboration (2007) http://www.cochranelibrary.com/Collaboration/.

Evidence-Based Medicine Working Group (1992) Evidence-based medicine. A new approach to teaching the practice of medicine. *Journal of the American Medical Association* 268: 2420–2425.

Feinstein AR (1968) Clinical epidemiology. The populational experiments of nature and of man in human illness. *Annals of Internal Medicine* 69: 807–820.

Haynes RB, Wilczynski NL, McKibbon KA, Walker CJ, and Sinclair JC (1994) Developing optimal search strategies for detecting clinically sound studies in MEDLINE. *Journal of the American Medical Informatics Association* 1: 447–458.

Holland W (1983) Inappropriate terminology. *International Journal of Epidemiology* 12: 5–7.

Laupacis A, Sackett DL, and Roberts RS (1988) An assessment of clinically useful measures of the consequences of treatment. *New England Journal of Medicine* 318: 1728–1733.

Paul JR (1938) Clinical epidemiology. *Journal of Clinical Investigation* 17: 539–541.

Sackett DL (1969) Clinical epidemiology. *American Journal of Epidemiology* 89: 125–128.

Sackett DL (1984) Three cheers for clinical epidemiology. *International Journal of Epidemiology* 13: 117–119.

Spitzer WO (1986) Clinical epidemiology. *Journal of Chronic Disease* 39: 411–415.

Straus SE (2002) Individualizing treatment decisions: The likelihood of being helped versus harmed. *Evaluation and the Health Professions* 25: 210–224.

Wu R and Straus SE (2006) Use of PDAs in health care: Systematic review of the literature. Evidence for handheld electronic medication records in improving care: A systematic review. *BioMedCentral Medical Informatics and Decision Making* 6: 26.

Further Reading

Cochrane AL (1999) *Effectiveness and Efficiency: Random Reflections on Health Services*, 3rd edn. London: Royal Society of Medicine Press.

Feinstein AR (1985) *Clinical Epidemiology; The Architecture of Clinical Research*. Philadelphia, PA: WB Saunders.

Fletcher RW and Fletcher SW (2005) *Clinical Epidemiology: The Essentials*, 4th edn. Philadelphia, PA: Lippincott Williams & Wilkins.

Guyatt GH and Rennie D (eds.) (2002) *User's Guides to the Medical Literature. A Manual for Evidence-Based Clinical Practice.* Chicago, IL: American Medical Association Press.

Haynes RB, Sackett DL, Guyatt GH, and Tugwell P (2006) *Clinical Epidemiology: How to do Clinical Practice Research.* Philadelphia, PA: Lippincott Williams & Wilkins.

Kramer MS (1991) *Clinical Epidemiology and Biostatistics.* Berlin, Germany: Springer-Verlag.

Paul JR (1966) *Clinical Epidemiology,* revised edn. Chicago, IL: University of Chicago Press.

Straus SE, Richardson WS, Glasziou P, and Haynes RB (2005) *Evidence-Based Medicine. How to Practice and Teach EBM,* 3rd edn. Edinburgh, UK: Elsevier Churchill Livingstone.

Weiss NS (2006) *Clinical Epidemiology: The Study of the Outcome of Illness,* 3rd edn. Oxford, UK: Oxford University Press.

Relevant Websites

http://www.cochranelibrary.com/ – Collaboration/Cochrane Collaboration.

http://www.cebm.utoronto.ca/ – Evidence-based medicine resources and clinical calculators.

http://www.inclen.org/ – International Clinical Epidemiology Network.

http://www.carestudy.com/CareStudy/Default.asp – International studies of the accuracy of the clinical examination.

Environmental and Occupational Epidemiology

N Pearce and J Douwes, Massey University, Wellington, New Zealand

In this article, we describe the key features of environmental and occupational epidemiology studies, the types of study designs, measurement of exposure, issues of bias, and interpretation of environmental and occupational epidemiology studies. We do not discuss methods of data analysis, and readers are referred to more detailed epidemiologic texts for more information (Rothman and Greenland, 1998).

Environmental epidemiology and occupational epidemiology are separate fields that are usually covered by separate textbooks (Steenland and Savitz, 1997; Checkoway *et al.*, 2004). However, the two fields often involve common exposures and there is therefore inevitably some overlap in the epidemiological methods that are used. For example, exposure to pesticides can be studied in the context of community exposures or exposures to pesticide production workers or commercial sprayers. These two different contexts of exposure provide the basis for the difference between environmental and occupational epidemiology. Each context has its own advantages and disadvantages in terms of conducting research, although in most instances studying such an exposure in the occupational context is easier and more valid scientifically than studying it in the environmental context.

Environmental Epidemiology

Environmental epidemiology is the use of epidemiology to investigate causes of disease that are found in the environment (Pearce and Woodward, 2004). A recent World Health Report estimated that 24% of the global disease burden and 23% of all deaths can be attributed to environmental factors (World Health Organization, 2006). Among children 0–14 years of age, the proportion of deaths attributed to the environment was estimated to be as high as 36%, with the largest proportion in developing countries. Diseases with the largest absolute burden included diarrhea, lower respiratory infections, other unintentional injuries including occupational injuries, and malaria. The most important risk factors contributing to disease and mortality are unsafe drinking water and poor sanitation and hygiene (diarrhea), and indoor air pollution related largely to household solid fuel use and possibly second-hand smoke as well as to outdoor air pollution (lower respiratory infections) (World Health Organization, 2006). In most developed countries, these risks are now largely controlled, with the exception of outdoor air pollution, through the provision of safe drinking water, adequate food, waste disposal, immunizations, and adequate health care. However, other diseases with suspected environmental causes such as cancer, cardiovascular disease, asthma, chronic obstructive pulmonary disease, and diabetes are still common and are in fact increasing in prevalence in many developed countries.

The term environment is very broad and includes epidemiological studies at the molecular, individual, population, and ecosystem levels. Analyses at the ecosystem level are unique to environmental epidemiology and often require research methods that are quite different from those used in other areas of epidemiologic research, including systems-based approaches such as complexity theory.

There are also some features of environmental epidemiology that provide particular challenges to researchers (Pearce and Woodward, 2004).

Firstly, environmental epidemiology is concerned generally with exposures that are, by definition, characteristics of the environment, not the individuals who live in that environment. Examples include infectious organisms in the water supply, features of the legislative environment (restrictions on smoking in bars for example), and air pollutants both indoors and outdoors. This means that the exposures that are being studied are typically widespread and not readily controlled by the individuals who are directly affected. What are the consequences for epidemiology? The fact that the exposures are widespread means that it may be difficult to find individuals who can act as an unexposed comparison group (for example, persons who are not exposed to air pollution). Sometimes the exposures are not only widespread, but also vary little within a given population (for example, air pollution levels in a neighborhood) compared with the differences between populations. In these circumstances, ecological studies – in which the unit of comparison is the group rather than the individual – may be particularly useful. An example of an ecological study of air pollution would be a study that compared the frequency of respiratory illnesses in different neighborhoods with the average levels of nitrogen oxide and ozone in those locations.

Secondly, environmental epidemiology often involves studying exposures at low levels. An example is environmental dioxin exposure. Exposures in the general environment from sources such as incinerators are usually orders of magnitude less than those that may be experienced in some occupational settings (such as workers in the incinerator, or workers producing chemicals contaminated with dioxin). One consequence is that environmental epidemiology is frequently searching for risks on the margin of detectability. However, this does not mean that the risks presented by low-level exposures in the general environment are necessarily unimportant. First, these exposures are typically involuntary (people who live close to incinerators, for example, have little choice over whether they are exposed to dioxin from the sites), and the public is far more sensitive to potential dangers of this kind than exposures that are seen to have an element of discretion about them. Second, the increase in risk for an individual may be small, but if exposures affect large numbers of people, then the overall burden of illness attributable to the exposure will be substantial. Relatively few people are exposed to dioxin at work, so although this may be an important personal health issue, the impact on the health of the population overall will be relatively small. On the other hand, if low-level environmental dioxin exposures do have health effects, then this would be a significant public health issue since the number of people at risk would be very large.

Thirdly, the measurement of exposure may be particularly difficult in environmental epidemiology studies. For example, if someone experiences spray drift from pesticides being sprayed on a farm near their home, it may be very difficult to determine how much exposure they received, if any.

Finally, studies of environmental causes of disease and injury tend to involve dispersed, heterogeneous populations. This provides particular challenges in recruitment of study participants and in the analysis of findings. It may be difficult to define the exposed population, weakening the confidence with which results can be extrapolated to other groups. The very mixed nature of the general population (in terms of age, health status, and co-exposures) means that an overall average risk estimate may mask considerable variations in the strength of effect in different subgroups. Consider for example a study of hospitalization rates in relation to ambient levels of air pollution in a major city. The population of the city will include a number of groups that are likely to be more susceptible than the average city inhabitant to the effects of pollution (such as the elderly, people with preexisting chest disease, outdoor workers). Typically, the numbers of susceptible individuals and the exposures they receive are not known, and caution must be applied in interpreting the relation observed between pollution levels and health outcome (e.g., numbers of hospital admissions per day). Exposure guidelines based on studies of this kind may not provide adequate protection to the most sensitive groups in the population, and this must be taken into account when epidemiological results are translated into public health policy (Woodward *et al.*, 1995).

Occupational Epidemiology

The major occupational health problems include cancer, heart disease, respiratory disease, musculoskeletal disease, neurological disease, hearing loss, and injury. Worldwide, 6000 people die each day as a result of their job, and of these deaths 15% are due to accidents and 85% to work-related disease. The picture is quite different when occupational morbidity is considered, with accidents accounting for about 90% of cases and nonfatal disease only about 10% (Driscoll *et al.*, 2004).

Studying exposures in the occupational context has many scientific advantages in comparison to studies of environmental exposures (Checkoway *et al.*, 2004).

Firstly, the exposures are generally well defined in time and space, rather than being ubiquitous in the environment. For example, in a study of occupational dioxin exposure, the exposure may be restricted to just a few departments within a factory, and workers in the other departments may serve as a nonexposed comparison group. Even if all workers in a particular factory receive some exposure, it is relatively straightforward to find a nonexposed comparison group from another factory or industry.

Secondly, as noted above, occupational exposures are typically at much higher levels than environmental exposures, and study power is therefore correspondingly greater.

Thirdly, the estimation of exposure is generally more straightforward in occupational studies. For example, in a study of pesticide production workers, even if individual exposure measurements were not available, it would be relatively straightforward to classify workers in categories of exposure on the basis of their work history (job titles and departments) and a Job-Exposure-Matrix (JEM) (Checkoway et al., 2004).

Finally, occupational populations are generally less heterogeneous than the communities that are studied in environmental epidemiology. For example, in studies of blue collar workers, there are usually few differences in lifestyle between exposed and nonexposed workers, so confounding by factors such as tobacco smoking and alcohol is usually weak. In addition, occupational populations do not usually include children or the elderly, two groups that may be particularly susceptible to some exposures. Furthermore, for many occupational exposures, it may be rare that the workforce includes pregnant women.

These differences between exposures in the occupational and environmental context mean that it is generally more straightforward, and more valid scientifically, to study the occupational context. On the other hand, there may be difficulties in extrapolating findings from occupational studies to more heterogeneous populations with lower levels of exposure. Furthermore, there are some environmental exposures (e.g., air pollution, pollen exposure) for which it is relatively difficult to find suitable occupational populations. Thus, for many exposures environmental studies provide a useful complement to occupational studies.

Types of Epidemiologic Studies

All epidemiologic studies are (or should be) based on a particular population (the study population, source population, or base population) followed over a particular period of time (the study period or risk period). The different epidemiological study designs differ only in the manner in which the source population is defined, and the manner in which information is drawn from this population (Checkoway et al., 2004).

Incidence Studies

The most complete approach involves utilizing all of the information from the source population in a cohort study (follow-up study, longitudinal study) of disease incidence. Follow-up may be prospective (which is more expensive and time-consuming but may enable better quality data to be collected), or it may be based on historical records.

The most common measure of disease occurrence is the incidence rate, which is a measure of the disease occurrence per unit time, and is the number of new cases of the outcome under study divided by the total person-time at risk. The usual approach is to compare the incidence rate in those exposed and those not exposed to a particular factor (e.g., air pollution) and to estimate the rate ratio. This may involve comparing the disease incidence in the exposed group (e.g., people living next to a factory which emits high levels of air pollution) with some nonexposed external reference population, such as another geographic area or the national population. Alternatively, if the source population involves both exposed and nonexposed persons (e.g., if some people are exposed and some are not exposed within the same geographical area), then a direct comparison can be made within this population.

Table 1 shows an example of an environmental epidemiology cohort study of the population exposed to dioxin after the 1976 accident in Seveso, Italy (Bertazzi et al., 2001). The accident took place in summer 1976 and exposed several thousand people in the neighboring area to substantial quantities of tetrachlorodibenzo-p-diozin (TCDD). Three contaminated zones (A, B, and R) were defined based on dioxin soil measurements along the direction of the prevailing winds. The study included all people living in these three zones at the time of the accident, or entering in the 10-year period after the accident. Vital status over the following 20 years was determined by contacting the vital statistics offices of the 11 study towns and of thousands of municipalities throughout the country to reach those subjects who had migrated (Bertazzi et al., 2001). The expected numbers of deaths were estimated based on the age, calendar period, and

Table 1 Cohort study of the population in zones A and B combined exposed to dioxin after the 1976 accident in Seveso, Italy

Years of follow-up	Observed	Expected	Relative risk	95% CI
All causes mortality				
0–4 years	103	109.4	0.9	0.8–1.1
5–9 years	113	104.1	1.1	0.9–1.3
10–14 years	95	105.7	0.9	0.7–1.1
15–19 years	127	117.3	1.1	0.9–1.3
Total (0–20 years)	438	436.2	1.0	0.9–1.1
All cancer mortality				
0–4 years	28	30.1	0.9	0.6–1.4
5–9 years	43	34.7	1.2	0.9–1.7
10–14 years	37	41.2	0.9	0.6–1.2
15–19 years	58	44.2	1.3	1.0–1.7
Total (0–20 years)	166	149.7	1.1	1.0–1.3

Modified from Bertazzi PA, Consonni D, Bachetti S, et al. (2001) Health effects of dioxin exposure: A 20-year mortality study. American Journal of Epidemiology 153: 1031–1044.

gender distribution of the population over the 20-year follow-up period. **Table 1** shows the findings for all-cause mortality and cancer mortality in the two most heavily exposed zones (A and B) in the 20 years following the accident. It shows that there was little evidence of an elevation in all-cause mortality, but there was a significant increase in cancer mortality, particularly for the period 15 years or more after the accident.

Incidence Case–Control Studies

Cohort studies are the most complete and definitive approaches to studying the occupational causes of disease, since they utilize all of the information in the source population. However, they often require large numbers and may be very expensive in terms of time and resources. The same findings can often be achieved more efficiently by using a case–control design. The key feature of case–control studies is that they involve studying all of the cases from the source population over the defined risk period (e.g., all cases of lung cancer in Rome during 2002), but only a sample of the non-cases are studied (e.g., a general population sample of people who do not currently have lung cancer). Exposure information is then collected for both groups. The aim is to obtain the same findings that would have been obtained with a full cohort study, but in a more efficient manner, because exposure information is collected only on the cases and a sample of controls, rather than on the entire population. For example, the earliest studies of smoking and lung cancer used the case–control design and the findings were subsequently confirmed in cohort studies.

In case–control studies, the relative risk measure is the odds ratio, which is the ratio of the odds of exposure in the cases (i.e., the number exposed divided by the number not exposed) and the odds of exposure in the controls. Gaertner *et al.* (2004) conducted a case–control study of occupational risk factors for bladder cancer in Canada. They identified incident cases of histological confirmed bladder cancer in adults aged 20–74 years identified through the provincial cancer registries in seven Canadian provinces, and selected 2847 controls from the general population of these provinces matched for age and gender. Cases and controls were sent postal questionnaires with telephone follow-up when necessary. **Table 2** shows the findings for auto mechanics, an occupation which involves exposure to exhaust fumes and lubricating oils, both of which can contribute to bladder cancer risk (Gaertner *et al.*, 2004). A higher proportion of cases than controls had worked as an auto mechanic (OR = 1.69, 95% CI 1.02–2.82) and there was a statistically significant association with duration of employment (**Table 2**).

Prevalence Studies

Incidence studies are usually conducted when studying fatal diseases such as cancer, since cases can be identified

Table 2   Case–control study of occupational risk factors for bladder cancer in Canada

Occupation	Cases	Controls	Odds ratio[a]	95% CI
Auto mechanic				
Never	851	2799	1.00[b]	1.02–2.82
Ever	36	48	1.69	0.66–2.83
1–5 years	15	25	1.37	0.76–4.88
5–15 years	9	14	1.93	0.97–6.34
>15 years	12	9	2.48	1.02–2.82

P-value for trend = 0.01.
[a]Adjusted for age, province, race, smoking, ex-smoking, and consumption of fruit, fried food and coffee, as well as for employment in nine suspect occupations.
[b]Reference category.
Modified from Gaertner RRW, Trpeski L, and Johnson KC (2004) A case–control study of occupational risk factors for bladder cancer in Canada. *Cancer Causes & Control* 15: 1007–1019.

through death registrations or cancer registrations. However, when studying nonfatal chronic disease such as asthma, it is difficult to detect incident cases without very intensive follow-up. Thus, it is more common to study prevalence rather than incidence. This can be defined as point prevalence estimated at one point in time, or period prevalence which denotes the number of cases that existed at any time during some time interval (e.g., 1 year). Prevalence studies represent a considerable saving in resources compared with incidence studies, since it is only necessary to evaluate disease prevalence at one point in time, rather than continually searching for incident cases over an extended period of time. On the other hand, this gain in efficiency is achieved at the cost of some loss of information, since it may be much more difficult to understand the temporal relationship between various exposures and the occurrence of respiratory disease. In particular, it is usually difficult to ascertain, in a prevalence study, at what age disease first occurred, and it is therefore difficult to determine which exposures preceded the development of disease, even when accurate historical exposure information is available.

Table 3 shows an example of a prevalence study. Ehrlich *et al.* (1998) conducted a cross-sectional study of kidney function abnormalities among 382 South African lead battery factory workers. Data on current and historical blood lead concentrations were available to categorize workers by exposure level. There were increasing prevalence trends of abnormalities of serum creatinine, serum uric acid, urinary N-acetyl-β-D-glucosaminidase with both current and historical cumulative blood levels.

Prevalence Case–Control Studies

Just as an incidence case–control study can be used to obtain the same findings as a full cohort study, a prevalence case–control study can be used to obtain the same

Table 3 Prevalence (%) of renal dysfunction in South African lead/acid battery production workers

Exposure Category	Serum creatinine $\geq 125\ \mu mol/l$ %	Serum uric acid $\geq 500\ \mu mol/l$ %	Urinary NAG[a] ≥ 5 u/g creatinine %
Current blood Lead ($\mu g/dl$)			
23–50	2.5	1.0	20.5
51–60	7.8	2.8	22.0
61–110	9.9	7.9	29.2
Cumulative blood Lead ($\mu g.y/dl$)			
7–520.0	4.1	4.1	19.1
520.1–2681	8.9	6.0	27.4

[a]N-acetyl-β-D-glucosaminidase.
Modified from Ehrlich R, Robins T, Jordaan E, et al. (1998) Lead absorption and renal dysfunction in a South African battery factory. *Occupational and Environmental Medicine* 55: 453–460; Checkoway H, Pearce N, and Kriebel D (2004) *Research Methods in Occupational Epidemiology*. New York: Oxford University Press.

findings as a full prevalence study in a more efficient manner. For example, if obtaining exposure information is difficult or costly (e.g., if it involves lengthy interviews or collection of serum samples), then it may be more efficient to conduct a prevalence case–control study by obtaining exposure information on all of the prevalent cases of disease and a sample of controls selected at random from the non-cases.

Table 4 shows an example of a prevalence case–control study. Studies of congenital malformations usually involve estimating the prevalence of malformations at birth (i.e., this is a prevalence rather than an incidence measure). Garcia *et al.* (1999) conducted a (prevalence) case–control study of occupational exposure to pesticides and congenital malformations in Comunidad Valenciana, Spain. A total of 261 cases and 261 controls were selected from those infants born in eight public hospitals during 1993–1994. For mothers who were involved in agricultural activities in the risk period (the month before conception and the first trimester of pregnancy), the adjusted prevalence odds ratio for congenital malformations was 3.2 (95% CI 1.1–9.0). There was no such association with exposure outside of this period, or with paternal agricultural work.

Measurement of Exposure

In studies of environmental and occupational causes of disease, the distinction must be made between exposure and dose. The term exposure refers to the presence of a substance (e.g., environmental pesticide exposure) in the external environment. The term dose refers to the amount

Table 4 Case–control study of parental agricultural work and congenital malformations

Agricultural work	Cases	Controls	Odds ratio[a]	95% CI
Mothers				
Never	127	134	1.0[b]	
Nonrisk periods	72	80	1.1	0.7–1.7
During risk period	15	7	3.2	1.1–9.0
Father				
Never	90	93	1.0[b]	
Nonrisk periods	66	78	0.9	0.5–1.5
During risk period	26	23	1.5	0.7–3.1

The risk period was defined as the month before conception and the first trimester of pregnancy.
[a]Adjusted for maternal and paternal confounders: spontaneous abortion (month), twins (index pregnancy), drug use during pregnancy (mother), heavy smoking during pregnancy (mother), education (mother), industrial work (father), and age >40 years (father).
[b]Reference category.
Modified from Garcia AM, Fletcher T, Benavides FG, et al. (1999) Parental agricultural work and selected congenital malformations. *American Journal of Epidemiology* 149: 64–74.

of substance that reaches susceptible targets within the body (e.g., concentration of a specific pesticide metabolite in the liver) (Checkoway *et al.*, 2004).

Epidemiological studies rarely have optimal exposure/ dose data and often rely on relatively crude measures of exposure. The key issue is that the exposure data need not be perfect, but that it must be of similar quality for the various groups being compared. Provided that this principle is followed, then any bias from misclassification of exposure will be nondifferential (see Information Bias), and will tend to produce false-negative findings. Thus, if positive findings do occur, one can be confident that these are not due to inaccuracies in the exposure data; on the other hand, if no association (or only a weak association) is found between exposure and disease, then the possibility of nondifferential information bias should be considered. In general, the aim of exposure assessment is to: (1) ensure that the exposure data are of equal quality in the groups being compared and (2) ensure that the data are of the best possible quality given the former restriction.

Subjective Measures of Exposure

More often than not exposure or dose cannot be measured directly; instead researchers have to rely on subjective methods of exposure assessment. This is particularly the case in historical cohort studies and in case–control studies focusing on diseases with a long latency period.

Traditionally, exposure to risk factors such as environmental tobacco smoke has been measured with questionnaires, and this approach has a long history of successful use in epidemiology. More recently, it has been argued that the major problem in epidemiology is the lack of adequate exposure data, and that this situation can be rectified by increasing use of molecular markers of exposure (Schulte and Perera, 1993). In fact, there are a number of major limitations of currently available biomarkers of exposures such as cigarette smoking, particularly with regard to historical exposures. Questionnaires have good validity and reproducibility with regard to current exposures and are likely to be superior to biological markers with respect to historical exposures.

In occupational epidemiology, exposure is often estimated simply on the basis of occupation and industry and is typically dichotomized as never/ever exposed. More recently there has been increased use of semi-quantitative exposure assessment covering the whole exposure period using the full work history, and applying quantitative job exposure matrices (JEM) and expert assessment (Checkoway et al., 2004). In the absence of more sophisticated methods, these approaches may provide an efficient and low-cost method of assessing exposure, but it may result in considerable (nondifferential) misclassification.

Exposure Monitoring

In addition to questionnaires, JEMs, and biological measurements, personal or environmental monitoring is commonly used to measure environmental or occupational exposures. Although this has the potential to provide a more valid and accurate exposure assessment, this may not always be the case and is strongly dependent on the chosen sampling strategy, which in turn is dependent on a large number of factors, including:

1. type of exposure and disease or symptoms of interest;
2. acute versus chronic health outcomes (e.g., disease exacerbation versus disease development);
3. population versus patient-based approaches;
4. suspected exposure variation both in time and space, and between the diseased and reference populations;
5. available methods to measure exposure;
6. costs of sampling and analyses.

Data collected for environmental or occupational monitoring purposes may be of limited value in epidemiological studies. For example, monitoring is often done in areas where exposures are likely to be highest, in order to ensure compliance with exposure limits. Epidemiological studies, by contrast, require information on average levels of exposure and it may therefore be necessary to conduct a special survey involving random sampling, rather than relying on data collected for monitoring purposes.

Personal Versus Area Sampling

In general, personal measurements best represent the etiologically relevant current exposures, and personal sampling is therefore preferred over area sampling. Modern sampling equipment is now sufficiently light and small to allow it to be used for personal sampling purposes, and several studies focusing on chemical air pollution, for example, have demonstrated its feasibility in both the indoor and outdoor environments (Checkoway et al., 2004). However, personal sampling may not always be possible due to practical constraints, i.e., it is too cumbersome for the study subjects, or there is no portable equipment to make the desired measurements (measurements of viable microorganisms, for example).

In situations where personal sampling is not possible, area sampling can be applied to reconstruct personal exposure using the microenvironmental model approach. In this model, exposure of an individual to an airborne agent is defined as the time-weighted average of agent concentrations encountered as the individual passes through a series of microenvironments. However, some exposures only occur episodically, and these patterns are not likely to be accurately captured by environmental area samplers. In addition, it is practically impossible to measure all the relevant microenvironments.

Sampling: When and How Often?

To the extent to which this is possible, samples should be taken such that they represent the true exposure at the appropriate time window. In the case of acute effects, exposure measurements taken shortly before the effects occurred would be most useful. For chronic effects, the situation is more complicated since exposure should ideally be assessed prior to the occurrence of health effects and preferably in the time window that is biologically most relevant, i.e., when the exposure is thought to be the most problematic or when subjects are most susceptible for these exposures. This is only possible in longitudinal cohort studies (or historical cohort studies where historical exposure information is available). Even then it is often not clear when people are most susceptible to the exposures of interest. In cross-sectional studies, exposure measurements can also be valuable in assessing retrospective exposures, particularly when the environment in which people live or work has not changed significantly.

Measures of exposure should be sufficiently accurate and precise, so that the effect of exposure on disease can be estimated with minimal bias and maximum efficiency. Precision can be gained (that is, measurement error can be reduced) by increasing the number of samples taken either by: (1) increasing the number of subjects in whom exposure is measured or (2) increasing the number of exposure measurements per subject. In population studies, repeated sampling within subjects is particularly effective with exposures that are known to vary largely over time within subjects relative to the variation observed between subjects with the same job title or in the same work force. If the within-subject variability is small compared to the variation between subjects, however, repeated measures will not significantly reduce measurement error. If within- and between-subject variation is known (from previous surveys or pilot studies, for example) the number of samples required to obtain a given reduction in bias of the risk estimate can be computed in the manner described by Boleij et al. (1995). For instance, in studies that involve airborne sampling of viable micro-organisms in the indoor environment a within- versus between-home variance ratio of 3–4 in concentration is not uncommon, due to high temporal variation in microbial concentrations, combined with very short sampling times. In this particular situation, 27–36 samples per home would be required to estimate the average exposure reliably for an epidemiological study with less than 10% bias in the relationship between some health endpoint and the exposure. For most other exposure situations, the within- versus between-subject variation is, however, substantially lower, and far fewer repeated samples are therefore required.

Exposure Grouping

In occupational epidemiology, a significant increase in validity may be achieved by using group mean exposure levels rather than individual levels since group-based exposure levels often (but not always!) vary less within job titles than within individuals. Exposure groups may be based on occupational categories, job title, work area, etc. Intragroup and intergroup variances and the pooled standard error of the mean can be calculated to evaluate the relative efficiency for various grouping procedures. Provided that reasonably homogeneous exposure groups can be defined with sufficient contrast between them, these same groups can be used to predict exposure levels of subjects for whom no exposure measurements are available, making this a very attractive option when limited resources are available to assess exposure. A similar approach may be employed for environmental exposures, but defining exposure groups with sufficient contrast is often not feasible because exposures often vary little within a given population. Ecological analyses may in those circumstances be more efficient (see Environmental Epidemiology).

Exposure Modeling

If the main factors that explain the variation in personal exposure are known, then mathematical models can be developed to predict individual exposure levels for those subjects where no or only limited exposure measurements are available (provided that valid information on determinants of exposure is available). Multiple regression models are most commonly employed, and can include variables such as tasks performed, type of production, environmental or climate characteristics, use of personal protective equipment, personal behavior, time spent in exposed areas, etc. Although these models can be very useful, they have limitations. In particular, the prediction model is generalizable only for the particular situation in which the data were collected. Extrapolation to other environments with the same exposure, or to the same environment at a different time point, may not be valid, and collection of new exposure data to update and/or validate the old model may be necessary (Boleij et al., 1995). Although exposure models to predict individual exposures have been used in environmental epidemiology, their use is more widespread (and perhaps more successful) in occupational epidemiology. Some examples of empirical exposure modeling include models to assess cadmium levels in blood in the general population, inhalation exposure to hydrocarbons among commercial painters, exposure to inhalable dust in bakery workers, and chemical and mutagenic exposure in the rubber industry. These types of exposure models have been shown to explain 50–80% of the variability in exposure, but models with poorer performance have also been described. For example, Van Strien et al. (1994) assessed the association between home characteristics and house dust mite allergen levels in mattress dust using multiple regression analyses, and this model explained 'only' 26% of the variance.

Although presented as separate strategies, often exposure assessment in occupational and epidemiological studies involve combinations of different approaches, for example a combination of subjective and objective measurements, or a combination of current personal sampling and the use of historical exposures collected for monitoring purposes.

Bias

Systematic error, or bias, occurs if there is a difference between what the study is actually estimating and what it is intended to estimate. Systematic error is thus distinguished from random error in that it would be present even with an infinitely large study, whereas random error can be reduced by increasing the study size.

There are many different types of bias, but three general forms have been distinguished (Rothman and Greenland, 1998): Confounding, selection bias, and information bias. In general terms, these refer to biases inherent in the source population because of differences in disease risk between the groups being compared (confounding), biases resulting from the manner in which study subjects are selected from the source population (selection bias), and biases resulting from the misclassification of these study subjects with respect to exposure or disease (information bias).

Confounding

Confounding occurs when the exposed and nonexposed groups (in the source population) are not comparable due to inherent differences in background disease risk, usually due to exposure to other risk factors. Similar problems can occur in randomized trials in that randomization is not always successful and the groups to be compared may have different characteristics (and different baseline disease risk) at the time that they enter the study. However, there is more concern about noncomparability in epidemiological studies because of the absence of randomization.

Confounding can be controlled in the study design, or in the analysis, or both. Control in the analysis involves stratifying the data into subgroups according to the levels of the confounder(s) and calculating a summary effect estimate that summarizes the information across strata. For example, in a study of environmental tobacco smoke (ETS) exposure and lung cancer, we might compare the risk of lung cancer in people exposed and people not exposed to ETS. We might make this comparison within five different age groups and in men and women, yielding ten (5×2) different comparisons; for each stratum, we would calculate the relative risk of lung cancer in those exposed to ETS, compared with those not exposed, and we would then average these relative risks across the strata, giving more weight to strata with larger numbers of people (and lung cancer cases).

Selection Bias

Whereas confounding generally involves biases inherent in the source population, selection bias involves biases arising from the procedures by which the study subjects are chosen from the source population. Thus, selection bias is not usually an issue in a cohort study involving an internal reference population and with complete follow-up, since this incorporates all of the available information from the source population. Selection bias is of more concern in case–control studies since these involve sampling from the source population. In particular, selection bias can occur in a case–control study if controls are chosen in a nonrepresentative manner, e.g., if exposed people were more likely to be selected as controls than nonexposed people.

Information Bias

Information bias involves misclassification of the study subjects with respect to disease or exposure status. Thus, the concept of information bias refers to those people actually included in the study (whereas selection bias refers to the selection of the study subjects from the source population, and confounding generally refers to noncomparability within the source population).

Nondifferential information bias occurs when the likelihood of misclassification of exposure is the same for diseased and nondiseased persons (or when the likelihood of misclassification of disease is the same for exposed and nonexposed persons). Nondifferential misclassification of exposure generally biases the effect estimate toward the null value. Thus, it tends to produce false-negative findings and is of particular concern in studies that find no association between exposure and disease (although it should be emphasized that nondifferential misclassification of a confounder can lead to bias away from the null if the confounder produces confounding towards the null).

Differential information bias occurs when the likelihood of misclassification of exposure is different in diseased and nondiseased persons (or the likelihood of misclassification of disease is different in exposed and nonexposed persons). This can bias the observed effect estimate in either direction, either toward or away from the null value. For example, in a lung cancer case–control study, the recall of exposures (such as pesticide exposure) in healthy controls might be different from that of cases with lung cancer. In this situation, differential information bias would occur, and it could bias the odds ratio toward or away from the null, depending on whether cases were more or less likely to recall previous exposures than controls.

As a general principle, it is important to ensure that the misclassification is nondifferential, by ensuring that exposure information is collected in an identical manner in diseased and nondiseased (and that disease information is collected in an identical manner in the exposed and nonexposed groups). In this situation, the bias is in a known direction (toward the null), and although there may be concern that negative findings may be due to nondifferential information bias, at least one can be confident that any positive findings are not due to information bias.

Interpretation of Environmental and Occupational Epidemiology Studies

The first task in interpreting the findings of an epidemiological study is to assess the likelihood that the study findings represent a real association, or whether they may be due to various biases (confounding, selection bias, information bias) or chance. If it is concluded that the observed associations are likely to be real, then attention shifts to more general causal inference, which should be based on all available information, rather than on the findings of a single study. A systematic approach to causal inference was elaborated by Bradford Hill (1965) and has since been widely used and adapted.

The temporal relationship is crucial; the cause must precede the effect. This is usually self-evident, but difficulties may arise in studies (usually case–control or cross-sectional studies) when measurements of exposure and effect are made at the same time (e.g., by questionnaire, blood tests, etc.).

An association is plausible if it is consistent with other knowledge. For instance, laboratory experiments may have shown that a particular environmental exposure can cause cancer in laboratory animals, and this would make more plausible the hypothesis that this exposure could cause cancer in humans. However, biological plausibility is a relative concept; many epidemiological associations were considered implausible when they were first discovered but were subsequently confirmed in experimental studies. Lack of plausibility may simply reflect current lack of medical knowledge.

Consistency is demonstrated by several studies giving the same result. This is particularly important when a variety of designs are used in different settings, since the likelihood that all studies are making the same mistake is thereby minimized. However, a lack of consistency does not exclude a causal association, because different exposure levels and other conditions may reduce the impact of exposure in certain studies.

The strength of association is important in that a strongly elevated relative risk is more likely to be causal than a weak association, which could be influenced by confounding or other biases. However, the fact that an association is weak does not preclude it from being causal; rather it means that it is more difficult to exclude alternative explanations.

A dose–response relationship occurs when changes in the level of exposure are associated with changes in the prevalence or incidence of the effect. The demonstration of a clear dose–response relationship provides strong evidence for a causal relationship, since it is unlikely that a consistent dose–response relationship would be produced by confounding.

Reversibility is also relevant in that when the removal of a possible cause results in a reduced disease risk, the likelihood of the association being causal is strengthened.

Of these criteria for causal inference, only the criterion of temporality is a necessary criterion for establishing causality, in that if the cause does not precede the effect then the association must not be causal. Furthermore, none of these criteria, either individually or collectively, is sufficient to establish causality with certainty, but causality may be assumed to have been established beyond reasonable doubt if these criteria are substantially met.

Acknowledgments

The Centre for Public Health Research is supported by a Programme Grant from the Health Research Council (HRC) of New Zealand. Jeroen Douwes is supported by an HRC-funded Sir Charles Hercus Fellowship.

See also: Demography, Epidemiology and Public Health; Social Epidemiology.

Citations

Bertazzi PA, Consonni D, Bachetti S, *et al.* (2001) Health effects of dioxin exposure: A 20-year mortality study. *American Journal of Epidemiology* 153: 1031–1044.

Boleij JSM, Buringh E, Heederik D, *et al.* (1995) *Occupational Hygiene of Chemical and Biological Agents.* Amsterdam, the Netherlands: Elsevier.

Checkoway H, Pearce N, and Kriebel D (2004) *Research Methods in Occupational Epidemiology.* New York: Oxford University Press.

Driscoll T, Mannetje A, Dryson E, *et al.* (2004) *The Burden of Occupational Disease and Injury in New Zealand: Technical Report.* Wellington, New Zealand: NOHSAC, 2004.

Ehrlich R, Robins T, Jordaan E, *et al.* (1998) Lead absorption and renal dysfunction in a South African battery factory. *Occupational and Environmental Medicine* 55: 453–460.

Gaertner RRW, Trpeski L, and Johnson KC (2004) A case–control study of occupational risk factors for bladder cancer in Canada. *Cancer Causes & Control* 15: 1007–1019.

Garcia AM, Fletcher T, Benavides FG, *et al.* (1999) Parental agricultural work and selected congenital malformations. *American Journal of Epidemiology* 149: 64–74.

Hill AB (1965) The environment and disease: Association or CAusation? *Proceedings of the Royal Society of Medicine* 58: 295–300.

Pearce N and Woodward A (2004) Environmental epidemiology. In: Cameron S, Cromar N and Fallowfield H (eds.) *Environmental Health in Australia and New Zealand*, pp. 3–19. Sydney, Australia: Oxford University Press.

Rothman KJ and Greenland S (1998) *Modern Epidemiology.* Philadelphia, PA: Lippincott-Raven.

Schulte P and Perera F (1993) *Molecular Epidemiology: Principles and Practices.* New York: Academic Press.

Steenland K and Savitz DA (eds.) (1997) *Topics in Environmental Epidemiology.* New York: Oxford University Press.

Teschke K, Olshan AF, Daniels JL, *et al.* (2002) Occupational exposure assessment in case–control studies: Opportunities for improvement'. *Occupational and Environmental Medicine* 59: 575–593.

Van Strien RT, Verhoeff AP, Brunekreef B, *et al.* (1994) Mite antigen in-house dust-relationship with different housing characteristics in the Netherlands. *Clinical and Experimental Allergy* 24: 843–853.

Woodward A, Guest C, Steer K, *et al.* (1995) Tropospheric ozone: Respiratory effects and Australian air quality goals. *Journal of Epidemiology and Community Health* 49: 401–407.

World Health Organisation (2006) *Preventing Disease Through Healthy Environments: Towards an Estimate of the Environmental Burden of Disease.* Geneva, Switzerland: WHO.

Further Reading

Armstrong B, White E, and Saracci R (1992) *Principles of Exposure Measurement in Epidemiology.* New York: Oxford University Press, 1992.

Pearce N, Beasley R, Burgess C, *et al.* (1998) *Asthma Epidemiology: Principles and Methods.* New York: Oxford University Press.

Steenland K (ed.) (1993) *Case Studies in Occupational Epidemiology.* New York: Oxford University press.

Social Epidemiology

L Myer, University of Cape Town, Cape Town, South Africa; Columbia University, New York, USA
E Susser and B Link, Columbia University, New York, NY, USA; New York State Psychiatric Institute, New York, USA
C Morroni, University of Cape Town, Cape Town, South Africa

Glossary

Discrimination The processes by which certain individuals or groups are placed at a systematic social and/or economic disadvantage on the basis of race, gender, or other characteristics.

Income inequality The degree of heterogeneity in income within a defined population, separate from the level of income in that population.

Levels of social organization The varying units of population at which the determinants of disease can be conceptualized, measured, and analyzed (e.g., individual, neighborhood, community, society).

Lifecourse approach An analytical perspective that views disease etiology as being shaped throughout an individual's lifetime rather than solely during adulthood; this includes the possibility of early life factors shaping adult health either independently or in conjunction with adult factors.

Risk factor epidemiology The paradigm of contemporary epidemiology in which determinants of disease and death are understood primarily as individual-level (rather than population-level) parameters.

Social networks The connections between individuals in a population that may influence health, for better (e.g., in providing psychological and/or material support) or worse (e.g., in facilitating communication of infectious agents and/or negative behaviors).

Socioeconomic position The economic and social situation of individuals or populations, commonly operationalized using the concepts of socioeconomic status or social class.

Introduction

Social epidemiology is the branch of epidemiology concerned with understanding how social and economic characteristics influence states of health in populations. Recently there has been a resurgence in interest among epidemiologists about the roles that social and economic factors play in determining health, leading to the recent publication of several volumes reviewing major developments in social epidemiology. This interest is by no means new: The study of socioeconomic conditions and health was a principal concern when epidemiology emerged as a formal discipline in Europe during the nineteenth century, and has remained at the forefront of thinking about population health in various quarters of the discipline since that time.

The renewed interest in social epidemiology has led to major advances in our understanding of the associations between social and economic inequalities and adverse health outcomes. There are consistent and compelling data from the United States and Europe indicating that individuals in the lowest income groups have mortality rates at least two to three times greater than those in the highest. Associations between social inequality and health have been demonstrated in prospective studies from a range of settings, and a number of distinct mechanisms have been postulated to explain the observed associations. As a result, many contemporary epidemiologists have come to recognize social inequalities, and socioeconomic position in particular, as among the most pervasive and persistent factors in determining morbidity and mortality. Though less definitive, there is also evidence to suggest that individuals with less social support suffer from greater morbidity and mortality than individuals with better developed social networks.

Along with these advances, the study of social factors and health has presented important challenges to epidemiology as a discipline. The conceptual and methodological approaches that characterize modern epidemiology are ideal for investigating causes of disease among individuals within populations. But this risk factor approach may be less well suited to research into social and economic factors – especially for understanding how factors operating at different levels of social organization influence the health of populations, or how dynamic temporal processes impact upon health across the lifecourse. Social epidemiologists are among the leaders in addressing these conceptual and methodological challenges, suggesting that social epidemiology has an important place in the future of the discipline.

History of Social and Economic Determinants Within Epidemiology

Although the term social epidemiology was coined only in 1950, observations of the association between the health of populations and their social and economic conditions can be traced back to the earliest examples of what we would today consider epidemiological thinking. As the discipline emerged formally in the nineteenth century, social factors were prominent in epidemiology's view of the determinants of population health. A brief overview of the history of social epidemiology demonstrates that although social issues ebbed from the forefront of epidemiological thinking during much of the twentieth century, their current popularity among epidemiologists is actually a rebirth of sorts.

Origins of Social Epidemiology

Early forerunners of epidemiology presented ideas that today resonate strongly with social epidemiologists, as the integrated nature of human health, lifestyle, and position within the social order lay close to the core of Western medical thinking through the late Renaissance. For example, during the late seventeenth century, Bernardino Ramazzini examined the links between particular occupations and specific health disorders. In addition to its seminal place in occupational epidemiology, his *De Morbis Artificum* (1700) may be considered among the earliest works on the link between occupational status, social position, and health.

Societal factors were prominently featured as determinants of health when epidemiology emerged as a formal discipline in Europe during the nineteenth century. In France, Louis Rene Villerme's study of mortality in Paris (1826) described the patterns of poverty and mortality across the city's wards; his finding of a continuous relationship between poverty and mortality – with poorer neighborhoods having worse health than wealthier ones across all levels of wealth – is the first evidence of the graded relationship that has since been widely documented (Kreiger, 2001). In England, William Farr analyzed the association between mortality and density of urban housing using statistical evidence; he ventured beyond basic descriptions to explore the mechanisms that may link poverty and health and how these may be intervened upon.

Social epidemiology traces a separate strand of its history to the origins of sociology in the late nineteenth century. The earliest sociologists made important contributions to thinking about how population-level characteristics could influence individual health outcomes. In *Suicide* (1897), Emile Durkheim investigated the social etiology of suicide with particular emphasis on the properties of societies that may operate independently of the characteristics of individuals within them (phenomena that he termed social facts), a topic that has received renewed interest among epidemiologists in recent years.

With the identification of infectious agents as the necessary causes of specific diseases beginning in the late nineteenth century, the focus of much of epidemiology began to shift away from societal factors. However, a number of landmark studies from this period demonstrated how socioeconomic conditions continued to act as critical determinants of population health. In their study of cotton mill workers in South Carolina during 1916–1918, Sydenstricker *et al.* (1918) developed insights into the role of family income in affecting risk of pellagra, and related this to nutrient intake rather than to the presence of an infectious agent. In their work on disease within birth cohorts, Kermack and McKendrick (1934) hypothesized the importance of early life experiences, including social class, in explaining patterns of morbidity and mortality in adulthood. The role of societal factors in mental health was a focus within sociology and related disciplines during this period, as Farris and Dunham's ecological studies of Chicago neighborhoods (1939) demonstrated that rates of hospitalization for certain mental illnesses appeared to increase with proximity to urban centers, leading to the hypothesis that social disorganization gives rise to increased risk of schizophrenia.

Socioeconomic Factors During the Modern Risk Factor Era

From the 1950s onward, the changing health profile of industrialized nations spurred a shift in the focus of mainstream epidemiology from infectious to chronic diseases. Social and economic conditions continued to receive attention during this time. The first departments of social medicine were established in Britain after World War II, as Jeremy Morris, Richard Doll, and others had begun to investigate the unequal distribution of chronic disease across social classes. It was during this period that the British 1946 National Survey of Health and Development, its sample stratified by social class, gave rise to a birth cohort that today continues to generate important insights into the perinatal and childhood determinants of adult health.

Although epidemiology was focused largely on the developed world during this time, important findings about the impact of social and economic conditions on health emerged from the developing world. In South Africa, Sidney Kark and his colleagues documented the social and economic structures that facilitated the spread of disease through impoverished populations. His *Social Pathology of Syphilis* (Kark, 1949) attributed the spread of sexually transmitted infections to migration patterns created by structural economic conditions, foreshadowing the devastating spread of the HIV/AIDS pandemic in recent times. Mervyn Susser, who was mentored by Kark, went on to join anthropologist William Watson in writing *Sociology in Medicine* (Susser *et al.*, 1962). This book drew examples from both the developing and developed worlds in investigating how the social, cultural, and economic features of populations combine to influence patterns in their health. Today, Kark and Susser are powerful influences on public health research in southern Africa, especially in the field of HIV/AIDS.

By the 1960s, the dramatic improvements in material conditions in the industrialized world, along with the establishment of national health-care systems across much of Europe, led many to believe that socioeconomic factors would become less critical in determining population health. As a result, epidemiologists, particularly in the United States, turned their attention to the role of specific behavioral and environmental factors in causing particular diseases; the archetypal work of this period was the identification of smoking as a cause of (or a risk factor for) lung cancer. Refinements over the last 50 years in epidemiological methods for the study of chronic diseases have propagated a focus on the role played by individual-level risk factors – environmental exposures, behaviors, genotypes – in disease etiology. The predominance of this risk factor approach saw less and less attention given to the study of social and economic factors in much of American epidemiology. This regression reached a low point during the 1980s, with one prominent epidemiology textbook commenting that socioeconomic position is "causally related to few if any diseases but is a correlate of many causes" (Rothman, 1986: 90).

Although social factors were generally not in the mainstream of epidemiology in the United States, the rise of the risk factor paradigm was nonetheless accompanied by several notable developments in the study of social and economic factors. Another South African and former student of Kark's, John Cassel, posited that the physiological and psychological stresses of modern society induced generalized vulnerability to disease. His seminal article, 'The contribution of the social environment to host resistance' (Cassel, 1976), did much to stimulate the modern body of work on the psychosocial mechanisms through which social and economic factors may influence health. Cassel's work, along with that of Leo Reeder, Leonard Syme, and others, blended perspectives from the social sciences with traditional epidemiology, producing work that would become the basis of the contemporary field of social epidemiology in the United States.

Recent Advances in Social Epidemiology

After a dormant period, there has been renewed interest in the influence of social and economic factors on health among epidemiologists in the United States during the last decade. This rejuvenation was sparked largely by research from Britain, where social epidemiology had remained at the forefront of public health thinking. The work of Jeremy Morris, Geoffrey Rose, and, later, Michael Marmot was crucial in demonstrating that, despite massive improvements during the second half of the twentieth century in standards of living and population health in the developed world, the social inequalities in health that had preoccupied the earliest epidemiologists a century before were still very much present.

During this recent, rapid expansion in epidemiological research on social inequalities and health, findings for the major associations linking specific socioeconomic factors with increased morbidity and mortality have been refined, and new areas of inquiry have emerged. The conceptualization and measurement of social and economic factors has evolved considerably, and in some instances, researchers have moved beyond documenting general associations toward developing testable hypotheses regarding the pathways involved. Given these far-reaching advances, a complete review of the breadth of social epidemiology is well beyond the scope of this article. Instead, we focus on three overlapping forms of social inequality that are at the heart of contemporary social epidemiology: Socioeconomic position, social networks, and discrimination; we include a discussion of the mechanisms that have been put forward by epidemiologists to explain these well-established associations.

Socioeconomic Position

The relationship between poverty and disease has been the primary focus of most contemporary social epidemiology, with considerable attention devoted to more detailed descriptions of and preliminary explanations for an association that has been noted for centuries. The general relationship is simple: There is a large body of literature that demonstrates that individuals who are of a higher socioeconomic position are generally healthier than individuals of a lower socioeconomic position. For example, Sorlie *et al.* (1995) analysis of the National Longitudinal Mortality Study, conducted in the United States between 1979 and 1989, showed that after adjusting for the effects of age, race, and education, the risk of death among men in the lowest income category was approximately three times that of men in the highest income category. However, the effect was slightly less among women.

Hundreds of studies have shown similar differences in morbidity and mortality according to absolute socioeconomic position across a range of different populations; by all historical accounts, this association has remained constant for at least several centuries, despite dramatic improvements in both population health and material wealth. This overwhelming consistency and persistence has led some researchers to comment that the association between socioeconomic position and health is the most reliable finding in all of epidemiology.

One important feature of the association between socioeconomic position and health is that it follows a clear monotonic curve. Rather than exhibiting a threshold effect, in which lower socioeconomic position is associated with poorer health only below a certain level of poverty, almost all of the available evidence indicates that lower socioeconomic position is associated with poorer health across all levels of socioeconomic position. This graded association has important implications for possible explanations of the link between socioeconomic position and health. While absolute material conditions may readily explain differences in health between the poorest and wealthiest members of a population, the factors that lead to the differences in health between the highest and second-highest socioeconomic strata are thought to be more complex.

Related to socioeconomic position, the link between occupational category and health is of particular interest in social epidemiology. Growing evidence suggests that systematic health differences exist between occupational groups, even among occupations with similar material working conditions and physical exposures, with workers of higher position generally enjoying better health. Important insights into the relationship between employment and health come from the Whitehall studies of British civil servants led by Michael Marmot and others. The original Whitehall study (Marmot *et al.*, 1984) demonstrated that the lowest grade of civil servants had approximately three times the risk of death compared to the highest grade (**Figure 1**).

This gradient was also apparent for cause-specific mortality and was explained only in part by traditional risk factors such as smoking, blood pressure, and plasma cholesterol. The second Whitehall study has suggested that occupational factors such as low job control are substantial predictors of the increased risk of coronary heart disease, stronger predictors, in fact, than many traditional coronary risk factors. The Whitehall studies are unique in that marked gradations in health are apparent within a relatively homogeneous population of office workers, suggesting that occupational and socioeconomic factors may impact health even within groups that are not exposed to material poverty.

Measurement of socioeconomic position and health outcomes

A wide array of measures of socioeconomic position has been employed by sociologists and epidemiologists, and underlying this are a number of different ways to conceptualize socioeconomic stratification. Among the many different approaches that have been used, a loose distinction can be drawn between approaches based on social class and those based on socioeconomic status.

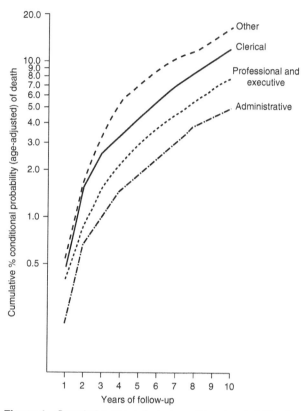

Figure 1 Cumulative age-adjusted conditional probability of death from all causes over 10 years, among British civil servants screened between 1967 and 1969. Adapted from Marmot MG, Shipley MJ, Rose G. Inequalities in death–specific explanations of a general pattern? *Lancet* 1984; 1(8384): 1003–1006.

The social class approach generally sees individuals as operating in different formal roles within a structured society, and these roles are reflected by well-defined class measures that tend to be categorical in nature and focus on the relation to means of economic production. To measure social class, preexisting occupational categories are commonly used, ranging from simple distinction between manual and nonmanual employment to complex class measures developed to facilitate international comparisons. Measurements based on socioeconomic status seek to incorporate several different dimensions of an individual's position within society; the most common measures focus on individual income (representing economic status), education (representing social status), and occupation (representing work prestige) as indicators of socioeconomic position. These three domains overlap substantially, and in many instances, one measure is used as a proxy for a broader construct of socioeconomic status.

In addition to variations in the conceptualization of socioeconomic position, the measures employed by epidemiologists are often adapted to the particular contexts of a given study population, with different measures considered more or less appropriate in specific settings.

One important example of this is the measurement of the assets of an individual or household, including resources owned (such as a television or refrigerator) or accessed (such as bank accounts). Households' assets may be summarized to form an asset index that provides a robust measure of wealth that is commonly used in developing country settings and for cross-country research (for instance, in Demographic and Health Surveys). The range of constructs and measurements used may also result from researchers' use of data collected for another purpose, limiting the ability to develop the most appropriate measurements of the construct of interest. Further, the diversity of measurements reflects the increasing complexity of the constructs themselves; as social and economic positioning in contemporary societies grows more intricate and dynamic, researchers develop new measures to adapt to this complexity. Ultimately, measures of socioeconomic position strike a balance between the data that are available, the most appropriate measures for the population under study, and investigators' underlying conceptualization of socioeconomic position.

A diverse set of health outcomes has been associated with socioeconomic position. Mortality is the most commonly used outcome; all-cause mortality is a robust indicator of health that is unlikely to be subject to some of the biases that may threaten the validity of epidemiologic studies. In addition, the association between socioeconomic position and cause-specific mortality and morbidity has been studied in detail for almost every class of disease. In some instances, the association has been extended to measures of subclinical disease, most notably for psychiatric and cardiovascular outcomes. Socioeconomic position has also been shown to be linked to negative health outcomes during pregnancy and infancy, as well as among the elderly, and the associations have also been documented using measures of physical disability and self-reported health.

It is important to note that there are variations in the association between socioeconomic position and particular health outcomes, including a handful of situations where particular diseases may appear more common among individuals of higher socioeconomic position. But despite these variations, the vast majority of the evidence points to parallel gradients of multiple measures of socioeconomic position and a range of adverse health outcomes. The strength and consistency of the overall association across this diversity of measures provides important evidence for the veracity of the overall effect.

Income inequality

A widely debated insight from the study of socioeconomic stratification and health is the possible role of the distribution of wealth within a population as a determinant of that population's health. Several researchers have used data from ecological studies (in which nations, counties, or other population groupings are the unit of analysis) to suggest that societies with less equitable distributions of wealth tend to be of poorer health, independent of the absolute wealth of the population, which is itself strongly linked to the health of populations. Richard Wilkinson's studies of the correlation between income inequality within industrialized nations and mortality rates (Wilkinson, 1996) are perhaps the most widely known example of this approach. Other researchers have investigated the association of income inequality and health in different settings using different units of population with mixed results. The most compelling support for the association between income inequality and health comes from analyses of income distribution and mortality among states and counties and cities within the Unites States (Lynch et al., 1998).

As with socioeconomic status in general, a number of measures have been used to gauge income inequality. The most common include the Gini coefficient (a unitless measure of the degree of income inequality in the population) and the Robin Hood Index (the proportion of all income that must be moved from the wealthiest households to the poorest in order to achieve perfect income equality); generally, these measures of income are highly correlated and do not generate substantially different results.

Part of the association between income inequality and health outcomes is accounted for by absolute income: Levels of absolute poverty are typically greater in societies with greater imbalances in income distribution. However, several studies have suggested that the association between income inequality and health persists after adjustment for individual-level income. It is important to note that, compared to the effects of socioeconomic position on health status, the impact of income inequality appears to be relatively small. Nonetheless, the study of income inequality and health is an important avenue of inquiry within social epidemiology, including research into social capital and the psychosocial impacts of socioeconomic conditions on health.

Explanations for the General Association

One of the principal challenges encountered by epidemiologists studying social and economic inequalities over the past 20 years has been to explain the observed links between socioeconomic inequalities, and socioeconomic position in particular, and health. Which pathways may account for the general association is much debated. Here we review the possibility of spurious relationships and then discuss three of the most prominent explanations.

In the first place, the observed associations may not be causal in nature. For example, some third variable or variables may confound the associations documented between various social inequalities and health. It is unclear, however, which factors could account for these associations across the range of exposure measures, health outcomes, geographic settings, and historical periods in which they have been demonstrated. Moreover, in most studies that adjust for numerous confounding variables, these associations persist. Another possible alternative explanation is that the observed associations are driven by social selection rather than causation: Morbidity leads to reduced socioeconomic position, rather than the other way around. While this may be particularly relevant for chronic illnesses or those with sustained subclinical forms, this explanation is rendered implausible by numerous prospective studies that examine social and/or economic conditions prior to the onset of disease (or death). Although it is important to recognize the potential for alternative explanations in evaluating the results of every study, neither confounding nor reverse causation appears capable of explaining the body of evidence linking socioeconomic position and health.

One common explanation for the association is that the increased frequency of particular individual-level risk factors in settings of low socioeconomic position, most notably behaviors and environmental exposures, leads to increased risk of disease and death. High-risk behaviors – such as smoking, poor diet, reduced physical activity, and increased alcohol consumption – frequently appear more common among poorer individuals. Indeed, in many settings, the pervasiveness of these lifestyle factors may lead to them being considered normative. Similarly, in many cases poorer communities are more commonly exposed to environmental agents involved in the etiology of particular diseases. But while high-risk behaviors and environmental exposures are important determinants of health, and are often strongly correlated with socioeconomic position, it seems unlikely that individual behaviors can adequately explain the observed associations between social inequalities and health. Empirically, the associations between social inequalities and health typically persist even after accounting for an array of individual-level behavioral risk factors, a finding that is seen most clearly in the Whitehall studies (discussed in the section titled 'Socioeconomic position'). An explanatory approach focused solely on individual behavior neglects the impact of social contexts on individual health and does account for the role that economic conditions may play in creating the material circumstances that shape individual action.

Looking beyond such explanations, several researchers have suggested that socioeconomic inequalities give rise to increased psychosocial stress, which induces increased physiological responses, which then contribute to poorer health. This line of thinking emphasizes the relative position of individuals within socioeconomic hierarchies as distinct from their absolute wealth or poverty. The epidemiological data supporting this mechanism is drawn from the ecological studies of income inequality and individual-level studies of relative socioeconomic position (such as the Whitehall studies) discussed in the section titled 'Socioeconomic position,' both of which suggest that location within a socioeconomic hierarchy makes an important contribution to health status. Based on this evidence, Wilkinson (1996) and others have hypothesized that perceptions of relative inequality increase psychosocial stress, which may affect physical health via various neuroendocrine mechanisms (sometimes referred to as allostatic load); individuals positioned lower in the hierarchy suffer greater psychosocial stress, leading to increased morbidity and mortality. This theory is supported by studies of nonhuman primates, suggesting that even when material and lifestyle factors are controlled in an experimental setting, individuals positioned lower in the hierarchy experience worse health. Although it represents an important avenue for future exploration, it is still unclear whether the etiological mechanisms related to psychosocial stress are important mediators of the effect of social inequalities.

A third set of approaches to explaining the observed association between socioeconomic inequalities and health emphasizes absolute socioeconomic position, and how this relates to the material conditions of individuals and populations. At the individual level, higher socioeconomic position (for instance, greater individual income) is important in reducing diverse risks associated with numerous adverse health outcomes. For example, increased socioeconomic position affords access to healthy diets, improved health care (including preventive health care, such as screening programs), better working conditions, and leisure time that may be used for exercise or relaxation. In addition to the individualistic effects of socioeconomic position on health, there are also contextual benefits associated with higher socioeconomic position that operate at the community- or population-level, such as improved public services and reduced community crime. The mechanisms that may be included here are diverse, from psychosocial elements, such as quality of residential life, to more traditional exposures, such as environmental toxins.

In understanding how absolute socioeconomic position and related material conditions may affect health, Link and Phelan (1995) have introduced the concept of socioeconomic status as a fundamental cause of adverse health outcomes. Citing the durability of the association of socioeconomic position and health through time despite radical changes in the health of populations and the major causes of disease, this explanation suggests that socioeconomic position embodies an array of material and social resources that could be employed in a range of manners and settings to avoid risks of morbidity and mortality. Despite changing health threats and the emergence of new health technologies, individuals of greater socioeconomic status are consistently better positioned to avoid risk factors for disease – both in terms of behaviors and environmental exposures – and receive better health care once disease occurs. The fundamental cause concept cuts across disease categories and may encompass a diverse range of potential pathways, including the behavioral and psychosocial explanations discussed above.

Social Connections

The way in which social connections and support systems affect health is a major avenue of inquiry within social epidemiology. The findings here are more varied, and perhaps more subtle, than in the case of socioeconomic position (where the general association is well-established); the precise nature of the association depends heavily on the social connections measured, the societal contexts of the populations studied, and the health outcomes involved. And while many social epidemiologists have focused on the positive impacts that increased social connections may confer on health status, the associations here appear to be far more complex than that.

A series of prospective studies conducted in the last 25 years have provided strong evidence that better developed social networks are associated with reduced all-cause mortality. Perhaps the best known of these is the Alameda County study of Berkman and Syme (1979). Between 1965 and 1974, individuals with reduced social integration (based on marital status, community group membership, and contacts with family and friends) were two to three times more likely to die than individuals with increased social integration; this association persisted after adjustment for various self-reported high-risk health behaviors. In a second landmark survey, House (1982) used composite measures of social relationships to show that individuals with reduced social ties when interviewed in the late 1960s were about twice as likely to die over the next 12 years, compared to individuals with increased social ties. Adjustment for biological health measures at baseline, including blood pressure, cholesterol, electrocardiogram results, and lung function, did not dispel this association. Similar results have been found in a number of other prospective studies from Europe, the United States, and Japan, despite the markedly different populations, background mortality rates, and causes of death across these studies (**Figures 2** and **3**).

In addition, more recent studies have shown that a paucity of social connections is associated with increased mortality from a range of specific causes, most notably cardiovascular disease and stroke. To quantify social networks and connections, a wide range of measures have been employed; some approaches have proved to be more broadly applicable than others. Given the highly context-specific nature of social ties, it is unlikely that any one set of measures can be employed universally across all research settings.

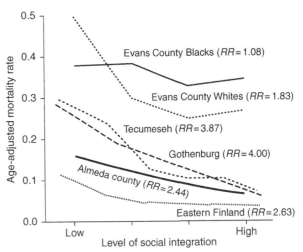

Figure 2 Level of social integration and age-adjusted mortality for males in five prospective studies: Relative risks of mortality at the lowest versus highest level of social integration. Reproduced from House JS, Landis KR, and Umberson D (1988) Social relationships and health. *Science* 241: 540–545. With permission from AAAS.

Although this evidence is highly suggestive of positive health benefits for social connectedness, several important questions of interpretation remain. In many instances, it is unclear whether the presence of strong social networks acts to prevent the onset of disease or to improve survival after onset. Typically the association appears to be stronger in men than in women and to vary according to urban or rural location. Moreover, exactly which aspects of social networks might confer health benefits is much debated. Psychosocial support, possibly conferring a reduction in the impact of stressful life events, has been the most widely discussed mechanism. Other potential pathways through which social networks lead to improved health status may include enhanced social influence and agency to prevent or treat illness, increased social stimulation and interaction, and/or increased access to material assistance in times of need.

Related to the research at the individual level into the positive impacts of social networks on health is a diverse body of work on how the collective social characteristics of a population (rather than the social characteristics of individuals within the population) impact on health. These group properties are sometimes referred to as social capital: "the ability to secure benefits through membership in networks and other social structures" (Portes, 1998: 8). While the term social capital is deployed in varying ways (and is by no means limited to public health), in the last few years, research findings have emerged that demonstrate a connection between the degree of social integration or cohesion that characterizes communities and the health of those communities. Kawachi and colleagues (1997) demonstrated that age-adjusted

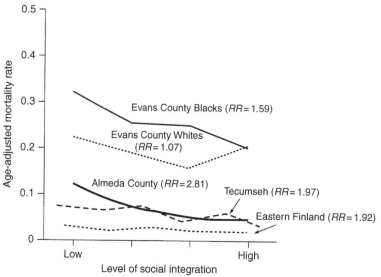

Figure 3 Level of social integration and age-adjusted mortality for females in five prospective studies: Relative risks of mortality at the lowest versus highest level of social integration. Reproduced from House JS, Landis KR, and Umberson D (1988) Social relationships and health. *Science* 241: 540–545. With permission from AAAS.

mortality rates among U.S. states were strongly correlated with measures of membership in voluntary civic groups, with perceptions of reciprocity in the community, and with perceptions of trust. The inverse relationship between mortality and perceptions of social trust – measured by the percentage of individuals surveyed who agreed that "most people would try to take advantage of you if they got the chance" – is among the most striking findings indicating that mortality is highest where there is little or no trust (or reciprocity) and vice versa.

Several studies have found that various measures related to the concept of social capital appear inversely related to income inequality, suggesting that decreased social capital may represent a pathway through which the unequal distribution of income influences health. However, it remains unclear whether group-level associations between social capital and population health are mediated by individual-level social connections.

As discussed here, social epidemiologists have focused primarily on the protective effects that social networks may have on health. However, it is important to note that social networks can have significant negative impacts on health, such as when networks promote exposure to infectious agents or high-risk behaviors (or both). Much of our understanding of the way in which social networks may have detrimental effects on the health of populations comes from the mathematical modeling of the spread of disease within populations. Social epidemiology and mathematical modeling have started to converge only recently; the confluence of these approaches to social networks and health, coupling the direct measurement of networks and individuals' positions within them along with the modeling of disease transmission within populations holds promise for the future.

Discrimination

The body of epidemiological research into the health disparities between different racial or ethnic groups has grown considerably in the past decade, providing powerful evidence that mortality rates within the United States are higher among African-Americans and other minority groups, relative to the general population. In one of the best-known analyses of race and health, McCord and Freeman (1990) showed that age-standardized death rates in Harlem (a predominantly African-American community in New York City) were more than twice that of Whites living in the United States. This finding was confirmed by the National Longitudinal Mortality Survey, which showed that mortality rates among African-Americans were appreciably higher than among Whites, despite statistical adjustment for employment, income, education, marital status, and household size; the differences are particularly pronounced among younger age groups. In addition to findings for mortality differences, similar associations have been demonstrated for a number of adverse health outcomes, including hypertension and cardiovascular disease as well as infant mortality and low birth weight. As in the case of the association between ethnicity and mortality, these disease-specific associations typically persist after adjustment for multiple indicators of socioeconomic position.

While differences in morbidity and mortality among ethnic groups are widely acknowledged, the explanations for these differences are far more contentious. Some researchers have argued that ethnic differences in health are due to genetic predispositions, but there is little evidence for this in any but a handful of conditions.

Others have pointed to shortcomings in epidemiological methods, suggesting that much of the observed association between race and health may result from the mismeasurement of, and subsequent inadequate statistical adjustment for, the effect of socioeconomic status on health. While this explanation may be plausible in some instances, the ubiquity of ethnic differences in health within socioeconomic strata as well as across time and place point to an independent association.

In explaining these differences in morbidity and mortality, Sherman James (1987), Nancy Krieger (1999) and others have taken a broader view of racial differences in health and posited ethnic discrimination (i.e., racism), rather than ethnicity itself, as the principal factor responsible for the observed associations between race and health. In this light, socioeconomic differentials may be part of the pathway through which racial discrimination affects health, rather than a confounder to be adjusted for in analysis.

Systematic discrimination and historical inequalities could act in several ways. Reduced access to and quality of health care are commonly cited explanations for the association between minority status and increased morbidity and mortality, particularly in the United States. Other mechanisms may include the increased stress and psychosocial burden associated with discrimination, as well as the reduced access to material resources among most minority groups. As epidemiological research into ethnic disparities in health expands, it is clear that the general association between racial categories and adverse health outcomes can provide only indirect evidence of the effects of racial discrimination. Further refinements in the conceptualization and measurement of discrimination are required to promote our understanding of the association between ethnicity and health.

Emerging Concepts Within Social Epidemiology

The recent advances within social epidemiology have been paralleled by a more general series of commentaries on epidemiological approaches under the risk factor paradigm. These critiques have focused primarily on the perceived preoccupation of contemporary epidemiology with how individual-level factors shape health and the subsequent difficulties epidemiologists face in researching determinants of health that are not easily reduced to individual-level terms (Schwartz et al., 1999). Although these commentaries refer to epidemiology as a discipline, they are especially relevant to, and have been motivated in part by, the study of social and economic inequalities. Here we focus on two particular areas of critique and the advances which have emerged from them: Levels of social organization and the diachronic processes shaping individual and population health.

Levels of Social Organization

Several commentaries have suggested that contemporary epidemiology is focused too much on etiologic factors that operate among individuals and too little on other, potentially relevant levels of social or biological organization. With respect to social epidemiology, this criticism challenges the focus on social and economic variables that are conceptualized and measured at the individual level (e.g., individual income or education). While important, this focus fails to account for the possibility that social inequalities operating at other levels of organization – such as the neighborhood, society, or even globally – may be of relevance in shaping health, separate from their individual-level counterparts. Different levels of social organization are often implicit within social epidemiological research, but most studies fail to specify the level(s) that are involved in conceptualizing and analyzing social inequalities. For instance, measures of average community income (e.g., income per capita) may be employed in some studies as a proxy for individual-level incomes within communities; in this case, a group-level variable is being used to capture an individual-level construct. Yet in other instances, the same measure of community income may be intended to reflect aspects of the wealth of the community – such as infrastructure development – that are distinct from (but may be related to) the individual-level measure of income. Other concepts in social epidemiology, such as social capital or income inequality, are inherently features of groups. In recognizing the different levels of social organization that are involved in their hypotheses and measurements, social epidemiologists are beginning to develop a framework for thinking about how social and economic characteristics of individuals, communities, and/ or societies may each contribute to health in unique ways; this line of thinking provides a more complex – and more fertile – conceptual approach than analyses focused exclusively at the individual level.

The ability to think across levels of social organization greatly expands epidemiologists' potential for understanding the determinants of individual and population health. For example, the course and outcome of schizophrenia varies markedly between developed and developing countries, with the disease appearing more benign (on average) in developing country settings. If the factors impacting the outcome of schizophrenia are viewed solely as the characteristics of individuals, this fact appears counterintuitive, as modern treatments with demonstrated efficacy are much more widely available in the developed world. In explaining this difference, epidemiologists have turned to the possibility that social and economic processes may help lead to improved schizophrenia outcomes in developing-country settings.

Considering the causes of disease operating across different levels of organization raises the possibility that groups may have features, beyond the aggregated characteristics of individuals within them, that can shape health outcomes, a phenomenon frequently referred to as emergent group properties. The ability to conceptualize social and economic factors as group properties that cannot be understood solely as individual-level variables represents an important vehicle for social epidemiologists. In a seminal paper, Sampson (1997) and colleagues demonstrated that the social features of Chicago neighborhoods helped to explain levels of violent crime, independent of the characteristics of the individuals living within them. In a similar vein, a growing number of epidemiological studies are investigating how the characteristics of particular social environments influence health outcomes independent of the characteristics of individuals living in those locations. Diez Roux (2001) demonstrated that the socioeconomic environment of neighborhoods was associated with substantially increased risk of both coronary heart disease and coronary events, even after statistical adjustment for individual-level socioeconomic status, smoking, blood pressure, and cholesterol levels. In the Alameda County study, Yen and Kaplan (1999) defined local social environments using area measures of socioeconomic status, the presence of commercial stores, and the condition of housing and the physical environment. They demonstrated that all-cause mortality and self-reported health status were associated with each of these parameters independently of individual-level risk factors. These and other studies have helped to show that communities or neighborhoods frequently encapsulate a range of structural properties that may influence health; however, researchers are only beginning to shed light on

how this is so, and approaches to understand these associations between social areas and health are at the cutting edge of social epidemiology.

Perhaps the most compelling evidence for the determination of health and disease at different levels of social organization comes from the global view of morbidity and mortality. As presented above, the bulk of epidemiologic research into socioeconomic position and health has focused within populations, and particularly within industrialized nations. While this approach has generated important insights, social epidemiology has largely ignored the global inequities that clearly demonstrate the effects of poverty on health (**Figure 4**).

As these inequalities in global health gain increasing political and economic attention, the need to better understand – and begin to address – them presents a central challenge to epidemiology. For social epidemiologists, this means moving beyond the simple characterization of individual-level exposure and outcome variables, toward incorporating varying units of social organization into research to understand the social and economic properties of communities, nations, and continents that help to determine morbidity and mortality.

Diachronic Processes

In parallel with the difficulties in recognizing various levels of social organization, epidemiology as a discipline has been challenged to understand how processes operating through time – historical and individual – shape the disease experience of populations and individuals. With respect to social epidemiology, this critique challenges the dominant

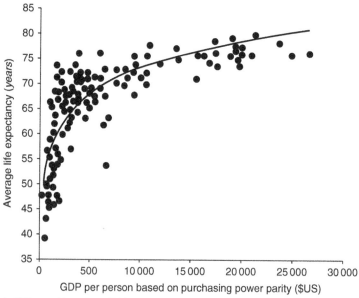

Figure 4   Life expectancy in 155 countries, circa 1993, and gross domestic product (GDP) per person in US dollars (adjusted for purchasing power parity). Adapted from Lynch JW, Smith GD, Kaplan GA, and House JS (2000) Income inequality and mortality: Importance to health of individual income, psychosocial environment, or material conditions. *British Medical Journal* 320 (7243): 1200–1204.

focus on social and economic factors, which are treated as static phenomena that are temporally proximate to disease, with researchers viewing social inequalities during adulthood as being of primary concern in understanding the causes of adult disease and death. There has been relatively little attention paid until recently to how social and economic forces at play earlier in life may shape later risk of morbidity and mortality.

In addressing this critique, epidemiologists are focusing increasingly on the potential impact of socioeconomic conditions in early-life on disease during adulthood. Cohorts in Britain and the United States have demonstrated links between social class at different stages of the lifecourse and adult mortality, as well as with a number of markers for cardiovascular disease. In some instances, these associations persist after accounting for adult socioeconomic position, though given the clear links between childhood and adult socioeconomic position, the appropriateness of traditional statistical adjustment for adult socioeconomic circumstances remains unclear. Debate as to how these effects may operate is considerable. Several researchers have suggested that insults during critical periods in early life initiate physiological processes culminating in later morbidity. Others have hypothesized that early life experiences help to shape adult circumstances, but do not have an independent impact on health outcomes. Bridging these views, Davey Smith and others have proposed a lifecourse approach, in which disadvantage in early life sets in motion a cascade of subsequent experiences that accumulate over time to produce disease in adulthood. To date, evidence exists to support each of these hypotheses. To discriminate between them, new conceptual and analytical approaches will be required.

Although social epidemiology is gradually rediscovering the importance of diachronic perspectives, psychiatric epidemiologists have made important advances in understanding the determinants of health operating over the lifecourse. For instance, there is a growing body of evidence to show that developmental antecedents in early childhood are strongly associated with a range of subsequent psychiatric symptoms. By developing testable hypotheses of the mechanisms that may mediate such associations, Sheppard Kellam (1997), Jane Costello, and others have advanced our understanding of how social contexts in early life shape later behaviors. In doing so, this body of research presents a useful model for social epidemiologists to explore how social contexts throughout the lifecourse may impact a range of health outcomes.

Conclusion

A diverse body of epidemiologic evidence leaves little doubt that economic and social inequalities are strong and consistent determinants of morbidity and mortality.

Recent advances have improved our understanding of the pathways through which these parameters affect health and refined how these inequalities are conceptualized and measured. As the full implications of the notion that human beings and their health states are constituted in both biological and social terms become more widely acknowledged within epidemiology, social epidemiology is likely to become an increasingly integral aspect of the broader discipline. The perspectives that social epidemiology brings to the study of the determinants of individual and population health are likely to continue to shape both the way in which epidemiology conceptualizes the causes of disease and how epidemiologists respond in practice to public health concerns.

See also: Cultural Epidemiology; History of Epidemiology.

Citations

Berkman LF and Syme SL (1979) Social networks, host resistance, and mortality: A nine-year follow-up study of Alameda County residents. *American Journal of Epidemiology* 109: 186–204.

Cassel J (1976) The contribution of the social environment to host resistance: The Fourth Wade Hampton Frost Lecture. *American Journal of Epidemiology* 104: 107–123.

Diez Roux AV, Merkin SS, Arnett D, *et al.* (2001) Neighborhood of residence and incidence of coronary heart disease. *New England Journal of Medicine* 345: 99–106.

Durkheim E (1951 [1897]) *Suicide: A Study in Sociology.* New York: The Free Press.

Farris RE and Dunham HW (1939) *Mental Disorders in Urban Areas.* Chicago, IL: University of Chicago Press.

House JS, Landis KR, and Umberson D (1988) Social relationships and health. *Science* 241: 540–545.

House JS, Robbins C, and Metzner HL (1982) The association of social relationships and activities with mortality: prospective evidence from the Tecumseh Community Health Study. *American Journal of Epidemiology* 116: 123–140.

James SA, Strogatz DS, Wing SB, and Ramsey DL (1987) Socioeconomic status, John Henryism, and hypertension in blacks and whites. *American Journal of Epidemiology* 126: 664–673.

Kark SL (1949) The social pathology of syphilis in Africans. *South African Medical Journal* 23: 77–84.

Kawachi I, Kennedy BP, Lochner K, and Prothrow-Stith D (1997) Social capital, income inequality, and mortality. *American Journal of Public Health* 87(9): 1491–1498.

Kellam SG and Van Horn YV (1997) Life course development, community epidemiology, and preventive trials: a scientific structure for prevention research. *American Journal of Community Psychology* 25: 177–188.

Kermack O, McKendrick AG, and McKinlay PL (1934) Death-rates in Great Britain and Sweden. Some general regularities and their significance. *Lancet* i: 698–703.

Krieger N (1999) Embodying inequality: a review of concepts, measures, and methods for studying health consequences of discrimination. *International Journal of the Health Services* 29: 295–352.

Krieger N (2001) Historical roots of social epidemiology: socioeconomic gradients in health and contextual analysis. *International Journal of Epidemiology* 30: 899–900.

Link BG and Phelan J (1995) Social conditions as fundamental causes of disease. *Journal of Health and Social Behavior* special issue, 80–94.

Lynch JW, Kaplan GA, Pamuk ER, *et al.* (1998) Income inequality and mortality in metropolitan areas of the United States. *American Journal of Public Health* 88(7): 1074–1080.

Lynch JW, Smith GD, Kaplan GA, and House JS (2000) Income inequality and mortality: Importance to health of individual income, psychosocial environment, or material conditions. *British Medical Journal* 320(7243): 1200–1204.

Marmot MG, Shipley MJ, and Rose G (1984) Inequalities in death–specific explanations of a general pattern? *Lancet* 1: 1003–1006.

McCord C and Freeman HP (1990) Excess mortality in Harlem. *New England Journal of Medicine* 322: 123–127.

Portes A (1998) Social capital: Its origins and applications in modern sociology. *Annual Review of Sociology* 24: 1–24.

Ramazzini B (1940 [original, 1700]) *De morbis artificum Bernardini Ramazzini diatriba, Diseases of workers: the Latin text of 1713 revised, with translation and notes.* Chicago, IL: University of Chicago Press.

Rothman K (1986) *Modern Epidemiology,* 1st edition. Philadelphia, PA: Lippincott Williams & Wilkins.

Rothman KJ (1986) *Modern Epidemiology.* Boston, MA: Little Brown and Company.

Sampson RJ, Raudenbush SW, and Earls F (1997) Neighborhoods and violent crime: a multilevel study of collective efficacy. *Science* 277: 918–924.

Schwartz S, Susser E, and Susser M (1999) A future for epidemiology? *Annual Review of Public Health* 20: 15–33.

Sorlie PD, Backlund E, and Keller JB (1995) US mortality by economic, demographic, and social characteristics: The National Longitudinal Mortality Study. *American Journal of Public Health* 85: 949–956.

Susser M, Watson W, and Hopper K (1985) *Sociology in Medicine,* 3rd edn. New York: Oxford University Press.

Sydenstricker E, Wheeler GA, and Goldberger J (1918) Disabling sickness among the population of seven cotton-mill villages of South Carolina in relation to family income. *Public Health Reports* 33: 2038–2051.

Villermé LR (1826) Rapport fait par M Villermé, et lu à l'Académie royal de Médicine, au nom de la Commission de statistique, sur une série de tableaux relatifs au mouvement de la population dans les douze arrondissements municipaux de la ville de Paris, pendant les cinq années 1817, 1818, 1819, 1820 et 1821. *Archives Générales de Médicine* 10: 216–247.

Wilkinson RG (1996) *Unhealthy Societies: The Afflictions of Inequality.* London: Routledge.

Yen IH and Kaplan GA (1999) Neighborhood social environment and risk of death: multilevel evidence from the Alameda County Study. *American Journal of Epidemiology* 149: 898–907.

Further Reading

Berkman LF and Kawachi I (eds.) (2000) *Social Epidemiology.* New York: Oxford University Press.

Diez Roux AV (2001) Investigating neighborhood and area effects on health. *American Journal of Public Health* 91: 1783–1789.

Evans RG, Barer ML, and Marmor TR (eds.) (1994) *Why Are Some People Healthy and Others Not?* New York: Aldine de Gruyter.

Krieger N (2001) A glossary for social epidemiology. *Journal of Epidemiology and Community Health* 55: 693–700.

Kuh D and Ben Shlomo Y (1997) *A Life Course Approach to Chronic Disease Epidemiology.* New York: Oxford University Press.

Leon D and Walt G (2001) *Poverty, Inequality and Health: An International Perspective.* New York: Oxford University Press.

Link BG and Phelan JC (2000) Evaluating the fundamental cause explanation for social disparities in health. In: Bird C, Conrad P and Fremont A (eds.) *The Handbook of Medical Sociology,* pp. 33–46. Upper Saddle River, NJ: Prentice Hall.

Marmot M (1999) *The Social Determinants of Health.* New York: Oxford University Press.

Myer L, Ehrlich R, and Susser ES (2004) Social epidemiology in South Africa. *Epidemiology Reviews* 26: 112–123.

Rose G (1992) *The Strategy of Preventative Medicine.* New York: Oxford University Press.

Relevant Websites

http://bmj.bmjjournals.com/cgi/collection/socioeconomic_determinants_of_health – BMJ.com Collection: Socioeconomic Determinants of Health.

http://www.macses.ucsf.edu/Default.htm – MacArthur Foundation Network on Socioeconomic Status and Health.

http://www.socialmedicine.org/ – Social Medicine Portal.

http://www.who.int/social_determinants/en/ – WHO Commission on the Social Determinants of Health.

Epidemiology of Inequity: Will Research Make a Difference?

H K Heggenhougen, Centre for International Health, University of Bergen, Norway; Department of International Health, Boston University School of Public Health, and Department of Global Health and Social Medicine, Harvard Medical School

This article is adapted from the presentation: "Research for Global Health. Can it stem the Tide of Inequity?", made to the 4th Students' Scientific Conference, Centre for International Health, University of Bergen, 13th of May 2004.

Introduction

Many are familiar with Ernest Hemingway's novel: *For Whom the Bell Tolls* and some may know the poem *Devotions Upon Emergent Occasions* written by John Donne in 1623 from which Hemingway derived his title:

> *No man is an island, entire of itself; every man is a piece of the continent, a part of the main; if a clod be washed away by the sea, Europe is the less, as well as if a promontory were, as well as if a manor of thy friends or of thine own were; any man's death diminishes me, because I am involved in mankind; and therefore never send to know for whom the bell tolls; it tolls for thee.*

This is a passionate reminder that, as human beings, we are not, or rather, we should not, be isolated individuals, selfishly greedy or alone and lost, but rather our nature, as human beings, ought to lead us to create and be a part of an inter-supportive human community by which we are connected both through care and responsibility.

Epidemiological research, including both biomedical and social determinants of health for different population groups, can guide the development process of creating such inter-supportive communities – healthier communities of equity and without poverty – the creation of which is after all the ultimate goal of all public health research.

One premise of this article is that international (global) epidemiological research is part of an overall development process, with particular attention to improving the health and general welfare of people living in poverty in different parts of the world. Equity, social justice and human rights issues are integral to this process since the degrees to which they are upheld as realities in people's lives are reflected in their epidemiology, in the patterns and prevalence of diseases. Thus, one function of epidemiology is to show this connection. Understanding, and contextualizing research in terms of these and other social (political and economic) determinants of health is paramount for formulating any effective intervention to improve health.

A further premise derives from a concern with the "so what?" question and with the importance of translating research results into policy and action. In sum, health research should be "translational". If this is done then research may reduce the modern public health plague, inequity, and the ill health which follows in its wake (Farmer, 1999; Wilkinson, 1996).

This kind of social epidemiological work has gained increasing adherents in recent decades. Yet, many, if not most, epidemiologists, and other public health researchers are against, or at best, ignore such efforts. They are deemed too broad to be meaningful, or, worse, they are opposed for taking attention and energy away from looking at immediate causes and making focused interventions which public health professionals are known to be good at (Satel and Marmor, 2001). I shall return to these conflicting perceptions of epidemiological and other public health research a little later. At this point I just wish to acknowledge this divide concerning what is an appropriate focus for epidemiological research, and to say I do not agree with Satel and Marmor (2001) and those who adhere to their position. Epidemiological efforts can make, and have made, a difference in the arena of social injustice affecting health and general human welfare as well as in reducing immediate disease risks. Further, I think it is not fruitful to present this in "either/or" terms. "Both/and" is a more productive and possible approach.

If we believe, if only partially, in the social determinants of health (Marmot, 2005), then we must focus on larger, fundamental factors as well as the more immediate ones (Link and Phelan, 1995). If we are serious about improving the health of the public we must of course carry on with the "traditional" public health research and interventions. But we must also focus and attempt to

guide social policy formulations and interventions on larger more fundamental issues. I believe such epidemiological research can make a difference.

Globalization and Its Consequences

With ever increasing globalization, including the Internet, supersonic travel and the internationally pervasive media, much of which can be seen in a positive light, in that, for example, human rights abuses and social injustices more easily come to light, the world is shrinking and we do, in many ways, live in *one* interactive world.

Unfortunately, this is only partially true. Tremendous benefits have been obtained by vast numbers of people throughout and between countries, for example, life expectancies have increased and infant mortality rates have fallen in many places, and millions now have clean water who did not have it only a few years ago. Yet, the good news is not universal. There is plenty of evidence that the theoretical concept of one inter-supportive world is flawed in practice. More and more voices – one of the most recent being that of Nelson Mandela speaking in Tromsø, Norway on June 12th, 2005 – are providing us with the "reality check" that the world really is not the mutually supportive home we would like it to be. We live in highly differentiated, local worlds both within and between countries.

While there are yet only a few who fear this may bring ruin upon us all, we all have an inkling of the fact that the benefit, or the misery, of one local world, is intimately linked with the misery or benefit of another, yet we seem to chose not to recognize *that as we rob others we unwittingly bankrupt ourselves.*

During a talk at the Harvard Medical School in 2001, Bernard Kouchner, the former French Minister of Health and founder of *Medecins sans Frontieres*, seriously asserted that the current state of intra- and international inequity (unjust inequality) affects the physical, social, economic and mental health of those on both the negative *and* the privileged sides of the equation (Kouchner, 2001). This is true, he claimed, not only when we, the privileged, are in close proximity to the destitute in the developed world, or when encountering street children in developing countries. And it affects us through the general knowledge we have nagging at the edges of our consciousness, and our conscience, of the deleterious consequences of inequity on the lives of billions. This profoundly affects our (mental) health. We know that the current state of the world is wrong, he noted. Even though we benefit from that state it constitutes a form of stress *because* we benefit from it.

It is important to distinguish between inequality and inequity; it is a matter of social justice. The fact that two groups are not equal may not be unjust but rather simply indicating difference, for example that men and women are biologically different. But inequity implies that the difference discussed is unjust, for example, that men and women are not paid the same for the same work, or have unequal power and opportunities in most countries in most societies: "Health inequities exist largely because people have unequal access to society's resources, including education, health care, job security and clean air and water – factors society can do something about" (Evans et al., 2001).

In his foreword to Paul Farmer's (2003) *The Pathologies of Power: Health, Human Rights and the New War on the Poor*, the Nobel economist Amartya Sen said: "The asymmetry of power can indeed generate a kind of quiet brutality. We know, of course, that power corrupts and absolute power corrupts absolutely. But inequalities of power, in general, prevent the sharing of different opportunities. They can devastate the lives of those who are far removed from the levers of control".

Mounting evidence shows globalization to be increasing the economic and social disparities between the rich and the poor with health opportunities being enhanced for the fortunate and inhibited for those at societies' margins (Evans et al., 2001; UNDP, 1999). In this regard, Frances Baum (2001), the Australian Professor of Public Health and author of the book, *The New Public Health* (Baum, 2002), says that "public health practitioners in rich countries have a responsibility to pose the question of how we can make the impact of economic globalization on health a top public health issue in the 21st Century".

In the next 25 years the world will have another 2 billion people. The great majority of these people will live in developing countries. As Wolfensohn, then head of the World Bank, put it in 2000: "Europe will be the same size in 25 years. But you will have this enormous move in developing countries, with all the attendant stresses *if* we are not able to deal with the question of poverty" (Wolfensohn, 2000). It was in October 2000, a year before the terrible events of the 11th of September, 2001, that Wolfensohn stated, quite prophetically, that, ". . . it is an issue not just of equity and social justice and morality. It really is an issue of peace, because it is unlikely that you will have stability in a world of inequity. People who have nothing, or have [very] little, or no place to go or no opportunity, react . . ."

More and more public health professionals are warning that a globalized world insufficiently tempered by human rights concerns and democratic principles must be amended. Not doing so will mean even more ill health and deprivation especially for the poor. Unfortunately, most of those who could do something about this may not be swayed by ethical arguments; essentially, that, as John Kenneth Galbraith (1994) said, "in the good society there cannot, must not, be a deprived and excluded underclass". Many may not even be particularly concerned with the creation of "the good society". But

the realization that inaction will not only affect the poor but will also have the much wider consequence of creating a breeding-ground for pandemic violence, as noted by Wolfensohn, has found receptive audiences.

In his book, *Infections and Inequalities* (Farmer, 1999), the infectious disease physician Paul Farmer asks, "If there is no role for any but the profiteers, what sort of 'health care environment' have we created?. . . By the crude calculus of modern public health, will self-protection become the sole justification for effective measures to contain the plagues of the poor?" (page 279). The answer, unfortunately, seems evident.

He goes on to suggest that the basic question which should occupy us is, how social forces, ranging from political violence to racism, come to be embodied in individual pathology (Farmer, 1999). Epidemiological evidence shows us that pathologies concentrate along the fault-lines of societies, among the most deprived and marginalized of the world.

Since the epidemiological evidence concludes that poverty, inequity and health are interlinked, a major focus and function of public health and encompassing epidemiological research must be to stem, and to reverse, the tide of inequity and resultant poor health, (Farmer, 1999; Wilkinson, 1996; Marmot, 2005; Farmer, 2003; Feachem, 2000; Kawachi et al., 1999; Leon and Walt, 2000; Marmot and Wilkinson, 1999; Navarro, 2000; Wilkinson, 1997; Wilkinson, 2005; World Health Organization, 2004a).

The Epidemiology of Poverty and Inequity

Let us look at some figures:

Between 1960 and 1998 the portion of income in the hands of the poorest 20% of the world's population dropped from 2.3% to 1.2%, while that of the world's richest 20% rose from 70.2% to 89% (UNDP, 1999). The richest 20% consume 160 times that of the poorest 20% (Rao and Lowenson, 2000).

At least one fifth of the world's population – 1.2 billion people – live in absolute poverty, surviving on US$1 or less a day, and half the world's population, 3 billion people, live in "moderate poverty", trying to survive on $2 or less a day (UNDP, 1999). It is not immediately clear how to define "moderate poverty" though it might indicate the possibility of having a house with a roof of metal sheeting rather than one of straw. Paul Farmer makes this distinction in terms of "decent" and "indecent" poverty.

Seventy percent of people living in absolute poverty are women. Indigenous communities suffer poverty at rates far above national poverty rates (Buvenic et al., 1996). There are an estimated 100 million street children worldwide (Desjarlais et al., 1995), and, according to the 2001 Human Development Report 24,000 people starve to death every day (UNDP, 2001).

The 2003 Human Development Report (UNDP, 2003) reports that 54 nations were poorer in 2003 than they were in 1990. Twenty of these countries are in sub-Saharan Africa, while 17 are in Eastern Europe and the Commonwealth of Independent States. The report documents "an unprecedented backslide . . . in some of the world's poorest nations". There are of course pockets of poverty and increasing inequity also in the world's richest countries, not least in the US. The aftermath of Hurricane Katrina and the fate of the astrodome refugees serves as a glaring example.

In Japan, female life expectancy is 85 years, in Sierra Leone it is 36. In Japan there is ample access to the best of health care while in Sierra Leone many never have access to either a doctor or a nurse. Lee Jong-wook, the WHO Director General, says that such gaps are unacceptable. These health gaps are of course symptoms of wider socioeconomic gaps.

When he accepted the 2002 Nobel Peace Prize, Jimmy Carter said the following: "I was asked to discuss, here in Oslo, the greatest challenge that the world faces. I decided that the most serious and universal problem is the growing chasm between the richest and poorest people on earth" (Carter, 2002).

It must be said again! The tide of inequity is increasing (both between and within nations) and this has significant health consequences for all segments of a society's population. Poverty, certainly, is linked with poor health, but it is particularly the combination of poverty and inequity which is lethal. And, surprisingly to some, the most devastating part of this equation is inequity. Epidemiological research continues to make this quite clear, pointing the way for required changes (Wilkinson, 1996; Marmot, 2005; Feachem, 2000; Kawachi *et al.*, 1999; Wilkinson, 2005; Halstead *et al.*, 1985; Macinko and Starfield, 2002).

Inequalities, Inequity and Structural Violence

Jim Kim, now at the WHO, and his coauthors showed in some considerable detail in the book *Dying for Growth* (Kim *et al.*, 2001) what scores of others have argued as well, namely, that while improved health is loosely tied to overall economic growth there is by no means a guarantee of such a connection.

Depending on the degree of social structural hierarchy, or degree of social cohesion and justice, economic growth in and of itself can mean even greater inequity, and for many, much worse health. The 1985 Rockefeller Foundation publication, *Good Health at Low Cost* (Halstead *et al.*, 1985), with examples of Costa Rica, Kerala State in India, Sri Lanka and elsewhere, showed much better health indicators in many poorer countries than in richer ones, precisely because of greater equity and more favorable social conditions.

Wilkinson (1997), in a study of 23 European countries found that mortality rates, for all social classes, were linked to income within countries rather than to absolute income differences between them. Lower mortality rates were shown in countries with smaller income differences. The study also found that long term rise in life expectancy appeared not to be related to long term economic growth rates.

China, which, in the last decade, has seen tremendous economic growth is an interesting example, showing a widening gap in health statistics for urban as compared to rural populations as well as between other population groups indicating that overall "economic growth alone is not sufficient for improvements in health status" (Liu *et al.*, 1999).

The socioeconomic divide is, of course, not the only form of inequity leading to poor health; racism and gender issues, to name but two others, have significant health consequences as indicated by a vast literature (Buvenic *et al.*, 1996; Östlin *et al.*, 2004). Again, to use China as an example, we learn that China suffers from pervasive gender inequity and that infant mortality for girls has increased since 1987. In 1995 it was more than 25% higher than for boys. China is also one of very few countries in the world where the suicide rate for women is greater than for men. It is 30% higher for Chinese women and, unlike in most other countries, the overall rate is higher in rural than in urban areas (Liu *et al.*, 1999).

Using such evidence, it is difficult to disagree with those who claim that inequity (not only inequity in access to health care services, but over-riding inequity leading to inequality in health) is the major modern plague. A claim which is made while being fully aware of the devastations and ravages of diseases such as HIV/AIDS, TB and Malaria.

The terms "structural violence" and "functional apartheid" (Farmer, 2004; Heggenhougen, 1995) are sometimes also used when referring to inequitable hierarchical social structures which, similarly, have devastating effect on people's health. The Population Health Forum defines structural violence as excess rates of poor health and death caused by the social and economic structures of society, by decisions about who gets what. They are violent because the harm caused to people are the result of human action (and inaction).

More direct forms of human violence, such as war and civil strife are of course not to be forgotten as lethal instruments of ill health. We should also note that the largest worldwide economic enterprise, by far, is the selling of arms, 85% of which is done by the five permanent members of the UN Security Council.

It was forty years ago that, as a warning against this growing inequity, Adlai Stevenson, the then US Ambassador to the UN, gave the impassioned "Space-Ship Earth" speech to the July, 1965, UN ECOSOC conference (Stevenson, 1965). It seems an even more apt warning today that allowing a growing divide to go unchecked spells ruin for us all – for those traveling in first class as well as those in steerage: "We travel together, passengers on a little spaceship, dependent upon its vulnerable reserves of air and soil, all committed for our safety to its security and peace, preserved from annihilation only by the care, the work, and I will say the love we give our fragile craft. We cannot maintain it half-fortunate, half-miserable, and half-free in the liberation of resources undreamed of until this day. No craft, no crew can travel safely with such vast contradictions. On their resolution depends the survival of us all" (Stevenson, 1965).

Research Challenges for Improving Global Health and the Role of Epidemiology

There are of course many ways to categorize global health research on equity and health: 1) Equitable research on the diseases that affect most of the world's population; 2) Research on equity of health care and services; 3) Research on more effective and better use of diagnosis, prevention, treatment and care; and 4) Research linking different social, political and economic population characteristics with different health indicators. And running through all four is an urgency to translate research knowledge into action, to use research as a guide for creating "the good society" (Galbraith, 1994).

The first kind of such global health research on the diseases affecting the majority of humanity has gained momentum in the past several years, especially as a result of the 10/90 problem raised by the Global Forum for Health Research (2004). Worldwide, only 10% of all resources for health research is spent on diseases that account for 90% of the total global disease burden. We must all be engaged in shifting this priority. The lives of millions could be saved and many millions more could live healthier and happier lives.

Further, we must focus on the second type of global health research to enhance the access to quality medical services for all segments of a country's population, but especially for the poorest and most marginalized. This may also be a matter of new biomedical knowledge for the relatively neglected diseases in the 10/90 debate, but equally important it requires researchers to point out the importance of creating equitable access to existing diagnosis, treatment and medications. This leads directly to the third type of research on more effective use of diagnoses and treatment. The importance of the fourth type of research, especially comparative epidemiology linking socioeconomic inequity with negative health outcomes, is, of course the main argument of this entire article.

These points are not novel (but they continue to be important) and not so different from some of the main points of the WHO, 2004, *World Report on Knowledge for*

Better Health (World Health Organization, 2004b): "Global health is characterized by persistent inequities ... effective interventions are often not reaching people who need them most ... Deep economic inequalities and social injustices continue to deny good health ... Positive change does not automatically result from sound evidence alone ... The notion of 'knowledge for better health,' therefore, must go beyond the production and passive dissemination of research".

Research is indispensable for reaching the Millennium Development Goals, of which good Health is both a central component and a result. This was the main message of the recent UK House of Commons (2004), Science and Technology Committee Report: *The Use of Science in UK International Development Policy*.

The 2002 *Annotated bibliography on equity in health, 1980–2001* by James Macinko and Barbara Starfield (2002), in the first issue of the *International Journal for Equity in Health*, concludes that there are three main types of approaches to health inequities: 1) Increasing or improving ... health services to those in greatest need, 2) restructuring health financing to aid the disadvantaged, and 3) altering broader social and economic structures to influence more fundamental determinants of health inequities. The authors state that there are few articles in the health literature which address the third approach. There is a need to do more.

Several public health specialists, while supporting the first kinds of global health equity research (for example, of challenging the persistence of the 10/90 divide) are strongly against the later, the more fundamental health equity research, indicating that such research is futile and simply done to be "politically correct" (Satel and Marmor, 2001). Such research, they say, is too broad for epidemiological and other public health researchers to tackle and takes attention and energy away from what public health researchers are really good at and "can do", such as improving water and sanitary conditions and increasing immunization uptake. Satel and Marmor conclude that while it may be seductive to partake in public debate on income distribution it will draw energies and resources away from "the vital issues that the public health profession has addressed so well in the past" (Satel and Marmor, 2001).

Granted, such work is easier said than done, but, as I stated earlier, it is unhelpful and inaccurate to present this as an "either/or" matter. A "both/and" approach would be more fruitful in the long run. Of course, epidemiologists and other public health researchers should focus on "traditional" topics, and on the "vital issues" which have been addressed in the past, but is also important that we focus on both the immediate and the fundamental risk factors (Link and Phelan, 1995) and that we see the interconnections between them.

It must be noted that focusing on the fundamental issues of social inequity and health is not a new effort.

Such an encompassing focus has existed since the time of Hippocrates, if not before, and received an impetus in the 19th century. And also within the last 25 years, through the Primary Health Care Declaration, the Ottawa Charter, the People's Health Charter, the New Public Health movement, and other recent initiatives such as the UN Commission on the Social Determinants of Health. If, as the mounting epidemiological evidence shows, inequity is a major (I would say, the major) factor contributing to differentiated ill health, and if public health professionals are to be serious then, difficult or not, we can not close our eyes to this obvious connection.

Sudhir Anand (2002), at Oxford, stated that there are at least two reasons for investigating inter-group inequalities in health: 1) It will enable us to identify groups at high risk so that public and health policy may be appropriately targeted to improve their health. The UK government's current initiative on inequalities in health is doing precisely this. 2) Inequalities in health which are particularly unjust will be revealed and group inequalities will show that they stem from social rather than natural factors – and may thus be avoidable.

Östlin *et al.* (2004) suggest that "ignoring factors such as socioeconomic class, race [ethnicity] and gender leads to biases in both the content and process of research … If the facts relating to the social distribution of health are not recorded, the problems remain invisible". Looking at these issues is not just a fad, or "politically correctness". Examination of inequitable social realities and related ill health are a necessary and central aspect of global public health (including epidemiological) research. We must use our research to point to ways in which inequity leads to poor health and also to ways in which it can be reduced, ways to advocate for change.

Researchers as Advocates for Change

Health research must be used to advocate for social changes, or for what Dr. Julio Frenk, the current Mexican Minister of Health, has called for, namely not only better health policies, but "healthier policies" in all arenas of society. I would suggest that it is within the remit of epidemiological researchers to influence broad social policy formulations as a means by which greater social, economic and political equity can be brought about. Also Dr. Harvey Fineberg, former Dean of the Harvard School of Public Health, and now the President of the U.S. Institute of Medicine, is said to have stated that "A school of public health is like a school of [social] justice" (as quoted in 3).

Research for change was the main theme of the October, 2004, issue of the *Bulletin of the World Health Organization* ("Bridging the Know-Do Gap in global Health"). While contributors dealt with translating research focusing on "immediate" factors, others, such as Sanders *et al.* (2004), focused on the larger social inequity

issues: "Most health researchers to date have only studied the world; the point, however, is to change it for the better".

Global health research must focus on ensuring that all have access to the requirements for good health. This is the right of all human beings as the 25th Article of the 1948 Universal Declaration of Human Rights reminds us: "Everyone has the right to a standard of living adequate for the health and well-being of himself and of his family, including food, clothing, housing and medical care and necessary social services, and the right to security in the event of unemployment, sickness, disability, widowhood, old age or other lack of livelihood in circumstances beyond his control".

And as instituted by Dr. Jonathan Mann, the first Director of the WHO AIDS Program and the founder of the Harvard Center for Health and Human Rights, at their graduation, all masters and doctorate graduates from the Harvard School of Public Health are handed the Universal Declaration of Human Rights along with their diplomas. Not only are health and human rights interlinked but public health research must lead to a change for a more universally recognized right to, and realization of, health.

Epidemiology has been, and can continue to be, in the forefront of demonstrating the social basis of ill health and showing not only that change needs to occur but also indicating what should be done, and how this can occur. The pathologist and physician Rudolph Virchow stated in Germany more than 150 years ago that "Medicine is a social science in its very bone and marrow". William Farr in England at approximately the same time, noticed that different classes had very different rates of mortality and he then became committed to social reform and in using social class and health statistics – epidemiological evidence – to advance these reforms. By epidemiological researchers showing evidence on socioeconomic inequity and ill health, there may be a chance of slowly beginning to affect fundamental factors, to stem the tide of growing inequity.

Public health professionals and social epidemiologists should not have to bring about such improved social conditions and consequent improved health alone. These are large development issues which also require a range of different actors, including development agencies and national policy makers. But the involvement of epidemiologists and public health professionals remains crucial and our research should not only be directed at formulating better health policies but 'healthier policies' in all domains. To return to the beginning we are reminded once again by John Donne and Ernest Hemingway that "No man is an island," that no one ought to be isolated and marginalized, and that we should "therefore never send to know for whom the bell tolls, it tolls for thee". We are irresponsible if our research does not (also) engage with this most problematic and prevailing public health issue: the plague of inequity.

References

Anand S (2002) The concern for equity in health. Harvard Center for Population and Development Studies Working Paper Series, vol. 12, No. 1.

Baum F (2001) Health, equity, justice and globalisation: Some lessons from the People's Health Assembly. *Journal of Epidemiology and Community Health* 55(9): 613–616.

Baum F (2002) *The New Public Health,* 2nd edn. Oxford: Oxford University Press.

Buvenic M, Gwin K, and Bates L (1996) *Investing in Women: Progress and Prospects for the World Bank.* Washington, DC: Overseas Development Council.

Carter J (2002) Nobel Peace Prize Speech, Oslo, 10 December.

Desjarlais R, Eisenberg L, Good B, and Kleinman A (1995) *World Mental Health – Problems and Priorities in Low-Income Countries.* Oxford: Oxford University Press.

Evans T, Whitehead M, Diderichsen Bhuiya FA, and Wirth M (2001) *Challenging Inequities in Health: From Ethics to Action.* Oxford: Oxford University Press.

Farmer P (1999) *Infections and Inequalities: The Modern Plagues.* London: University of California Press.

Farmer P (2003) *Pathologies of Power: Health, Human Rights, and the New War on the Poor.* Berkeley, CA: University of California Press.

Farmer P (2004) An anthropology of structural violence. *Current Anthropology* 45(3): 305–325.

Feachem RG (2000) Poverty and inequity: A proper focus for the new century. *Bulletin of the World Health Organization* 78(1): 1–2.

Galbraith JK (1994) The good society considered: The economic dimension. *Journal of Law and Society* 3–4 (Annual Lecture: St. David's Hall, Cardiff Law School, 26 January, 1994).

Global Forum for Health Research (2004) Health Research for Policy, Action and Practice – Resource Modules.

Halstead S, Walsh J, and Warren K (1985) Good health at low cost. *Proceedings of a Conference Held at the Bellagio Conference Center,* Bellagio, Italy, 29 April–3 May.

Heggenhougen HK (1995) The epidemiology of functional apartheid and human rights abuses. *Social Science & Medicine* 40(3): 281–284.

Kawachi I, Wilkinson RG, and Kennedy BP (eds.) (1999) *Income Distribution and Health: A Reader.* New York, NY: New Press.

Kim J, Millen J, Gershman J, and Irwin A (eds.) (2001) *Dying for Growth.* Monroe, ME: Common Courage Press.

Kouchner B (2001) Personal Communication.

Leon DA and Walt G (eds.) (2000) *Poverty, Inequality and Health: An International Perspective.* Oxford: Oxford University Press.

Link BG and Phelan J (1995) Social conditions as fundamental causes of disease. *Journal of Health and Human Behavior* 80–94.

Liu Y, Hsiao WC, and Eggleston K (1999) Equity in health and health care: The Chinese experience. *Social Science & Medicine* 49(10): 1349–1356.

Macinko JA and Starfield B (2002) Annotated bibliography on equity in health, 1980–2001. *International Journal for Equity in Health* 1(1): 1–39.

Marmot M and Wilkinson RG (eds.) (1999) *Social Determinants of Health.* Oxford: Oxford University Press.

Marmot M (2005) Social determinants of health inequalities. *Lancet* 365(9464): 1099–1104.

Navarro V (ed.) (2000) *The Political Economy of Social Inequalities: Consequences for Health and the Quality of Life.* Amityville, NY: Baywood.

Östlin P, Sen G, and George A (2004) Paying attention to gender and poverty in health research: Content and process issues. *Bulletin of the World Health Organization* 82(10): 740–745.

Population Health Forum. Advocacy for action toward a healthier society, Structural Violence, http://depts.washington.edu/eqhlth/pages/issues.html#income.

Rao M and Lowenson R (2000) *The Political Economy of the Assault on Health. Discussion Papers Prepared by the Peoples' Health Assembly's Drafting Group.* Savar, Bangladesh: Gonoshasthaya Kendra.

Sanders D, Labonte R, Baum F, and Chopra M (2004) Making research matter: A civil society perspective on health research. *Bulletin of the World Health Organization* 82(10): 757–763.

Satel S and Marmor TR (July 16, 2001) Does inequality make you sick? The dangers of the new public health crusade. *The Weekly Standard.*

Stevenson A (1965) Space Ship Earth Speech to the ECOSOC Meeting in July 1965.

UNDP (1999) *Human Development Report.* Oxford: Oxford University Press.

UNDP (2001) *Human Development Report.* New York, NY: Oxford University Press.

UNDP (2003) *Human Development Report.* New York, NY: Oxford University Press.

United Kingdom, Government of House of Commons Science and Technology Committee (2004) The Use of Science in UK International Development Policy. Thirteenth Report of Session 2003–2004, vol. 1, p. 107.

Wilkinson RG (1996) *Unhealthy Societies: The Afflictions of Inequality.* London: Routledge.

Wilkinson RG (1997) Health inequalities: Relative or absolute material standards? *BMJ* 314: 591–595.

Wilkinson RG (2005) *The Impact of Inequality, How to Make Sick Healthier.* London: Routledge.

Wolfensohn JD (2000) Poverty and development. The world development report 2000/2001. Keynote Address at the Conference on World Poverty and Development: A Challenge for the Private Sector, Amsterdam, 3 October.

World Health Organization (2004a) *The World Health Report.* Geneva: WHO.

World Health Organization (2004b) *World Report on Knowledge for Better Health: Strengthening Health Systems (Summary).* Geneva: WHO.

Cultural Epidemiology

J A Trostle, Trinity College, Hartford, CT, USA

Introduction

The field of cultural epidemiology is a set of methods and theoretical rationales for linking culture to human health at the population scale. It includes efforts to conceptualize aspects of culture as harmful or protective of human health; to combine textual and numerical or statistical accounts of health and disease; to unpack and further explore causal pathways between pathogens, behaviors, or psychological states and disease; and to describe the assumptions and practices of the discipline of epidemiology as a cultural practice and way of knowing. Many of these efforts have been undertaken by cultural anthropologists, and more specifically by medical or biocultural anthropologists, but they have also been undertaken by epidemiologists, psychologists, and sociologists. The following sections describe the relevance of culture for epidemiology; contrast social and cultural epidemiologies; review historical precedents; describe contemporary challenges of theory and method facing those working in this domain; and conclude with approaches and steps addressing those challenges.

The Centrality and Complexity of the Concept of Culture

The term culture has been defined in many ways over the past century. Contemporary anthropologists emphasize that culture comprises systems of meaning and patterns of behavior, but that these systems and patterns are locally determined, often contested, temporally specific, unequally distributed, sometimes contradictory, and strongly influenced by power and protest. The term society, in contrast, refers to groups of people who live together, interact in specific ways, and form rules that govern their behavior such as institutions of marriage, work, family life, law, and religion. The field of social epidemiology emphasizes the effects of such rules and institutions on human health, looking at categories such as social inequality, income, class, occupation, religious affiliation, and gender. Compared to social epidemiology, the field of cultural epidemiology is at once more reflexive and self-critical. Cultural epidemiology measures how meaning and belief are relevant to and visible in health and disease, but also examines the assumptions behind measures and variables, and the variability in measures and in measuring across populations. Cultural epidemiology and social epidemiology have complementary but different objectives, with cultural epidemiology asking not only about causal linkages, but also about the origins and cross-cultural validity of the concepts and measures developed in any particular academic context and disciplinary domain.

Consider the difference between social and cultural explanations for the differential survival following the sinking of the passenger ship Titanic on its first voyage in 1912, data used in many introductory epidemiology courses to teach about mortality. **Table 1** summarizes these data in terms of the percentages of different groups that survived the accident, showing the joint effects of economic status, age, and gender.

The conventional story told with these data is that survival was higher for women than men, for children than adults, and for high- than low-status passengers. This differential survival shows a social effect of class: High-status passengers had privileged access to cabins near the lifeboat deck and to the lifeboats that ensured survival. But even though higher economic status is associated with higher survival (with other referring to the

Table 1 Survival percentages by economic status, age, and gender

Gender		Age	
		Adult	Child
Male			
Economic status	High	32.6% of 175	100% of 5
	Medium	8.3% of 168	100% of 11
	Low	16.2% of 462	27.1% of 48
	Other	22.3% of 862	–
Female			
Economic status	High	97.2% of 144	100% of 1
	Medium	86.0% of 93	100% of 13
	Low	46.1% of 165	45.2% of 31
	Other	87.0% of 23	–

crew), a larger percentage of females than males, and children than adults, survived within each economic status group. These data thus also show the importance of a cultural rule, namely women and children first, that people use to regulate access to lifeboats in maritime accidents. Social epidemiology explains the tragedy in terms of class stratification and ideas about the relative value of rich versus poor, and cultural epidemiology explains the tragedy in terms of ideas about the relative value of women and children compared to men and adults in maritime accidents. These are complementary accounts.

Why Cultural Epidemiology Matters

The literature and rhetoric on global health challenges is increasingly filled with references to the critical importance of phenomena such as migration, urbanization, ethnic conflict, rapid travel, trade, and poverty. These and similar forces clearly represent human decisions and actions. Even disease-enhancing forces that might more commonly be called natural than social, such as climate change or antibiotic resistance or even the so-called natural history of disease itself (see **Figure 1**), have had their human contributions revealed.

Figure 1 displays a model of the natural history of disease as used in an epidemiology text published by the U.S. Centers for Disease Control and Prevention. The model has a timeline of events (marked by arrows above the timeline) that take place inside human bodies, and also names a set of stages (labeled between bars below the timeline). The text below the CDC diagram identifies places where social and cultural forces influence the timing and outcome of these so-called natural events, making the natural history of disease look instead quite contingent and strongly influenced by human behavior and belief. For example, exposure to pathogens is influenced by occupation and cultural practices such as cooking. Symptoms such as pain are differentially perceived and classified by different peoples. Diseases may be labeled as acute or chronic,

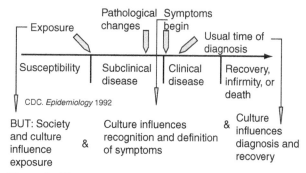

Figure 1 The natural history of disease according to the CDC.

curable or incurable, natural or divine, depending on the terminology of local medical systems. Outcomes of recovery, infirmity, or death depend at least partly upon the availability and efficacy of treatments such as pills, injections, poultices, and/or surgical techniques.

As epidemiologic research has spread worldwide as a form of scientific research, it has uncovered dramatic differences in the distribution and impact of the forces that create disease in different contexts. This is perhaps best exemplified in the literature about the epidemiologic transition, which predicted that as nations, as well as areas within nations, industrialize, they will move from morbidity and mortality profiles characterized by acute and infectious diseases such as respiratory infections, diarrheal diseases, and measles, to profiles characterized by chronic and noncommunicable diseases such as diabetes, cardiovascular diseases, cancer, and asthma (Omran, 1971). These kinds of epidemiologic conclusions about general links between human behavior and human health are accompanied by specific evidence of the range and variability of such associations.

But variability in causation requires variability in intervention, so with respect to treatment or prevention, broad epidemiologic conclusions also need to be accompanied by locally valid strategies. For example, epidemiological conclusions about the importance of high cholesterol in causing heart disease must be supplemented by work that translates that finding into meaningful messages. Those messages must be relevant to different groups of people who consume different kinds of foods and who cook with different techniques. Cultural epidemiology, because of its attention to local context and contingent meaning, can assist intervention designs in ways that more global and generic epidemiologic findings cannot (Caprara, 1998). It can thus contribute to global health by improving both the specificity and applicability of epidemiologic results.

Cultural epidemiology is used to increase the validity of public health research by mixing observational and unstructured interview methods with more conventional population surveys or health record reviews. It is also used

to promote more appropriate choice and definition of causal frameworks and research variables.

Researchers within the domain of cultural epidemiology produce etiologic clues relevant to untangling the causes of disease. A dramatic illustration occurred in the early 1960s, when researchers found that the mortuary practice of consuming human brain tissue spread a mortal disease called kuru among the Fore people in New Guinea. The pathogen is now known in biomedicine as a prion. Such clues are seen today in larger connections between cultural consonance (the extent to which an individual lives and espouses core cultural values) and blood pressure, or access to social capital and prevention of infectious disease transmission, or presence of plantation agriculture and the prevalence of both malaria and sickle cell trait. There is a rich historical precedent for this work.

Early Schools of Epidemiology and Their Past and Present Relevance to Cultural Epidemiology

Early (mid-nineteenth century) epidemiology has been divided into biological, sociological, and geographical domains (Ackerknecht, 1948). Late in the nineteenth century, a psychological domain could be added. The roots of cultural epidemiology extend to all of them, but run most deeply into the biological, sociological, and psychological realms discussed below.

Biological Epidemiology

The importance of fieldwork

Cultural epidemiology has antecedents in the biological school of mid-nineteenth century epidemiology. Researchers interested in disease causation employed a variety of theories – such as those of miasma or contagion – to guide their choice of methods. They did extensive fieldwork in specific communities in an effort to link customs and behaviors with generalizations about disease causation. The tradition of fieldwork in epidemiology has been called shoe leather epidemiology. The writings of Peter Panum on measles in the Faroe Islands, of John Snow on cholera in London, and of Rudolf Virchow on famine and typhoid in Upper Silesia (now Poland) are some of the best-known examples. These researchers compiled detailed ethnographic descriptions drawn from their own observations and personal experience over time, and they combined them with broad statistical or geographic conclusions about disease prevalence and differential risk. Virchow paid particular attention to the social and political causes of the typhoid epidemic and is considered a critical early contributor to cultural epidemiology.

The ethnographic tradition continues to be used in investigating particular disease outbreaks. It is also used by anthropologists to reveal or distangle the causes of disease, often in collaboration with epidemiologists. This was seen in studies of chronic diseases such as hypertension and diabetes in the 1960s and in cross-cultural research on the causes of diarrheal diseases and respiratory infections in the 1970s and 1980s. Beginning in the 1980s, research on the causes and prevention of HIV/AIDS used ethnographic methods and insights that could be called cultural epidemiology, and that work continues today.

Sociological Epidemiology

The importance of inequality and social disruption

The sociological school of epidemiology in the nineteenth century was linked to struggles by reformers who sought to improve the health of factory workers, the conditions of urban slums, and the extent to which health itself was a focus of social concern and legislation. A variety of statistical studies were undertaken, especially in France, Germany, the United Kingdom, and the United States, showing that social and economic conditions were important predictors of human health.

Two major figures in sociological epidemiology are Rudolf Virchow and Emile Durkheim. Virchow's contribution in terms of applying his fieldwork observations was described above, but he also espoused a theoretical model that acknowledged social inequality and powerlessness as relevant to disease status. He spoke of the need to increase education, freedom, and prosperity as lasting solutions to the challenges of famine and disease. Emile Durkheim, the French sociologist, also made an important contribution to cultural epidemiology by showing that a seemingly individual act such as suicide had a series of stable and quantifiable attributes when viewed as a collective social phenomenon. Durkheim was a theoretical and methodological pioneer in sociological epidemiology, envisioning and demonstrating the importance of collective and unseen social forces in the deaths of individuals.

Attention to social causes of morbidity and mortality diminished at the beginning of the twentieth century, overshadowed by studies emphasizing single (often infectious) rather than multiple causes of disease. But with the spread of the epidemiologic transition (Omran, 1971) and the growing importance of diseases such as cancer, heart disease, and diabetes, single-cause models no longer provided the same explanatory power, and the social environment began to return as a factor worthy of investigation.

The importance of the social and cultural environment

Research and intervention in South Africa and in the state of North Carolina in the United States are some of the most important – but certainly not the only – innovative projects to have addressed the social and cultural environment.

In South Africa beginning in the late 1930s, Sidney Kark and colleagues embarked upon more than a decade of interdisciplinary work that brought social scientists, clinicians, and epidemiologists together to study local beliefs and practices as well as the health of rural communities as a whole, and to combine these in novel forms that took account of cultural differences in the design of health interventions. The growing apartheid policies of South Africa stopped this program and caused many of its participants to leave the country, but this also allowed many of the critical components of this experiment to take new shape in sites as widespread as Israel, Uganda, Kenya, England, and the United States (Trostle, 1986).

John Cassel was one of those who left, and his research group at the University of North Carolina at Chapel Hill became one of the most important centers of cultural epidemiology. It was Cassel, in his early work in South Africa, who described how important it was to link knowledge of cultural beliefs to knowledge of epidemiological risk factors in the design of effective public health interventions (Trostle, 1986). He and his colleagues pioneered studies of how urbanization affected heart disease mortality and how the social environment might influence host resistance or susceptibility to disease. His group also published some of the first studies that tried to separate the influence of cultural systems from social systems.

Psychological–Psychiatric Epidemiology

Social and cultural causes and patterning of symptoms

The origins of contemporary interest in the epidemiology of psychological dysfunction, and the relevance of culture to such dysfunction, extend back to the early twentieth century, to an interdisciplinary expedition sent from Cambridge University to the Torres Straits, between Australia and New Guinea. A psychologist and physician on that expedition, W.H.R. Rivers, developed and disseminated the idea that medical systems could be studied as social institutions, which has since become a central tenet in the field of medical anthropology. With respect to cultural epidemiology, Rivers pioneered the theories and methods that led to important discoveries about cross-cultural differences in perception.

Other important population-based studies of mental functioning were first developed by a group associated with Cornell University in the 1950s and 1960s. The first project directors were Alexander and Dorothea Leighton, psychiatric epidemiologists who held joint appointments in the Cornell Anthropology Department. Together with a large group of students and staff, the Leightons undertook more than a decade of ethnographic fieldwork in a group of Canadian communities labeled Stirling County. They used those data to contextualize the prevalence and symptom patterns of psychiatric dysfunction in communities they categorized along a spectrum from social health to social disintegration. This project has clear connections to studies of the health-related effects of the social environment, its primary difference being its focus on mental rather than physical health outcomes.

There are now at least two modern components of cultural epidemiology related to psychology and mental disorder. One is the distribution of psychological symptoms in the community and their relationship to the social environment, work which continues that of the Leightons (e.g., Murphy, 1994). The other describes the cultural patterning of psychological symptoms as well as other local representations of distress (e.g., Guarnaccia and Rogler, 1999; Weiss, 2001). This latter domain bears some resemblance to what is called lay epidemiology, described in a later section titled 'Popular and Lay Epidemiology.' There are many parallels between cultural epidemiology as applied to physical and as applied to mental conditions, including concerns about sampling, case definition, and symptom classification, as well as causal frameworks that attend to both individual and group-level effects.

The Relationship Between Technology, Epidemiology, and Anthropology

The contributions of individuals and interdisciplinary teams highlighted in the prior sections took place within a context of rapid changes in science, legislation, and values. Advances in both epidemiology and the social sciences have been fuelled by a broad variety of technologies, and their impact has taken very different forms at different historical moments. Epidemiology is based on the ability to compare cases of disease (a numerator) to a measured population at risk (a denominator). Its attention to numerators was moved forward in the eighteenth century by the invention of institutions such as the hospital, which facilitated the recognition and counting of cases, as well as by the invention in the nineteenth century of observational technologies such as the stethoscope, microscope, laryngoscope, and even tissue staining, which facilitated the isolation of causes of disease. Epidemiology's attention to denominators was greatly improved by the invention of systems of record keeping and vital statistics, including censuses.

Industrial technologies, and the working conditions and labor migration they precipitated, increased the interest and attention that social scientists devoted to human health, and especially their attention to the health consequences of rapid social change. New forms of travel and communication, and expansion of industrial empires overseas, also facilitated the access colonial anthropologists had to previously unknown human groups, and increased governmental and academic interest in collecting information about such groups.

In the twentieth century, these forces continued to push the frontiers of anthropology and epidemiology, as well as their joint application in cultural epidemiology. Administrative processes that help enroll or trace study participants are important here, as are the explosive growth of computers and ready access to statistical analysis software. Complex databases can contain quantitative, qualitative, or combined types of study information. Digital photography, satellite imagery, magnetic resonance imagery, and genetic maps allow complex new research questions to be studied even as they force research teams to be interdisciplinary.

Contemporary Challenges

Unpacking variables

An important contribution of cultural epidemiology is to critique accepted public health concepts and research variables. Considerable recent effort has been invested in unpacking common epidemiologic variables such as race, class or status, and time. Some of this work has demonstrated that familiar anthropological processes (e.g., identity change) are visible in vital statistics. For example, a study that compared race and ethnicity at birth and death showed that these categories change, and change more often for minority than majority classifications (Hahn et al., 1992). Other work has shown how the association of disease transmission with culturally defined seasons of the year can influence Tanzanian locals to be willing to use bednets in some seasons but not others, even though the risk of malaria transmission from mosquito bites is fairly constant throughout the year (Winch et al., 1994). Febrile illnesses are thought to be caused by malaria only during some seasons. In the case of race and ethnicity, unexpected variability is shown in variables that have been used to define identity for health purposes; in the second, this variability is shown in local concepts of time. In traditional epidemiologic practice, neither of these is assumed to exhibit much change over time or by place. The process of unpacking variables can lead to more accurate and complete causal models, can reduce inappropriate generalization of study results, and can improve measurement.

Measuring

Cultural epidemiology attempts to maintain a close tie between the process of data collection and the objectives of data analysis. Unlike traditional epidemiology, where acquisition of a data set is often the first step in research, a cultural epidemiologist will first be concerned to understand how data have been, or might best be, collected. Cultural epidemiologists are likely to stress that the process of collecting data is often a process of cultural exchange, and that therefore conveying information involves a set of exchanges of goods and services (e.g., money, patient referrals, authorship on scientific articles), or sentiments (e.g., pride, loyalty, altruism), that must be recognized and fulfilled. These exchanges take place between data bank managers and researchers, between doctors and professors, between patients and doctors, and between community members and survey researchers. One set of contributions to measurement from cultural epidemiology includes understanding what kinds of topics and questions will be perceived as sensitive in different areas and by different groups of people, how best to learn about sensitive behaviors or attitudes, when observation is required and when interviews will suffice, and what kinds of interviewers are likeliest to elicit valid responses from other specified types of respondents. In sum, culture influences data collection and measurement strategies by influencing who is willing to participate in a study, how accurately they will respond to tests or questions, and how their answers will be categorized.

Surveillance

Another aspect of measurement concerns what sources of data are taken as valid and authoritative. This is especially important for disease surveillance, when bureaucracies seek to monitor the health of the people. Classical epidemiology tends to rely upon the formal resources of a health system: Disease surveillance takes place in hospitals, clinics, doctors' offices, and the other components of an official vital statistics system. However, cultural epidemiology proposes relying on the more pervasive informal resources of a health system, either as a validity check on formal reports or as an alternative to such reports. For example, a Brazilian study showed the utility of soliciting mortality data from coffin-makers and other community members who might have knowledge about infant and child deaths that would modify official estimates based on death certificates (Nations and Amaral, 1991). This is consistent with an anthropological concern for the similarities and differences between local and higher-level processes, also a topic of contemporary concern in epidemiology.

Measuring Culture

Anthropologists have periodically been challenged by epidemiologists to explain why they have not done more to use culture and/or cultural identity as a variable predicting disease. For example, epidemiologists have asked anthropologists to "prepare maps and draw boundaries so that cultural areas can be identified where certain beliefs are widely if not universally subscribed" (Murphy, 1994: 243). More recently, a contributor to *The International Journal of Epidemiology* (Eckersley, 2005: 263) proposed that the contribution to global stress and mental disorder of

cultural values such as individualism and materialism was under-researched. Responding to anthropologists who criticized his effort as being too broad and insufficiently nuanced, the author denied that the only way to study the effects of culture on health was "to focus on the details of population patterning and distribution, individual and group differences, and culture as local knowledge, and to explore culture's health impacts at this level." He argued instead that cultural effects should also be capable of being studied – and seen – at global scales. One of the fundamental challenges to cultural epidemiology thus consists of showing the importance of local cultural effects without making it easy to generalize inappropriately about the usefulness of culture as a predictive variable.

One such approach to this challenge involves defining culture as a set of models for behavior and of beliefs that are approximated to varying extents by individuals in a given social group. The extent to which any individual's behavior or belief duplicates the prevailing models is called cultural consonance, and the degree of cultural consonance itself is used as a health predictor, with increasing consonance associated with increasing health (Dressler, 2005). This is one example of a set of research studies conducted among migrants moving internationally or domestically from one context to another, and within groups of individuals who face social discrimination that limits their ability to progress as they desire. This research does not label cultural content as positive or negative, rather it explores the stressful (and therefore health-related) effects of prolonged inability to live in the way one believes one should.

Multilevel Analysis

During the final decades of the twentieth century, some epidemiologists grew increasingly critical of epidemiological explanations that relied on single causes or that measured risk at just one level of abstraction. An important commentary suggested that the metaphor of Chinese boxes (implying interlocking or nested levels of causality) be substituted for that of black boxes (implying complex but uncertain etiology in risk factor analysis) (Susser and Susser, 1996). This critique turned on the issue of whether epidemiology had successfully developed the tools needed to analyze disease transmission in human populations where statistical assumptions about independence of exposure often fail, and where the definition and measurement of group or neighborhood effects is difficult. Building on a theoretical focus developed a century earlier in sociological epidemiology, the new multilevel paradigm investigates the intertwining health effects of individual behavior, neighborhood influences, and other larger contexts. Rather than summing individual behaviors and calculating a grouped level of risk, the most effective multilevel research investigates how the behavior of the collective adds additional force to the behavior of any individual in that collective. Its analyses are nonlinear as well as linear, and it models as much as it estimates risk.

Multilevel approaches pose clear challenges to a cultural epidemiology. This is because anthropological approaches to multilevel analysis often involve synthesizing and presenting data from individuals, groups, social movements, and global economic contexts to draw comparisons even where those different levels do not comprise the same individuals. A more epidemiological approach to multilevel analysis would involve combining data on individuals, groups of those same individuals, and village and higher-level variables relevant to those same groups that may be invisible at the individual level. The first approach is a synthetic but still at heart comparative approach, while the latter builds multiple narratives across linked levels. This kind of linking is most feasible and appropriate where sampling strategies allow populations to be aggregated and disaggregated for different analytic purposes. Thus cultural epidemiologic research that aspires to multilevel analysis needs to employ epidemiological sampling strategies.

Popular and Lay Epidemiology

There are two additional alternatives to traditional epidemiology practiced by professionals using the biomedical model of disease. Popular epidemiology is defined as "the process by which laypersons gather scientific data and other information, and also direct and marshal the knowledge and resources of experts in order to understand the epidemiology of disease" (Brown, 1992: 269–270). This label recognizes the role that community residents can play in recognizing clusters of health problems, linking those clusters to environmental or other local causes, organizing their own as well as other formal professional investigations, and negotiating with supportive and opposing groups in government, academe, and industry. It is still the application of standard diagnostic categories, sampling strategies, and theories of disease causation, although it is controlled by people in the community rather than professionals or consultants.

Lay epidemiology is defined as "a scheme in which individuals interpret health risks through the routine observation and discussion of cases of illness and death in personal networks and the public arena, as well as from formal and informal evidence arising from other sources, such as television and magazines" (Frankel *et al.*, 1991: 428). It is another way of conceptualizing the use of epidemiology to include illness labels and health-related concerns that are not addressed or not accepted by the professional medical community. While this definition does not explicitly mention cross-cultural difference, one could readily extend it to cases where local communities perceive themselves as suffering from maladies not recognized by medical professionals. This was the case with many of the studies mentioned earlier in the section titled 'Psychological–psychiatric epidemiology': the objective of both lay epidemiology and of the epidemiological study of patterns of mental distress is to apply the same types of epidemiologic concepts and methods to nonbiomedical as to biomedical categories.

Returning Data to Communities

Cultural epidemiology has a potentially strong but often unrealized role to play in helping research results to be shared with local communities. Especially in areas with high illiteracy and low schooling, the challenge of converting quantified scientific results into intelligible products is not trivial. But the challenge is even more profound in areas where the basic assumptions of scientists and of the lay public are very different, if not diametrically opposed. In these areas, not only would translation be required from statistics into visual displays and oral accounts, but also cultural translation from the assumptions of science into those of religion and/or popular belief. Success depends upon in-depth knowledge of local vocabularies and belief systems, as well as knowledge of local desires and local uses for information.

Anthropology of Epidemiology

Epidemiology is a culture in itself, with its own assumptions, practices, and social relations, but it has not, as yet, been the source of much empirical work as an object of study for anthropologists. Anthropologists have conducted research in doctor's offices, hospitals, sorceror's huts, healer's clinics, and international health organizations, but few have worked in epidemiological offices, laboratories, or field studies. A few recent exceptions to this generalization include research on the work of Contract Research Organizations (CROs) that recruit human subjects and perform clinical trials of pharmaceuticals in developing countries (Petryna, 2005) and on laboratories involved in genetic epidemiology research (Montoya, 2007). Work like this is especially important because it helps reveal new ways that emerging global administrative processes (in the case of CROs) or new technologies applied to inherited forms of classifying human difference (in the case of genetic epidemiology) create and shape human knowledge.

Conclusion

Making progress on the challenges listed above, not to mention resolving them, requires more awareness of their importance as well as better training and more research. Yet these needs are not easy to satisfy: Joint training in both disciplines is not yet standard, postdoctoral training is rare, and publication outlets and research funding relatively inaccessible. There are signs of movement, for example the U.S. National Institutes of Health has issued a series of requests for research grant proposals building on a report titled 'Toward Higher Levels of Analysis: Progress and Promise in Research on Social and Cultural Dimensions of Health' (National Institutes of Health, 2001), but neither it nor national health research funding institutions in other countries have specific review bodies dedicated to the kinds of research described here. The institutional site that perhaps most closely sponsors and reviews cultural epidemiology would be the World Health Organization's Special Programme on Research and Training in Tropical Diseases, especially its Social, Economic and Behavioural Research group.

Some progress continues to be visible: Academic training appears to be responding to opportunities for better cross-fertilization between social scientists and epidemiologists. It is increasingly common and easy for doctoral students in anthropology to receive a Master's degree in public health with a specialization in epidemiology as part of their course of study. It is also more common, though not yet prevalent, for epidemiology students to take basic social science courses during their training, or to undertake postdoctoral work in social sciences related to health. Medical anthropologists also hold a number of important positions both in national health organizations and in the World Health Organization. For example, while as of 1996 there were 19 anthropologists working at the U.S. Centers for Disease Control and Prevention, at the end of 2005 there were 55, and they occupied senior positions in many different divisions (James Carey, personal communication, January 2006). Local traditions of cultural epidemiology are growing in sites where the boundaries between social science and medicine are more porous, including important research from Canada, Brazil, Ecuador, Peru, Mexico, South Africa, Thailand, England, Germany, Israel, Kenya, and Pakistan.

The term cultural epidemiology is but one label for a variety of types of work now being undertaken individually and jointly by anthropologists and epidemiologists. Some described here as doing cultural epidemiology might instead label their work as cross-cultural psychiatry, anthropological epidemiology, ethnoepidemiology, biocultural anthropology, and a host of other terms, because the label is not yet commonly accepted as a subfield within epidemiology or public health, and thus does not yet have status equivalent to social epidemiology. Nonetheless, no matter what label is used, there is increasing attention being paid to understanding the health-related effects of society and culture, with many important areas still to be developed and explored.

See also: Demography, Epidemiology and Public Health; Health Surveys; History of Epidemiology; Re-emerging Diseases; Social Epidemiology.

Citations

Ackerknecht EH (1948) Anticontagionism between 1821 and 1867. *Bulletin of the History of Medicine* 22: 562–593.

Brown P (1992) Popular epidemiology and toxic waste contamination: Lay and professional ways of knowing. *Journal of Health and Social Behavior* 33: 267–281.

Caprara A (1998) Cultural interpretations of contagion. *Tropical Medicine and International Health* 3: 996–1001.

Dressler WW (2005) What's *cultural* about bio*cultural* research? *Ethos* 33: 20–45.

Eckersley R (2005) Author's response: Culture can be studied at both large and small scales. *International Journal of Epidemiology* 35: 263–265.

Frankel S, Davison C, and Davey Smith G (1991) Lay epidemiology and the rationality of responses to health education. *British Journal of General Practice* 41: 428–430.

Guarnaccia PJ and Rogler LH (1999) Research on culture-bound syndromes: New directions. *American Journal of Psychiatry* 156: 1322–1327.

Hahn RA, Mulinare J, and Teutsch SM (1992) Inconsistencies in coding of race and ethnicity between birth and death in US infants: A new look at infant mortality, 1983 through 1985. *Journal of the American Medical Association* 267: 259–263.

Montoya MJ (2007) Bioethnic conscription: Genes, race, and Mexican ethnicity in diabetes research. *Cultural Anthropology* 22: 94–128.

Murphy JM (1994) Anthropology and psychiatric epidemiology. *Acta Psychiatrica Scandinavica Supplement* 385: 48–57.

National Institutes of Health (2001) *Toward Higher Levels of Analysis: Progress and Promise in Research on Social and Cultural Dimensions of Health. Executive Summary.* Washington DC: NIH Publication No. 21–5020. http://obssr.od.nih.gov/Documents/Publications/HigherLevels_Final.PDF (accessed September 2007).

Nations MK and Amaral ML (1991) Flesh, blood, souls, and households: Cultural validity in mortality inquiry. *Medical Anthropology Quarterly* 5: 204–220.

Omran AR (1971) The epidemiologic transition: A theory of the epidemiology of population change. *Milbank Quarterly* 49: 509–538.

Petryna A (2005) Ethical variability: Drug development and globalizing clinical trials. *American Ethnologist* 32: 183–197.

Susser M and Susser E (1996) Choosing a future for epidemiology: II. From black box to Chinese boxes and eco-epidemiology. *American Journal of Public Health* 86: 674–677.

Trostle J (1986) Anthropology and epidemiology in the twentieth century: A selective history of collaborative projects and theoretical affinities, 1920–1970. In: Janes CR, Stall R, and Gifford SM (eds.) *Anthropology and Epidemiology*, pp. 59–94. Dordrecht, the Netherlands: D. Reidel.

Weiss MG (2001) Cultural epidemiology: An introduction and overview. *Culture & Medicine* 8: 5–29.

Winch PJ, Makemba AM, Kamazima SR, *et al.* (1994) Seasonal variation in the perceived risk of malaria: Implications for the promotion of insecticide-impregnated bed nets. *Social Science and Medicine* 39: 63–75.

Further Reading

Briggs CL and Mantini-Briggs C (2003) *Stories in the Time of Cholera: Racial Profiling During a Medical Nightmare.* Berkeley, CA: University of California Press.

Cassel JC, Patrick RC Jr, and Jenkins CD (1960) Epidemiologic analysis of the health implications of culture change. A conceptual model. *Annals of the New York Academy of Sciences* 84: 938–949.

DiGiacomo SM (1999) Can there be a "cultural epidemiology"? *Medical Anthropology Quarterly* 13: 436–457.

Frankenberg R (1993) Risk: Anthropological and epidemiological narratives of prevention. In: Lindenbaum S and Lock M (eds.)

Knowledge, Power, and Practice: The Anthropology of Medicine in Everyday Life, pp. 219–242. Berkeley, CA: University of California Press.

Hopper K (1991) Some old questions for the new cross-cultural psychiatry. *Medical Anthropology Quarterly* 5: 299–330.

Inhorn MC and Whittle KL (2001) Feminism meets the "new" epidemiologies: Toward an appraisal of antifeminist biases in epidemiological research on women's health. *Social Science & Medicine* 53: 533–567.

Janes CR, Stall R, and Gifford SM (eds.) (1986) *Anthropology and Epidemiology*. Dordrecht, the Netherlands: D. Reidel.

Kark SL and Steuart GW (eds.) (1962) *A Practice of Social Medicine: A South African Team's Experiences with Different African Communities*. Edinburgh: E & S Livingstone.

Kunitz SJ (1994) *Disease and Social Diversity: The European Impact on the Health of Non-Europeans*. Oxford, UK: Oxford University Press.

Lindenbaum S (1978) *Kuru Sorcery: Disease and Danger in the New Guinea Highlands*. New York: McGraw-Hill.

Sobo EJ (1995) *Choosing Unsafe Sex: AIDS-Risk Denial Among Disadvantaged Women*. Philadelphia, PA: University of Pennsylvania Press.

Trostle J (2005) *Epidemiology and Culture*. Cambridge, UK: Cambridge University Press.

Trostle J and Sommerfeld J (1996) Medical anthropology and epidemiology. *Annual Review of Anthropology* 25: 253–274.

Genetic Epidemiology

H Campbell and N Anderson, University of Edinburgh Medical School, Edinburgh, UK

Introduction

It is clear that genetic factors are an important determinant of most if not all human diseases and thus investigation of these factors should be an essential element of any epidemiological study of disease causation or variations in disease frequency. Familiarity with research strategies in genetic epidemiology should therefore be a requirement in the training of all epidemiologists and clinical scientists studying disease mechanisms. Although the ability to study specific genetic factors directly is relatively recent, the advances in the Human Genome Project and related genetic laboratory methods now mean that it is possible to measure these factors with considerably greater precision and validity and less expense than for most environmental exposures.

By understanding the basic mechanisms of physiological pathways and pathological processes implicated in disease etiology through the identification of genetic factors underlying these processes, it is hoped that new treatments and disease prevention strategies will be developed. A secondary aim is to identify increased genetic susceptibility within individuals where this risk has been shown to be reversible through genetic manipulation or amenable to reduction by some other intervention.

Khoury *et al.* (1993) have suggested a hierarchy of research hypotheses in genetic epidemiology, addressing questions such as:

- Does the disease cluster in families?
- Is the clustering due to genetic or environmental factors?
- If there is evidence for a genetic factor, can a specific mode of inheritance be identified?
- Can the genetic risk factor be identified?

- Can the risk of disease associated with the genetic risk factor be quantified?
- Do environmental factors modify the expression of the genetic factor?

In the following sections, we consider how we may attempt to provide answers to these questions. For those readers unfamiliar with basic genetics, **Figure 1** provides a schematic of a pair of chromosomes in order to define some key genetic concepts and **Table 1** provides a glossary of some other commonly used terms.

Research Strategies

Currently little is known about the genetic architecture underlying complex diseases. This makes it difficult to be certain which approach is likely to be the most successful in identifying genetic factors. Important issues include:

- Number of loci involved: Animal models suggest that the genetic basis of many complex diseases and traits is polygenic (many genes with small effects) rather than oligogenic (a small number of genes with large effects).
- Genetic diversity: Experience from published studies of Mendelian disorders and monogenic forms of complex disease suggests that extreme locus and allelic heterogeneity is the rule. There are few data on locus and allelic complexity in common disorders, although most published examples show substantial heterogeneity.
- Frequency of variants: Most variation in the human genome is considered to be due to common alleles

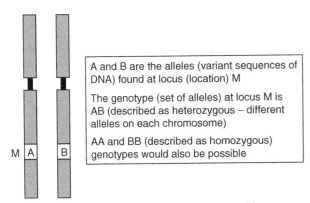

A and B are the alleles (variant sequences of DNA) found at locus (location) M

The genotype (set of alleles) at locus M is AB (described as heterozygous – different alleles on each chromosome)

AA and BB (described as homozygous) genotypes would also be possible

Figure 1 Schematic of a pair of chromosomes, with an explanation of some fundamental concepts.

(present at a minor allele frequency of >1%). Less frequent variants include the primary causes of the rare, Mendelian genetic diseases. Common variants may contribute significantly to genetic risk for common diseases (common variant–common disease hypothesis). The alternative, common disease–rare variant hypothesis holds that late-onset diseases are due to large numbers of rare variants at many loci with the contribution of most individual variants being very small (perhaps too small to further our understanding of disease).

• Heterogeneity in gene expression and due to interactions: Other levels of complexity include heterogeneity in expression patterns of different alleles in the same gene and the presence of gene–gene and gene–environment interaction effects. These issues are important since most current statistical methods are based on an oligogenic model of complex disease, with a single risk allele in each gene.

Some consideration of these issues is important in selecting the most appropriate study design. For example, substantial allelic heterogeneity considerably reduces the power of association methods and favors family-based association or linkage approaches. Since the genetic architecture of complex diseases is largely unknown, it is important that the selected analytic methods are robust and perform well under a variety of models.

A further important consideration is the choice of study population in order to minimize the effects of environmental or lifestyle and cultural factors, so as to maximize genetic effects and the relationshipx between the genetic markers and disease phenotypes under study.

First Step: Detecting the Influence of Genes

Genetic epidemiology requires a substantial commitment of time and resources, so that it is important first

Table 1 Glossary of some genetics terminology

Term	Definition
Complex disease	A condition thought to result from a mixture of genetic and environmental risk factors, rather than a mutation in a single gene (a Mendelian disorder)
Gene	A sequence of DNA responsible for coding protein structures
Genome	An organism's complete sequence of DNA, contained within one full chromosomal set
Haplotype	The set of alleles present on a single chromosome at two or more loci that are physically close (linked) to each other
Linkage disequilibrium	Association between the alleles of two different loci at a population level that results from the loci being physically close (allowing the same genetic material to be inherited intact in successive generations)
Marker	A sequence of DNA (that may or may not be a gene) that is identifiable by molecular biological techniques and thus has a known position within the genome
Meioses	Cell divisions within germ cells that result in offspring with random assortments of parental DNA
Pedigree	A collection of genetically related individuals, most often an extended family group
Phenotype	An observable manifestation (such as a physical measurement or a disease state) of the action of one or more genes. Sometimes referred to as a trait
Population stratification	A form of confounding: varying rates of disease and allele frequencies within subgroups of the population induce a disease–marker association at the level of the whole population
Single nucleotide polymorphism (SNP)	A locus at which the DNA sequence between individuals will differ by only one base pair but may still function as a marker

to show a clear influence of genetic factors on variation in a complex trait or on disease frequency. Subsequently, these data can be used to estimate the size of the genetic contribution to disease susceptibility. Evidence suggestive of a genetic influence can be found in the presence of genetic syndromes, e.g., familial polyposis coli leading to colon cancer, or from animal models of disease shown to have a clear genetic basis. More quantitative estimates of genetic contribution are typically obtained from family studies by analysis of pedigrees. Family history information is of limited utility for estimating familial aggregation. However, two specific measurements are useful:

- Lambda sib (λ_s) describes the increase in risk of disease in a sibling of an affected individual compared to the general population risk. It provides a summary of evidence for genetic factors in complex disease and is an important determinant of power. Note, however, that its value could also be due in part to shared environmental exposure, that λ_s relates to the total genetic effect and not of individual factors, and that results are specific to a given population with a particular pattern of environmental exposure.

- Heritability is defined as the proportion of disease variation directly attributable to genetic differences among individuals relative to the total variation in the population (genetic and nongenetic). As above, the estimate is always population-specific.

More definitive evidence can be found in twin and adoption studies. Studies of disease or trait value concordance rates in twins provide an alternative estimate of the size of the genetic component that is less confounded by environment. Evidence in favor of the importance of genetic variants is given by:

- high level of monozygotic twin concordance;
- monozygotic twin greater than same sex dizygotic twin concordance (both affected or unaffected by disease);
- monozygotic twin concordance same when twins reared apart.

Evidence from these studies is, however, limited by ascertainment bias: Concordant monozygotic twins are more likely to self-refer or to be referred by a doctor and monozygotic twins are likely to experience more similar environmental factors than dizygotic twins.

Adoption studies are able to estimate separately genetic and environmental contributions to disease risk by comparing disease rates in true parents of affected and nonaffected adopted children (who share genetics, but not environment) or disease rates in the adopted children of affected and nonaffected true parents (who share environment but not genetics), which allows an estimate of heritability to be made. However, there are limited opportunities to conduct these studies and the utility of the results is limited by small numbers, selection biases, and problems in determining true parental status.

Second Step: Gene Discovery

Most gene discovery studies utilize DNA-based methods and statistical genetic mapping techniques that use recombination events to determine genetic distance between two loci. Two major approaches, linkage and association, can be used: linkage studies use information from observed meioses and association studies use information from the unobserved meioses that connect pedigrees historically.

Linkage Analysis

Linkage studies test whether a disease and a genetic variant are inherited together in a pedigree by identifying coinheritance of chromosomal regions. It assesses whether genetic variants (markers) segregate with the disease according to Mendelian patterns of inheritance in large pedigrees with multiple affected individuals. This approach has proven to be very effective for rare Mendelian single-gene disorders and Mendelian forms of common complex disease. Thus it is the main strategy for identification of genetic variants of large effect. However, the same large genetic effect results in selection against these genes and so by definition they cause rare diseases or rare forms of common diseases. It has much less power to detect genetic variants with small effects and so may be much less effective for common complex diseases.

Most common disorders show a complex segregation pattern in which the type of inheritance is not clear, so simpler pedigrees are studied. The most common unit of study consists of two affected siblings and their parents, with increased sharing of markers providing evidence that the marker is genetically linked to a nearby gene that affects susceptibility to the disease. However, this approach is relatively inefficient and to provide strong evidence large numbers of such families must be studied and hence international collaboration is usually required. This approach is robust to the genetic heterogeneity that is typically found in different affected sib pairs and can provide information on the approximate localization of genetic variants. This approach can also be used to identify loci underlying quantitative traits (usually abbreviated to QTL – quantitative trait locus or loci) by correlating the degree of phenotypic similarity between affected relatives with the number of alleles shared at a locus that causes disease.

Association Studies

Association studies measure differences in the frequency of genetic variants between unrelated affected individuals (cases) and controls (unaffected individuals who are unrelated to any cases or controls in the sample). They thus study recombination and transmission of genes in populations over large timescales and are affected by the relatedness of populations, the effect of mutation and genetic drift on allele frequencies, migration, and gene–gene and gene–environment interaction. Association studies are premised on the hypothesis that common genetic variants underlie susceptibility to common diseases and take one of two main forms: Direct or indirect.

Direct association

In direct association studies, genetic variants in selected genes that are believed to cause disease are studied. This, however, requires the genetic variant of interest to be known and markers in or close to the gene to have been identified. Studies of these so-called candidate genes have been successful in identifying genetic variants affecting disease susceptibility. These studies are most meaningful when applied to functionally significant variants with a clear biological relation to disease mechanisms or the trait under study.

Indirect association

Indirect association studies investigate the association between a disease and neutral variants located near disease susceptibility variants. The association is therefore a result of allelic association (linkage disequilibrium or LD) between the marker and risk allele. This approach can also be considered as the identification of segments of the genome that are shared by people because they are inherited from a common ancestor. Among individuals affected by the disease, these segments may harbor susceptibility genes. The average size of shared segments is set by the number of generations separating two individuals from their common ancestor and this governs the number of markers needed to discover them. A few hundred markers are sufficient when the common ancestor is recent (as in siblings), but hundreds of thousands of markers are required to discover very ancient gene variants. The markers of choice are single nucleotide polymorphisms (SNPs) because of their high frequency, low mutation rates, and amenability to automation. A very comprehensive SNP database and massive genotyping capacity are thus required for these genome-wide association studies.

Association studies should follow the principles of good study design established in traditional epidemiological case–control studies as a means of improving the validity of study findings by reducing the opportunities for chance, bias, or confounding to account for study results. Technological advances such as the availability of SNP databases and affordable, very high-throughput genotyping are set to extend the potential and improve the efficiency of association approaches. However, the very large number of genetic variants in the human genome and the lack of detailed knowledge about the molecular and biochemical processes involved in the etiology of complex diseases suggest that it is very likely that many spurious associations will be found and reported. The great majority of reported associations have not led to new insights into complex disease or drug response

mechanisms and are now considered to be false-positive results. These positive associations could be due to:

- artifacts such as differences in handling, storage, or genotyping between cases and controls;
- chance, with multiple association studies performed with publication of only those that show positive results (multiple testing with publication bias);
- chance, with multiple testing of markers, each with low prior probability of causing disease (inappropriate significance levels chosen);
- bias in the estimate of association due to poor study design, particularly in the choice of controls;
- confounding due to population stratification or other (unrecorded) differences between cases and controls.

Association studies can be population-based (case–control) or family-based, in which transmission of alleles from parents to affected and unaffected offspring is studied (see **Figure 2**). Family-based association studies offer some advantages in the ability to assign haplotypes and the ability to look at parent-of-origin effects, as well as protecting against confounding via population stratification. A number of alternative genomic control approaches have been described which utilize data from unlinked DNA markers to measure and adjust for population substructure effects in population-based association studies.

Third Step: Gene Characterization

Key questions to be addressed after the identification of a genetic variant's role in a disease process or variation in a trait associated with health or disease are:

- What is the prevalence of gene variants in different populations?

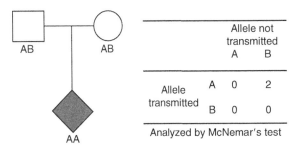

Figure 2 Example of a family-based association analysis – the transmission/disequilibrium test (TDT). Shown for a single family trio (out of the larger trio collection actually needed) of two heterozygous parents (father = square, mother = circle) and one child (diamond = either sex, shaded = affected by disease), with each individual genotyped for a single marker with two possible alleles. The A allele is transmitted twice, once by each parent, and AA (the child's genotype) forms a pseudo-case. The two B alleles are never transmitted, so BB is a pseudo-control. Data are analyzed by the 2 × 2 table shown.

- What is the risk (relative and attributable) of disease associated with these variants?
- What is the contribution of gene variants to the occurrence of disease in different populations (population-attributable risk)?
- What is the risk of disease associated with gene–gene and gene–environment interactions?

The prevalence of gene variants (allele frequencies) can be estimated from large unselected cohorts or large randomly sampled control series in different populations. Absolute risks can be measured in population-based cohort studies and relative risks in cohort or genetic association studies (which measure an odds ratio). The attributable risk expresses the size of excess risk to an individual due to the presence of a particular genetic variant. The population-attributable risk estimates the overall contribution of the genetic factor to a disease in a specific population, but depends not only on the relative risk (or odds ratio) but the allele frequency of the variant. In environmental epidemiology, population-attributable risk can be used to express the reduction in incidence of disease that would be achieved if exposure to the factor in the population were eliminated. This has less meaning with respect to genetic variants and disease. However, it may be useful when considering pharmacogenetics and the potential for the reduction in side effects that may be achieved if genetic testing could identify all those genetically predisposed to a certain drug adverse effect and prescriptions were avoided in those found to carry that variant.

Mendelian Randomization

Genetic epidemiology has the potential to improve the understanding of environmental as well as genetic determinants of disease. During gamete formation and conception, a random assortment of genes is passed from parents to offspring. In those offspring, if a genetic variant directly influences the level of an intermediate trait, which in turn alters disease risk, then the relationship between the variant and disease risk should be consistent with the associations between the variant and the intermediate trait and that trait and disease. If the trait level is directly influenced by an environmental exposure, this Mendelian randomization approach will provide data on the relationship between the environmental exposure and disease, but may reduce or avoid the confounding that is inherent in observational epidemiology studies. It may thus improve the ability to determine the causal nature of some environmental exposures, because the association between a disease and a genetic variant that mimics the biological link between a proposed environmental exposure and disease is not susceptible to reverse causation or confounding.

Future Perspectives

There is likely to be a move from the focus on gene discovery to include the need to understand function, biochemistry, and physiology before causal pathways can be understood and eventual public health benefits can be realized. The explosion of genomic technological capability and information is therefore the start and not the end of the path leading to the development of new drugs or other interventions.

In the short term, this will involve studies that integrate data on genetic variants, expression microarrays and pathophysiological phenotypes in order to define variants that influence mRNA expression levels and QTL so that casual pathways can be studied. Increasingly, the phenotypes will include protein intermediates measured by proteomic technologies. This systems biology approach will involve huge complexity and great computing power and new analytic approaches (such as clustering algorithms to classify genes into hierarchical sets, genes with similar expression patterns grouped together) will be required to analyze and interpret these data.

This will require greater collaboration between research groups in order to share data for meta-analysis and to increase power. Increasing partnership between governments, the pharmaceutical industry, medical research charities, and universities will become the norm for future genetic epidemiological research.

Citation

Khoury MJ, Beaty TH, and Cohen B (1993) *Fundamentals of Genetic Epidemiology.* Oxford, UK: Oxford University Press.

Further Reading

Balding DJ (2006) A tutorial on statistical methods for population association studies. *Nature Reviews: Genetics* 7: 781–791.

Burton PR, Tobin MD, and Hopper JL (2005) Key concepts in genetic epidemiology. *The Lancet* 366: 941–951.

Campbell H and Rudan I (2002) Interpretation of genetic association studies in complex disease. *The Pharmacogenomics Journal* 2: 349–360.

Campbell H and Rudan I (2007) Study design in mapping complex disease traits. In: Hastie N and Wright AF (eds.) *Genetics and Common Disease*, pp. 92–112. Edinburgh, UK: Churchill Livingstone.

Davey Smith G and Ebrahim S (2005) What can mendelian randomisation tell us about modifiable behavioural and environmental exposures? *British Medical Journal* 330: 1076–1079.

Hattersley AT and McCarthy MI (2005) What makes a good genetic association study? *The Lancet* 366: 1315–1323.

Hirschorn JN and Daly MJ (2005) Genome-wide association studies for common diseases and complex traits. *Nature Reviews: Genetics* 6: 95–108.

Hopper JL, Bishop DT, and Easton DF (2005) Population-based family studies in genetic epidemiology. *The Lancet* 366: 1397–1406.

Nitsch D, Molokhia M, Smeeth L, DeStavola BL, Whittaker JC, and Leon DA (2006) Limits to causal inference based on mendelian randomization: A comparison with randomized controlled trials. *American Journal of Epidemiology* 163: 397–403.

Ott J (1991) *Analysis of Human Genetic Linkage*. Baltimore, MD: Johns Hopkins University Press.

Palmer LJ and Cardon LR (2005) Shaking the tree: Mapping complex disease genes with linkage disequilibrium. *The Lancet* 366: 1223–1234.

Risch NJ (2000) Searching for genetic determinants in the new millennium. *Nature* 405: 847–856.

Thomas DC (2004) *Statistical Methods in Genetic Epidemiology*. Oxford, UK: Oxford University Press.

Wang WYS, Barratt BJ, Clayton DG, and Todd JA (2005) Genome-wide association studies: Theoretical and practical concerns. *Nature Reviews: Genetics* 6: 109–118.

Wright A, Charlesworth B, Rudan I, Carothers A, and Campbell H (2003) A polygenic basis for late-onset disease. *Trends in Genetics* 19: 97–106.

Relevant Websites

http://linkage.rockefeller.edu/ – Genetic Analysis Resources at Rockefeller University.

http://www.cdc.gov/genomics/hugenet – Human Genetic Epidemiology Network.

http://pngu.mgh.harvard.edu/~purcell/ – University of Harvard, Psychiatric & Neurodevelopmental Genetics Unit, Center for Human Genetic Research, Massachusetts General Hospital.

http://www.kumc.edu/gec/geneinfo.html – University of Kansas Medical Center, Information for Genetic Professionals.

http://csg.sph.umich.edu/ – University of Michigan Centre for Statistical Genetics.

http://watson.hgen.pitt.edu/ – University of Pittsburgh Department of Human Genetics.

http://www.well.ox.ac.uk – Wellcome Trust Centre for Human Genetics.

Dental Epidemiology

P G Robinson and Z Marshman, School of Clinical Dentistry, Sheffield, UK

Introduction

Dentistry boasts a long tradition of studying the distribution of oral disease and its determinants. There are also countless examples where epidemiological data have been directly translated to shape health policy and interventions. Observations that dental disease was a large barrier to recruiting young men to serve in the British army during the Boer war prompted the formation of the first school dental service and national surveys of oral health. Later, Trendley Dean used newly developed measures to link the concentration of fluoride in drinking water to both mottling of the teeth and lower levels of dental caries (tooth decay). His 21 cities study identified the optimum concentration of fluoride in water to be 1 part per million. This figure is still used as the benchmark some 65 years later.

Nowadays, oral epidemiology is used to describe the oral health of populations and establish their dental treatment needs. Repeated monitoring of oral health provides information of effects of interventions. More analytical research has demonstrated links between oral and other diseases and randomized controlled trials provide robust evidence of the effectiveness of new materials and treatments.

Oral epidemiology shares many features of other branches of the discipline, but can be complicated by specific features of the mouth and by the low reliability of some of the measures. The last 30 years have shown huge decreases in the burden of some dental diseases in the developed world, but profound social and geographical trends persist. This article will review some key features of the methods of oral epidemiology including the outcomes used and potential risk factors that are confounders and mediators for oral disease, and outline some procedures essential in oral epidemiology. The second half of the article will review the distribution of oral conditions of public health importance (caries, periodontal diseases, oral cancers and dental trauma) in relation to geographic, age, temporal, socioeconomic, and ethnic trends.

Measurement of Oral Health

The Presence and Number of Teeth

The most easily understood measures of dental status are the number of standing teeth and the proportion of the population with no natural teeth (edentulous). In the absence of affordable dental treatment and the lack of interest among people to save their teeth, dental extraction is often the principal form of dental treatment. Teeth may require extraction because they are decayed or affected by severe periodontal disease, or they may be extracted because nobody has the interest or resources to save them. Historically, edentulousness affected large numbers of adults in the developed world, but this trend has reduced with more people retaining some natural teeth. Consequently, the proportion of the population edentulous is dwindling along with the value of this measure.

Dental Caries

Dental caries is the repeated demineralization of tooth substance by bacterial acids. It can be successfully treated by application of fluoride, by removing the demineralized tissue and obturating the cavity with a filling, or by extracting the tooth.

The Decayed, Missing and Filled index (DMF for permanent teeth and dmf for deciduous or milk teeth) can be used with the number of affected teeth as the numerator (dmft) or the number of affected surfaces (dmfs). As it is (more accurately) an index of disease and treatment experience, it is sensitive to the treatment decisions of dentists and being cumulative and irreversible, it is sensitive to the age of the people examined. Nor does the index distinguish between a small filling that might never have been necessary and a severe lesion that has resulted in the extraction of the tooth. Finally, the index is unresponsive to secondary disease or retreatment of the same site, so its use to measure caries increments in the same individuals over time is complicated unless careful treatment records of the interim period are available. Other variants of DMF account for the presence of fissure sealants that may be indistinguishable (and indeed may serve the same purpose) from small fillings.

For the reasons above, dmf and DMF are of greatest value in young people, but in any circumstance the data must be age-specific. The ages between 6 and 12 years are often avoided because children of this age will have a mixed dentition of deciduous and permanent teeth. Surveys are typically conducted on children aged 5 (when they may be readily sampled at school) and 12 years. The mean DMFT of 12-year-olds is used as the standard to compare dental health in many publications including the World Health Organization (WHO) Oral Health Databank (World Health Organization, 2001). Adults are usually compared in 10-year age bands (e.g., 35- to 45-year-olds).

Another approach is to create a less precise version of the index to describe the dental status of adults as the proportion with 20 or more teeth or the proportion with 20 or more sound and untreated teeth. Despite these limitations, DMF has proved an invaluable index for many years. It is widely understood and has intuitive meaning. Moreover, to entirely dispense with it now would prevent consideration of temporal changes by comparison with historical data.

As understanding of dental disease has grown and our treatments have become more focused, there has been a need for more refined indices. Variants of DMF now have different thresholds for recording whether caries is only evident visually or whether it has caused cavitation and whether it remains limited to enamel, has penetrated into the dentine or to the pulp of the tooth. Research using different thresholds for dental caries

provides strong evidence that the role of fluoride is to inhibit the progression of early carious lesions as much as preventing new disease.

Three other indices can be derived from DMF data to ascertain patterns of care. The care index records the amount of restorative care received as the proportion of the DMF that is filled teeth (F/DMF), whereas the restorative index considers the amount of disease that has been treated restoratively by expressing the filled component as a proportion of the decayed and filled teeth (F/DF). Recognizing that the distribution of caries is skewed, the Significant Caries Index was introduced to bring attention to the individuals most prone to caries (Bratthall, 2000). It is the mean DMFT for the third of the population with the highest caries experience.

One other measure of dental caries is required. With more people retaining their teeth into longer life, there is accompanying recession of the gums (gingivae) either by periodontal diseases or by abrasion with tooth cleaning aids, which exposes the roots of the teeth. Unprotected by highly mineralized enamel, their surfaces are susceptible to root caries, which can be recorded separately.

Periodontal Diseases

Periodontal diseases affect the supporting structures of the teeth and arise from the interaction of the host's immune system with the bacteria of dental plaque. Gingivitis (inflammation of the gums) is exceedingly common. In a smaller proportion of cases, there is loss of attachment between the tooth and the adjacent tissues. This condition (periodontitis) is irreversible and may be manifest as a pocket between the tooth and the gingiva and/or by recession of the tissues (hence getting long in the tooth). As more tissue is lost, the teeth may become mobile. In addition, some plaque may calcify with mineral deposits from saliva to create calculus (tartar), which can hamper oral hygiene efforts.

All these variables – plaque, gingivitis, pocket depth, recession, attachment loss, mobility, and calculus – are studied in periodontology. Research is complicated by the plethora of indices available for each one. For example, in 42 trials found for a Cochrane review of powered toothbrushes, plaque was recorded using ten different indices and gingivitis with nine.

These indices are considered in many standard texts (Lindhe, 2003) and so will be covered only briefly. Specific choice of index should be governed by the usual criteria of the purpose and conditions of the research, the reliability and precision required, and by feasibility.

Plaque indices used for field epidemiology tend to record either the thickness of the plaque or the proportion of each tooth covered by it. In some cases, the tooth surface is divided into smaller areas to allow for more precise assessment. In nearly all cases, these indices are ordinal and contain a subjective element. Reliability can be enhanced by reducing precision, so that the plaque index of Silness and Loe records the thickness of plaque present on a scale of 0 to 3. Calculus indices share common characteristics with those for gingivitis. Gingival indices tend to consider swelling, redness, bleeding, and ulceration, although many use a combination of these indicators. Again the indices are subjective and are necessarily imprecise. While one sign is objective (bleeding on probing), it is very sensitive to the pressure applied (typically 25 g) and to recent disturbance of the tissues.

Perhaps the most important measure of periodontitis experience is lost probing attachment (LPA). It records the position of the gingival crest and the base of the periodontal pocket relative to the junction between the cement and enamel to permit calculation of the pocket depth and total amount of lost attachment. Probes of standard thickness are passed into the pockets to feel for the junctions. The probes have gradations to allow measurement. Some indices record only pocket depth, which is simpler, but may underestimate the amount of lost attachment if the gingivae have receded. Gingival recession is seen both with age and in tobacco smokers.

Measurement of LPA is surprisingly difficult. It is sensitive to the pressure with which the probe is applied as well as its position and angle. Attempts to overcome these difficulties include the use of smaller, lighter, and flexible probes, which help to prevent the application of excess pressure. Splints (stents) that can be attached to the teeth to guide the probe into the same place for repeated measurements are useful in longitudinal research but are too resource-intensive for field epidemiology. These complexities allow for substantial random measurement error. For example, trained periodontal epidemiologists aim to achieve 90% of LPA measurements within 1 mm of each other. That represents a 2-mm range for a disease that causes results in only 6 mm of lost attachment over a lifetime in only 10% of people. This problem is further complicated because LPA is the legacy of a lifetime's experience of disease and does not indicate current disease activity. Therefore, analytical research in periodontology is best served with longitudinal data, even though many changes in LPA will be masked by measurement error. Large sample sizes and elaborate statistical approaches are used to meet these challenges, but the lack of reliable measures continues to hamper periodontal research.

There are several aggregate indices that should be used with great care. Russell's Periodontal Index (1956) combines etiological factors and signs of disease, yet calculates mean scores that have no intrinsic meaning. The Community Periodontal Index of Treatment Need was developed to estimate treatment needs of the population as a function of the numbers of people who fell

into each category. This approach was roundly criticized as unrealistic and because it did not correspond to the stages of periodontal diseases or their treatment. However, disaggregated the categories within the index (now called Community Periodontal Index) provide reasonable descriptors of population periodontal health (the proportions with gingivitis, mild pocketing, and moderate pocketing), but its use beyond simple descriptive epidemiology is limited.

Tooth Wear

Tooth wear is loss of tooth tissue not caused by dental caries. It is often due to several etiological factors including attrition, abrasion, or erosion. The most widely used index is the Tooth Wear Index developed by Smith and Knight (1984). A score is given for each tooth surface from 0 to 4, depending on the severity of the wear.

Dental Opacities

Indices of dental opacities fall into two categories, those that record the severity of the defects associated with dental fluorosis and those that are simply descriptive. Proponents of the fluorosis indices argue that the indices have a history of construct validity proven by repeated and effective use and that the indices correspond well to the microscopic changes in the enamel. Those who favor the principal descriptive index (the Developmental Defects of Enamel, DDE) are concerned that there are other causes of anomalies and that fluorosis is not distinguishable from other types. Their intention to describe the defects, rather than relate them all to changes first described in fluorosis, is laudable, but DDE rates the severity of the defects on four different scales for different colors and morphology, thus complicating both scoring and analysis of the data. It may be that 'a rose by any other name would smell as sweet' and that the fluorosis indices will suffice for all forms of defect.

Subjective Assessments

The growth in the use of quality of life as an outcome in dentistry mirrors that in general health and is probably more apposite, as survival is rarely a concern in relation to oral health (with the exception of oral cancers). A variety of generic oral health-related quality-of-life measures are available. Two, the Oral Health Impact Profile (OHIP) and the Oral Impacts of Daily Performance (OIDP), were developed from a well-conceived model of health and have been translated and validated for use in many settings. Short forms of the OHIP have been developed for specific situations. These measures have been put to a range of uses, including assessing the psychosocial impacts of oral conditions, exploring models of oral health and evaluating health-care interventions. Other condition-specific measures have also been developed (Slade, 1997).

Risk Factors for Oral Health and Disease

Although oral diseases have a limited number of primary etiologic factors, a range of determinants and predisposing factors may confound and mediate these relationships. Failure to fully account for these factors has led to overestimations of relationships in analytical epidemiology. For example, early research associating periodontal diseases and heart disease led to considerable conjecture about the causative pathways between periodontal pathogens and the heart, yet both diseases share important risk factors (for example, socioeconomic status and tobacco smoking). More accurate accounting for these factors suggests that many links are due to confounding. The effects of these factors are dose-related and so precise measures reduce residual confounding. **Table 1** provides a brief summary of factors that should be considered in the design and analysis of epidemiological studies of oral conditions. Exposure to dental treatment also plays a role in the etiology and progression of some of these conditions.

Procedures

The use of the measures described in the previous section is very susceptible to changes in the conditions of the oral examination. The position and power of the lighting source, the relative placement of examiner and examinee, the specifications of the instruments used, and whether or not the teeth are dried beforehand will all affect the results. There are two sets of protocols in common use throughout the world.

First, Oral Health Surveys: Basic Methods by the WHO (WHO, 1997) provides comprehensive and easy to follow advice on its recommended measures, coding systems, recording sheets and examination protocols. Within the WHO Pathfinder Methodology, the WHO will provide examination sheets and then provide descriptive statistical analysis of data collected using its protocols. Second, the other widely used criteria are those of the British Association for the Study of Community Dentistry (Pitts, 1997).

As several of the measures described in this review are subjective and the methods are carefully standardized, there is a need for careful calibration and training of epidemiological examiners before data are collected.

One important aspect of oral epidemiology is the multiple values for each individual. Some periodontal measures can be recorded at six sites for every standing tooth. With up to 32 teeth and several variables, hundreds of measurements may be taken for each person. Partial recording indices can be used to record only half the mouth, a smaller number of specified teeth, or the worst score in each sextant of the mouth. Researchers must trade the potential loss of data against the time and costs to be saved by using partial recording indices.

Other consequences of multiple measures arise during data analysis. Measures from the same mouth are subject to many common factors and do not fulfill the requirements for independence in straightforward statistical tests. Moreover, the use of mean scores within a mouth may swamp differences associated with localized areas of disease (for instance those seen in HIV infection). One solution is to create a summary measure at the level of the individual such as the presence of a particular condition, the worst score per mouth (severity), or the number of sites above a stated threshold (extent of disease). The use of multilevel modeling shows great promise in this regard, as it is a powerful statistical technique that may account for factors within a population, within an individual, and then within a particular area of the mouth (Tu *et al.*, 2004).

Trends

Wide variation exists between countries in the amount and quality of dental epidemiological data and consequently in the ability to monitor trends in disease prevalence. For example, in Denmark a computer-based system tracks the oral health status of each child every year. In contrast, in other countries, the only data that are available are small surveys of populations in a single area.

Dental Caries

There are differences in the prevalence and severity of dental caries between and within countries. Oral disease

Table 1   Determinants and risk factors for oral conditions

Disease	Determinants and risk factors
Dental caries	Exposure to fluoride, socioeconomic status, age, dietary sugars
Periodontal diseases	Tobacco use, plaque, age, diseases affecting the immune system
Oral cancers	Tobacco use, alcohol, exposure to sunlight, leukoplakias
Dental trauma	Age, alcohol use, gender
Dental anomalies	Exposure to fluoride, trauma, systemic disease or tetracycline use during tooth development
Tooth wear	Habits, occupational and dietary exposure to acid, gastric reflux and vomiting

surveillance systems introduced by the WHO in the 1960s allow comparisons between countries. From the year 2000, the database includes 184 countries. The WHO and the Fédération Dentaire Internationale jointly set a global goal for 2000 of no more than three decayed, missing, and filled teeth for 12-year-olds (World Health Organization/Fédération Dentaire Internationale, 1982). This was achieved by 68% of countries.

Children

Generally in low-income countries, the prevalence of dental caries is relatively low, with a mean DMFT in 12-year-olds of approximately 1.9. In middle-income countries, the DMFT is about 3.3, and in high-income countries about 2.1 (World Health Organization, 2001).

While a general decline in dental caries has been seen in 12-year-old children in many industrialized countries since the early 1970s, evidence from some Western European countries suggests no further reductions are occurring among 5-year-olds, and caries levels may be slightly increasing (Marthaler et al., 1996). For example, in Norway the mean dmft in 5-year-olds increased from 1.1 in 1997/1998 to 1.5 in 2000. In some developing countries, particularly in Africa, an increase in the prevalence of caries in children may be apparent as the consumption of sugars has increased and sufficient amounts of fluoride have not been introduced (Petersen, 2003). However, the quality of the data preclude firm conclusions being drawn.

While data from national surveys are useful, they often mask within-country differences. For example, the UK Child Dental Health Survey 2003 reported levels of dental caries in permanent teeth to be the lowest ever recorded (Office for National Statistics, 2004). However, local surveys revealed at least a sevenfold difference in the mean dmft of 5-year-olds in areas with the lowest and highest caries experience in 5-year-olds (dmft in Maidstone Weald = 0.47, dmft in North Kirklees = 3.69).

Adults

Lifetime experience of caries in adults approaches 100%, although fewer surveys of adult caries levels are conducted than for children. In terms of dental caries experiences, most industrialized countries and some countries of Latin America show high mean DMFT levels (i.e., 14 or more) with much lower caries experience in developing countries of Africa and Asia.

The proportion of adults with no natural teeth varies with age and in developed countries rises steeply from the age of 70 onward. There has been a trend in industrialized countries over the past 30 years for fewer adults to become edentulous. For example, data from the UK Adult Dental Health Surveys show a reduction from 37% edentulous in 1968 to 13% in 1998; this trend is likely to continue as the predicted extrapolation to 2028 shows (**Figure 1**).

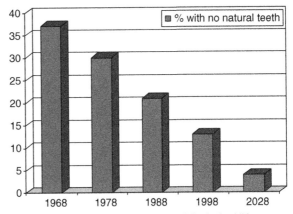

Figure 1 Percentage of edentulous adults in the UK.

Examining the data in more detail reveals an age-related cohort effect of caries experience in adults in industrialized countries. Those brought up in the 1960s, 1970s, and 1980s have benefited from fluoride toothpaste, the introduction of affordable dental care, and a more preventative approach to the management of dental caries. This has resulted in a cohort of people with more unrestored teeth and high expectations to maintain not just the presence of their own teeth, but also a high standard of dental appearance.

The earlier generation, born in the 1930s, 1940s, and 1950s, still retain their natural teeth to a far greater extent than their parents' generation, but have more heavily restored dentitions. This cohort was brought up at a time of higher risk of developing caries and it was not until the mid-1960s and early 1970s that a more conservative approach to restoring teeth was advocated. Consequently, this age group needs repeated placement and replacement of restorations with progressive loss of tooth structure and weakening of the tooth. As well as a huge volume of restorations, this cohort also has high expectations of retaining their teeth, which will have implications for dental care needs for at least the next 30 years.

A third group, those born before the 1930s, have relatively high levels of edentulousness and are vulnerable to health problems such as stroke and dementia, which make denture wearing problematic. Where all teeth are lost, there is a significant impact on diet and general well-being.

Disparities

For all age groups, there are marked differences in dental caries experience due to disparities in socioeconomic status, whether indicated by income, education, or occupational prestige. Using the United States as an example, poor children have twice as much caries as higher income children, with more chance of the caries remaining untreated. This is also the case in adults, with the proportion of untreated caries being higher in poor people. Low-social-class or low-income adults are also more likely to become edentulous (Department of Health and Human Services, 2000).

Studies around the world have been conducted to establish the role of ethnicity in disparities in caries experience. No consensus has been reached. Disagreements about the role of ethnicity are largely related to confounding between ethnicity and socioeconomic status. The data are complicated by several other factors such as different findings between the deciduous and permanent dentitions and assignment of ethnicity, religious differences, and maternal literacy.

Periodontal Diseases

Like dental caries, periodontal diseases are common with the vast majority of adults affected by gingivitis at any one time. Periodontal disease of the most severe level (which may result in tooth loss) varies between countries, affecting between 5 and 15% of adults worldwide.

At all ages, men are more likely than women to have severe disease. A significant relationship between periodontal disease and socioeconomic status exists, with low income or low education contributing to poor periodontal status (Petersen and Ogawa, 2005). Interestingly, smoking has been shown to be more important than socioeconomic variables in the etiology of periodontitis. However, smoking is strongly related to socioeconomic status in many developed countries. In the UK, people in routine and manual households are more likely to smoke than those in managerial and professional households (31% compared with 18%), and tobacco use accounts for more than half of periodontitis in adults (Department of Health and Human Services, 2000). There is also evidence from developing countries of the importance of smoking in the etiology of periodontitis.

Periodontal disease can also be associated with systemic diseases including diabetes and HIV/AIDS. The risk of destructive loss of attachment is three times higher among diabetics than nondiabetics. Approximately 177 million people worldwide have diabetes mellitus, and this number is predicted to double by 2030, which is likely to increase the incidence of periodontal disease.

Severe and unusual forms of periodontal diseases, including necrotizing ulceration, are associated with HIV infection and cause a significant burden where the underlying infection is common.

While tooth loss is the most severe consequence of periodontal disease, there is one type of gingival inflammation, noma, which can progress from the supporting tissues of the tooth to orofacial gangrene. WHO has suggested a global incidence of 140 000 cases. It is rare in developed countries and most common in sub-Saharan Africa, particularly among children under 5 years. If noma is not treated early with antibiotics it can progress to severe disfigurement and functional problems. It is estimated that less than 10% of affected people seek treatment and there is a mortality rate of 70–80% for those without proper treatment.

Oral Cancer

Oral cancer includes cancer of the lip, tongue, salivary glands plus other sites in the mouth. Oral cancer is the eighth most common cancer worldwide, with an estimated 405 318 newly diagnosed cases in 2002. Overall incidence worldwide for males has been estimated at 6.42 per 100 000 population (7.55 for more developed countries compared to 5.98 for less developed countries). There is large variation in incidence between countries. For example, within Asia, the incidence per 100 000 population is 12.6 in India, where oral cancer accounts for up to 40% of all malignancies among men. This is compared to 4.6 in Thailand and 0.7 in China (World Health Organization, 2001). There are also discrete pockets in some countries with high incidence such as the Bas-Rhin department of France with 62.1 per 100 000. The worldwide mortality rate for males has been estimated at 3.09 per 100 000 with a higher mortality rate in less developed countries compared to more developed countries (3.25 and 2.78, respectively).

Trends over time in oral cancer incidence vary by country and for different subgroups of the population. There has been a trend for increased incidence in some European countries such as Denmark, France, Germany, and the United Kingdom and to a lesser extent in Australia, Japan, New Zealand, and the United States.

The incidence of oral cancer increases with age, with most cases occurring in people over 60 years. In the UK, people under 45 years account for only 6% of all oral cancer cases. However, there is now evidence of an increased incidence in those less than 45 years and it has been suggested that oral cancer in the young may be a distinct entity that acts in an aggressive manner (Conway *et al.*, 2006).

In most countries, oral cancer is more common in males than females. In the United States, the incidence in males is 15.8 per 100 000 compared to 5.8 per 100 000 for women. This gender difference has narrowed slightly: in 1950 the ratio was approximately 6:1 (Silverman, 1998).

Incidence rates vary by ethnic group. In the United States, rates are higher for black people than white (12.5 and 10.0 cases per 100 000 people, respectively). Asians and Pacific Islanders, American Indians, Alaska Natives, and Hispanics all have a lower incidence than white and black people. Black people also have lower 5-year survival rates than whites (34% compared to 56%), possibly due to late presentation and diagnosis associated with low access to care (Department of Health and Human Services, 2000).

The main risk factors for oral cancer are tobacco use and excessive alcohol consumption, with these factors accounting for an estimated 90% of all oral cancers. Tobacco use, including both smoked and smokeless (e.g. chewing tobacco, snuff, paan), varies widely between countries. Chewing of areca nuts, betel nuts, paan, and gutka are common in South Asian populations and can be mixed with tobacco products.

Dental Trauma

The most commonly occurring type of dental trauma is fractured enamel. In children, damage to primary teeth most often occurs between 2 and 4 years of age and 7–10 years for the permanent dentition. Data on dental trauma from many countries, particularly developing countries, are unavailable or unreliable. Some countries in Latin America report dental trauma in about 15% of schoolchildren, whereas prevalence of 5–12% have been found in children aged 6–12 years in the Middle East. In the UK, 11% of 12-year-olds and 13% of 15-year-olds had some damage (Office for National Statistics, 2004; Petersen *et al.*, 2005). Data on trends over time are also inconsistent. Generally, it is more common among males than females.

A significant proportion of dental trauma relates to sports, unsafe playgrounds or schools, road accidents, or violence. Causes differ between countries, particularly with respect to leisure activities, with football injuries being a common event in Brazil and ice-skating injuries occur more frequently in Scandinavian countries. Most traumatized front teeth in children and adolescents remain untreated. Research from Brazil suggests children with fractured teeth involving dentine were 20 times more likely to report impacts on their daily lives than children without fractured teeth (Cortes *et al.*, 2002).

Future Trends

Better data are needed to monitor trends in oral disease especially on ethnicity and socioeconomic status to allow analysis for population subgroups.

An important future consideration for trends in dental disease is the growing proportion of older people worldwide. Currently about 600 million people are aged 60 years and over, and this figure is expected to double by 2025. Managing dental diseases in this cohort is complicated by their already heavily restored dentitions, vulnerability to root caries, and the difficulty maintaining oral cleanliness as their manual dexterity reduces with age. Monitoring of oral disease among older adults in terms of tooth loss, dental caries, periodontal disease, and oral cancer will be required to meet the challenge of preventing and managing poor oral health in this growing population subgroup.

See also: Observational Epidemiology.

Citations

Bratthall D (2000) Introducing the Significant Caries Index together with a proposal for a new global oral health goal for 12-year-olds. *International Dental Journal* 50: 378–384.

Conway DI, Stockton DL, Warnakulasuriya KAAS, Ogden G, and Macpherson LMD (2006) Incidence of oral and oropharyngeal cancer in United Kingdom (1990–1999): Recent trends and regional variation. *Oral Oncology* 42: 586–592.

Cortes M, Marcenes W, and Sheiham A (2002) Impact of traumatic injuries to the permanent teeth on the oral health-related quality of life in 12- to 14-year-old children. *Community Dentistry Oral Epidemiology* 30: 193–198.

Department of Health Human Services (2000) Oral Health in America: A report of the Surgeon General. Washington, DC: Department of Health and Human Services.

Lindhe J, Karring T, and Lang NP (2003) *Clinical Periodontology and Implant Dentistry*. London: Blackwell Publishing.

Marthaler TM, O'Mullane DM, and Vrbic V (1996) The prevalence of dental caries in Europe 1990-1995. *Caries Research* 30: 237–255.

Office for National Statistics (2004) Dental health survey of children and young people 2003. http://www.statistics.gov.uk/ssd/surveys/cdhs.asp (accessed November 2007).

Petersen PE (2003) *The World Oral Health Report*. Geneva, Switzerland: World Health Organization.

Petersen PE and Ogawa H (2005) Strengthening the prevention of periodontal disease: the WHO approach. *Journal of Periodontology* 76: 2187–2193.

Petersen PE, Bourgeois D, Ogawa H, Estupinan-Day S, and Ndiaye C (2005) *The Global Burden of Oral Diseases and Risks to Oral Health*. Geneva, Switzerland: World Health Organization.

Pitts N (1997) The BASCD coordinated NHS Dental Epidemiology Programme caries prevalence surveys 1985/6-1995/6. *Community Dental Health* 14(supplement 1): 1–51.

Silverman S (1998) *Oral cancer*. Hamilton, Ontario: American Cancer Society.

Slade GD (1997) *Measuring Oral Health and Quality of Life*. Chapel Hill, NC: University of North Carolina-Chapel Hill.

Tu YK, Gilthorpe MS, Griffiths GS, *et al.* (2004) The application of multilevel modeling in the analysis of longitudinal periodontal data–Part I: Absolute levels of disease. *Journal of Periodontology* 75: 127–136.

World Health Organization (1997) *Oral Health Surveys: Basic Methods*, 4th edn. Geneva, Switzerland: World Health Organization.

World Health Organization (2001) *Global Oral Health Data Bank*. Geneva, Switzerland: World Health Organization.

World Health Organization/Fédération Dentaire Internationale (1982) Global goals for oral health by the year 2000. *International Dental Journal* 32: 74–77.

Further Reading

Daly B, Watt R, Batchelor P, and Treasure E (2002) *Essentials of Dental Public Health*. Oxford, UK: Oxford University Press.

Pine C (1997) *Community Oral Health*. Bath, UK: Wright.

Relevant Websites

http://www.statistics.gov.uk/ssd/surveys/cdhs.asp – National Statistics, 2003 Dental Health Survey of Children and Young People.

http://www.who.int/oral_health/en/ – World Health Organization, Oral Health.

Cancer Epidemiology

P A Wark, London School of Hygiene and Tropical Medicine, London, UK
J Peto, London School of Hygiene and Tropical Medicine, London, UK and Institute of Cancer Research, Sutton, UK

Cancer Distribution Worldwide

Cancer is a major public health problem throughout the world, causing more than a quarter of all deaths in many countries. Cancer accounted for approximately 7 million deaths worldwide in 2002, one in eight of all deaths. In the same year, 11 million people were diagnosed with cancer and nearly 25 million people diagnosed with cancer over the previous 3 years were still alive (Parkin *et al.*, 2005). The absolute number of people diagnosed with cancer is increasing steadily because of continuing increases in life expectancy and world population, and it has been estimated that there will be 15 million new cases per year by 2020.

Lung (1.4 million cases), breast (1.2 million cases), and colorectal (1 million cases) cancer are the most commonly diagnosed cancers, whereas lung cancer (1.2 million cancer deaths), stomach cancer (700 000 deaths), and liver cancer (600 000 deaths) are the most common causes of cancer death (Parkin *et al.*, 2005).

Numbers of new cancer cases (incidence) and deaths (mortality) in 2002 are presented in **Figure 1** for developed and developing countries. The ratio of mortality to incidence reflects the fatality rate of the cancer. Pancreas and liver cancer, for instance, have similar incidence and mortality because their prognosis is poor. Breast cancer has a relatively good prognosis, so mortality is much lower than incidence, particularly in developed countries.

Many types of cancer vary in incidence by more than one order of magnitude between different populations, and every type is rare in some part of the world (Doll and Peto, 1981). The convergence toward local cancer rates seen among immigrants (**Figure 2**) excludes a genetic explanation of these differences. By the 1960s, cancer epidemiologists had therefore concluded that most cancers are in principle preventable and many could be avoided by a suitable choice of lifestyle and environment. Many specific causes of cancer are now known, the most important being smoking, obesity, and a few cancer-causing (oncogenic) viruses, but a large proportion of global variation for common cancers such as breast, prostate, colon, and rectum remains unexplained.

Age-specific cancer incidence and mortality rates have fallen for some cancer sites, while other cancers have become more common, reflecting changes in relevant exposures, diagnosis, treatment, and screening. Increases

in cigarette smoking since the 1950s caused large increases in death rates for smoking-related cancers, but overall mortality from cancers not caused by smoking has generally decreased or remained stable in most Western countries (Peto *et al.*, 2006).

Effect of Cancer Screening on Incidence and Mortality

Cancer screening programs can reduce mortality by early detection of the disease and hence earlier treatment, but for some cancers the benefit may be too small to justify the costs. Well-organized cervical screening prevents the majority of cervical cancers by detecting and treating premalignant disease, but for breast and prostate cancers mortality is reduced while cancer incidence is increased by screening, because early cancers are detected that would never have become symptomatic. Widespread prostate specific antigen (PSA) testing from around 1986 onward has caused an enormous increase in the incidence of prostate cancer in the United States, followed a few years later by smaller increases in other countries, but has had only a small effect on mortality.

Population screening for colorectal cancer has recently been introduced in some Western countries, but its long-term impact on mortality and morbidity in a population setting will not be known for many years. Studies on the benefits of lung cancer screening are ongoing. Some screening programs are targeted at individuals at high risk, particularly people with a strong family history of the disease.

Environmental and Lifestyle Causes of Cancer

Carcinogenic Effects of Tobacco

The most important discovery in the history of cancer epidemiology is the carcinogenic (cancer-causing) effect of tobacco. Lung cancer incidence increases rapidly among continuing smokers, but remains roughly constant in ex-smokers. The risk is therefore greatest in those who begin to smoke when young and continue throughout life. Second-hand, or environmental, tobacco smoking is also carcinogenic, but it is hard to quantify the magnitude of the risk.

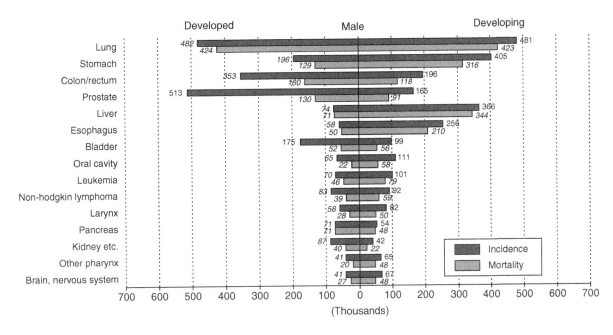

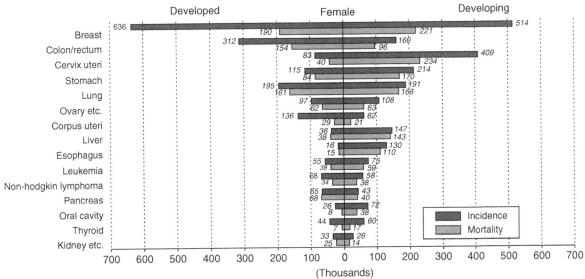

Figure 1 Estimated numbers of new cancer cases (incidence) and deaths (mortality) in 2002. Data shown in thousands for developing and developed countries by cancer site and sex. Reproduced from Parkin DM, Bray F, Ferlay J, and Pisani P (2005) Global cancer statistics, 2002. *CA: A Cancer Journal for Clinicians* 55: 74–108.

The large increase in male cigarette smoking in most developed countries that occurred during the first half of the twentieth century caused an unprecedented epidemic in the lung cancer rate several decades later. A reduction in tar levels in cigarettes combined with decreases in smoking has subsequently reduced the lung cancer rate in many developed countries. Women in most Western countries began smoking later than men and fewer have stopped, so their lung cancer rates are either still increasing or falling less rapidly.

For many years, the carcinogenic effects of tobacco were thought to be restricted largely to the lung, pancreas, bladder, and kidney, and (synergistically with alcohol) the larynx, mouth, pharynx (except nasopharynx), and esophagus. More recent evidence indicates that stomach, liver, cervix, myeloid leukemia, and probably colorectal cancer are also increased by smoking. This makes smoking the most important known risk factor for cancer.

The relative importance of different smoking-related diseases varies widely between populations, as smoking usually multiplies the background rate due to other factors. In China, where liver cancer is common, smoking causes more premature deaths from liver cancer than from heart disease, while in the United States liver cancer is rare even in smokers (**Figure 3**).

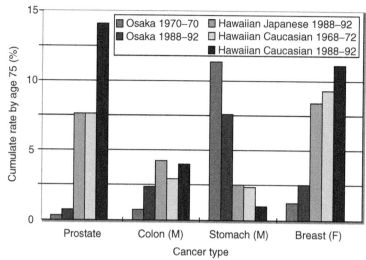

Figure 2 Cancer rates in migrants become similar to those in the local population. Cancer rates in 1990 among Japanese migrants to Hawaii, and around 1970 and 1990 in Japan (Osaka) and in Hawaiian Caucasians. Local rates for prostate, colon, and breast cancer increased over time (due partly to increased completeness of diagnosis and registration, particularly for prostate cancer in Hawaiian Caucasians) and stomach cancer decreased; but the effects of migration were larger.

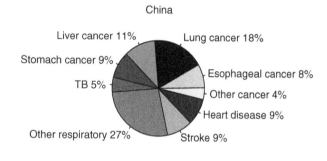

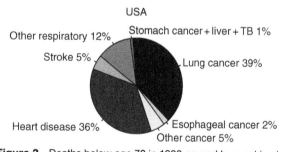

Figure 3 Deaths below age 70 in 1990 caused by smoking in China and the United States. Other cancers are mouth, pharynx, larynx, bladder, and pancreas. Data on China are derived from Liu BQ, Peto R, Chen ZM, *et al.* (1998) Emerging tobacco hazards in China: 1. Retrospective proportional mortality study of one million deaths. *British Medical Journal* 317: 1411–1422, and data on the United States are derived from Peto R, Lopez D, Boreham J, *et al.* (1994) *Mortality from Tobacco in Developed Countries, 1950–2000.* Oxford: Oxford University Press.

The Effects of Diet and Overweight

Nutritional epidemiology is notoriously complex owing to the variety of foods and their many constituents and to intercorrelations and temporal changes in their patterns of use. Cancer risks in old age may also depend as much on diet in early life as on current habits.

Most dietary factors do not show a strong and consistent enough effect to establish them unequivocally as important carcinogens or anticarcinogens. Exceptions are drinking alcohol, consumption of various foods contaminated with aflatoxin, and a few local customs (such as feeding Chinese-style salted fish to infants, which causes nasopharyngeal cancer). Extensive research during the past two decades has shown that rates for various cancers correlate fairly consistently with certain aspects of diet, but opinions still differ on the strength of the evidence. In the 1980s, nutritional epidemiology focused mainly on meat, fat, and total energy intake as potential risk factors, and on dietary fiber, fruits, and vegetables, vitamins A, C, and E, and β-carotene as protective factors. More recent research has concentrated on red and processed meat as risk factors, and on folate and other B vitamins, vitamin D and calcium, selenium and specific non-nutrient components of fruits, vegetables, and whole grains (e.g., phytoestrogens and isothiocyanates present in cruciferous vegetables) as protective factors. The overall evidence that fats are hazardous and fruits and vegetables are protective seems less convincing than initially thought, and more specific compounds and mechanisms are being investigated. Fat is classified according to its source (animal or vegetable fat) and its different subtypes (e.g., saturated fat). A high intake of n-3 fatty acids, derived from fatty fish, may prove to be beneficial. The evidence on diet and cancer has been systematically reviewed and summarized by the World Cancer Research Fund/American Institute for Cancer Research in 2007.

Dietary supplements may not have the same effects as the foods that contain them, and some may even be harmful. For example, β-carotene appeared to be associated with reduced risk of cancer in observational studies, but 12 years of treatment in a large randomized trial showed no benefit, and in two shorter trials the lung cancer risk was higher in those who received β-carotene supplements (Greenwald *et al.*, 2007). Aspirin probably reduces colorectal cancer incidence but may take a decade or more to do so.

Most reports conclude that about one-third of cancer deaths might be avoidable by dietary change. However, dietary recommendations differ, and Doll and Peto (2005) concluded that only cancers due to obesity are definitely avoidable. Radical changes in national dietary habits would not be easy to achieve even if there were a consensus on which foods are relevant.

There is now a consensus that cancer is commoner in those who are overweight. The evidence on weight is strongest for postmenopausal breast cancer and cancers of the endometrium, gallbladder, and kidney, but several other sites contribute to the observed overall cancer risk. A large prospective cohort of nonsmokers in America, where obesity is particularly common, provides the strongest evidence on the association between body mass index (BMI; weight divided by the square of height) and cancer mortality (Calle *et al.*, 1999). The authors did not calculate an attributable fraction, but if the observed excess mortality reflects a direct effect their data suggest that approximately 10% of all cancer deaths among American nonsmokers (7% in men and 12% in women) would be avoided if no one's BMI exceeded 25 kg/m^2. It is, however, not clear how much the risk can be reduced by weight reduction in those who are already overweight. Mortality from nonmalignant diseases is increased in those who are either too thin or too fat. Since obesity is an increasing problem in Western societies, the number of weight-related cancers will inevitably increase in the years to come.

Reproductive and Hormonal Factors

The effects of reproductive factors on breast and ovarian cancer have long been assumed to reflect underlying hormonal processes, and this is confirmed by the effects of both endogenous and exogenous hormones. Breast cancer incidence is transiently increased by pregnancy and while estrogens are administered as oral contraceptives or hormone replacement therapy (HRT), and is permanently lowered by late menarche, early menopause, early first childbirth, and high parity. Endometrial cancer incidence is also transiently increased by HRT. Combined estrogen and progestin HRT has a larger effect than estrogen alone for breast cancer, but a smaller effect for endometrial cancer. Ovarian cancer incidence declines with increasing parity, and both endometrial and ovarian cancers are less common in oral contraceptive users. Both oral contraceptives and HRT appear to reduce colorectal cancer incidence.

The Western diet is associated both with earlier age at menarche and with postmenopausal obesity, which increases endogenous estrogen production. Breast cancer incidence is much higher in most Western countries than in many developing countries, and this is partly (and perhaps largely) accounted for by these dietary effects combined with later first childbirth, lower parity and shorter breastfeeding. The development of cancers of the testis and prostate may also depend on hormonal effects, but apart from the increased risk in an undescended testis, no behavioral or reproductive correlate is strongly predictive of these diseases.

Viruses, Bacteria, and Parasites

Important discoveries of the past 30 years in cancer epidemiology relate to the carcinogenic effects of infectious agents. Recent estimates of the global cancer burden caused by specific viruses, bacteria, and parasites (Parkin, 2006) imply that about 20% of all cancers worldwide are caused by known infections (**Table 1**).

Helicobacter pylori, a chronic gastric bacterial infection that can cause gastric ulcers, is a major factor in the development of stomach cancer, accounting for an estimated 63% of all stomach cancers and 5.5% of all cancers worldwide. The evidence is particularly strong for noncardiac gastric cancers, which comprise more than 80% of gastric cancers. *H. pylori* is common in developed and developing countries, and more than half of all stomach cancers might be prevented if *H. pylori* could be eradicated.

More than 100 human papillomaviruses (HPVs) have been identified, and DNA from a subgroup of sexually transmitted HPVs that includes HPV16, HPV18, and HPV45 is detectable in virtually all cervical cancers worldwide. These and other HPVs are also found in other anogenital cancers, and in some cancers of the mouth and pharynx. HPV vaccines are now available, but their long-term effect on overall cervical cancer incidence remains to be established. At present, the high cost of HPV vaccines precludes their widespread use in developing countries that lack the resources for organized cervical screening, where their potential impact is greatest. Their effect in countries that already have effective screening is unclear. They are only effective against specific HPV types, so they will not prevent all cervical cancers; they are unlikely to be effective in women who have already been infected; and vaccinated women may be less likely to participate in cervical screening, which is known to be very effective.

The contribution of hepatitis B virus (HBV) to liver cancer in high-incidence regions has long been recognized, and the hepatitis C virus (HCV) is similarly carcinogenic.

Table 1 Carcinogenic infectious agents and the percentage of the global cancer burden they account for

Agent	Organism	Cancer	Percentages caused by organism	
			% of this cancer	% of global cancer burden
Helicobacter pylori	Bacterium	Stomach	63	5.5
Human papillomaviruses (HPV)	Virus	Cervix	100	4.5
		Other anogenital	56	0.5
		Mouth, pharynx	4	0.1
Hepatitis B and C virus (HBV, HCV)	Virus	Liver	85	4.9
Epstein-Barr virus (EBV)	Virus	Nasopharynx	98	0.7
		Hodgkin lymphoma	46	0.3
		Burkitt's lymphoma	82	0.1
Human immunodeficiency virus/Herpes virus 8 (HIV/HHV8)	Virus	Kaposi sarcoma	100	0.6
		Non-Hodgkin lymphoma	12	0.3
Schistosomes	Parasite	Bladder	3.0	0.1
Human T-cell lymphotropic virus I (HTLV-1)	Virus	Leukemia	1.1	0.03
Liver flukes	Parasite	Liver	0.4	0.02
Total			–	17.8

Adapted from Parkin DM (2006) The global health burden of infection-associated cancers in the year 2002. *International Journal of Cancer* 118: 3030–3044.

Hepatitis B infection is common in developing countries, and together with hepatitis C it accounts for 85% of all liver cancers worldwide (Parkin, 2006). The incidence of several virally induced cancers is further increased by specific cofactors such as salted fish (nasopharynx), smoking (liver and cervix), aflatoxin (liver), and malaria (the major cofactor with EBV for Burkitt's lymphoma in Africa). There is also strong epidemiological evidence for an infective etiology in childhood leukemia, but no specific pathogen has been implicated. Therapeutic immunosuppression causes a marked increase in the incidence of non-melanoma skin cancer and some virally induced cancers. The discovery that many other epithelial cancers are also increased by immunosuppression (Buell *et al.*, 2005) suggests that unidentified viruses may be important in these cancers as well. The alternative is the long-standing but equally speculative theory that many nonviral cancers are normally kept in check by the immune system.

Occupational and Environmental Carcinogens

Roughly a dozen specific occupational exposures and several complex mixtures, particularly the combustion products of coal, have caused high risks of certain cancers (predominantly lung cancer) in heavily exposed workers. Exposure levels for many industrial hazards have been progressively reduced in many Western countries since the 1930s, and by the late 1970s it was assumed, probably correctly, that the occupational exposure levels then current would contribute a very small proportion of future cancer incidence. But uncontrolled asbestos use had been widespread in the construction industry in Western countries from the 1950s to the mid-1970s, when public concern led to a rapid reduction. The resulting epidemic of mesothelioma in building and other workers born after 1940 did not become apparent until the 1990s because of the long latency of the disease. Incidence rates are still rising, and asbestos exposure prior to 1980 may eventually cause 250 000 mesotheliomas and a similar number of lung cancers in Western Europe. Chrysotile (white asbestos) causes a much lower mesothelioma risk than other types, but all forms of asbestos cause cancer.

This tragic episode was largely avoidable, as the carcinogenic effects of asbestos were known by 1960; but it illustrates the major weakness of epidemiology as an early warning system. The increase in cancer incidence caused by increased exposure to a carcinogen might not be detectable for several decades, and laboratory testing must remain the first line of defense against potentially dangerous new agents, particularly those affecting endocrine or paracrine signaling that could be biologically active at very low levels.

Epidemiological studies of markers such as DNA adducts in the lung or chromosomal aberrations in lymphocytes might also provide early warning of a potential hazard. But such direct or indirect measures of mutagenic or transforming potency have never detected an important carcinogen and even today cannot provide quantitative estimates of risk.

Epidemiological data on human cancer rates still provide the only reliable evidence that the cancer risks caused by long-established activities such as working in an oil refinery or living near a high-voltage power line are not large. There is as yet little evidence of a link between mobile phone use and cancer risk, but it may be too early for an effect to be detected. Apart from melanoma and other (usually nonfatal) skin cancers due to excessive exposure to sunlight, the only substantial and widespread cancer risk known to be caused by an avoidable environmental factor in developed countries is the further increase in lung cancer among smokers caused by indoor radon escaping from the ground or from building materials, although both indoor and outdoor air pollution from fossil fuels may also contribute to the risk in smokers. The risk to nonsmokers is relatively trivial in developed countries, but burning fossil fuels indoors without adequate ventilation certainly contributes to the high lung cancer rates, even in nonsmokers, seen in parts of China.

Genetic and Molecular Epidemiology of Cancer

An inherited mutation that predisposes carriers to cancer often involves a gene that is mutated or deleted during the transformation of a normal cell to cancer in people who have not inherited a defective gene. Some of these genes affect metabolism of carcinogens, but many are involved in normal cellular mechanisms such as detection and repair of DNA damage, control of the cell cycle, or apoptosis (programmed cell death). They have been discovered in many ways, notably by laboratory studies of such pathways, linkage in families with cancer syndromes such as hereditary retinoblastoma, DNA sequence homology with oncogenic viruses, and recently by direct comparison of normal and tumor DNA, which is now being done systematically throughout the genome for a few cancers.

Polymorphisms in Candidate Genes

There have been many studies comparing the prevalence in cancer patients and unaffected controls of differences in DNA sequence in genes involved in the metabolism of external or endogenous mutagens or in the production or processing of sex hormones or their analogs. A few polymorphisms in such genes seem to alter the risk substantially, such as the N-acetyltransferase 2 (*NAT2*) variant underlying the slow acetylator phenotype, which increases the risk of bladder cancer, particularly in workers heavily exposed to certain aromatic amines. But systematic meta-analysis reveals little or no effect for most such single polymorphisms, and the pooled data for the minority that are statistically significant usually suggest carrier:noncarrier risk ratios of less than two, and often much less.

There have been various reports of statistically significant gene–environment interactions, such as a much larger lung cancer risk due to passive smoking in women with glutathione S-transferase μ1 (GSTM1) deficiency, or an increased breast cancer risk due to smoking in postmenopausal women that was confined to NAT2 slow acetylators. In these examples, however, the estimates of the risk in susceptibles (although not their lower confidence limits) were inconsistent with the much lower overall effect of passive smoking on lung cancer or of smoking on breast cancer (which is nil) in larger studies. Many apparently significant gene–gene or gene–exposure interactions will arise by chance, but some will be real. The reported interaction between a polymorphism in the methylenetetrahydrofolate reductase (*MTHFR*) gene and dietary folate in colorectal cancer is a biologically plausible mechanism with epidemiological support.

Familial Risks for Common Cancers

Hereditary cancer syndromes caused by an inactivating mutation in a single crucial gene such as hereditary breast cancer (*BRCA1* or *BRCA2*), polyposis coli (*APC*), Li-Fraumeni syndrome (*TP53*), and familial retinoblastoma (*RB1*) are very rare, and most familial cancers seem to be the result of a spectrum of genetic risk in the population, varying continuously from very low to very high, because of the combined effects of dozens or even hundreds of low-penetrance variants in different genes, each with a very small effect. The people at highest risk are those who happen to inherit a large number of such variants. This has been studied most extensively for breast cancer. The high risk in patients' identical twins indicates that susceptible women contribute a high proportion, and perhaps even the majority, of overall breast cancer incidence. This must be due mainly to low-penetrance genes, as only about 2% of all cases are attributable to inactivating mutations in *BRCA1* or *BRCA2*. Such polygenic susceptibility conferring a site-specific lifetime risk the order of 30–50% in those at highest risk may underlie many cancers. The effects of such variants in combination with each other and with environmental risk factors could be substantial, but their total contribution to cancer incidence will not be known until data on risk factors and extensive genotyping are available for very large numbers of patients and controls. Recent studies have focused on inactivating mutations or polymorphisms in genes involved in cellular mechanisms of cancer development rather than carcinogen metabolism. This is now a major area of research, and several low-penetrance genes have already been discovered. Inactivating mutations in several genes that interact with *BRCA1* or *BRCA2* (*ATM*, *CHEK2*, *BRIP1*, *PALB2*) increase the breast cancer risk by approximately twofold, and some polymorphisms in such genes also confer a moderately increased cancer risk. An example is the I1307K single nucleotide polymorphism (SNP) in the *APC* gene, which is carried by about 1 in 20 Ashkenazi Jews and almost doubles their colon cancer risk.

Genomewide Studies

Complete genetic information on cancer patients and healthy controls will ultimately require sequencing of the whole genome in many thousands of individuals. This is not yet feasible, but a million known SNPs throughout the genome can now be analyzed simultaneously, and very-large-scale studies involving protein and RNA expression profiles or DNA methylation at specific sites are also being carried out. Genomewide SNP studies have identified common haplotypes (ancient DNA sequences that may be carried by 10% or more of the population) associated with prostate, colorectal, and breast cancer risk. These associations sometimes identify a specific gene, but some are in noncoding regions, and their significance is not yet understood. A SNP that is commoner in cancer patients may cause the specific alteration in a protein that produces the increased cancer risk, but most merely identify a region containing an unknown susceptibility locus, and discovering the relevant sequence variant and its effects may require extensive further research.

Mechanisms of Carcinogenesis

Age-incidence patterns for non-hormone-dependent carcinomas, and the effects of timing and dose level of various agents alone and in combination (particularly smoking, alcohol, ionizing radiation, and some occupational carcinogens), are parsimoniously explained by the multistage model of carcinogenesis. This was developed many years before the identification of any of the hypothesized sequence of heritable events in human carcinogenesis and has led to several important conclusions,

notably the epidemiological and experimental evidence that somatic aging processes *per se* play little or no role in carcinogenesis (**Figure 4**).

The incidence rate of cancer is presumably proportional both to the rate of the final rate-limiting step in carcinogenesis and to the number of premalignant cells that have undergone all but this final step. The rapid increase in the lung cancer incidence rate among continuing smokers ceases when they stop smoking, the rate remaining roughly constant for many years in ex-smokers. The fact that the rate does not fall abruptly when smoking stops indicates that the mysterious final event that triggers the clonal expansion of a fully malignant bronchial cell is unaffected by smoking, suggesting a mechanism involving signaling rather than mutagenesis. Such data are still generating new mechanistic hypotheses.

The Future of Cancer Epidemiology

Over the next decade, cancer epidemiologists will be increasingly preoccupied with genetically susceptible subgroups. Comparison of the DNA in cancerous and normal cells from the same patient may lead directly to the identification of most of the genes that are commonly mutated in carcinogenesis. Candidate genes are also being identified on the basis of structural homologies from the human genome sequence. Extensive sequence or SNP comparisons between affected relatives and between cancer patients and controls may define combinations of polymorphisms or inherited defects in such genes that identify a few percent of the population whose average lifetime risk may be as high as 50% for a particular cancer.

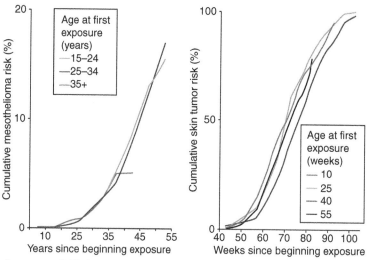

Figure 4 Age has no effect on susceptibility to some carcinogens. Left panel, cumulative mesothelioma risk in US insulation workers. Right panel, cumulative skin tumor risk in mice treated weekly with benzo(a)pyrene. Mesothelioma rates in humans and skin tumor rates in mice depend on time since first carcinogenic exposure but not on age, suggesting an initiating effect of these carcinogens. Lung cancer incidence in smokers depends on duration of smoking but not on age, and stops increasing when smoking stops, indicating both early- and late-stage effects. Radiation-induced cancer incidence increases with age at exposure above age 20, suggesting predominantly late-stage effects.

An alternative possibility is that many susceptibility genes will be discovered by studying phenotypic characteristics such as mammographic density or chromosomal instability that correlate with cancer risk. Assays for defective DNA repair correlate consistently with substantially increased susceptibility, and chromosomal aberrations predict increased cancer risk irrespective of carcinogenic exposure.

Once they are identified, susceptible people might benefit disproportionately from screening or prophylaxis, while those at low risk would be reassured. But there will also be penalties. A different susceptible minority will be identified for each disease, and a high proportion of the population may eventually suffer the consequences of being classed as genetically susceptible to some major risk. The hazards of screening for cancer susceptibility are illustrated by the widespread introduction of testing for prostate-specific antigen in the United States, which has reduced prostate cancer mortality only marginally but has led to a sharp increase in recorded incidence and considerable postoperative psychosexual and physical morbidity. Striking gene–environment interactions may be discovered, but most causes of cancer are likely to increase the risk by a smaller amount but a similar factor in those who are less susceptible. If smokers are less likely to stop smoking on discovering that their lifetime lung cancer risk is only 10%, the population death rate might even be increased by such knowledge.

Advances in genetic and molecular understanding will increasingly enable epidemiologists to quantify the relationships between risk factors and specific events in carcinogenesis. Direct monitoring of changes in the genes that underlie carcinogenesis or their products is likely to provide sensitive and specific measures that can be correlated both with cancer incidence and with exposure to carcinogenic agents or activities. Characteristic mutations in DNA from subclinical cancers or their precursor lesions can already be quantified, and serum levels of hormones such as estrogen and prolactin, or growth factors such as insulin-like growth factor-I, as well as chromosomal damage itself, are predictive of increased risk for certain cancers. The effects of some carcinogens are seen mainly in histological subtypes of cancer. For example, smoking increases the risk for squamous cell cervical cancer, but not for the adenomatous type. Such research is now extended through the identification of subtypes of cancer that develop through different pathways by analysis of their patterns of gene alterations or protein expression.

The most significant developments in cancer epidemiology may result from discoveries in virology and tumor immunology. The speculation that unidentified viruses (perhaps including some animal viruses) are associated with many human cancers is consistent with the large increase in overall cancer rates seen in immunosuppressed patients (Buell, 2005). The difficulty is that an unknown virus might mimic the epidemiological effects of dietary or genetic mechanisms. Thus, for example, the migrant

patterns for prostate cancer (**Figure 2**) might be due partly to an endemic infection, as they are for stomach cancer. Viruses usually act synergistically with other carcinogens and therefore provide alternative approaches to risk reduction. The crucial issue is which of the increased cancer risks in immunosuppressed patients reflect an unknown viral etiology and which reflect immunosurveillance targeted at nonviral tumor markers. Some cancers may well be preventable by vaccination with tumor-specific antigens or by some less specific immunostimulation.

Current Priorities in Cancer Prevention

The large differences in the pattern of cancer incidence between developed and developing countries (**Figure 1**) imply different priorities for prevention, but at an individual level the most important difference is between smokers and nonsmokers, particularly in developed countries. **Table 2** shows approximate percentages of future cancer deaths in the United States that would be avoided by successively removing the effects of smoking, known infections, alcohol, current occupational and environmental pollution, inactivity, and obesity. Whether sunlight increases or reduces overall cancer mortality is not yet established. The additional effect of specific dietary recommendations such as those of the American panel (American Institute for Cancer Research/World Cancer Research Fund, 1997) is much more speculative. Avoidance of overweight and prevention or treatment of oncogenic infections are the most important aims for

Table 2 Approximate percentages of future cancer deaths among smokers and nonsmokers in the United States that would be prevented by successive elimination of smoking, known infections, alcohol, sun exposure, current levels of workplace and air pollution, lack of exercise, and obesity

Cause	Deaths (%) after removing preceding causes	
	Current smokers	Nonsmokers
Smoking	60	–
Known infections	2	5
Alcohol	0.4	1
Sunlight[a]	?	?
Air pollution	0.4	1
Occupation	0.4	1
Lack of exercise	0.4	1
Diet		
Overweight (BMI>25 kg/m^2)	4	10
Other dietary factors[b]	4–12?	10–30?
Presently unavoidable	About a quarter	At least half

[a]Sunlight is the main source of vitamin D and hence may prevent more deaths from other cancers than it causes through melanoma and other skin cancers.
[b]The effects of specific dietary factors in people of normal weight are still uncertain.

nonsmokers; but it is absurd for smokers in the West to worry about anything except stopping smoking.

Tobacco causes one-third of all cancer deaths in developed countries. About one in five of cancers worldwide are caused by known infectious agents. HBV alone causes almost as many cancers as smoking in China, and can be prevented by vaccination. HPV vaccines may eventually prevent almost all cervical cancers, and if the prevalence of *H. pylori* can be reduced, many stomach cancers would be avoided. The belated elimination of asbestos by many Western countries will eventually prevent the great majority of mesotheliomas and many lung cancers. Various cancer screening tests are partially effective, and cervical screening is very effective.

Acknowledgments

This article is based on an earlier review (Peto J (2001) Cancer epidemiology in the last century and the next decade. *Nature* 411: 390–395), which includes references to original work. We are grateful to Cancer Research UK for support.

See also: Clinical Epidemiology; Environmental and Occupational Epidemiology; Genetic Epidemiology.

Citations

American Institute for Cancer Research/World Cancer Research Fund (2007) *Food, Nutrition and the Prevention of Cancer: A Global Perspective*. Washington, DC: American Institute for Cancer Research/World Cancer Research Fund.

Buell JF, Gross TG, and Woodle ES (2005) Malignancy after transplantation. *Transplantation* 80: S254–S264.

Calle EE, Thun MJ, Petrelli JM, Rodriguez C, and Heath CW (1999) Body-mass index and mortality in a prospective cohort of US adults. *New England Journal of Medicine* 341: 1097–1105.

Doll R and Peto R (1981) The causes of cancer: Quantitative estimates of avoidable risks of cancer in the United States today. *Journal of the National Cancer Institute* 66: 1191–1308.

Doll R and Peto R (2005) Epidemiology of cancer. In: Warrell DA, Cox T, Firth J, and Benz EJ Jr (eds.) (2005) *Oxford Textbook of Medicine*, 4th edn., pp. 193–218. Oxford, UK: Oxford University Press.

Greenwald P, Anderson D, Nelson SA, and Taylor PR (2007) Clinical trials of vitamin and mineral supplements for cancer prevention. *American Journal of Clinical Nutrition* 85: 314S–317S.

Liu BQ, Peto R, Chen ZM, *et al.* (1998) Emerging tobacco hazards in China: 1. Retrospective proportional mortality study of one million deaths. *British Medical Journal* 317: 1411–1422.

Parkin DM, Bray F, Ferlay J, and Pisani P (2005) Global cancer statistics, 2002. *CA: A Cancer Journal for Clinicians* 55: 74–108.

Parkin DM (2006) The global health burden of infection-associated cancers in the year 2002. *International Journal of Cancer* 118: 3030–3044.

Peto R, Lopez D, Boreham J, *et al.* (1994) *Mortality from Tobacco in Developed Countries, 1950–2000*. Oxford, UK: Oxford University Press.

Peto R, Watt J, and Boreham J (2006) *Deaths from Smoking*. Geneva, Switzerland: International Union Against Cancer (UICC).

Further Reading

Adami H-O, Hunter DJ, and Trichopoulos D (2002) *Textbook of Cancer Epidemiology*. Oxford, UK: Oxford University Press.

Buffler PE (1997) *Mechanisms of Carcinogenesis: Contributions of Molecular Epidemiology*. Lyon, France: International Agency for Research on Cancer.

Dos Santos Silva I (1999) *Cancer Epidemiology: Principles and Methods*. 2nd edn. Lyon, France: International Agency for Research on Cancer.

Peto J, Carbone M (eds.) (2004) Cancer epidemiology. *Oncogene* 23: 6327–6540

Schottenfeld D and Fraumeni JF (2006) *Cancer Epidemiology and Prevention*, 3rd edn. New York: Oxford University Press.

Stewart BW and Kleihues P (2003) *World Cancer Report*. Lyon, France: IARC Press.

Relevant Websites

http://www.cancer.org – American Cancer Society.
http://www.cancer.gov/ – American National Cancer Institute.
http://www.cancerresearchuk.org/ – Cancer Research UK.
http://www.deathsfromsmoking.net/ – Deaths from smoking. Estimates of the number of deaths caused by smoking, for each of 40 developed countries (and five groupings of countries).
http://www-dep.iarc.fr/ – International Agency for Research Cancer, which includes worldwide cancer incidence and mortality data.

Psychiatric Epidemiology

G S Norquist, University of Mississippi Medical Center, Jackson, MS, USA
K Magruder, Medical University of South Carolina, Charleston, SC, USA

Overview

Background

Epidemiology (derived from the Greek *epi* meaning upon, *demos* meaning people, and *logos* meaning study) is the study of factors that influence the occurrence, distribution, prevention, and control of diseases and other health-related events in human populations. It provides a framework that helps public health officials identify important health problems, their magnitude and causative factors.

Epidemiology has been traditionally an observational science of populations but more recently newer areas in the field (e.g., clinical epidemiology) have initiated interventions in populations. By determining the personal characteristics and environmental exposures that increase risk for disease, epidemiologists identify individual risks and assist in the development of public health policy to alleviate personal and environmental exposures. They have helped to understand the factors that influence the risk of developing chronic diseases such as schizophrenia.

A variety of types of studies are used in epidemiology. The most common found in mental health are cross-sectional (prevalence) studies. Data from such studies have been used to determine levels of need, to identify groups that are at highest risk for disease, and to determine changes over time in the occurrence of disorders. Such data are particularly informative in public policy for allocating resources and developing public health prevention strategies. More recently, psychiatric epidemiology has focused on determining better ways to classify people into more homogeneous disease groups to focus interventions into populations in which they will be most successful. In addition, the field has sought to determine risk factors (including biological and social) for the development of disorders to promote future efforts at prevention. One of the key issues is identification of the factors that are responsible for the occurrence of a particular mental health problem.

The purpose of this article is to provide a general overview of epidemiology in the mental health area. The term mental health in this article refers to conditions defined in the *Diagnostic and Statistical Manual of Mental Disorders* (DSM) and the *International Statistical Classification of Diseases and Related Health Problems* (ICD) *Classification of Mental and Behavioral Disorders*. Thus, it will refer to disorders that are sometimes called psychiatric or neuropsychiatric (including substance use disorders). The article presents key examples of methods and assessment instruments used in mental health epidemiology. However, a detailed review and discussion of epidemiologic methods and instruments is beyond the scope of this article. For such details, the reader is referred to several textbooks on mental health epidemiology listed in the 'Further reading' section.

History

The early period of epidemiology is marked by a focus on health issues related to the growing industrial revolution in Europe. Public health officials were concerned with general social reform and the effects of overcrowding in urban industrial areas, with an emphasis on sanitary conditions. In the mental health area, there was concern that environmental toxins were the cause of disorders. For example, mercury was considered a cause of psychosis and lead exposure was suspected as a contributor to mental disorders. One of the early founders of epidemiology, William Farr, was among the first to study mental illnesses. He studied the physical condition of inmates in English asylums in the early part of the nineteenth century. During this time, many thought there was a virtual epidemic of mental illness but another important figure in epidemiology, John Snow, insisted the increase was more likely the result of an increase in detection rather than a true increase in incidence.

The second period in the development of epidemiology began around the start of the twentieth century and focused on germs as a cause of disease. Epidemiology became virtually synonymous with the study of infectious diseases. One of the causes of insanity identified during this time was the late effects of syphilis. Discovery of the spirochete that causes this illness led to the development of the first medication to stop this infectious agent (Salvarsan 606). Although emphasis was placed on finding infectious agents, there were some epidemiologists at this time who studied other causes of disease. One notable finding during this time was the association of nutritional deficiency with the occurrence of pellagra. Initially it was thought to be due to an infectious agent but studies in institutionalized populations (including those in mental institutions) led to the association with nutritional deficiency.

After the Second World War, infectious diseases started to decline in the higher-income countries. However, those countries realized the increasing importance of noncommunicable diseases such as cardiovascular disease. This led to a move away from consideration of single etiologic factors and to the consideration of various risk factors that could lead to disease development. New methods such as cohort and case-control designs were developed to identify these risk factors. Mental illnesses were also considered to be chronic noncommunicable disorders, but initial epidemiological work in psychiatry focused more on counting disease in community surveys rather than the study of risk factors. Thus, there were very few cohort or case-control studies in the early part of this era that focused on mental illnesses. Most of the studies in mental health during the initial years of this period were unstructured face-to-face field surveys with poor reliability.

In the late 1970s during the Carter administration in the United States, a special commission on mental health called for a study to obtain information on mental illness across the United States. Around the same time, the third edition of the *Diagnostic and Statistical Manual* (DSM-III) was published in the United States. It moved toward use of explicit criteria to make a diagnosis and increased the reliability of making such diagnoses. This standard nomenclature made it possible to develop measures that could be used in large community surveys.

Substance abuse had for some time not been considered a true disorder but rather a weakness of character or a personality disorder. However, after the Second World War it was recognized as a major public health problem, and the field sought to quantify it through assessments that focused on alcohol and drug use disorders. As a result of this effort, the significant impact of such disorders has now been recognized as well as the frequent comorbidity with other psychiatric disorders.

In recent years, mental health epidemiology has expanded to include attention to genetics and the molecular basis of disease. This has brought more attention to determination of biological risk factors through the field of genetic epidemiology. Attention has also been focused on social processes that can affect exposure to risk factors. This field of social epidemiology seeks to understand how social factors might influence differences in health status across populations.

Methods

Issues for Mental Health

One of the major problems in psychiatric epidemiology has been the difficulty in measuring mental and substance abuse disorders reliably and validly. Determination of a case is made on the basis of symptoms and not clear objective signs like a biopsy result. Because diagnosis is dependent on symptom reports from individuals there can be significant problems with biased reporting (both over- and underreporting). A key concern is the lack of objective, well-defined biological markers of mental illness.

There are continuing debates in the field about how to define the presence of an illness and whether there should be categorical definitions or use of a dimensional model. A dimensional approach focuses on a collection of symptoms and involves a quantitative assessment of the number of symptoms a person has from a few to many. Another approach is to define pathology in terms of a syndrome. In this scheme, a pattern of symptoms may include essential symptoms and others associated with the syndrome. This type of scheme takes the duration of symptoms into consideration and may include severity of the symptoms and resulting disability. Depending on the types of symptoms present, the duration and disability, a syndrome may be considered to be present or absent. Thus, this becomes a dichotomous measure (present or absent) and the resulting conditions are placed into categories of disorders.

Other problems in making diagnoses in mental health are the changes in symptoms over time, even without treatment, and the potential for recall bias (i.e., failure to remember past symptoms). The latter is a particular problem when trying to assess lifetime diagnoses. Stigma may also affect what a person reports about his/her behavior. Some people may not want to report symptoms due to embarrassment and may not come forward for treatment.

Terms

Below are listed some common terms used in psychiatric epidemiological studies. Familiarity with these will aid the reader in understanding such studies. A more detailed description of the various epidemiologic terms can be found in resources listed in the section titled 'Further Reading.'

- Case: This represents the presence of a mental or substance abuse disorder in a person.
- Case registry: A database of people with a defined mental and/or substance use disorder. It may include other data such as demographic and clinical treatment information.
- Comorbidity: This is the presence in a person of at least two different disorders. It may be used to represent the occurrence of somatic or psychiatric disorders and simultaneous or lifetime occurrence.
- Control group: This is a group of people who are used as a basis for comparison to another group. Depending on the study design, control subjects do not receive the experimental intervention or are healthy and do not possess the disorder or risk factor in question.
- Incidence: This represents the number of new cases or events that occur during a particular period of time.
- Odds ratio (OR): A measure of the odds of an event/disorder occurring in one group compared to the odds of the event/disorder occurring in another group. Thus, an odds ratio of one (1) means that the event/disorder is equally likely to occur in both groups. If the odds ratio is greater than one (>1), then the event/disorder is more likely to occur in the first group. If less than one (<1), then the event/disorder is less likely to occur in the first group.
- Predictive value of a test: The positive predictive value of a test or screen is the proportion of all people who test positive on a screen who actually have the disorder being screened. The negative predictive value is the proportion of all people who test negative on a screen who do not have the disorder being screened.
- Prevalence: This represents the number of cases/events that exist during a particular period of time. This figure would include both new cases (incidence) and those that were already present but still existed during the defined period of time. It is expressed in terms of the period of time defined to contain the cases or events. Thus, point prevalence would be the prevalence at a specific point in time. Period prevalence would expand the time over which cases or events could be present. For example, one might have one month, 6 months, 12 months (1 year), or lifetime prevalence. Period prevalence is used more often these days in mental health epidemiology because the diagnosis of mental disorders requires the occurrence of symptoms over periods of time.

- Risk factor: This is something that increases the chance for development of a disorder or the occurrence of an event. It is important to note that it is not necessarily causal but rather associated with the disorder or event. There may also be more than one risk factor for a given disorder and a particular combination of such factors may be necessary before a disorder develops. Risk factors can be inherent in the individual (e.g., age and gender) or they may represent an exposure (e.g., substance abuse, economic status).
- Reliability: This is the degree to which any particular measure produces consistent results even among different raters of the measure. Reliability is often a problem in making diagnoses of mental and substance abuse disorders.
- Sensitivity: This represents the proportion of people with a disorder in a population who are identified correctly by a screen or test as having a disorder.
- Specificity: This represents the proportion of people without a disorder in a population who are identified correctly by a screen or test as not having a disorder.
- Validity: This is the extent to which any given indicator of a disease actually represents the presence of that disease. In psychiatry, the gold standard against which validity is most often measured is the diagnosis made by a clinician.

Assessment

Background

The field of psychiatric epidemiology has developed various ways to assess and diagnose mental disorders. Some early studies used direct observation and assessment by clinicians. However, with the growing need for larger community surveys, it became too expensive to use clinicians to make every assessment. As a result, survey instruments were developed that could be used by either clinicians or trained lay interviewers to provide reliable diagnoses of mental illnesses.

Before considering the specific instruments used to measure mental disorders, it is important to understand how such disorders are determined. In psychiatric epidemiological studies, disorders are assessed usually through a set of defined questions. The set of questions is known as an instrument or test and can be divided into two types: A scale or schedule. An instrument can be administered through direct observation by a clinician, through trained lay interviewers, or self-report by the subject.

A scale is sometimes called a screen and usually focuses on the dimensional aspect of pathology. Responses to items or questions on a scale are given individual values and when added provide a score. The presence of pathology is determined by this overall score.

A schedule is more comprehensive and complex than a scale and determines various diagnoses through a structured set of questions. Some instruments have been designed to be administered by trained lay people (i.e., nonclinicians) in community settings. In addition, schedules determine if the symptoms are present at the time of the interview or occurred at some other point in time. They are designed to contain a variety of disease modules so one can opt to assess a selected number of diagnoses. Some are designed so a respondent who answers negatively to certain stem questions for a particular disease can skip the rest of the module.

Concern has been raised about the validity of schedules used in epidemiological studies. They may overestimate the prevalence of disorders, especially if compared to assessments made by clinicians. However, some recent studies seem to indicate clinician assessments may actually result in a larger number of identified cases (i.e., a higher prevalence) unless one looks only at recent symptoms when clinician assessments may have lower estimates of pathology. In addition to concerns about reliability and validity, a major issue is whether dimensional or categorical measurement is better. The concern is that categorical measurement is too restrictive and human behavior is not so easily divided into strict categories. Yet, dimensional measures such as scales often use cut points and thus create categories, while categorical measures involve some dimensional qualities. Most branches of medicine use categorical diagnoses; thus such approaches are compatible with general medical diagnostic practice.

Instrument development

During the Second World War, several scales were developed to assess psychopathology such as the Maudsley Personality Inventory in the United Kingdom. The first structured interviews were conducted in two community surveys shortly after the Second World War. These were the Stirling County Study and the Midtown Manhattan Study. They used the Health Opinion Survey and the Twenty-Two Item Scale, respectively. Yet, the studies did not rely on the instruments for final diagnoses. Instead, they had psychiatrists review the results from the instruments. In spite of some differences in the way the two studies assessed psychiatric conditions, they both reported that about 20% of people had a mental disorder.

President Carter's Commission on Mental Health called for national information on psychiatric disorders and use of mental health services in the United States at the start of the 1980s. This led to the development of the Epidemiologic Catchment Area (ECA) study, the first national epidemiologic survey for psychiatric conditions in the United States. The Diagnostic Interview Schedule (DIS) was developed for use in the ECA. It was the first complex diagnostic schedule designed to be used in a community study and set the stage for future epidemiologic surveys around the world.

Around the time of the ECA study, the WHO collaborated with the U.S. Alcohol, Drug Abuse and Mental

Health Administration to assess the state of international diagnosis and classification. A product of this collaboration was the development of a new instrument, the Composite International Diagnostic Interview (CIDI). This instrument is highly structured and does not allow interviewers to interpret responses, as was allowed in some early international studies that used the Present State Examination (PSE) developed in the United Kingdom. One version of the CIDI, the UM-CIDI, was used in the U.S. National Comorbidity Survey (NCS). The CIDI has been used in a variety of international epidemiologic surveys, including national surveys in Australia and Norway. The latest version is being used in the World Mental Health Project, which is attempting to provide an international estimate of mental disorders and the disability associated with them.

Instruments have also been developed for use in various clinical settings (e.g., primary care settings). The most prominent of these is the General Health Questionnaire (GHQ). Other instruments designed for this setting are the Personal Health Questionnaire, the Patient Health Questionnaire, the Medical Outcomes Study 36-Item Short Form Health Survey (SF-36), and the Primary Care Evaluation of Mental Disorder (PRIME-MD).

Other instruments have been designed to allow clinicians to make reliable assessments of patients in clinical settings. Among the most prominent of these is the Hamilton Rating Scale for assessment of depressive symptoms. Others include the Schedule for Affective Disorders and Schizophrenia (SADS) and the Structured Clinical Interview for DSM-III-R (SCID).

The selection of an instrument depends on what one wants to do with it. For example, if one wants to compare community data to those being collected around the world the choice at this time is the CIDI as it is being used in the largest international study to date.

Study Designs

Here are described the common study designs and examples of each related to mental health and substance abuse. The most common design used in traditional mental health epidemiological studies is the cross-sectional (prevalence) survey.

Nonexperimental or observational

In these types of studies, an investigator does not have control over exposure to an intervention or risk factor in any particular group. There are three basic types summarized here.

Cross-sectional (prevalence) surveys

In this type of study, one selects a population and determines the presence or absence of a disease or exposure to a risk factor by assessing the subject at a single point in time. The subject may be asked about past events but is not followed for any period of time. The classic epidemiological surveys in psychiatry have been cross-sectional in design (e.g., the ECA study). These studies are useful in determining the mental health status and service needs of community populations. A variety of techniques are used to sample community populations for such studies (e.g., stratified random sampling). A few of these cross-sectional studies have had additional follow-up interviews with subjects (e.g., the Stirling County Study). Such studies with a repeated assessment could be considered a hybrid design.

In addition, the type of instrument used in a cross-sectional survey can vary. One might create a case registry such as that used by the National Health Insurance in the United Kingdom. These could use assessments by both clinicians and individually administered instruments. However, a typical design is to administer an instrument to every subject from a survey population. A less expensive option is a two-stage design in which people are first given a short instrument (e.g., a scale) and those who test positive are then given a more thorough instrument to assess psychopathology.

Case-control study

In this type of study, one selects two different groups to compare. One is a group of people with the condition one wants to study (cases) and the other is a group of people who are as similar as possible to those people with the condition, except they do not have the condition (controls). One looks back in time to determine whether the two groups had different exposure to risk factors of interest. Although these types of studies are subject to potential biases (e.g., selection bias), they are relatively inexpensive and can be conducted quickly. For rare disorders, it is an efficient study design. If a case-control study indicates a finding of interest it can be tested through more rigorous methods such as a cohort study.

Cohort study

In this type of study, people are selected to be observed over time. These are usually conducted in a prospective (forward) fashion with disease-free subjects but can be done in a retrospective (backward) time fashion as long as the temporal sequence of exposure predating disease onset can be established. In contrast to case-control studies, groups are not defined by the presence of a disease, but rather by the presence of a risk factor or exposure and subjects are followed over a period of time. During the time of study, one looks for the development of new cases (incidence) and attempts to connect exposure to certain risk factors with the development of the disorder. These studies require large numbers of people since only a small number are likely to develop the condition of interest and thus can be quite costly and take long periods of time.

Nevertheless, cohort studies can establish without question that risk factors predated disease onset and are an important strategy in epidemiology.

Experimental
Clinical trials
These types of studies are also known as randomized controlled clinical trials (RCTs). In this type of study, people are allocated randomly to either a group that receives an experimental intervention or a group that does not receive the intervention. Thus, the investigator can control both the distribution of subjects into comparison groups and the experimental condition for a group. By using random assignment, one can reduce greatly or eliminate the potential for selection bias. In addition, raters are usually blinded to the experimental intervention and in many studies placebos are used. Some recent clinical trials have utilized hybrid designs in which subjects are given some choice of the intervention and no placebo is used.

Studies and Results

Listed below are the designs of some of the most influential recent epidemiological studies in mental health. This is followed by a summary of results from these and some other studies. The reader is referred to the published full reports of the studies for comprehensive details and results.

Recent Studies

Epidemiologic Catchment Area Study
The Epidemiological Catchment Area (ECA) Study, funded by the U.S. National Institute of Mental Health, was launched in the early 1980s to assess the prevalence of mental and substance use disorders in the United States and the use of mental health services. Instead of a national probability sample, the ECA used five specific geographic regions in the U.S. to select population samples. Two waves of data were collected from subjects. The first wave started around 1980 and the second wave was collected 1 year later, with the last site finishing in the mid-1980s. The first wave had a combined sample size of a little over 20 000 people and the second wave was not able to assess about 21% of the first sample. It used the Diagnostic Interview Schedule (DIS) to obtain diagnoses for the major DSM-III diagnoses through trained lay interviewers in face-to-face community interviews. This was a ground-breaking study in that it was the first to use structured complex diagnostic interview schedules to obtain estimates of community mental health.

National Co-Morbidity Survey-Replication
This study is a replication of a similar study (National Co-Morbidity Survey) conducted in the early 1990s on a national sample in the United States. The National Co-Morbidity Survey-Replication (NCSR) is part of the World Mental Health Surveys described in the next section and was funded by the U.S. National Institute of Mental Health. It is a nationally representative (United States), cross-sectional household survey of people aged 18 and older. Interviews were conducted in person from 2001 to 2003 by trained lay interviewers using the WMH-CIDI. The response rate was approximately 71%, and the sample size was a little over 9200 people.

National Epidemiologic Survey on Alcohol and Related Conditions
The U.S. National Institute of Alcohol Abuse and Alcoholism launched a nationally representative survey of people 18 years and older in 2001. The National Epidemiologic Survey on Alcohol and Related Conditions (NESARC) study has two waves of data collection with the first wave completed in 2001–02. Although the survey is of noninstitutionalized populations, it did make an effort to include people who live in housing units more likely to have higher substance use patterns (e.g., shelters and group homes). The response rate for the first wave (81%) was much higher than previous surveys.

The survey used the Alcohol Use Disorder and Associated Disability Interview Schedule-DSM-IV version (AUDADIS-IV). This is a state of the art structured diagnostic interview that is designed to be used by lay interviewers. This instrument was designed to be more accurate than previous instruments in assessing alcohol and substance use disorders. The survey conducted face-to-face interviews with over 43 000 people across the United States.

WHO World Mental Health Surveys
In 1998 the WHO established the World Mental Health Survey (WMH) Consortium to address the limitations of previous surveys of mental health disorders around the world. Prior surveys were unable to adequately assess severity of disorders, interviews used in the surveys were not standardized to allow cross-national comparisons, and the majority of surveys were in high-income countries, thus limiting their generalizability to other areas of the world. The Consortium expanded the CIDI (WMH-CIDI) to include questions that would assess severity, impairment, and treatment. Surveys were then launched in 28 countries in each region of the world, including low-income countries.

Each area is using the WMH-CIDI, a fully structured diagnostic interview that uses trained lay interviewers to obtain information. Age of subjects varies by country, but the most common range is 18 and older. Sample sizes vary by country but all used multistage household probability sampling. Response rates have varied so far from lows around 45% to highs of about 88%. There are differences in the demographics, with some sites having young and less educated populations.

Global Burden of Disease

In the early 1990s, the WHO supported a study that was the first to use epidemiologic data and projections of disability from various disorders to estimate the public health burden of various medical disorders. The purpose of the study was to quantify the years of healthy life lost as a result of disease in the various countries of the world. The identified measure for this is known as DALYs (disability-adjusted life years) and incorporates death and disability from a disorder. This study, known as the Global Burden of Disease (GBD) study, had a significant influence on the perception of the impact of various disorders. Prior estimates had indicated infectious diseases were the most important causes of public health problems. However, this study, which considered not only mortality from a disease but the burden imposed by living with disability from the disease, changed the perception of which diseases were the most important in terms of impact on public health. Chronic diseases with significant effects on long-term disability (e.g., major depression) now were considered more important from

a public health perspective than had previously been projected. There were a number of criticisms about the methodology of the study and concerns about miscalculations of the impact of certain diseases (e.g., HIV/AIDS).

These projections were updated recently by the WHO to consider more current epidemiological data on burden of disease and mortality. In addition, the update moved from considering projections by only the eight regions of the world to project at the country level and then aggregated the results into regional and income-level groups. The various diseases and injury causes were grouped into three levels: Group I (communicable, maternal, nutritional causes), Group II (noncommunicable diseases), and Group III (injuries).

Data on Mental Illness and Substance Use Disorders

Table 1 shows a comparison of data from the three most prominent studies in the United States and a meta-analysis of studies conducted in Europe and the initial findings of the European component of the WHO World Mental Health Surveys. It is important to note that one cannot make clear comparisons across these studies as the time of data collection was different, the samples are obviously

Table 1 Twelve-month prevalence of mental and substance use disorders (percent of study population)

	ECA	NCS-R	NESARC	Europe[e]	ESMeD[g]
Any mood disorders	9.5	9.5	9.3	9.1	4.5
Major depression	5.0	6.7	7.2	6.9	4.1
Dysthymia	[a]	1.5	1.8		1.1
Mania	1.2	0.6	1.7	0.9	
Any anxiety disorders	12.6	18.1	11.1	12.0	8.4
Panic disorder	1.3	2.7	2.1	1.8	0.7
Social phobia	2.1	6.8	2.8	2.3	1.6
Specific phobia	10.9	8.7	7.1	6.4	5.4
Generalized anxiety disorder	[b]	3.1	2.1	1.7	0.9
Any substance use disorder	9.5	3.8	9.3	3.4[f]	
Any alcohol use disorder	7.4	3.1[c]	8.5		1.0
Any drug use disorder	3.1	1.4[d]	2.0		
Any disorder	28.1	26.2		27.4	11.5

[a]All sites did not assess 12-month prevalence for dysthymia.
[b]All sites did not assess generalized anxiety disorder.
[c]Alcohol abuse only; see text.
[d]Drug abuse only; see text.
[e]Figures are median values from meta-analysis of multiple studies.
[f]Dependence only (excludes abuse).
[g]Figures are from recent update analysis except dysthymia and alcohol use which are from original analysis.
Data from: Regier DA, Narrow WE, Rae DS, et al. (1993) The de facto US mental and addictive disorders service system: Epidemiologic catchment area prospective 1-year prevalence rates of disorders and services. *Archives of General Psychiatry* 50: 85–94 (ECA); Kessler RC, Chiu WT, Demler O, et al. (2005) Prevalence, severity, and comorbidity of 12-month DSM-IV disorders in the national comorbidity survey replication. *Archives of General Psychiatry* 62: 617–627 (NCS-R); Grant BF, Stinson FS, Dawson DA, et al. (2004) Prevalence and co-occurrence of substance use disorders and independent mood and anxiety disorders. *Archives of General Psychiatry* 61: 807–816 (NESARC); Wittchen HU and Jacobi F (2005) Size and burden of mental disorders in Europe – A critical review and appraisal of 27 studies. *European Neuropsychopharmacology* 15: 357–376 (Europe); Alonso J and Lepine J (2007) Overview of key data from the European study of the epidemiology of mental disorders (ESEMeD). *Journal of Clinical Psychiatry* 68: 2, 3–9 (ESMeD).

Table 2 Twelve-month prevalence of mental and substance abuse disorders (percent of population) by region

Region	Anxiety	Mood	Substance	Any
Americas	6.8–18.2	4.8–9.6	2.5–3.8	12.2–26.4
Europe	5.8–12.0	3.6–9.1	0.1–6.4	8.2–20.5
Africa	3.3–11.2	0.8–6.6	0.8–1.3	4.7–16.9
Asia	2.4–5.3	1.7–3.1	0.5–2.6	4.3–9.1

Data from: WHO World Health Survey Consortium (2004) Prevalence, severity and unmet need for treatment of mental disorders in the World Health Organization world mental health surveys. *Journal of the American Medical Association* 291: 2581–2590.

different, and the methods varied. However, despite these differences, it is remarkable that estimates are very close in some diseases. The obvious exception is the report from the ESMeD study, which has lower 12-month prevalence estimates. It is not clear why this would be the case, but it represents a summary of data from several European countries and if one looks at the range for those countries (**Table 2**) there is significant variation. In addition, there were some initial problems in the survey implementation in these countries that could have resulted in lower estimates. The meta-analysis represented in the column labeled Europe presents median estimates and the range is variable for these, especially alcohol dependence, depression, and specific phobia. For substance abuse, the figures from the NCS-R study are probably low because the module used to obtain these diagnoses did not consider responses to questions about dependence in those who did not respond positively to abuse questions.

Table 2 shows the first data from the WHO-Mental Health Survey (WMH). The estimates vary across countries despite similar methodology. However, there are likely to be cultural differences in the interpretation of the questions and the concept of mental illness. In addition, the stigma attached to mental illness and substance abuse may be greater in some areas and impede responses to such questions. An issue that often arises in any mental health survey is a concern that the disorders reported do not represent significant clinical problems. Thus, recent surveys such as the WMH have attempted to measure severity and disability. The WMH initial reports show variation in severity and disability but in some settings more than 50% of the cases are of serious or moderate severity. Days out of work are much higher for those with serious disorders than those classified as having mild severity.

Data on Comorbidities

Among the interesting findings from recent studies is the recognition that mental disorders and substance use disorder are comorbid at higher levels than was previously expected. The NESARC study found that 20% of people with a current substance use disorder also had a mood disorder. These disorders appear to be independent and

Table 3 Leading causes of DALYs (world)

2002	2030
1. Perinatal conditions	1. HIV/AIDS
2. Lower respiratory tract infections	2. Unipolar depressive disorders
3. HIV/AIDS	3. Ischemic heart disease
4. Unipolar depressive disorders	4. Road traffic accidents
5. Diarrheal disease	5. Perinatal conditions
6. Ischemic heart disease	6. Cerebrovascular disease
7. Cerebrovascular disease	7. COPD
8. Road traffic accidents	8. Lower respiratory tract infections
9. Malaria	9. Hearing loss, adult onset
10. Tuberculosis	10. Cataracts

From Mathers CD and Loncar D (2006) Projections of global mortality and burden of disease from 2002 to 2030. *PLoS Medicine* 3: 11: e442.

not substance induced. Such findings on co-morbidity are important as they point to the need to assess and provide services for both mental and substance abuse disorders when a person is seen initially for one or the other disorder. There are no current data to clarify this increased co-morbidity among mental and substance abuse disorders. One may lead to the onset of the other type of disorder, there may be common genetic or environmental causes or the methods used to assess these disorders may overestimate co-morbidity. An understanding of these linkages could aid in development of preventive and treatment interventions for co-morbidity.

Burden of Disease Data

One can see in **Table 3** that noncommunicable diseases (Group II) are the most important causes of disease burden. By the year 2030, Group II causes are expected to have a greater impact on overall burden of disease around the world than Group I (communicable) causes. **Table 4** shows that major depression becomes a significant factor in the overall burden of disease regardless of a country's income level.

Although these updated projections address some of the criticism of the original Global Burden of Disease Study, there are still limitations to the study. Recent epidemiological

Table 4　Leading causes of DALYs (2030) by country income ranking

High income	Middle income	Low income
1. Unipolar depressive disorders	1. HIV/AIDS	1. HIV/AIDS
2. Ischemic heart disease	2. Unipolar depressive disorders	2. Perinatal conditions
3. Alzheimer and other dementias	3. Cerebrovascular disease	3. Unipolar depressive disorders
4. Alcohol use disorders	4. Ischemic heart disease	4. Road traffic accidents
5. Diabetes mellitus	5. COPD	5. Ischemic heart disease
6. Cerebrovascular disease	6. Road traffic accidents	6. Lower respiratory tract infections
7. Hearing loss, adult onset	7. Violence	7. Diarrheal diseases
8. Trachea, bronchus, lung cancers	8. Vision disorders, age-related	8. Cerebrovascular disease
9. Osteoarthritis	9. Hearing loss, adult onset	9. Cataracts
10. COPD	10. Diabetes mellitus	10. Malaria

From Mathers CD and Loncar D (2006) Projections of global mortality and burden of disease from 2002 to 2030. *PLoS Med* 3: 11: e442.

studies such as the WHO-WMH study have improved what data are available for mental health, but there are still problems in the quality of such epidemiological data across regions. In addition, measures of disability are not ideal and projections are based on present data and various assumptions about future disease that could change with time. Thus, although data such as these are helpful for planning distribution of future health services, they must be interpreted with caution.

Service Use Data

Many of the epidemiological studies have assessed use of mental health services. As can be seen in **Table 5**, large numbers of people with a mental disorder during a 1-year period do not seek medical care for such services. Obviously, such data will differ according to the ability to access such services and the stigma attached to using them. However, it is interesting to note that even within countries that provide universal coverage there is still a large amount of unmet need (low use in those with disorders). The studies also looked at the use of a variety of other service sectors (including nontraditional providers). Such data show that even though significant numbers of people use other service sectors for mental health care there are still large numbers of people with a disorder who do not seek care anywhere. Those least likely to use services are the elderly, men, people without resources such as insurance, and those living in rural areas where care is not readily available.

Future Needs

Assessments and Methods

The field of mental health epidemiology has come a long way in the past 100 years, with tremendous growth since the end of the Second World War. Key to this expansion has been the development of explicit criteria for diagnostic assessment. These have increased reliability in

Table 5　Prevalence of 12-month use of mental health services (percent of those with mental disorder)

Sector	ESMeD	ECA	NCS-R
Mental health specialist	31.4	12.7	21.7
General medical physician	34.1	12.7	22.8

Data from Alonso J and Lepine J (2007) Overview of key data from the European study of the epidemiology of mental disorders (ESEMeD). *Journal Clinical Psychiatry* 68: 2, 3–9 (ESMeD); Regier DA, Narrow WE, Rae DS, et al. (1993) The de facto US mental and addictive disorders service system: Epidemiologic catchment area prospective 1-year prevalence rates of disorders and services. *Archives of General Psychiatry* 50: 85–94. (ECA); Wang PS, Lane M, Olfson M, et al. (2005) Twelve-month use of mental health services in the United States. *Archives of General Psychiatry* 62: 629–640 (NCS-R).

making diagnoses and facilitated the development of instruments that can be used in large-scale community surveys. However, a number of issues still confront the field. Among the most prominent is the issue of diagnostic validity. Efforts are underway currently to update the DSM and ICD classification systems. That process has initiated discussions about the best ways to classify mental and substance abuse disorders and whether a more dimensional approach should be considered. Given the growing findings from basic neuroscience and genetics about potential biological causes of mental disorders, there is a need to connect this information with future diagnostic classifications. Collection of biological data in epidemiological studies could help to further this connection.

In addition to classification by symptoms, more attention should be focused on other aspects of disorder such as disability. A number of efforts are already underway in this area, but better assessments of severity, disability, and quality of life are needed. For many people with mental and substance abuse disorders, the most important end points in treatment are improvement in functional status and quality of life, not just a reduction in symptoms.

Previous studies have focused on cross-sectional looks at populations with very few cohort studies. Although they are less costly and perhaps easier to conduct, these prevalence studies have major limitation when trying to determine risk factors for development of disorders. Thus, the field needs to launch large cohort studies that would help delineate the various risk factors (biological, individual, environmental, and social) and the interplay among them. Only more comprehensive information is likely to lead us to a better understanding of the natural history of mental disorders and the various etiological factors that are involved in their development.

More international collaboration would be helpful. Previous studies have shown the importance of mental and substance abuse disorders as public health problems throughout the world. There is much to learn from different regions and standardization of assessments and classification systems together with collaborative large multinational studies would move the field much further.

Topics

A number of recent studies have looked at the interface between mental disorders and other medical disorders such as cardiovascular disease. More work in this area would help to delineate the impact of mental health on other medical disorders and vice versa. This could lead to new interventions for the prevention and early intervention of medical disorders that are co-morbid with mental health disorders.

Given the increasing attention to genetic factors in disease, genetic epidemiological studies in mental health offer an opportunity to understand the complex linkage between genes and environment. Recent work has shown that the presence of certain genes together with certain environmental exposures increases the risk for development of depression. Studies that address the impact of genes on response to pharmacological or psychotherapeutic interventions in the presence of particular environmental exposure would help to revolutionize treatments in mental health.

Epidemiological studies have tremendous potential to inform the allocation of public health resources. However, previous studies have tended to focus on specific individual factors that affect use of resources (e.g., insurance status, availability of services). Studies that address both individual factors and macro-level environmental factors (e.g., organization of services, public mental health policies) at the same time would strengthen the ability to make more informed public policy decisions for the provision of health-care services. This could lead to better systems of care, ensuring that limited services reach those most in need of them.

See also: Genetic Epidemiology; Observational Epidemiology.

Citations

Alonso J and Lepine J (2007) Overview of key data from the European study of the epidemiology of mental disorders (ESEMeD). *Journal Clinical Psychiatry* 68: 2–9.

ESEMeD/MHEDEA 2000 Investigators (2004) Prevalence of mental disorders in Europe: Results from the European Study of the Epidemiology of Mental Disorders (ESEMeD) project. *Acta Psychiatrica Scandinavica Supplementum* 109 (supplement 420): 21–27.

Grant BF, Stinson FS, Dawson DA, *et al.* (2004) Prevalence and co-occurrence of substance use disorders and independent mood and anxiety disorders. *Archives of General Psychiatry* 61: 807–816.

Hughes CC, Tremblay MA, Rapoport RN, and Leighton AH (1960) *People of Cove and Woodlot: Communities from the Viewpoint of Social Psychiatry. Vol. 2, Stirling County Study of Psychiatric Disorder and Sociocultural Environment*. New York: Basic Books.

Kessler RC, Chiu WT, Demler O, *et al.* (2005) Prevalence, severity, and comorbidity of 12-month DSM-IV disorders in the national comorbidity survey replication. *Archives of General Psychiatry* 62: 617–627.

Mathers CD and Loncar D (2006) Projections of global mortality and burden of disease from 2002 to 2030. *PLoS Med* 3(11): e442.

Regier DA, Narrow WE, Rae DS, *et al.* (1993) The de facto US mental and addictive disorders service system: Epidemiologic catchment area prospective 1-year prevalence rates of disorders and services. *Archives of General Psychiatry* 50: 85–94.

Wang PS, Lane M, Olfson M, *et al.* (2005) Twelve-month use of mental health services in the United States. *Archives of General Psychiatry* 62: 629–640.

WHO World Health Survey Consortium (2004) Prevalence, severity and unmet need for treatment of mental disorders in the World Health Organization world mental health surveys. *Journal of the American Medical Association* 291: 2581–2590.

Wittchen HU and Jacobi F (2005) Size and burden of mental disorders in Europe – A critical review and appraisal of 27 studies. *European Neuropsychopharmacology* 15: 357–376.

Further Reading

Kessler RC, Demler O, Frank RG, *et al.* (2005) Prevalence and treatment of mental disorders, 1990 to 2003. *New England Journal of Medicine* 352(24): 2515–2522.

McDowell I (ed.) (2006) *Measuring Health: A Guide to Rating Scales and Questionnaires*. Oxford, UK: Oxford University Press.

Mezzich JE, Jorge MR, and Salloum IM (1994) *Psychiatric Epidemiology: Assessment of Concepts and Methods*. Baltimore, MD: Johns Hopkins University Press.

Murphy JM, Laird NM, Monson RR, *et al.* (2000) A 40-year perspective on the prevalence of depression. *Archives of General Psychiatry* 57: 209–215.

Murray CJL and Lopez AD (eds.) (1996) *The Global Burden of Disease: A Comprehensive Assessment of Mortality and Disability from Diseases Injuries and Risk Factors in 1990 and Projected to 2020*. Cambridge, MA: Harvard University Press.

Prince M, Stewart R, Ford T and Hotopf M (eds.) (2003) *Practical Psychiatric Epidemiology*. Oxford, UK: Oxford University Press.

Regier DA, Kaelber CT, Rae DS, *et al.* (1998) Limitations of diagnostic criteria and assessment instruments for mental disorders. *Archives of General Psychiatry* 55: 109–115.

Robins LN and Regier DA (eds.) (1991) *Psychiatric Disorders in America: The Epidemiological Catchment Area Study*. New York: Free Press.

Susser E, Schwartz S, Morabia A and Bromet EJ (eds.) (2006) *Psychiatric Epidemiology*. Oxford, UK: Oxford University Press.

Tsuang MT and Tohen M (eds.) (2002) *Textbook in Psychiatric Epidemiology*. New York: A John Wiley & Sons Inc.

US Department of Health, Human Services (1999) *Mental Health: A Report of the Surgeon General*. Rockville MD: US Department of Health and Human Services.

US Department of Health and Human Services (2001) *Mental Health: Culture Race, and Ethnicity: A Supplement to Mental Health: A Report of the Surgeon General*. Rockville MD: US Department of Health and Human Services.

World Health Organization (2001) *Mental Health: New Understanding New Hope*. Geneva, Switzerland: World Health Organization.

http://www.hcp.med.harvard.edu/icpe – International Consortium in Psychiatric Epidemiology.

http://www.sinica.edu.tw/~ifpe – International Federation of Psychiatric Epidemiology.

http://www.niaaa.nih.gov – National Institute on Alcohol Abuse and Alcoholism.

http://www.nida.nih.gov – National Institute on Drug Abuse.

http://www.nimh.nih.gov – National Institute of Mental Health.

http://www.who.int – World Health Organization.

http://www.wparet.org – World Psychiatric Association.

Relevant Websites

http://www.cdc.gov – Centers for Disease Control and Prevention.

Perinatal Epidemiology

L S Bakketeig and P Bergsjø, Norwegian Institute of Public Health, Oslo, Norway

Introduction

It is well established that events during pregnancy and childbirth influence the health and development of the newborn baby. In recent years, we have come to realize that events occurring in pregnancy and early childhood may also affect health into adult life. Even events occurring before pregnancy and intergenerationally can affect reproduction. Population-based studies of these relationships are called perinatal epidemiology, which has evolved into a major subspecialty of epidemiology. Events or exposures may affect both mother and child; those affecting the mother are labeled maternal, while the term perinatal refers to the child.

Perinatal surveillance has been established through a system of medical registration of births in a number of countries. In Norway, medical registration of births was established in 1967. The main reason was the thalidomide catastrophe in Europe some years earlier. The other Nordic countries followed suit: Denmark in 1968, Iceland in 1972, and Sweden in 1973. Finland established its registry somewhat later, in 1987. The registries have served several other purposes than monitoring the frequency and type of congenital malformations. The data, which contain civic and medical information on the child, parents, and family, have been extensively used for perinatal research, of which several examples will be given. In Norway, mother, father, and child are identified by unique individual registration numbers. This facilitates linkage of successive births to the same mother with the same father or different fathers and linkage across generations. The medical birth registries can also be linked to other health-related registries, for example the cancer registries.

Traditionally, perinatal epidemiologists have focused on exposures and outcomes that occur in the perinatal period, which for research purposes covers the period from conception through birth and the first part of life. For perinatal surveillance and statistical comparisons of mortality and morbidity between regions and countries, a more specific definition is used.

Definitions and Definitional Pitfalls

According to *Webster's New World Medical Dictionary*, the perinatal period "starts at the 20th to 28th week of gestation and ends 1 to 4 weeks after birth." By international convention, strict limits are defined in the tenth revision of the *International Statistical Classification of Diseases and Related Health Problems* (ICD-10), stating that the perinatal period commences at 22 completed weeks (154 days) of gestation (the time when birth weight is normally 500 g), and ends 7 completed days after birth. The lower limit is arbitrarily chosen to represent the time when a fetus is potentially viable; before this time a terminated pregnancy would be labeled miscarriage or abortion, after this time it is a birth. However, the ICD-10 definition of birth does not take gestational age into account; it only distinguishes between live birth and fetal death (deadborn fetus).

The ICD-10 definition is not as straightforward as it looks at first glance. Gestational age is variously defined. According to ICD-10, it should be based on the date of the first day of the last normal menstrual period, or on the best clinical estimate if this date is not available (or uncertain). With the advent of second-trimester ultrasound dating, sonographic biometry has increasingly replaced menstrual dates in countries where ultrasound is an integral part of prenatal care. Seven completed days has three logical interpretations: 168 h from the hour of birth, the date of birth plus 6 completed days and the date of birth plus 7 completed days, which are all in use. Since the incidence of early neonatal death tapers off toward a minimum during the first week after birth, these different definitions do not seriously affect international comparisons.

In many countries, civil notification of stillbirth starts at 28 completed gestational weeks, which precludes the enumeration of stillbirths between 22 and 28 weeks. International perinatal comparisons are therefore most often restricted to births beyond 28 weeks. To avoid enigmatic definitions of gestational length, age is in some instances replaced by birthweight of 1000 g or more. The different limits for compulsory notification of stillbirths entails another source of error in comparisons, since births shortly past the time limit tend to be underreported. In a concerted European comparison of perinatal mortality, it was found that adjustment for different cut-off points for birthweight and gestational age would reduce the differences in perinatal mortality by between 14% and 40% in the different countries and regions (Graafmans *et al.*, 2001).

Perinatal Mortality

Perinatal mortality is defined as the number of fetal deaths past 22 (or 28) completed weeks of pregnancy plus the number of deaths among live-born children up to 7 completed days of life, per 1000 total births (live births and stillbirths). A joint interagency expert meeting on global indicators of sexual and reproductive health organized by WHO, UNICEF, and UNFPA in 2000 recommended perinatal mortality rate (PNMR) to be one of 17 chosen indicators. To avoid the problem of determining gestational age, the expert group advised that for comparative purposes 500 g and 1000 g should replace the time limits (World Health Organization, 2001). It goes without saying that PNMR will be higher when the 22-week limit or 500-g limit is used, because of the added number of stillbirths between 22 and 27 weeks. **Figure 1** shows perinatal death rates in Norway in four time periods by gestational age. There has been substantial improvement in survival of extremely preterm births since 1967; in 1997–2004 there were 48% perinatal deaths among those born between 22 and 27 weeks, compared to 91% in 1967–76 (Skjærven, 2006). Norway was chosen for the example because there is compulsory notification of all births (stillbirths and live births) from 16 weeks onwards, which ensures nearly complete coverage. The remarkably enhanced survival over a span of 40 years is largely ascribed to better neonatal intensive care, which is of course related to those born alive. During the same period, the stillbirth rate in Norway past 28 weeks fell from 11.2 in 1967 to 2.9 per 1000 births in 2004. It is difficult to sort out the causes, but better overall maternal health status is thought to play an important part.

Using PNMR for global monitoring pinpoints the wide gap in reproductive health between rich and poor countries. Perinatal death is more common than maternal death, by a factor of about 100. Local registration will serve as an impetus to perinatal audit, which in turn may induce measures for improvement. **Figure 2** shows perinatal mortality in the WHO regions of the world over a

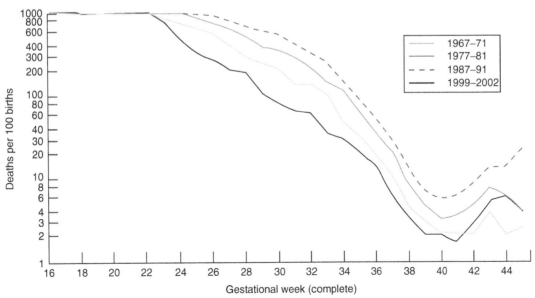

Figure 1 Perinatal mortality rates in Norway in four time periods during 1967–2002, by gestational age. Data from the Medical Birth Registry of Norway.

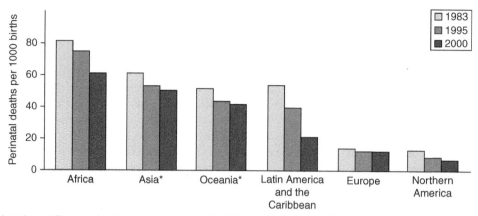

Figure 2 Perinatal mortality rates in three time periods by WHO Regions. *Australia, New Zealand, and Japan have been excluded from regional estimates but are included in the total for developed countries. From World Health Organization (2006) *Neonatal and Perinatal Mortality. Country, Regional and Global Estimates.* Geneva: World Health Organization.

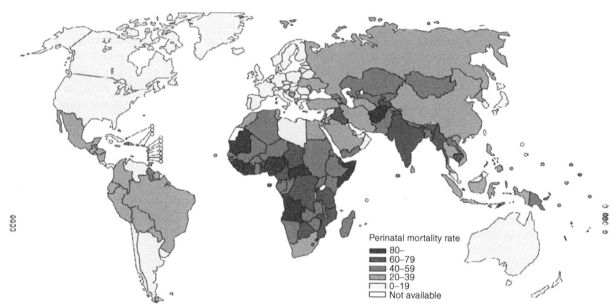

Figure 3 Perinatal mortality rates by country, 2000. From World Health Organization (2006) *Neonatal and Perinatal Mortality. Country, Regional and Global Estimates.* Geneva: World Health Organization.

span of 18 years and **Figure 3** gross country estimates in the year 2000. With a PNMR of 62 per 1000 births, Africa at present ranks higher than the Nordic countries did more than 100 years ago. However, a local population-based study in rural Northern Tanzania came up with an optimistically lower figure, 27 per 1000 births, for which no scientific explanation was found (Hinderaker *et al.*, 2003). In developing countries, the ratio of stillbirths to first-week deaths is approximately 50/50. In Europe, stillbirths have the higher share, while in Northern America it is lower, the PNMR in both regions being around 10 per 1000 births (**Table 1**). In all likelihood, these latter differences are caused by registration shortfalls.

Causes of Perinatal Death

To monitor perinatal mortality over time and make comparisons between countries and regions, one needs to know the causes of death. This implies a classification system that is clearly defined and fit for the purpose of introducing corrective measures. Various systems have been presented, with different emphasis on maternal and fetal or newborn conditions and complications. To determine the cause of death in a stillborn fetus as a rule requires an autopsy; this in practice is an exception rather than a standard procedure.

Table 2 is an example of causes of perinatal death in districts of rural Tanzania in 1995–96, grouped according

Table 1   Global estimates of stillbirths, early neonatal deaths and perinatal mortality by WHO region in 2000

Region	PNM rate	Still birth rate	ENMR
Africa	62	32	31
Asia	50	27	24
Europe	13	8	4
Latin America	21	10	12
North America	7	3	4
Oceania	42	23	19

From World Health Organization (2006) *Neonatal and Perinatal Mortality. Country, Regional and Global Estimates.* Geneva: World Health Organization.

Table 2   Causes of death in 136 cases of perinatal death in rural Tanzania, 1995–96

	All cases	Avoidable
Total	136	34
Infections	53	19
Asphyxia-related conditions	32	9
Immaturity-related conditions	20	1
Other causes/unclassifiable	16	2
Congenital conditions	9	0
External causes of death	2	0
Sudden death	1	0
Specific conditions	1	1
No information	2	2

Adapted from Hinderaker SG, Olsen BE, Bergsjø PB, *et al.* (2003) Avoidable stillbirths and neonatal deaths in rural Tanzania. *International Journal of Obstetrics and Gynecology* 110: 616–623.

Table 3   Selected neonatal conditions and interventions in Norway 2004. Numbers and proportions per 1000 births. The total number of births was 58 041

Condition	Number	Proportion per 1000
Respiratory distress syndrome	563	9.7
Intracranial hemorrhage	134	2.3
Fractured limbs	234	4.0
Facial paresis	35	0.6
Brachial plexus injury	136	2.3
Hip joint dysplasia, treated	572	9.9
Conjunctivitis, treated	442	7.6
Systemic antibiotics treatment	1363	23.5
Hyperbilirubinemia, treated	5431	93.6

Perinatal Morbidity

Perinatal epidemiologists also study diseases, injuries, and genetic aberrations diagnosed *in utero*, at birth, or in the early neonatal period, and their short- or long-term consequences. They can be classified in much the same way as the causes of death in **Table 2**. The Medical Birth Registry of Norway routinely reports incidence rates of a number of specified neonatal conditions, shown in **Table 3**. The most common of these conditions was treated neonatal hyperbilirubinemia (or jaundice), which occurred in almost 10% of the newborns. Treatment for the majority of these was phototherapy. Systemic antibiotic treatment was given to 2.4%, while hip joint dysplasia and respiratory distress syndrome were diagnosed each in about 1% of the newborns (Skjærven, 2006).

Perinatal Audit

Perinatal audit is defined as "the systematic, critical analysis of the quality of perinatal care, including the procedures used for diagnosis and treatment, the use of resources and the resultant outcome and quality of life for women and their babies" (Dunn and McIlwaine, 1996). Peer review is another label. The definition covers a variety of quality assessment activities, with the implicit understanding that audit feedback should lead to changes to improve services. In this context, audit should be a formal procedure, with a multidisciplinary panel consisting of professionals of high standing, chosen among people of the same ranks and positions as those who cared for the cases to be audited, but preferably with no links to their departments. We have previously given a more detailed account of our experiences of perinatal audit through 20 years (Bergsjø *et al.*, 2003) and will only give a few examples in this brief outline.

Audits of perinatal deaths have been used to advantage in both developing and developed countries. An example of the former is given in **Table 2**, which provides the

to a classification system developed by the International Collaborative Effort (ICE) on Birth Weight, Plurality, Perinatal and Infant Mortality (Cole *et al.*, 1989). The data derive from a prospective population-based study. Of the deaths recorded, 46% were stillbirths. Some of the neonates died more than 1 week after birth. Infection-related deaths dominated. Malaria was diagnosed in 20 out of 53 cases (Hinderaker *et al.*, 2003).

Besides the direct cause of death, a number of other factors have been shown to influence the incidence of perinatal mortality. Gestational age and birth weight are obvious. Maternal age, parity, and a number of maternal conditions and diseases such as diabetes, the antiphospholipid syndrome, preeclampsia, and smoking are risk factors to varying degrees. In multiple pregnancies, the second in a set of twins carries the higher risk. More boys than girls die in the perinatal period. Isoimmunization due to blood group incompatibility has largely been eliminated following the introduction of anti-rhesus-gammaglobulin, but is still a risk factor. Intrapartum events (breech and transverse fetal presentation, mode of delivery, maternal hemorrhage) may threaten the baby's life. In rich countries with decreasing PNMRs, congenital conditions take an increasing share of perinatal deaths.

Table 4 Summary results of audit of selected types of perinatal deaths in some Western European countries and regions

Country	Unavoidable		Potentially avoidable		Total graded
	Number	%	Number	%	Number
Belgium	92	48.9	96	51.1	188
Denmark	127	48.8	133	51.2	260
England	100	46.5	115	53.5	215
Finland	111	68.1	52	31.9	163
Greece	51	48.6	54	51.4	105
The Netherlands	81	51.6	76	48.4	157
Norway	84	60.4	55	39.6	139
Scotland	42	49.4	43	50,6	85
Spain	57	55.9	45	44.1	102
Sweden	83	64.3	46	35.7	129
Total	828	53.7	715	46.3	1543

Most countries are represented by regions (provinces).
Adapted from the EuroNatal study, Richardus JH, Graafmans WC, Verloove-Vanhorick SP, and Mackenbach JP (2003) Differences in perinatal mortality and suboptimal care between 10 European regions: Results of an international audit. *BJOG: An International Journal of Obstetrics and Gynaecology* 110: 97–105.

added information that one of four cases was considered to be possibly avoidable. In a similar exercise covering ten European countries or regions, a multinational and multidisciplinary panel decided that between 35% and 54% of selected cases of perinatal death were potentially avoidable (**Table 4**). The cases had been selected among groups in which care and treatment were most likely to have a significant impact on the outcome, and the figures therefore only indicate relative differences in standards between countries and regions (Richardus *et al.*, 2003). If all of the perinatal deaths within each birth population had been reviewed, the proportion of potentially avoidable cases would have been considerably lower.

Perinatal Risk Factors

Birth registries serve as important surveillance systems allowing description of relevant factors associated with pregnancies and childbirth. For example, the frequencies of interventions such as cesarean section and adverse outcome of birth such as perinatal death. The associations between maternal age and parity and preterm birth are shown in **Table 5**. With the exception of teenaged mothers, the incidence of preterm birth is consistently lower among those who have given birth previously.

Another example is the association between the length of maternal education and preterm birth in different time periods, as shown in **Table 6**. Mothers with a low education level had increased risk of preterm birth in all three time periods, 1967–76, 1977–86, and 1987–98.

Table 7 shows the association between the risk of preterm birth by sex of the fetus, previous preterm birth, and previous fetal death. It can be seen that male fetuses have 20% increased risk of being born preterm (6.5% vs. 5.4%). A previous preterm birth increases the incidence

Table 5 Age, parity, and preterm birth

Maternal age and preterm birth		Proportion of preterm births (%)
Para 0	Age < 20 years	7.4
	Age 20–24	5.3
	Age 25–29	5.4
	Age 30–34	6.5
	Age 35+	8.9
	All ages	5.8
Para 1+	Age < 20 years	9.0
	Age 20–24	4.8
	Age 25–29	4.0
	Age 30–34	4.5
	Age 35 +	6.1
	All ages	4.6

Based on data from Skjærven R (2006) Forekomst av og overlevelse blant ekstremt premature barn. In: *Fødsler i Norge 2003–2004. Årsrapport/Annual Report.* Bergen, Norway: Medisinsk fødselsregister/Medical Birth Registry of Norway, pp. 199–205 ($n = 1\,680\,994$).

from 5.2% to 11.4% ($RR = 2.19$) and a previous fetal death increases the risk from 5.6 to 8.1 ($RR = 1.45$).

Time trends of preterm births of less than 37 completed weeks' gestational age in Norway 1967–98 are shown in **Table 8**. It appears that little change in the frequency has occurred over this time period, in spite of considerable changes in habits of living (diet and smoking), in vitro fertilization, ultrasound dating of pregnancies, and a more interventional obstetric practice. Perinatal survival has improved considerably for these tiny babies, as shown in **Figure 1**. The causation of preterm birth is mainly unknown, although a significant part of the causation is linked to genes from both parents. The genetic and environmental components of the causation call for innovative research in order for decision makers to develop effective preventive strategies.

Table 6 Frequency of preterm birth (%) by level of maternal education in three periods in Norway

Maternal education	1967–76 %	1967–76 RR	1977–86 %	1977–86 RR	1987–98 %	1987–98 RR
Low	5.9	1.40	5.6	1.47	6.6	1.43
Medium	4.8	1.20	4.6	1.21	5.4	1.17
High	4.0	1.00	3.8	1.00	4.6	1.00
Unknown	6.8	1.70	6.7	1.76	7.0	1.52
Total	5.1		4.7		5.4	

Based on data from Skjærven R (2006) Forekomst av og overlevelse blant ekstremt premature barn. *Fødsler i Norge 2003–2004. Årsrapport/Annual Report*, pp. 199–205. Bergen, Norway: Medisinsk fødselsregister/Medical Birth Registry of Norway (n = 1 680 994).

Table 7 Percentage preterm births by sex of the fetus and by previous pregnancy outcomes

Sex and previous outcomes		Preterm birth (%)
Sex of fetus	Male	6.5
	Female	5.4
Previous preterm birth	Yes	11.4
	No	5.2
Previous fetal death	Yes	8.1
	No	5.6

Based on data from Skjærven R (2006) Forekomst av og overlevelse blant ekstremt premature barn. In: *Fødsler i Norge 2003–2004. Årsrapport/Annual Report*. Bergen, Norway: Medisinsk fødselsregister/Medical Birth Registry of Norway, pp. 199–205, 1967–98 (n = 1 680 994).

Analytical Studies

In searching for risk factors, two major approaches are employed within perinatal epidemiology. The individuals may be defined according to a specific outcome variable, for example preterm birth. Risk factors can be related to this outcome by the case–control approach. Is the risk factor more prevalent among the cases than among the controls? Control cases can be matched to the cases for one or more variables, such as age and parity. Alternatively, the total cohort can be used for the comparisons, in which case it is called a case–cohort study. The other approach involves identification of individuals according to the presence of the risk factor under study and following the individuals over time and recording the outcome(s) in question. This is called a prospective, or cohort, study. Recently, huge cohorts of pregnancies have been established allowing cohort analyses, or so-called nested case–control studies, which mean case–control studies within the cohort material.

During the 1960s, diethylstilbestrol (DES) was widely used to prevent abortion or preterm birth (on scanty evidence, later shown to be invalid). An investigation

Table 8 Time trends of preterm births of less than 37 completed weeks' gestational age (%) in Norway, 1967–98

Gestational age (weeks)	Time periods 1967–76	1977–86	1987–98
16–27	0.5	0.5	0.6
28–32	0.8	0.7	0.8
33–36	3.8	3.6	4.0
Total <37	5.1	4.8	5.4
Total number of births <37 completed weeks	390 021	467 752	623 221

Based on data from Skjærven R (2006) Forekomst av og overlevelse blant ekstremt premature barn. In: *Fødsler i Norge 2003–2004. Årsrapport/Annual Report*. Bergen, Norway: Medisinsk fødselsregister/Medical Birth Registry of Norway, pp. 199–205, 1967–98 (n = 1 680 994).

that started in Boston in 1971 (Herbst et al., 1977) is a classical example of a case–control study in perinatal epidemiology. Three physicians at the Vincent Memorial Hospital reported a striking association between maternal use of DES during the first trimester of pregnancy and the development 15–20 years later of vaginal cancer in daughters born of these mothers. Seven young women were diagnosed with this cancer that was rarely seen in young women. Because of this clustering of cases (seven within 4 years), it was decided to conduct a case–control study comparing these seven cases plus an additional one from another hospital and their families with an appropriate comparison group (controls) in order to identify factors that might explain the appearance of the cancers. Four matched controls were selected among young women who did not have vaginal cancer (matched for age and place of birth). Thus the study consisted of eight cases and 32 controls. As shown in **Table 9**, seven of the eight women with vaginal cancer had mothers who had been exposed to DES in their pregnancies compared to none of the 32 controls. No other differences between cases and controls were found. This was such a strong observation that causality was suspected. Thus a previously unknown cause of a disease was disclosed.

Most studies that use data from the medical birth registries use a cohort design where both exposure and outcome variables are collected from the registry. A recent example concerns fetal and infant survival following preeclampsia. The study showed that fetal and infant survival in preeclamptic pregnancies have improved over the past 35 years in Norway. However, the selective risk of neonatal death following a preeclamptic pregnancy has not changed over time (Basso et al., 2006).

Some researchers combine data from a medical birth registry with data from other registries. Fosså et al. linked data from the patient registry of the Norwegian Radium Hospital and from the Norwegian Cancer Registry with data from the Birth Registry of Norway. They examined

Table 9 Exposure to diethylstilbestrol (DES) among mothers of eight young women with cancer of the vagina, compared to 32 matched controls

		Cancer vaginalis	
		+	−
DES	+	7	0
	−	1	32
Total		8	32

Based on data from Herbst AL, Ulfelder H, and Poskanzer D (1971) Adenocarcinomas of the vagina association of maternal stilbestrol therapy with tumor appearance in young women. *New England Journal of Medicine* 284: 878–881.

the parenthood in successive births after adult cancer. Female cancer survivors delivered more preterm births and low-birth-weight infants than women in a matching noncancer population. Male cancer survivors, on the other hand, did not differ from noncancer fathers in the outcome of successive births (Fosså *et al.*, 2005).

Recurrence Risk

Sibling studies became possible because the Norwegian Medical Birth Registry employs the unique individual identification system, whereby it is possible to link successive births to the same mothers. Bakketeig (1977) presented the first data showing the strong tendency to repeat low birth weight, preterm birth, and small for gestational age (SGA) birth. **Table 10** shows the relative prediction of adverse outcomes among second births based on the outcome of the mothers' first birth. For example, the prediction of low birth weight (LBW) is 5.6 times as strong if the elder sibling was also LBW as opposed to having appropriate birth weight. The risk of preterm birth was 4.0 times higher if the mother's first birth was also a preterm delivery, compared to a nonpreterm birth. A similar risk was shown for a SGA second birth where the first birth was also SGA compared to not being SGA. This tendency to repeat was later confirmed in much larger data sets (Bakketeig *et al.*, 1979). Mothers somehow appeared to be programmed to produce births of a certain gestational age and size. If they departed from this pattern the offspring was at a greater risk of perinatal death (Bakketeig and Hoffman, 1983).

The tendency to report birth outcomes was found to be cumulative. As shown in **Table 10**, two preterm births increased the risk of a subsequent preterm birth nearly eightfold compared to the two first births not being preterm.

The risk of preterm birth is dependent on whether the mother or the father, or both parents, were born preterm, as shown in **Table 11**.

Skjærven *et al.* (1988) examined whether the birth weight and perinatal mortality of second birth were

Table 10 The cumulative tendency to repeat preterm birth (< 37 weeks)

Previous births			Subsequent births preterm birth	
First	Second	No	%	RR
N		461 052	3.9	1.0
P		29 278	16.3	4.18
N	N	155 417	4.1	1.0
N	P	7081	14.8	3.61
P	N	9912	9.2	2.24
P	P	1960	32.3	7.88

Based on the first 7-year period of the Medical Birth Registry of Norway, 1967–1973 (a total of 464 067 births). Skjærven R (2006) Forekomst av og overlevelse blant ekstremt premature barn. In: *Fødsler i Norge 2003–2004. Årsrapport/Annual Report.* Bergen, Norway: Medisinsk fødselsregister/Medical Birth Registry of Norway, pp. 199–205. P, gestational age <37 weeks; N, gestational age ≥37 weeks.

Table 11 Preterm birth (<37 weeks) by parental gestational age at birth

Mother	Father	Total number of births	Outcome preterm births (%)
N	N	83 191	6.5
P	N	3310	9.1
N	P	4441	7.1
P	P	204	11.3
Total		91 146	

P, preterm; N, not preterm.

conditional on the weight of the first birth. They showed that a woman's successive offspring tend to have similar birth weights. Mean birth weights among second births differ by as much as 1000 g depending on the weight of the first birth. Also, the survival of the second baby at a given weight is strongly affected by its weight relative to the first baby's weight. A baby may be average size compared to the population norm, but small compared to its elder siblings. Such a baby has increased mortality that goes with being relatively small. For example, an infant weighing 3250 g is relatively large if the mother's previous baby weighed 2250 g, but relatively small if the previous birth weighed 4250 g. In the first case, the perinatal mortality risk of the 3250-g baby is 2.2 per 1000 while in the second case the baby with the same weight has perinatal mortality of 9.0 per 1000 (or four times higher).

Focusing on mothers with two births Vatten and Skjærven (2003) showed that women who changed partners between their pregnancies had an increased risk of preterm birth, birth with low birth weight, and increased risk of infant mortality, compared with women with the same partner in their pregnancies.

Mjelve *et al.* (1999) studied mothers' two first singleton births. They showed that siblings' gestational ages were significantly correlated ($r = 0.26$) and that the risk of having a preterm birth was nearly ten times higher among mothers whose firstborn had been delivered before 32 weeks' gestation compared to mothers whose first birth had been at 40 weeks' gestation. They also found that the perinatal mortality in preterm second births was significantly higher among mothers whose first infant was born at term compared with mothers whose first born child was delivered at 32–37 weeks. They concluded that since perinatal mortality among preterm births is dependent on gestational age in the mother's previous birth, a common threshold of 37 weeks' gestation for defining preterm birth as a risk factor for perinatal death may not be appropriate for all births.

Generational Studies

Skjærven et al. (1997) focused on whether a baby's survival is related to its mother's birth weight. They linked births during 1981–94 to data on all mothers born from 1967 onwards, thereby forming 105 014 mother–offspring units. The mother's birth weight was strongly associated with the weight of her baby. Mortality among small babies was much higher where the mothers were born large. For example, babies weighing between 2500 and 3000 g had a threefold higher perinatal mortality if their mothers' birth weight was 4000 g or higher, compared to those whose mothers had been small at birth (between 2500 and 3000 g).

Magnus et al. (1993) examined the correlation of gestational age and birth weight across generations. Based on linkage of 1967–69 births and 1986–89 births, they obtained 11 072 pairs of mother–firstborn offspring. A low correlation coefficient (0.086) was found for gestational age across generations, whereas the correlation between maternal and offspring birth weight was 0.242. Mothers with birth weight below 2500 g had a significantly increased risk (OR = 3.03, 95% CI 1.79–5.11) of having a low weight baby compared with mothers with birth weight above 4000 g. On the other hand, if the mother was born before 37 weeks' gestation, the risk of having a preterm birth was not significantly increased (OR = 1.48, 95% CI 0.96–2.21) compared with mothers born at term. The authors concluded that in contrast to birth weight, variation in human gestational age does not appear to be influenced by genetic factors to any large degree.

Record Linkage to Registries Outside Medical Birth Registries

In a study focusing on preeclampsia and subsequent breast cancer Vatten et al. (2002) showed that women with preeclampsia and/or hypertension in their first pregnancy had a 19% (95 CI, 9%–29%) lower risk of breast cancer compared to other parous women. This was based on data from the Medical Birth Registry of Norway linked to the Cancer Registry of Norway. The results indicate that pathophysiology surrounding preeclampsia and gestational hypertension plays a role in breast cancer etiology.

Maternal and Child Cohorts

Large cohorts of pregnancies have been established for research purposes in Denmark and Norway. Pregnant women have been included from early on in their pregnancies. Information has been collected as well as biological material (blood, urine) from the women and partly from their partners (Norway). These cohorts are important additional sources for further studies on maternal and child health. To exemplify, one can establish case–control (or case–cohort) studies within the cohort on its scientific strength. We may want to test a specific hypothesis on causation of a certain type of cancer. Each of these cohorts contains a variety of information on, for example, lifestyle of the mother when the patient was a fetus or baby, in addition to biological material collected during pregnancy, which would allow for testing of a specific hypothesis on causation.

Citations

Bakketeig LS (1977) The risk of repeated preterm or low weight delivery. In: Reed DM and Stanley FJ (eds.) *The Epidemiology of Prematurity.* Baltimore, MD: Urban and Schwarzenberg.

Bakketeig LS, Hoffman HJ, and Harly EE (1979) The tendency to repeat gestational age and birth weight in successive births. *American Journal of Obstetrics and Gynecology* 135: 1086–1103.

Bakketeig LS and Hoffman HJ (1983) The tendency to repeat gestational age and birth weight in successive birth related to perinatal survival. *Acta Obstetricia et Gynecologica Scandinavica* 62: 85–92.

Basso O, Rasmussen S, Weinberg CR, Wilcox AJ, Irgens LM, and Skjærven R (2006) Trends in fetal and infant survival following preeclampsia. *Journal of the American Medical Association* 296: 1357–1362.

Bergsjø P, Bakketeig LS, and Langhoff-Roos J (2003) The development of perinatal audit: Twenty years' experience. *Acta Obstetricia et Gynecologica Scandinavica* 82: 780–788.

Cole S, Hartford RB, Bergsjø P, and McCarthy B (1989) International Collaborative Effort (ICE) on Birth Weight, Plurality, Perinatal, and Infant Mortality: III. A method of grouping underlying causes of infant death to aid international comparisons. *Acta Obstetricia et Gynecologica Scandinavica* 68: 113–117.

Dunn PM and McIlwaine G (eds.) (1996) Perinatal audit. *Prenatal and Neonatal Medicine* 1: 160–194.

Fosså SD, Magelssen H, Melve K, Jacobsen AB, Langmark F, and Skjærven R (2005) Parenthood in survivors after adulthood cancer and perinatal health in their offspring. A preliminary report. *Journal of the National Cancer Institute Monographs* 34: 77–82.

Graafmans WC, Richardus J-H, Macforlane A, et al. (2001) Comparability of published perinatal mortality rates in Western Europe: the quantitative impact of differences in gestational age are birthweight criteria. *BJOG: An International Journal of Obstetrics and Gynecology* 108: 1237–1245.

Herbst AL, Ulfelder H, and Poskanzer D (1971) Adenocarcinomas of the vagina association of maternal stilbestrol therapy with tumor appearance in young women. *New England Journal of Medicine* 284: 878–881.

Hinderaker SG, Olsen BE, Bergsjø PB, *et al.* (2003) Avoidable stillbirths and neonatal deaths in rural Tanzania. *International Journal of Obstetrics and Gynecology* 110: 616–623.

Magnus P, Bakketeig LS, and Skjærven R (1993) Correlations of birth weight and gestational age across generations. *Annals of Human Biology* 20: 231–238.

Mjelve KK, Skjærven R, Gjessing HK, and Øyen N (1999) Recurrence of gestational age in sibships: Implication of perinatal mortality. *American Journal of Epidemiology* 150: 756–762.

Richardus JH, Graafmans WC, Verloove-Vanhorick SP, and Mackenbach JP (2003) Differences in perinatal mortality and suboptimal care between 10 European regions: Results of an international audit. *BJOG: An International Journal of Obstetrics and Gynaecology* 110: 97–105.

Skjærven R (2006) Forekomst av og overlevelse blant ekstremt premature barn. *Fødsler i Norge 2003–2004. Årsrapport/Annual Report*, pp. 199–205. Bergen, Norway: Medisinsk fødselsregister/Medical Birth Registry of Norway.

Skjærven R, Wilcox AJ, and Russel D (1988) Birthweight and perinatal mortality of second births conditional on weight of the first. *International Journal of Epidemiology* 17: 830–838.

Skjærven R, Wilcox AJ, Øyen N, and Magnus P (1997) Mothers' birth weight and survival of their offspring: Population-based study. *British Medical Journal* 314: 1376–1380.

Vatten LJ and Skjærven (2003) Effects on pregnancy outcome of changing partner between first two births: Prospective population study. *British Medical Journal* 327: 1138.

Vatten LJ, Romundstad PR, Triohopulos D, and Skjærven R (2002) Pre-eclampsia in pregnancy and subsequent risk of breast cancer. *British Journal of Cancer* 87(9): 971–973.

World Health Organization (2001) *Reproductive Health Indicators for Global Monitoring. Report of the second Interagency meeting*. WHO, Geneva 17–19 July 2000. WHO/RHR/01.19. Geneva, Switzerland: World Health Organization.

World Health Organization (2006) *Neonatal and Perinatal Mortality. Country, Regional and Global Estimates*. Geneva, Switzerland: World Health Organization.

SECTION 3
EPIDEMIOLOGY OF SPECIFIC DISEASES

Epidemiology of Diabetes Mellitus

J K Bardsley and H E Resnick, MedStar Research Institute, Hyattsville, MD, USA

Introduction: Types of Diabetes

Diabetes is a chronic, progressive disorder characterized by abnormalities in carbohydrate, fat, and protein metabolism and hyperglycemia. Chronic hyperglycemia is associated with damage to large and small blood vessels in the eyes, kidneys, nerves, and heart. Heart disease, high blood pressure, stroke, kidney failure, amputations, and blindness are common among persons with diabetes. Complications often begin 10–15 years after disease onset, depending in part on glucose control. The four clinical classes of diabetes are type 1 diabetes, type 2 diabetes, gestational diabetes, and other. In addition, prediabetes is a recognized clinical state that is associated with elevated risk of diabetes.

Type 1 Diabetes

Type 1 diabetes results from autoimmune beta cell destruction, leading to absolute insulin deficiency. It is characterized by abrupt onset of hyperglycemia and a strong propensity for ketoacidosis. Type 1 diabetes comprises only 5–10% of all diabetes cases. Genetic factors are associated with type 1 diabetes, although no single genetic factor is known to be the cause.

Type 2 Diabetes

Type 2 diabetes, comprising approximately 85% of diabetes cases, has a multihormonal pathophysiology in which either the body does not produce enough insulin or the cells are resistant to the biological effects of insulin, resulting in hyperglycemia. This disease typically progresses from insulin resistance to postprandial hyperglycemia to clinical diabetes requiring pharmacologic intervention.

Gestational Diabetes Mellitus

Gestational diabetes mellitus (GDM) is diabetes that is first diagnosed during pregnancy. In GDM, pregnancy hormones block the action of maternal insulin, causing insulin resistance and hyperglycemia. Women with a history of GDM are at increased risk of developing Type 2 diabetes.

Other Types of Diabetes

Up to 5% of cases of diabetes have other specific causes and include diabetes that results from the mutation of a single gene or chromosomal abnormality and drug- or chemically induced diabetes. These include maturity onset diabetes of the young, latent autoimmune diabetes of aging, Down syndrome, Klinefelter's syndrome, and Turner's syndrome.

Prediabetes

Prediabetes (or impaired glucose tolerance, IGT) is a condition that raises the risk of developing type 2 diabetes, heart disease, and stroke. In prediabetes, blood glucose levels are between the normal and diabetic ranges. Progression to diabetes among those with prediabetes is not inevitable: Obesity and physical inactivity are modifiable factors that affect risk of type 2 diabetes.

The remainder of this article will focus on type 2 diabetes, the most common form.

Worldwide Prevalence of Type 2 Diabetes

Some 194 million people worldwide have diabetes. In the past 30 years, diabetes has evolved from a relatively mild ailment of older people to a major cause of premature morbidity and mortality. Complications from diabetes result in increased disability, reduced life expectancy, and considerable health-care costs worldwide.

Risk of type 2 diabetes is linked to an increasing prevalence of obesity. This results from unfavorable changes in dietary and lifestyle patterns, particularly an increase in fatty foods and reduction in physical activity at home, work, and school. Replacement of traditional diets rich in fruits and vegetables by high-calorie diets high in animal fats and low in complex carbohydrates is happening in all but the least-developed countries.

Heredity

Diabetes prevalence is growing at different rates in different populations. Researchers believe that genes affecting various aspects of carbohydrate metabolism contribute to the development of type 2 diabetes. For example, in the United States, African Americans, Hispanic/Latino Americans, American Indians, Asian Americans, and Pacific Islanders are at a higher risk than the rest of the population. The increase of type 2 diabetes prevalence in children was first reported among the Pima Indians in the western United States, a population with the world's highest recorded prevalence of type 2 diabetes in adults, as well as high rates of obesity. Among people of European ancestry, the age-adjusted prevalence of diabetes is 5%, whereas among some indigenous populations, the prevalence rate is 40% or higher. Although genetic background explains the susceptibility to this chronic disease, modernization and urbanization have brought about the changes that are contributing to obesity and diabetes reported in indigenous populations.

Diabetes in Developing Countries

Throughout the world, economic development, urbanization, and affluence are accompanied by adoption of a diet high in nutritionally poor carbohydrates. In developing countries, people are moving from rural areas to cities. These cultural changes affect the number of people at risk because people living in cities tend to be less physically active and heavier. People who are heavier have a higher risk of diabetes (**Figures 1** and **2**).

In developing countries, the majority of people with diabetes are adults of working age. According to the World Health Organization, the number of people with diabetes in developing countries is expected to rise by 150% in the next 25 years.

Diabetes in Developed Countries

In economically developed countries, diabetes is the fourth or fifth leading cause of death, affecting mostly people who are older than 65. In addition, it is the poor people who get diabetes. Poverty limits access to fresh fruits and vegetables, leisure time for exercise, and health care.

A transformation has occurred in farming, food processing and distribution, transportation, and shopping practices (Beaglehole *et al.*, 2003). Food is often consumed outside the home. Alterations in food production, preparation, and consumption have fueled epidemics of noncommunicable diseases, such as diabetes, and threaten economic development. For example, the invention of microwave ovens created a market for frozen foods that are quick and easy to prepare and also high in fat and sodium.

Link with Obesity

Childhood obesity has reached epidemic proportions. Worldwide, approximately 22 million children younger than age 5 are overweight. Type 2 diabetes, once virtually unknown in adolescence, now accounts for as many as half of all new diagnoses of diabetes in some populations (Pinhas-Hamiel and Zeitler, 2005). Childhood obesity is linked to abnormalities in blood pressure, lipid, lipoprotein, and insulin levels in adults, as well as to the risk of coronary artery disease and diabetes (Freedman *et al.*, 2001).

A close relation exists between rates of type 2 diabetes in adults and the appearance of the disorder in adolescents. Type 2 diabetes in children was reported earliest in countries with the highest rates of adult type 2 diabetes. As diabetic children age, they experience earlier onset of diabetes complications relative to persons who develop

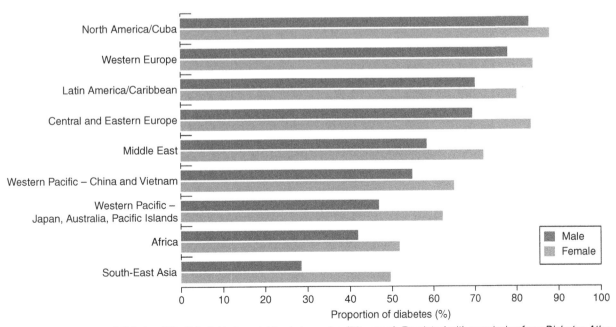

Figure 1   Proportion of diabetes (%) attributable to weight gain by region (30+ years). Reprinted with permission from *Diabetes Atlas*, 2nd edn. (2003) International Obesity Task Force. http://www.iotf.org/popout.asp?linkto=http://www.eatlas.idf.org/ (accessed December 2007).

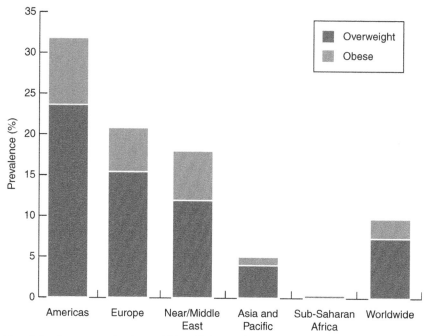

Figure 2 Overweight and obesity among school-age children (5–17 years). Reprinted with permission from *Diabetes Atlas*, 2nd edn. (2003) International Obesity Task Force. http://www.iotf.org/popout.asp?linkto=http://www.eatlas.idf.org/ (accessed December 2007).

diabetes in adulthood. In India and China, diabetes prevalence is expected to double by 2030, due in part to a rise in type 2 diabetes among children and young adults. In the past several decades, children's lifestyles have changed dramatically in developed countries, as reflected in unhealthy dietary habits and inactivity.

Causes: Societal Changes

Inactivity

Economic development has reduced the frequency of work-related physical activity. Leisure time physical activity is also low. Little time is spent outdoors, and traveling in cars has replaced walking in many developed countries. The reduction in sidewalks and increase in paved roads seem to facilitate these trends.

Technology

The advances in technology that accompany economic development further reduce the need and opportunity for physical activity. Television exposes children and adults to hours of commercials for nutritionally poor foods. The following list presents some technologies and their effects on inactivity:

- Cars. No need to walk to the store, work, or bus stop.
- Television. A typical child watches approximately 40 000 commercials on television each year, a number that has doubled during the same time that the rate of pediatric overweight has increased dramatically. Television viewing

among children is correlated with a higher intake of nutritionally poor foods and a lower intake of fruits and vegetables (Ritchie *et al.* 2005). Not only do children sit still while they watch television; they often passively consume high-calorie foods at the same time.

- Video games. Time children spend playing video games is sedentary time.
- Internet shopping. No need to walk from the car to the store and back.
- E-mail. No need to walk to deliver a message.
- Personal digital assistants. No need to walk to the computer; it's now in your pocket.
- Cell phones. No need to walk to a phone; it's in your pocket, too.

Changes in Diet

Economic development is associated with Westernization of diet in non-Western countries. As a result, diabetes is now appearing in India and Africa. Some factors contributing to obesity and diabetes in the developed countries are listed below:

- Eating out. Portions are large, and additional fats are added.
- Not eating as a family; poorly balanced meals.
- Television viewing during mealtime, which is inversely associated with consumption of products not typically advertised, such as fruits and vegetables.
- High fructose corn syrup: The rise in type 2 diabetes closely parallels increased use of sweeteners, particularly high-fructose corn syrup.

Europe

In Europe, diabetes is prevalent among the older people. A third of this region's population is age 50 or older, a proportion that is expected to increase to >40% by 2025. Thus, the number of people with diabetes and prediabetes will likely increase despite an expected overall reduction in the European population (**Table 1**). This will place an increasing financial burden on the declining working age population to provide resources for the rising number of older people with diabetes complications.

As in other economically developed countries, the prevalence of obesity in Europe has been rising and is now 15–20% among adults. Rates of childhood overweight and obesity in England have increased between 2.0-fold and 2.3-fold over ten years. As in other developed regions, diabetes rates are rising along with obesity prevalence.

North America

The rise in diabetes prevalence in North America follows the rise in obesity. In the United States, from 1980 to 2004, the number of people with diabetes more than doubled (from 5.8 million to 14.7 million). According to the Centers for Disease Control and Prevention, data from a 2003–2004 survey show that 66% of U.S. adults are overweight or obese.

The mean age at diagnosis of type 2 diabetes in the United States has decreased from 52 years in 1988–94, to 46 years, reported in 1999–2000 (Centers for Disease Control, 2005). People age 65 years or older account for almost 40% of the population with diabetes. In Canada, 10% of people 65 and older have the disease, compared with 3% of those in the 35–64 age group.

While the prevalence of overweight and obesity has increased in all segments of the U.S. and Canadian populations, it is particularly common among minority groups. African Americans, Hispanic/Latino Americans, American Indians, Asian Americans, and Pacific Islanders are at a higher risk for type 2 diabetes than are U.S. Whites. The increase in type 2 diabetes in children was first reported among the Pima Indians in central Arizona. In Canada, the problem is particularly apparent in indigenous populations, including children, and especially among women and girls. In some Canadian indigenous communities, the prevalence of type 2 diabetes among girls 10–12 years old has been reported to be 3.6%.

Among U.S. and Canadian youth, obesity, physical inactivity, and intrauterine exposure to maternal hyperglycemia have become widespread and may contribute to the increased development of type 2 diabetes during childhood and adolescence. Among U.S. children and teens ages 6–19, 16% are overweight according to 1999–2002 data, triple the 1980 percentage. Some 2 million U.S. adolescents (or one in six overweight adolescents) age 12–19 have prediabetes. A study by the Centers for Disease Control and Prevention estimated that one in three U.S. children born in 2000 will develop diabetes in their lifetime.

More than 60% of U.S. adults do not achieve the recommended amount of regular physical activity. In fact, 25% of adults are not active at all. This habit of inactivity tends to be perpetuated by their children.

In Mexico, a high prevalence of diabetes is associated with low levels of education. Sudden changes in traditional lifestyles, as seen in newly arrived migrants to large cities, result in diabetes in this genetically susceptible population. Mexico has one of the world's highest rates of soft drink consumption. The earlier age of onset of diabetes in Mexicans and the limited access of migrants to optimal medical and preventive care precipitate diabetes complications.

South and Central America

In conjunction with economic development, the South and Central America region is undergoing a nutritional transition. Obesity rates have increased markedly during the past 10–15 years and have become a public health problem in most countries. Obesity is prevalent in the adult population, especially among women with limited education and among the urban poor (Uauy *et al.*, 2001). Dietary changes

Table 1   Growing worldwide diabetes epidemic (numbers are in millions unless otherwise specified)

	Europe	North America	South & Central America	Asia	Africa	Eastern Mediterranean & Middle East	Western Pacific	Worldwide
Population								
2003	871.8	441.7	422.8	1251.4	666.6	544.6	2110.7	6.3×10^9
2025	862.6	533.8	544.6	1629.7	1107.4	839.2	2445.7	8.0×10^9
Adults with diabetes (ages 20–79 years)								
2003	48.4	23.0	14.2	39.3	7.1	19.2	43.0	194
2025	58.6	36.2	26.2	81.6	15.0	39.4	75.8	333
Adults with impaired glucose tolerance								
2003	63.2	20.3	18.5	93.4	21.4	18.7	78.6	314
2025	70.6	29.6	29.5	146.3	39.4	36.5	120.2	472

Data are from the International Diabetes Foundation.

and increasing inactivity help explain these trends. As income increases in transitional countries, so does the consumption of high-fat foods, including industrially processed hydrogenated fats. A study conducted in the city of Santiago, Chile, showed that the principal components of food expenditure among the poor are bread, meat, and soft drinks. As intake of these foods has increased to the detriment of grains, fruits, and vegetables, rates of obesity, insulin resistance, and type 2 diabetes have increased.

In Santiago in 1970, about 75% of the population lived in urban areas; in 1997 this figure was 87%. The number of cars increased from 363 150 in 1970 to 1 969 128 in 1997. Televisions numbered 12 170 in 1970 and increased to >2 million in 1997. Some 90% of school-age children in Santiago watch television on weekdays, and of these, 20% watch more than 3 h daily. Data from several urban centers, including Santiago, show that television viewing and television commercials have a direct relationship to snack food consumption and other food purchased by children at school (Uauy et al., 2001).

As malnutrition rates fall in this region, the need to prevent overweight and obesity should be considered as important as the eradication of undernutrition, which sometimes occurs in the same households. Supplementary feeding programs are widespread throughout this region. A survey of 19 Latin American countries found that more than 20% of the population receives food assistance. Nutrition programs have become a social benefit expected by individuals living in poverty. Despite the benefits (i.e., the significant reductions in underweight and wasting), these programs can affect obesity rates. While food supplements benefit some, the provision of high-fat foods can be detrimental for others.

In response, supplemental food programs are now adapting the food provided to fit the nutritional profile of the preschool population. Sugar and saturated fat content of the ration have been lowered, fat-free milk is being provided, and additional fresh fruits and vegetables have been added.

Asia

The expected increase in diabetes prevalence in Asia is due in part to increased life expectancy in India. The adult population of India comprises 85% of the population of this region. As in other developing countries, diabetes prevalence in India is higher among the affluent, suggesting that economic growth will continue to escalate diabetes prevalence.

India currently has the world's largest diabetic population, with an estimated 35 million. This number is expected to reach 73 million by 2025. This region has the world's highest prevalence of IGT, further evidence of the coming increase in diabetes prevalence in this area.

Various Asian populations may be particularly susceptible to the health risks of central obesity (fat carried in

the abdominal area). Consequently there is an increasing focus on waist circumferences, which may predict diabetes risk better than does body mass index.

The incidence of diabetes in adults in this region is growing at an alarming rate. By 2025, China is expected to show an increase of up to 68%.

Among Japanese schoolchildren, the incidence of type 2 diabetes increased from 0.2 to 7.3 per 100 000 children per year between 1976 and 1995 – an increase attributed to changing dietary patterns and increasing rates of obesity. In some areas of Japan, type 2 diabetes has become the dominant form of diabetes in children and adolescents.

Africa

As in other developing countries, in parts of sub-Saharan Africa, obesity exists alongside undernutrition. According to the International Diabetes Foundation, the prevalence of type 2 diabetes is low in both rural and urban African Bantu communities but is ten times higher in African Muslim and Hindu communities in Tanzania and South Africa and in the Chinese community in Mauritius.

The current rate of diabetes in Africa is reaching epidemic proportions and is predicted to increase by more than 90% by 2010, predominantly affecting individuals of working age.

Foot complications are a major problem for people with diabetes in Africa. In Africa, diabetic foot infections lead to amputation in 25–50% of cases and often result in death. Not only are amputations life-threatening; they often cause life-long dependence and inability to work.

Common practices such as walking barefoot and wearing inappropriate footwear contribute to injuries that can lead to infection in the foot and result in amputations. Late referral to hospitals, as well as poor knowledge of and access to foot care, play a major role in the high amputation rate in Africa.

Of the world's 49 least developed countries, 33 are in sub-Saharan Africa. Incomes in these countries do not allow for the purchase of insulin and other supplies to manage diabetes. Lack of access to insulin and diabetes supplies frequently occurs as a result of natural disasters, civil unrest, or national financial crises. The widespread lack of access to insulin, refrigeration, and health care threatens the lives of people with diabetes in sub-Saharan Africa.

Eastern Mediterranean and Middle East

Diabetes prevalence in some countries of the Eastern Mediterranean and Middle East is among the highest in the world. During the past 30 years, major social and economic changes have occurred in this region. These include urbanization, decreasing infant mortality, and increasing life expectancy. The aging of the population, along with socioeconomic and lifestyle changes, has resulted in a dramatic increase in type 2 diabetes. In Iran, obesity rates vary from rural to urban populations, rising to 30% among women in Tehran.

Rapid economic development, especially in wealthy oil-producing countries, has been associated with alterations in nutrition, decreased physical activity, and increased obesity. The United Arab Emirates, Bahrain, Kuwait, and Oman have diabetes prevalence rates that are among the world's highest, as are their IGT prevalence rates. As in other countries with high diabetes prevalence, the onset of type 2 diabetes is occurring in relatively young people. This trend is following the rising rates of obesity. In Egypt, childhood overweight and obesity have increased 3.9-fold in 18 years.

Western Pacific

The link between obesity and type 2 diabetes is most manifest in the Western Pacific area, which has some of the highest levels of adult obesity. Obesity prevalence rates of 60–80% are found among adults on some islands, including Samoa and Nauru. In Tonga, 60% of the adult population is obese, and 12% of men and nearly 18% of women have type 2 diabetes, a doubling of the rate in 25 years. A further 20% have prediabetes.

Adolescents from minority groups in Australia (Aboriginal) and New Zealand (Maori) have a high prevalence of type 2 diabetes. Data from Australia indicate that 40–50% of the diabetes patients there are from immigrant groups (Pakistan, Turkey, South America, South Asia, India, Middle East), and analyses suggest that adoption of a Westernized lifestyle is strongly associated with type 2 diabetes in these populations (Pinhas-Hamiel and Zeitler, 2005).

The high prevalence of diabetes in the affluent cities indicates that in this region as well, diabetes prevalence is increasing along with economic and urban expansion.

Global Trends

According to the World Health Organization, the number of people with diabetes will more than double over the next 25 years, reaching 366 million by 2030. Most of this increase will occur as a result of a 150% rise in developing countries.

The greatest increases are expected in the Middle East, sub-Saharan Africa, and India (**Figures 3** and **4**). The biggest demographic change in global terms will be an increase in diabetes among people older than age 65.

In developing countries, most people with diabetes are in the 45–64 age group. In developed countries, the majority of people with diabetes are older than age 64. By 2030, it is estimated that the number of people with diabetes who are older than age 64 will be more than 82 million in developing countries and more than 48 million in developed countries (Wild *et al.*, 2004).

Strategies for Prevention

Large, population-based studies in China, Finland, and the United States have demonstrated the possibility of preventing or delaying diabetes in overweight people with prediabetes. These trials have shown that changes in diet and physical activity, resulting in a 5–7% weight loss, can reduce the risk of developing type 2 diabetes.

Studies have shown that people with prediabetes can prevent or delay the onset of diabetes. This can be accomplished through 30 min or more of physical activity most days of the week and a nutritious diet. In all the studies conducted in people at high risk, lifestyle changes have been more effective than the use of drugs to prevent diabetes.

The scale of the diabetes epidemic requires global initiatives to reduce obesity and increase physical activity. Informed policy decisions on urban design and on food pricing and advertising can help reduce the population-wide risks of developing type 2 diabetes.

The following steps, categorized by place of action, can be implemented to help stop this epidemic.

Home

- Restrict children's screen time (i.e., time spent watching television and playing video games).
- Eat dinner as a family. Family dinners are associated with more fruits and vegetables, fewer fried foods, less soda, less fat, and more micronutrients.
- Be active as a family. Exercising together creates norms and expectations about regular physical activity.

School

- Support 'walking school bus' programs in which adults accompany children walking to and from school.
- Suggest that schools provide healthful food, ban soda and candy sales, and teach appropriate nutrition and activity habits. Advocate for parenting and healthful cooking classes in high schools and adult education programs in order to have an impact on the next generation (Ritchie *et al.*, 2005).
- Have recess and gym class more often (or every day) at school.

Urban Design

- Build sidewalks to promote walking.
- Promote mixed land use so that people can walk to school and work.

Health Care

- Instead of relying on endocrinologists, rely on nutritionists, nurses, and diabetes educators.

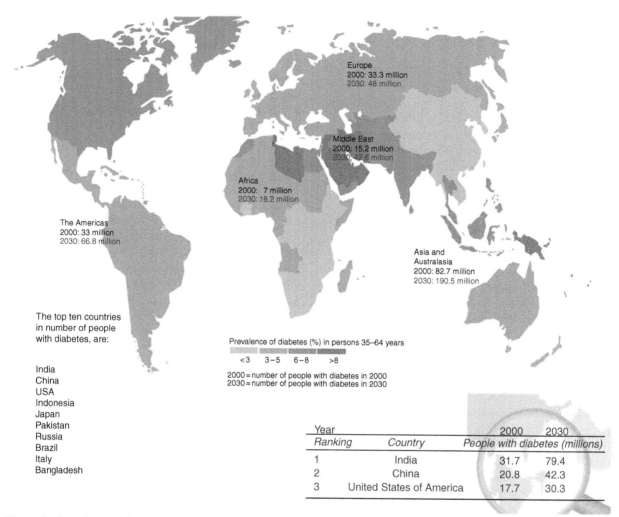

The top ten countries in number of people with diabetes, are:

India
China
USA
Indonesia
Japan
Pakistan
Russia
Brazil
Italy
Bangladesh

Prevalence of diabetes (%) in persons 35–64 years

<3   3–5   6–8   >8

2000 = number of people with diabetes in 2000
2030 = number of people with diabetes in 2030

Year		2000	2030
Ranking	Country	People with diabetes (millions)	
1	India	31.7	79.4
2	China	20.8	42.3
3	United States of America	17.7	30.3

Figure 3 Prevalence of diabetes worldwide. Reprinted with permission from http://www.who.int/diabetes/facts/en.

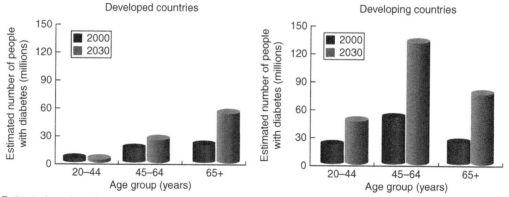

Figure 4 Estimated number of people with diabetes in developed versus developing countries, 2000 and 2030. Reprinted with permission from http://www.who.int/diabetes/facts/en/.

- Direct efforts toward diabetes prevention. View diabetes as a chronic rather than an acute disease.
- Teach healthy people how to stay healthy via daily exercise and nutritious food; concentrate on teaching mothers and children because habits are established early.

Marketing and Media

- Regulate advertising of foods aimed at children.
- Encourage restaurants to provide smaller portion sizes and more healthful options.

Policy

- Limit the addition of high-fructose corn syrup to foods.
- Incorporate physical activity into jobs.
- Encourage a diet based on unprocessed foods.
- Direct preventive activities at the entire population via community intervention programs and integrate them with measures directed against other diseases, such as hypertension and cardiovascular disease.

Conclusion

The number of people with diabetes is increasing due to population growth, aging, urbanization, and increasing prevalence of obesity and inactivity. As more countries become economically developed and their populations adopt a high-fat, nutritionally poor diet, the epidemic of diabetes can be expected to continue.

Acknowledgments

We gratefully acknowledge the assistance of Rachel Schaperow, Medstar Research Institute, in the research and writing of this article.

Citations

Beaglehole R and Yach D (2003) Globalisation and the prevention and control of non-communicable disease: The neglected chronic diseases of adults. *Lancet* 362: 903–908.

Centers for Disease Control and Prevention (2005) *National diabetes fact sheet: general information and national estimates on diabetes in the United States, 2005*. Atlanta, GA: U.S. Department of Health and Human Services, Centers for Disease Control and Prevention.

Freedman DS, Khan LK, Dietz WH, Srinivasan SR, and Berenson GS (2001) Relationship of childhood obesity to coronary heart disease risk factors in adulthood: The Bogalusa Heart Study. *Pediatrics* 108: 712–718.

Pinhas-Hamiel O and Zeitler P (2005) The global spread of type 2 diabetes mellitus in children and adolescents. *Journal of Pediatrics* 146: 693–700.

Ritchie LD, Welk G, Styne D, Gerstein DE, and Crawford PB (2005) Family environment and pediatric overweight: What is a parent to do? *Journal of the American Dietetic Association* 105(5 Suppl 1): S70–S79.

Uauy R, Albala C, and Kain J (2001) Obesity trends in Latin America: Transiting from under– to overweight. *Journal of Nutrition* 131(3): 893S–899S.

Wild S, Roglic G, Green A, Sicree R, and King H (2004) Global prevalence of diabetes: Estimates for the year 2000 and projections for 2030. *Diabetes Care* 27: 1047–1053.

Further Reading

Ebbeling CB, Pawlak DB, and Ludwig DS (2002) Childhood obesity: Public-health crisis, common sense cure. *Lancet* 360: 473–482.

Gorman C (2003) Why so many of us are getting diabetes. *Time Magazine* December 8, 59–69.

James PT, Leach R, Kalamara E, and Shayeghi M (2001) The worldwide obesity epidemic. *Obesity Research* 9(suppl. 4): 228S–233S.

Kleinfield NR (2006) Diabetes and its awful toll quietly emerge as a crisis. *New York Times*, January 9.

Pinhas-Hamiel O, Dolan LM, Daniels SR, Standiford D, Khoury PR, and Zeitler P (1996) Increased incidence of non-insulin-dependent diabetes mellitus among adolescents. *Journal of Pediatrics* 128 (5 Pt 1): 608–615.

Santora M (2006) East meets West, adding pounds and peril. *New York Times*, January 12.

Urbina I (2006) In the treatment of diabetes, success often does not pay. *New York Times*, January 11.

Relevant Websites

http://www.diabetes.org – American Diabetes Organization.
http://www.cdc.gov – Centers for Disease Control and Prevention.
http://www.idf.org – International Diabetes Federation.
http://www.phac-aspc.gc.ca/new_e.html – Public Health Agency of Canada.
http://www.who.int/diabetes – World Health Organization Diabetes Programme.

Epidemiology of Injuries

E T Petridou and C N Antonopoulos, Athens University Medical School, Athens, Greece
D-M Alexe, London School of Hygiene and Tropical Medicine, London, UK

Terminology and Definitions

Injuries: The Theoretical Definition

A clear definition is essential in pursuing the etiology of any given pathological entity. According to Haddon's energy-release theory of causation, injuries result from tissue damage caused by transfer of energy (mechanical, electrical, thermal, chemical, radiation) to the body produced in the course of energy exchanges that have relatively sudden discernible effects. Two important considerations that should be taken into account in the definition of injuries are the identification of the causal event as well as the assessment of the subsequent pathological outcome. Indeed, some somatic lesions that are not related to a traumatic process may occur (e.g., injuries following septic shock), whereas contact of some physical agents with the human body may not always result in a physical injury (e.g., road crashes from low-speed rear impacts may sometimes leave no visible mark) (Langley and Brenner, 2004).

Haddon's definition covers both the etiology and the outcome of injury, but it does not cover all terminological aspects. For example, an injury can occur from the lack of energy following, for example, the sudden decrease in the energy supplies to the human body, such as oxygen or heat in cases of drowning and frostbite, respectively, contrary to Haddon's definition. While this dimension has been recently included in the definition, concerns with regards to other aspects still remain, given that death itself, irrespective of its cause, is defined as the lack of energetic resources and activities.

Other controversial issues relate to some forms of tissue damage caused during medical procedures. For instance, a surgical incision is the result of intentional transfer of mechanical energy and this transfer results in tissue damage; yet traditionally surgical incisions are not included in counts of intentional injuries. On the contrary, other types of injury that result in no pathological lesions, such as ingestion of foreign bodies into the digestive track, are commonly characterized as injuries. It should also be noted that Haddon's definition does not include the psychological dimension of injury, namely the relatively recently identified posttraumatic stress disorder or those suffering from depression following, for example, a sexual assault.

A widely debated issue with regards to injury terminology has focused on why it is appropriate to use the word accident, given the inherent connotation of fate as the underlying mechanism leading to an injury. Etymologically, the word accident comes from the Latin word *accidentum*, which means that something unfortunate has happened by chance, without one's foresight or expectation. It has been argued that the use of this word in the context of injuries may deter injury prevention efforts, as an event that is due to chance cannot be predicted or prevented. In an effort to strengthen the importance of injury prevention measures and precautionary interventions, a radical attitude has been adopted by one of the most prestigious medical journals, the *British Medical Journal*, whose editors have decided to ban the word accident from the columns of the journal. This move has raised a lively debate in the scientific community, as a more appropriate approach seems to be defining distinctive features in the terms injury, lesion, trauma, and accident, so that the preventability of injuries is clearly stated. Therefore it has been recommended to use injury, lesion, or trauma in describing the result caused to the human body instead of the term accident. The term accident, however, is often used by lay people to describe both the unintentional event leading to an injury as well as the

resulting lesion. The tyranny of words is not the issue at stake, however. Instead, the distinction between the unintentional event that has led to the body lesion (accident) and the body lesion itself should be clearly made. It is important to provide detailed information associated with the description of the event and its external cause, concentrate on how to raise awareness, and channel all human potential and how to combat this contemporary epidemic, irrespective of cultural and terminological deviations.

Injuries: The Operational Definition

According to the etiological mechanism, unintentional injuries are classified on the basis of their external cause in the following categories of the ICD-10 version 2006:

1. Motor vehicle traffic accidents;
2. Other transport accidents;
3. Accidental poisoning;
4. Accidental falls;
5. Accidents caused by fire and flames;
6. Accidental drowning;
7. Accidents caused by machinery, cutting, piercing instruments;
8. Accidents caused by firearm missile;
9. All other accidents, including late effect.

Another category of injuries concerns those produced by drugs, medications causing adverse effects in therapeutic use, while the sizeable category of intentional injuries is divided into those resulting from suicide and self-inflicted injuries and those from homicide and injury purposely inflicted by another person. Lastly, the category encompassing other external causes includes legal interventions and operations of war and other injuries.

Commonly Used Terms in Injury Research and Prevention

Safety is a term frequently used in injury research and prevention, referring to the condition of being protected against failure, damage, error, accidents, or harm. This term comes from Latin (*salus, salube,* and *solidus,* all used to define a status of good health or otherwise being healthy). Injury prevention refers to measures that are being taken in order to reduce the incidence and severity of injuries and focuses on the implementation of safety promotion measures in an effort to provide a safer environment as well as on how to tackle risk-taking behaviors. Injury prevention measures are separated into active and passive behaviors, depending on whether an individual is expected to intentionally undertake an action aiming to maximize the effect of a prevention measure (for example wearing a seatbelt vs. enjoying the protection provided by built-in air bags in the event of road traffic injuries).

In conclusion, the definitions of injury and other related terms have been significantly improved during the last decades, both in terms of theoretical and practical applications. Fine-tuning these definitions, however, with a view to providing a common understanding, would substantially facilitate international and time trend comparisons through the development of injury indicators and contribute to etiological injury research. High-quality injury surveillance systems are prerequisites for setting priorities and actions for injury prevention as well as for monitoring the effectiveness of projects aiming to ultimately lead to the reduction of the burden of injuries.

Classifications, Coding Systems, and Injury Categories

Classifications and Coding Systems

Understanding how injuries occur, what the underlying risk factors are, and assessing the magnitude of the problem is necessary in any decision-making effort aiming to reduce their burden. Time trends showing reduction of the incidence of injury following specific interventions can ideally be used to identify good practices and select appropriate prevention strategies as well as to gain support for a chosen injury prevention strategy or to evaluate injury prevention programs.

Mortality data represent only the top of the injury pyramid, but they are available virtually worldwide and coded under the International Classification of Diseases (ICD), established in 1900. ICD is designed to promote international comparability in the collection, processing, classification, and presentation of mortality data reported either by physicians, medical examiners, and coroners or collected from death certificates. Mortality data are also collected from physicians' offices and hospital inpatient and outpatient records. The ICD Clinical Modification (CM) is the main system used to code nonfatal injury data from medical records, such as hospital records, emergency department records, and physician's office data.

Apart from the codes describing the nature (N) of the body lesion (e.g., femoral fracture), injury-related fatalities were until recently coded in the 9th revision of the ICD (ICD-9) based on the external (E) cause of injury from E800.0 to E999.9. E codes described the underlying circumstances of an injury death of unintentional intent and were grouped by injury type:

1. Motor vehicle traffic accidents;
2. Other transport accidents;
3. Accidental poisoning;
4. Accidental falls;
5. Accidents caused by fire and flames;
6. Accidental drowning and submersion;
7. Accidents caused by machinery and by cutting and piercing instruments;
8. Accidents caused by firearm missile;
9. All other accidents, including late effects;
10. Drugs, medicaments causing adverse effects in therapeutic use.

Intentional injuries were grouped into three categories, namely:

1. Suicide and self-inflicted injury;
2. Homicide and injury purposely inflicted by other persons;
3. Other external causes including those fatal injuries of undetermined intent or those related to legal interventions and operations of war.

Revisions in the ICD coding reflect advances and/or changes in the understanding of the underlying mechanisms and terminology and are designed to maximize the amount of information that a code can provide. In the latest ICD revision (ICD-10), the E codes for fatalities were replaced with V, W, X, and Y codes along with special reference (U codes) for injuries due to terrorism. Thus, the underlying external cause of death is indicated by the U01–U03, V01–Y36, Y85–Y87, or Y89 codes, whereas the nature of injury codes corresponds to the S00–T78 and T90–T98 of the Injury and Poisoning chapter of the ICD-10 manual. Conversion tables between the ICD-9 and ICD-10 codes for injuries (**Table 1**) are available but the different philosophy in the development of ICD-10 requires some caution in their use (WHO, 2004).

Consideration of multiple causes of death in the analysis of injury mortality ICD-10 data provides a more comprehensive assessment of the genuine number of deaths by type of injury. For instance, a poisoning-related death from carbon monoxide can be identified by using both the underlying cause of injury code X47 and the nature of injury diagnosis code T58 in the multiple cause data. Other changes refer to the terminology of intentional injuries. Thus, the term homicide has been changed in the new code to assault and the term suicide to intentional self-harm. Regarding drowning, more details are given for the type of water sources involved (e.g., bathtub, swimming pool, natural water), whereas in the ICD-9, the emphasis was on the activity being undertaken at the time of the event (e.g. swimming, diving), resulting in loss of

Table 1 ICD-9 and corresponding ICD-10 codes for injuries

Category	ICD-9	ICD-10
All Injury	E800–E999	U01–U03, V01–Y36, Y85–Y87, Y89
Unintentional	E800–E869, E880–E929	V01–X59, Y85–Y86
Suicide	E950–E959	U03, X60–X84, Y87.0
Homicide	E960–E969	U01–U02, X85–Y09, Y87.1
Undetermined	E980–E989	Y10–Y34, Y87.2
Legal intervention	E970–E978	Y35–Y36

information in the new version. Water transportation-related drowning codes (e.g., V90 and V92) are included in the other transport codes rather than with drowning codes. External cause codes for poisoning are substantially less detailed and have to be combined with the multiple cause-of-death poisoning codes to regain poisoning details. Transport accidents are given by the characteristics of the injured person (e.g., pedestrian, pedal cyclist, car occupant), whereas in ICD-9, they were given by type of vehicle involved in the accident (e.g., railway, water transport accidents). The subcategory of Bites and Stings in the ICD-9 framework was dropped from the ICD-10 matrix. Lastly, in ICD-10, bitten by has been combined with contact with and/or struck by for some relevant codes. Lastly, because the introduction of the ICD-10 classification can cause distortion in the time trend analyses, several options have been recommended in order to account for the changes and limitations introduced by the new code, e.g., noting in the graphs the time where ICD-10 was implemented, using comparability ratios, or specifically examining the codes and deciding whether the likelihood of error is substantial.

Major Categories of Injuries

Overall, injuries are grouped into five major categories. Three of these categories comprise unintentional acts, namely motor vehicle, home and leisure, and occupational injuries, and another two intentional acts, namely suicides/self-inflicted injuries and interpersonal violence. It should be noted, however, that the intent is not always evident or easy to determine, which is why a considerable proportion of injuries may be unclear or inadvertently misclassified.

Motor vehicle injuries

Motor vehicle injuries (also called road traffic injuries or road crashes) account for a vast proportion of fatal injuries. The estimated annual toll is 1.2 million out of a total of 5 million fatal injuries worldwide. In other words, more than 3000 people die every day in road crashes, while approximately 30 000 are seriously injured. They are defined as a collision involving at least one vehicle in motion on a public or private road that results in at least one person being injured or killed (WHO, 2004). Sometimes a road traffic injury may also refer to an automobile striking a human or animal. Therefore, prevention strategies may differ by type of road user.

Specifically, road traffic injuries may concern:

1. Passengers, occupants of vehicles other than the driver or rider; passengers of hackneys, cars, motor caravans, cars used as taxis, minibuses, buses, and pedal cycles;
2. Pillion passengers (passengers on mopeds or motorcycles);
3. Pedestrians (e.g., children on scooters, roller skates or skateboards, children riding toy cycles on the footpath,

persons pushing bicycles or other vehicles or operating pedestrian-controlled vehicles, persons leading or herding animals, occupants of prams or wheelchairs, people who alight safely from vehicles and are subsequently injured, persons pushing or pulling a vehicle, persons other than cyclists holding on to the back of a moving vehicle;

4. Pedal cyclists, such as drivers/riders of pedal cycles, including children riding toy cycles on the road;
5. Motorcyclists: Drivers/riders of mopeds and motorcycles;
6. Drivers of motor vehicles (e.g., drivers of hackneys, cars, motor caravans, cars used as taxis, minibuses, and buses);
7. Other road users (drivers and passengers of invalid/three-wheelers, tractors, ridden horses, other motor vehicles, and other nonmotor vehicles).

Vulnerable road users is a term specially referring to those participants in the traffic environment who are not protected by an outside shield, namely pedestrians and two-wheelers, as they carry a greater risk of injury in any collision against a vehicle and are therefore highly in need of protection against such collisions. Among vulnerable road users, the elderly, the disabled, and children are considered even more vulnerable.

Home and leisure injuries

The realization that the majority of injuries occur at home or during leisure time, and that this type of injury results in a high proportion of job absenteeism, disability, and injury costs, has motivated injury prevention organizations and world organizations to incorporate consumer protection into their agendas. Given the high numbers of new consumer products introduced on the market every year, research, assessment and management of the health risks and safety hazards associated with them relies on the availability of injury data; hence, additional classification systems were developed to account for and detail consumer products that might have been involved in the causation of the injury.

Introduction of these surveillance systems has been instrumental in supporting the development of safety standards and guidelines; in enforcing legislation by conducting investigations, inspections, seizures, recalls, and prosecutions; in testing and conducting research on consumer products and providing importers, manufacturers, and distributors with hazard and technical information; in publishing product advisories, warnings, and recalls; and in promoting safety and the responsible use of products because all these sectors rely on the availability of data generated by ongoing routine health data collection sources. Alternative sources for data collection were sought, for example by the Consumer Product Safety Commission in the United States or the European Home and Leisure Accident Surveillance System (EHLASS) in the European Union, the latter relying on reporting from sentinel systems located in hospital accident and emergency departments. Among other types of injury derived from these systems, those related to sport and school activities were found to deserve special consideration.

Occupational injuries

A sizeable proportion of injuries in the working population used to be of occupational origin. They are usually defined as events that happen during a paid activity and have resulted in at least 3 days of absence from work for medical care, according to Eurostat. All injuries in the course of work outside the premises of someone's business are covered by this definition, even if they are caused by a third party (on a client's premises, on another company's premises, in a public place or during transport, including road traffic injuries) as well as cases of acute poisoning. Injuries on the way to or from work (commuting accidents) are excluded, as well as cases of medical origin such as a heart attack at work and occupational diseases. A fatal injury at work is defined as an injury that leads to the death of a victim within 1 year of its occurrence.

As a rule, migrants and young workers are particularly vulnerable for occupational injuries, with young age and inexperience considered as important risk factors. Through concerted and sustainable efforts, occupational injuries have been substantially reduced over time, at least in the developed parts of the world, and the underlying reasons for this long-term success have to be explored. It is worth noting, however, that a substantial part of injuries still occurs among young children who work in mostly unpaid small family business and farms and they are not formally included in the occupational injuries.

Suicide and self-inflicted injuries

Suicide is the result of a complex, multicausal human behavior and in several parts of the world is associated with severe social stigmatization. It accounts for a high burden of injury fatalities, and in some parts of the world deaths by suicide have surpassed those resulting from road crashes. The realization of this fact has led some political bodies, such as the Division of Public Health of the European Union, to prioritize the fight against suicide high on their agendas. Special emphasis is put on the prevention and promotion of mental health. Indeed, clinical or subclinical depression accounts for more than two-thirds of suicides. Several other risk or protective factors for suicide have been identified. Poor mental health in general as well as a history of other major mental disorders, in particular the presence of a prior suicide attempt, is among the widely spread but modifiable risk factors for attempted or successfully committed suicide.

Interpersonal violence

Violence is defined as the

> intentional use of physical force or power, threatened or actual, against another person or a group of people that results in or has a high likelihood of resulting in injury, death, psychological harm, maldevelopment or deprivation. (WHO, 2002)

Intentional injuries resulting from interpersonal violence include homicide, assaults, child abuse and neglect, intimate partner violence, elder abuse, and sexual assault.

A specific type of violence, known as intimate partner violence, occurs in the context of intimate relationships of either heterosexual or homosexual types. It involves any threatened or actual use of physical force against an intimate partner that either results in or has the potential to result in injury, harm, or death. Such violence may lead to lethal consequences (murder) or nonlethal offences (domestic violence, spouse abuse, woman battering, courtship violence, sexual violence, date rape, and partner rape) (WHO, 2002). Child abuse or maltreatment is another type of intentional injury and refers to all forms of physical and/or emotional ill-treatment, sexual abuse, neglect, or negligent treatment or commercial or other exploitation, resulting in actual or potential harm to the child's health, survival, development, or dignity in the context of a relationship of responsibility, trust, or power and is grouped in four types: Physical abuse, sexual abuse, emotional abuse, and neglect.

The incidence and prevalence of intimate partner violence are severely underestimated. In the United States, the problem has begun to be recognized only since the 1970s, while in Europe researchers have started to address this important social, legal, and public health issue relatively recently. Intimate partner violence is regarded as a social taboo; therefore, disclosure is extremely difficult, especially in traditional societies. Health-care providers are rarely provided formal training concerning the recognition, assessment, and referral of victims, and resources to assist victims and perpetrators of abuse and provide them with support are limited. To this end, substantial efforts have been undertaken by several major bodies such as WHO, whereas screening tools specifically designed for the identification of intimate partner violence in primary health settings and hospital emergency departments have to be developed. The most commonly observed pattern includes younger injured women and older men, presenting on their own at the emergency department during the late evening and night hours with certain types of injuries, notably multiple facial injuries (Petridou *et al.*, 2002).

Injury Data Collection and Data Sources

The major source for injury mortality data is the Home State Office of Vital Statistics or Vital Records. As a rule, injury mortality data are collected at the county level, reported to the state or federal government, and then presented to the WHO Statistical Information database (WHOSIS). More user-friendly information is provided by web-based injury statistics query and reporting systems that provide customized injury-related mortality data, e.g., WISQARS (Web-based Injury Statistics Query and Reporting System) for the United States, developed by the National Center for Injury Prevention and Control, or the CDC Wonder Database for county, state, and national injury mortality data in the United States. More recently, a pilot Injury Statistics Portal for injury mortality data in the European Union of 25 Member States (EU-25) has been developed, aiming to provide readily available information with regard to mortality from injuries. Valuable information on severe nonfatal injuries could have been made available through E-coded hospital discharge data. At present, the low and uneven, at least among EU member states, proportion of E-coded hospital discharge data hinders the development of respective query systems for injury morbidity data.

Data on deaths due to injury are of high and satisfactory quality in most countries. However, the reliability of data collected in certain situations in countries with a strong religious background surrounding the taboo of dying through suicide is sometimes questionable. Therefore, deaths from suicide may instead be reported as due to unintentional causes in these countries. Nevertheless, the variation in suicide rates in different parts of the world is so great that these mortality data must be monitored for cross-country disparities as well as the effect of different prevention strategies.

Specific injury-type data recording systems are also in place, including fatal and nonfatal road traffic injuries, such as the International Road Traffic Accidents Database (IRTAD), the National Highway Transport Safety Administration (NHTSA) in the United States, and the European Union Community Road Traffic Database (CARE). Similarly, data on occupational injuries are assembled by the EUROSTAT in the European Union and by the U.S. Department of Labor in the United States. Lastly, the United Nations Disability database may prove useful in providing information on disability related to accidents, obtained through national surveys in some countries.

Measures of Injury Burden

Epidemiologic Indices

Traditional epidemiologic principles and indices are also used in injury epidemiology to measure and monitor the burden of injuries. Thus, injuries are frequently described in terms of mortality (fatal injuries) or morbidity (nonfatal injuries), the latter mainly assessed via hospital discharge or emergency department visitation data or non-health-care

sources providing cause-specific data, such as the road traffic police or those reported by insurance companies. Overall and cause-specific incidence and prevalence figures are necessary for evidence-based policy making. During the last few decades, newly developed indices, such as years of potential life lost or years lived with a disability are utilized to quantify the consequences of injuries. The most commonly used terms are synoptically defined in the following sections.

Incidence and prevalence of injuries

The incidence rate refers to the number of new cases of injured persons occurring in a population during a specific time interval. For instance, injury incidence rates (which include fatalities before 1992) declined 39% during 1976–2001, from 8.9 cases per 100 full-time workers in 1976 to 5.4 cases in 2001. In order to calculate the respective yearly incidence rate, one has to divide the number of observations (injuries) by the population of all countries of the WHO Region of Europe during the same year and then to multiply by 100 000 (or another appropriate multiplier). This calculation is actually an estimate of the crude injury rate and has the advantage of being a simple, easily calculated measure, which gives a broad picture of the magnitude of injuries in a particular area in a particular time period. This rate does not adjust, however, for the possible confounding effect of the age structure of a population; thus, it does not reflect the variation in the risk of disease due to factors such as age, which also affect injury risk. For this purpose, age-standardized injury rates are used. To obtain standardized rates, statistical methods are applied, so as to neutralize the influence of certain characteristics to the disease factor and to make two populations with different demographic characteristics comparable.

Mortality rate is the most commonly used and most widely available index for cross-country and time trend comparison and refers to the number of injury deaths in a given population. The corresponding mortality rate in the WHO Region of Europe was almost 61 unintentional injury deaths per 100 000 people.

Fatality measures how lethal a type of injury is. Thus, most fatal injuries are those that produce the highest number of deaths among those who have sustained an injury. Specifically, in work-related roadway crashes in the United States during 1992–2001, approximately one fatality per 100 000 full-time equivalent (FTE) workers was recorded, with 1.6 deaths per 100 000 FTE among workers aged 55–64 years, 3.8 among those aged 65–74 years, and 6.4 among those aged more than 75 years according to CDC.

Prevalence refers to the total number of injuries recorded in a defined population at a specified moment in time. It is expressed as the percentage of the population suffering from respective injuries in the total population at that moment. For example, in a recent U.S. study, the prevalence of reported acute trauma due to intimate partner violence among women attending hospital emergency departments ranged between 2 and 14% for physical or sexual abuse experienced at some point during the past year, whereas the lifetime prevalence was 37% (Sethi *et al.*, 2004).

Injury risk

Absolute risk defines a person's chance of developing a specific disease over a specified time period; therefore, it is actually a measure of the cumulative incidence. Thus, the risk of dying from injuries in the European Union is about 5% for residents of southern and northern countries and 7.5 in New Member States (WHO mortality data analyzed by CEREPRI, 2004, unpublished data).

Relative risk compares two populations in terms of the injury risk associated with being exposed versus unexposed to a specific risk factor. It refers to the number of people experiencing injuries in the exposed population versus those in the unexposed population and quantifies the risk associated with that specific factor under investigation. The relative risk is described as the rate ratio obtained from comparing the incidence of injuries in the two groups or risk ratio, resulting from the cumulative risk in the exposed population reported to that of unexposed people. Basically, odds ratio and risk ratio both represent expressions of relative risk.

The rate difference or attributable risk refers to the difference in the injury incidences between two groups of people (exposed vs. unexposed) and indicates the number of cases in a given population that occurred due to exposure to the studied risk factor.

The attributable risk percentage is the proportion of injury cases in the exposed group (population) that is attributable to the exposure or the incidence of injury in the exposed individuals that would be eliminated if the specific exposure were to be eliminated (Last, 2000).

Measures of the Impact of Injuries on Life Expectancy and Quality of Life

Years of life lost (YLL) is an estimation of premature mortality, defined as the number of years of life lost among persons who die before the conventional cut-off year of age, usually 65 or 75. YLLs are calculated from the number of deaths multiplied by a standard life expectancy at the age at which death occurs (WHOSIS, 2006).

Years lived with a disability (YLD) measures the years of healthy life lost by living in a state of less than full health.

Disability-adjusted life years (DALYs) for a disease are the sum of the years of life lost due to premature mortality in the population and the years lost due to disability for incident injury cases. The DALY is a health gap measure that extends the concept of potential years of life lost due to premature death (PYLL) to include equivalent years of

healthy life lost in a state of less than full health, broadly termed disability. One DALY represents the loss of 1 year of equivalent full health (WHOSIS, 2006).

Health-adjusted life expectancy (HALE) is defined as the number of years that a newborn can expect to live in full health based on current rates of ill health and mortality (WHOSIS, 2006).

All these indicators are useful tools in quantifying and monitoring injuries at the population level as well as in estimating the effectiveness of prevention measures by assessing their time trends and making cross-country comparisons.

Measures of Injury Severity

Clinical Measures

From the clinical point of view, injury severity can be evaluated by use of specific scales, which address (1) the anatomical location and extent of an injury (anatomical scales) and/or (2) the functional consequences of an injury (functional severity scales).

Anatomical measures

Abbreviated Injury Scale

The Abbreviated Injury Scale (AIS) is an anatomical scoring system that was first introduced in 1969. Injuries are ranked in a scale ranging from 1 to 6 (1 corresponding to an injury of minor severity, 5 to a severe one and 6 to a fatal injury). This scale was meant to measure the immediate threat to life associated with an injury and was developed to provide a more comprehensive measure of injury severity.

Injury Severity Score

The Injury Severity Score (ISS) is an anatomical scoring system that provides an overall score for patients with multiple injuries. Each injury is assigned an AIS score and is allocated to one of six body regions (head, face, chest, abdomen, extremities (including pelvis), and external). Only the highest AIS score in each body region is used. The three most severely injured body regions have their score squared and added together to produce the ISS score. The ISS score ranges from 0 to 75. It is virtually the only anatomical scoring system in use and correlates linearly with mortality, morbidity, hospital stay, and other measures of severity.

Anatomic Profile

The Anatomic Profile (AP) was introduced to overcome some of the limitations of the ISS. It is based on the AIS but comprises four specific body regions (head/brain/spinal cord, thorax/neck, all other serious injury, and all nonserious injury).

Trauma and Injury Severity Score

The Trauma and Injury Severity Score (TRISS) calculator determines the probability of survival from the ISS and the Revised Trauma Score (RTS), taking into account the patient's age. ISS and RTS scores can be input independently or are calculated from their base parameters.

A Severity Characterization of Trauma

A Severity Characterization of Trauma (ASCOT), introduced by Champion *et al.* (1990), is a scoring system that uses the Anatomic Profile to characterize injury instead of ISS. ASCOT has been shown to outperform TRISS, particularly for penetrating injury.

Therapeutic Intervention Scoring System

The Therapeutic Intervention Scoring System (TISS) was developed to quantify severity of illness among intensive care patients and it is based on the type and amount of treatment received. The underlying philosophy was that the sicker the patient, the greater the number and complexity of treatments provided.

Functional severity scales
Revised Trauma Score

The Revised Trauma Score (RTS) is one of the more common scores aimed at measuring the functional consequences of an injury (Boyd *et al.*, 1987). It uses three specific physiologic parameters: (1) the Glasgow Coma Scale (GCS), (2) systemic blood pressure (SBP), and (3) the respiratory rate (RR). RTS is heavily weighted toward the GCS to compensate for major head injury without multisystem injury or major physiological changes and correlates well with the probability of survival.

Glasgow Coma Scale

The Glasgow Coma Scale (GCS) is a neurological scale aiming to provide a reliable, objective way of recording the conscious state of a person, both for initial and continuing assessment of the patient, which has a special value in predicting the ultimate outcome. Generally, comas are classified as severe, with GCS ≤ 8, moderate, GCS 9–12, and minor, GCS ≥ 13.

APACHE I, II, III systems

APACHE I is a severity of disease/injury classification system. Its name stands for Acute Physiology and Chronic Health Evaluation. APACHE II was introduced as a simplified modification of the original APACHE. The APACHE II score consisted of three parts: 12 acute physiological variables, age, and chronic health status. The APACHE III system was designed to predict an individual's risk of dying in a hospital. It compares each individual's medical profile against nearly 18 000 cases in its memory before reaching a prognosis that is, on average, 95% accurate.

The aforementioned scales of injury severity are used in triaging injured people. Their adequacy in correlating injuries and the clinical and laboratory results of an injured person with the chances he or she has for survival has been substantiated. They are dynamic scales, which regularly undergo revisions, whereas trauma scoring systems play a central role in the provision of trauma care.

Descriptive Epidemiology: Burden of Injuries

The Public Health Burden of Injuries

The burden of injuries worldwide

Injuries are responsible for an appalling number of deaths worldwide. Annually, more than 5 million people lose their lives due to injuries, a figure corresponding to almost 14 000 recorded deaths per day or 570 every hour. In other words, one in ten deaths worldwide are due to injuries, with unintentional injuries representing two-thirds of this burden and intentional injuries the remaining one-third. Injuries affecting a large segment of the population are those related to motor vehicle accidents, falls, suicide, and self-inflicted injuries. Road traffic injuries, for instance, account for one-quarter of this burden (WHO, 2002).

Deaths are only part of the picture. It is estimated that more than 100 million injury cases are severe enough to require medical attention (about 2500 per 100 000 people) and there are more than 60 million years lost due to disability from injuries. When looking at the causes of years of life lost (YLL) due to premature morbidity, injuries rank third (more than 1900 YLL per 100 000 people) after infectious diseases and cardiovascular illnesses (WHO, 2002). In contrast, the resources devoted to injury prevention are scarce. One 1996 report from the WHO indicates that funding for the prevention of these injuries is less than $1 per disability adjusted life compared to the $26 for HIV/AIDS at the top of the relevant list (WHO, 1996). This figure, however, refers exclusively to WHO funding for injury prevention and should be treated with caution. In truth, we simply do not have a good estimate of the total resources devoted to injury prevention, as funding is provided across many different sectors.

Injuries are not uniformly distributed across countries: Low- and middle-income countries account for almost 90% of the total burden of fatal injuries, whereas more developed regions, as a rule, are safer both in terms of the possibility of sustaining an injury as well as eventually dying due to an injury. More specifically, the African and the South-Asian Regions are the WHO regions experiencing the highest injury rates (**Figure 1**). The European Union of 25 Member States, however, accounts for only 30% of the fatal injury burden in the WHO European Region, whereas the age-standardized injury mortality rate in the EU is approximately

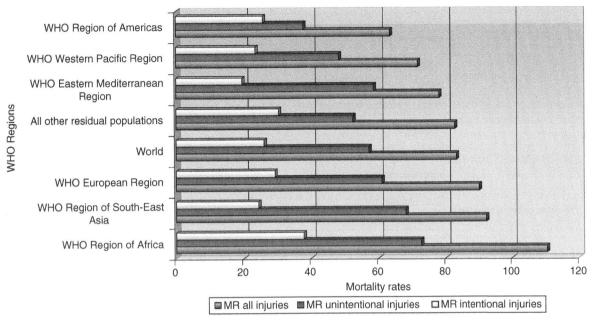

Figure 1 Injury mortality rate (deaths per 100 000) by intent in the WHO Regions. Data from WHO Burden of Diseases Project, estimates for 2002, data analyzed by CEREPRI, University of Athens, Greece.

half of the average rate worldwide. Most road traffic injuries occur in the African and South-Asian regions. It is of interest to note, however, that the WHO Europe Region has the highest mortality rate due to poisonings, probably due to alcohol intoxication and falls (**Figure 2**).

Injury risk by age group and gender

Additional information can be obtained by examining the injury mortality rate within age groups and genders and by type of injury. Globally, the probability of dying from injuries is twice as high for men as for women, but the risk varies at different ages. In the EU for example, road traffic injuries are the leading cause of death among males and young people aged 15–44 years in most parts of the world, while at older ages, falls account for a large number of deaths (**Figure 3**).

In the United States, motor vehicle crashes are the leading cause of death for children ages 1–3, with drowning being the second cause (CDC, 2004). In 2003, one-third of children aged 4 and younger who died in motor vehicle crashes were unrestrained. In the 4–11 age group, nearly 3 200 000 children were nonfatally injured. Unintentional falls were the most common cause, while homicide was the fourth leading cause of death, taking the lives of 250 children in 2002. Adolescents have the highest risk for motor vehicle crashes and are four times more likely to crash per mile driven than older drivers. As regards the 20–49 age group, 13 600 000 adults were nonfatally injured, with falls being the most common cause (CDC, 2004). Injuries in older adults follow the same pattern, with 14 000 estimated deaths due to falls in 2002, corresponding to 2 700 000 recorded injuries in 2003 (CDC, 2004).

As regards DALYs, road traffic injuries in the year 2002 were the eighth leading cause of DALYs for all age groups, while self-inflicted injuries were the 17th leading cause. In particular, road traffic injuries (22%), falls (11%), self-inflicted violence (11%), and interpersonal violence (9%) were the main injury-related causes of DALYs (WHO, 2002).

Time trends

Past injury records reveal substantial variation in injury rates. For instance, road traffic injury mortality rates peaked around 1990 in all country groups, then fell from 25 per 100 000 people in 1991 to 16 per 100 000 in 1997 and then more or less leveled off at 18 per 100 000 (WHO, 2005). By the year 2020, a dramatic injury increase is expected to occur and road traffic injuries, interpersonal violence, war, and self-inflicted injuries will rank among the 15 leading causes of death if current trends continue. Notably, this increase is predicted for low- and middle-income countries, while high-income countries will record a 30% drop in injury fatalities. Road traffic injuries are the main cause of this rise and they are expected to rank third in terms of disease burden by the year 2020 (WHO, 2005).

Much research has inevitably concentrated on fatal injuries because of the greater availability of data. Much less is known about the long-term consequences of nonfatal injuries. These have significant resource consequences and a more systematic method of measuring such injuries would be welcome. In Greece, for example, for every injury fatality, an estimated 36 people are hospitalized, whereas 380 require outpatient treatment in

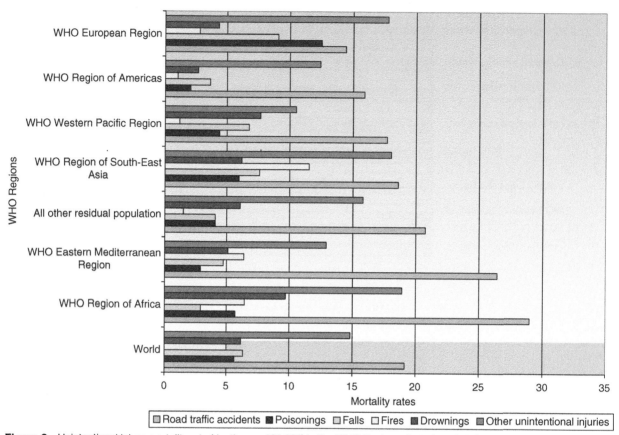

Figure 2 Unintentional injury mortality rate (deaths per 100 000) in the WHO Regions. Data from WHO Burden of Diseases Project, estimates for 2002, data analyzed by CEREPRI, University of Athens, Greece.

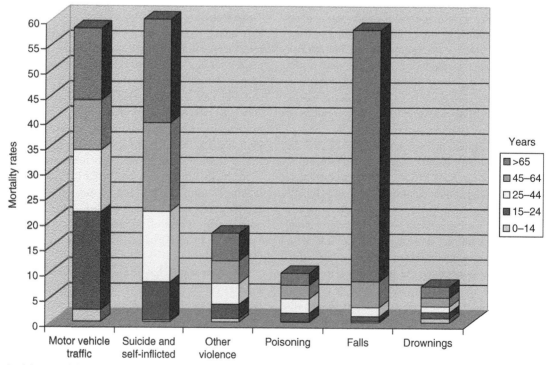

Figure 3 Injury mortality rates for selected types of injury (deaths per 100 000) by age group, both genders, in the EU-25. Data from WHOSIS 2004, data analyzed by CEREPRI, University of Athens, Greece.

hospital emergency departments. By quantifying the above ratio, it is estimated that the 4486 injury fatalities recorded in the EU correspond to 161 800 nonfatal injuries per year that require hospitalization and 1 700 000 emergency department consultations. Many more people seek help from their general practitioner or treat themselves and even more suffer from short- or long-term disabilities as a result of their injuries. The corresponding ratios may differ by age, region, and health delivery system, but these figures are indicative of the high prevalence of serious injuries and testify to the resulting drain on health resources and productivity lost (**Figure 4**).

Estimating the preventable fraction of injuries

Improvement of emergency medical care services and treatment modalities has contributed considerably to the reduction of injuries over the last few decades in several parts of the world. Much greater and possibly more cost-efficient gains can be expected through dedicated injury prevention and safety promotion practices. Several studies have recently attempted to quantify the potential for prevention of injuries. Basically, the variance in the country-specific injury mortality rates can be attributed to the different strategies and levels of prevention efforts that have been undertaken in different countries; then, using alternative theoretical scenarios, an attempt can be made to estimate the potential for prevention if all countries being considered were to achieve the lowest overall or injury-specific rates.

The main aim of this exercise is to encourage interested parties and government officials to undertake specific action and formulate national plans that can monitor progress toward combating the injury epidemic. A study by Petridou concerning the preventable fraction of childhood injuries

showed that half of childhood lives lost could have been saved if all member states in the European Union of 15 Member States (EU-15) had matched the accomplishments of the country with the lowest mortality rate. What is more, injuries stem from a variety of causes and EU countries show considerable variability, making it all the more difficult for every country to meet the ideal country's criteria. Some countries have been more effective in combating mortality from certain categories of injuries, whereas others have been more successful with respect to other types of injuries. Only by achieving the lowest childhood mortality rates in every single injury category can the proportion of deaths due to injuries that could have been prevented be eliminated (Petridou *et al.*, 2000) (**Table 2**). The importance of establishing widely accepted national prevention programs can be evidenced by the northeast region of the United States, which has developed such prevention strategies and reduced childhood mortality rates. It is estimated that if every region of the United States had the same injury rate as the Northeast, one-third of all unintentional childhood injuries would not have occurred (Philippakis *et al.*, 2004). As regards intentional injuries, over 73% of all intentional injury deaths could have been avoided if all EU countries matched the country with the lowest intentional injury mortality rate. This corresponds to 600 fewer

Table 2 Age-adjusted childhood (0–14 years) mortality rates per 100 000 person-years in EU member states (1984–93) and four major geographic regions of the United States circa 1990 and 1997

| Regions | Mortality rates per 100 000 during specified periods | | | |
	1984	1989–1991	1993	1996–1998
U.S. regions				
Midwest U.S.		13.2		10.6
Northeast U.S.		9.8		6.4
South U.S.		16.3		13.1
West U.S.		12.8		9.6
Total U.S.		13.5		10.5
EU Regions				
Austria	14.5		8.9	
Belgium	13.6		10.5	
Denmark	9.8		6.8	
Finland	8.0		7.1	
France	14.4		8.5	
Germany	13.8		7.6	
Greece	13.2		9.1	
Ireland	12.3		8.3	
Italy	8.4		6.7	
Netherlands	10.1		6.3	
Portugal	24.9		15.1	
Spain	12.2		10.4	
Sweden	6.4		5.0	
UK	10.2		5.4	

From Philippakis A, Hemenway D, Alexe DM, *et al.* (2004) A quantification of preventable unintentional childhood injury mortality in the United States. *Injury Prevention* 10: 79–82.

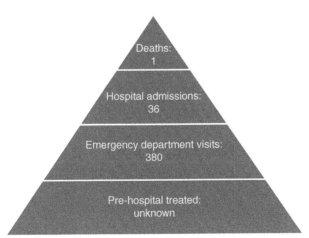

Figure 4 The injury pyramid for all causes of injury, all ages in Greece (average number for 1998–2001). Data from National Statistical Service of Greece, average number for 1998–2001 and EDISS (Emergency Department Injury Surveillance System), data 1998–2001.

intentional injury deaths in children, approximately 40 000 fewer adult deaths, and over 14 000 fewer intentional injury deaths in the elderly.

Etiological Considerations: Risk Factors and Vulnerable Population Groups

The role of individual risk factors for injury as well as the contribution of the physical and social environment in the causation of injury have been intensively studied over the last few decades, mainly in Australia, Canada, the United States, and several members of the European Union, notably in regions where injury reduction has been more effective. The study of modifiable or nonmodifiable characteristics has been considered essential for the subsequent planning and monitoring of targeted prevention efforts and orientation of human and financial resources.

Sex and Age

Males have a higher risk of sustaining injuries, both fatal and nonfatal, than women. Interestingly, gender differences in the mortality and morbidity rates are evident from the first years of life and peak during adolescence, pointing to underlying inherent or biological factors. Injury is the leading cause of death in children aged 1–14 years, adolescents, and young adults. Injury mortality

rates increase steadily with advancing age and peak among the more fragile elderly (**Figure 5**). Although cardiovascular diseases and cancer surpass injury as a cause of death among the elderly, in most developed parts of the world, injury mortality rates among the elderly almost triple compared with that among middle-aged adults.

Socioeconomic Factors

As a rule, all types of injuries are more common among the more disadvantaged population groups, with family income and per capita gross domestic product (GDP) strong predictors of injury risk. In the European Union, for example, injury mortality rates have been found to correlate significantly at the country level. The mostly low- and middle-income new EU Member States have higher mortality rates compared with EU countries of higher GDP for all types of injury (**Figure 6**).

At the community and family level, poverty may influence the risk for injury through several mechanisms, such as poor housing and problematic traffic and road structures. Specifically, children living in these areas are more likely to be living in houses that have close proximity to busy roads; therefore, the risk of sustaining a traffic injury is significantly higher. Moreover, when an accident occurs, the medical support in these areas is often deficient, with further consequences in the outcome of an injury. Other socioeconomic factors that have been studied in relation to

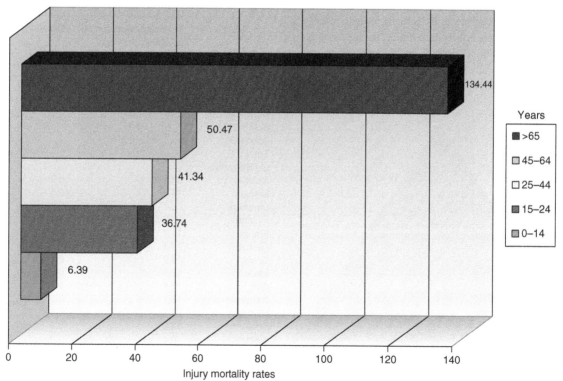

Figure 5 Age-specific injury mortality rates (deaths per 100 000) in the EU-25. Data from WHOSIS 2004, data analyzed by CEREPRI, University of Athens, Greece.

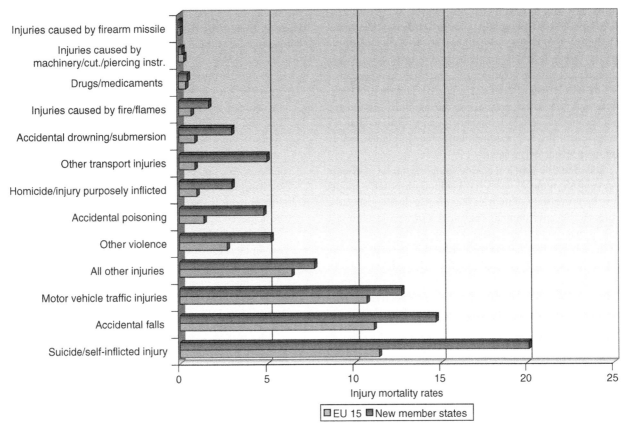

Figure 6 Type of injury-specific mortality rates in the EU-15 and the EU new Member States. Data from WHOSIS 2004, data analyzed by CEREPRI, University of Athens, Greece.

the risk for injury are poor educational background and family structural factors such as single parenthood, young age of the mother, crowding, and poor living conditions.

Correlations between injuries and tobacco, alcohol, and/or drug use have also been reported. It has been estimated that alcohol is involved in about 40% of all road traffic injuries. Moreover, even though physical exercise has immense benefits to human health, participation in professional sports activities as well as vigorous exercise has been shown to increase injury risk (e.g., overuse injuries). It has been reported that people undertaking very high levels of exercise are twice as likely to sustain an injury as those who do not undertake any exercise. It is of interest to note, however, that being overweight seems to be a risk factor for sustaining an injury.

Risk-Taking Behavior

There seems to be an inherited tendency to develop violent behaviors, whereas being prone to injuries is a more complex process. The interactions of these characteristics with environmental factors, including social surroundings, seem similarly complex. There is no doubt, however, that risk-taking behavior is linked with the causation of injury and that it also influences the severity of the outcome once

the injury occurs. The probability of a person manifesting a violent temper, for instance, has been associated with certain biological characteristics such as a low resting heart rate. Several childhood social, family, and psychological characteristics such as antisocial behavior as a child, impulsivity, low intelligence and achievement, family criminality, poverty, and poor parental child-rearing behavior, have also been correlated with violence in later life. Moreover, specific human behaviors, such as using a cell phone while driving a car, speeding, and alcohol intake and driving, in other words, not complying with safety rules and regulations, have been repeatedly correlated with a high risk for injury. The underlying mechanisms have not been fully explored, but the Human Genome Project is an ambitious step in this direction.

From Theory to Practice: What Works in Injury Prevention?

Haddon's Injury Prevention Model

It is now clear that injury is a major epidemic today that requires the input of multidisciplinary teams reflecting on a theoretical background that could enable scientists and practitioners in the field to focus on and maximize the impact of actions to remedy this scourge. Progress in the field has always been slow and painful and the major challenge is how to most effectively use the results of injury research for the implementation of injury prevention projects. In this context, it is essential that the nature of injuries be clearly defined, that risk factors be identified, and that their progression be carefully monitored and evaluated based on agreed-upon criteria, so that the most cost-efficient methodologies be implemented in injury-prevention projects.

Based on the classical epidemiological model of disease prevention, some 35 years ago Haddon proposed a model for the prevention of injuries that clearly distinguishes the role of the environment (physical and socioeconomic), the human factor (host), and the role of the vector/agent of the energy exchange in the etiology of an accident. The model aimed to specifically address the role of each of these factors in the etiological chain of events leading to injury and provide a framework for the respective prevention measures. According to this model, different factors seem to interact and eventually determine the occurrence and the severity of the injury during the pre-event, the event, and the post-event phases of an accident. Therefore, completion of a matrix could assist in the exploration of the potential underlying factors and the different time periods during which they might have exerted their effect. A version of the Haddon matrix principle applied to the problem of injuries to children falling on playgrounds is shown in **Table 3** (Runyan, 2003).

Injury prevention measures can primarily target each one of these specific levels or address all of them. Thus,

the basic injury prevention principles derived from the Haddon theory for road traffic injury prevention can be delineated as follows (WHO, 2006):

1. Prevent the initial aggregation of the particular energy form. This is usually done by discouraging the use of vehicles and designs that are particularly hazardous and by encouraging alternate travel modes.
2. Reduce the amount of energy aggregated. Examples are setting speed limits on roads, making engines that are not very powerful, and installing speed limiters on existing vehicles.
3. Prevent the inappropriate release of energy. This can be achieved by designing vehicles and the environment such that road users do not make mistakes easily, for example, through the use of better brakes, safer intersections and roundabouts, and skid-resistant roads.
4. Alter the rate or spatial distribution of energy release from its source. Making pointed and sharp surfaces rounded and flatter distributes the forces over a larger area during an impact and thus reduces stresses on the body. Vehicles meeting appropriate crashworthiness criteria will transfer less energy to occupants.
5. Separate susceptible structures from the energy being released by means of space or time. Separate lanes for bicycles and pedestrians reduce the probability of the riders or walkers being hit by motor vehicles. Daytime curfews for trucks in cities reduce the number of crashes involving pedestrians.
6. Interpose a material barrier to separate the released energy from susceptible structures. Examples are

Table 3 An example of the Haddon matrix applied to the problem of injuries to children falling in playgrounds

Haddon matrix

	Host (children in the playground)	Agent/vehicle (specific playground equipment and devices)	Physical environment (overall playground design)	Social environment (community norms, policies, rules)
Pre-event (before the fall)	Teach children to follow safety rules in the playground (e.g., no crowding on the climbing equipment)	Construct equipment with tacky grips, sized to children's hands, to reduce the risk of hands slipping	Build sliding boards into hillsides so children do not have to climb to heights	Foster social norms that encourage adults to help maintain orderly play on the playground
Event (during the fall and time of impact)	Teach children to fall in ways that reduce injury	Reduce the number of protrusions on equipment so falling children do not hit sharp components	Ensure the presence of resilient surfacing	Organize community-watch systems to monitor playground safety (e.g., maintaining surfacing)
Post-event (after the child is injured by the fall)	Teach children how to summon help when injuries occur (e.g., using emergency call boxes)	Avoid equipment in which children can fall into areas not easily reached by rescue personnel	Provide benches for supervisors that afford good visibility of all playground areas to facilitate noticing when children are injured	Ensure funding for adequate emergency personnel appropriately equipped to deal with pediatric emergencies

From Runyan WC (2003) Introduction: Back to the future – Revisiting Haddon's conceptualization of injury epidemiology and prevention. *Epidemiologic Reviews* 25: 60–64.

physical road dividers on highways, and bollards and fences between pedestrian paths and roads.

7. Modify contact surfaces or basic structures that can be impacted. Padded interiors and absence of sharp objects prevent injury. Examples include softer car and bus fronts, breakaway poles on highways, and use of helmets by two-wheeler riders.

8. Strengthen human beings who are susceptible to injury by the energy transfer. An example is treatment for osteoporosis of older road users.

9. Quickly detect and evaluate injury and prevent its continuation or extension. Injury can be limited by efficient systems for extraction of victims from vehicles, emergency care, and management of crash sites.

10. Carry out all necessary measures between the emergency period immediately following injury and ultimate stabilization of the process. Such measures include intermediate and long-term repair and rehabilitation.

The primary and secondary Es of injury prevention

Since the mid-1970s, a plethora of injury prevention programs have been designed and implemented; yet there is still a debate about what works best in injury prevention and how to facilitate the connection between what seems to be theoretically effective and what works in everyday life. Thus, effective prevention can be described at three levels:

1. Theoretical, which requires optimal performance of the proposed or experimentally tested measures (e.g., the theoretical effectiveness of car restraints in simulation crashes could exceed 80%); this level does not provide for the effect of human errors and of faulty equipment.

2. Pragmatic, the realistically attainable effect of injury-preventive measures, were all equipment to perform as expected and were all individuals willing to use the measures provided (e.g., the pragmatic effectiveness of car restraints is approximately 60% because of suboptimal quality controls or maintenance of the equipment or unpredictable use of car restraints).

3. Population-based, i.e., the net effect of a preventive program taking into account the uptake of the measure by the population and any possible barriers and financial obstacles (e.g., the population-based effectiveness of car restraints may be less than one-third when the usage rate is only one in two).

Nowadays, a vast array of measures – principally passive prevention – are available for almost all types of injury, which could yield considerable gains in injury prevention if they were to be widely accepted at the population level. Thus, the challenge in injury prevention may be rather how to minimize the difference between their pragmatic and population-based effectiveness than how to introduce a new preventive measure of high theoretical effectiveness.

One conceptual framework aiming to facilitate policy makers and practitioners in the field to conceptualize the injury prevention theory that has already been promoted since the 1950s is to utilize all three Es – education, enforcement, and engineering – when implementing a program. In subsequent years, secondary Es were added to the primary Es – evaluation, environment, enactment, economics, empowerment – emphasizing additional components that should be taken into account and the complexities encountered in program implementation.

By combining information on both the costs and the effectiveness of different policies and interventions, economic techniques such as cost-effectiveness or cost–benefit analyses can provide decision makers with data aiming to inform and assist decisions on how to make the best use of available resources to maximize benefits. It is a valid argument, for example, to ask a policy maker to support a car restraint loan scheme, in which for a modest rental fee (15 euros) for a child car restraint, the equivalent gain per life year saved would amount to over 400 euros, while the cost for each prevented casualty would be approximately 32 000 euros.

Several systematic reviews have been undertaken aiming to assess the effectiveness of injury prevention measures and best practices in the implementation of projects. It seems, however, that what might prove to be a best practice in a certain community or population group may not be as effective when implemented in another; therefore, it has been recommended that the term best practice be replaced by the term good practice. With regards to the reduction of road traffic injuries, most gains stem from vehicle and environmental changes, whereas attempts to improve safe behaviors clearly lag behind. It seems, however, that as we are reaching the stage of diminishing returns with regards to investments in further improvements in the host and the environment components of the injury triangle or when there are practically no passive prevention measures available (e.g., prevention of childhood drowning in a water environment), safer behavior and attentive childhood supervision become of paramount importance. The state of the art with regard to methodological questions on technology transfer, behavioral maintenance, and evaluation of effective behavioral modification projects is presented in *Injury Prevention: Behavioral Science Theories, Methods and Applications* (Gielen *et al.*, 2006).

Injury Prevention Approaches

During the last few decades, injury prevention has evolved as a distinct public health discipline comprising (1) theoretical principles, (2) etiologic research, namely epidemiology, biomechanics, and basic science, (3) application methods, namely, prevention programs, product research, environmental design, and clinical trials, and (4) outcome research, i.e., injury rate and severity, cost effectiveness, quality of care, and health-related quality of life. Despite the great losses in human lives, however, community involvement in injury prevention fades compared to the participation that can be mustered for presumed environmental threats. This paradox was already recognized several years ago when Surgeon General Everett Koop commented: "If a disease were killing our children at the rate that unintentional injuries are, the public would be unbelievably outraged and demand that this killer be stopped" (Girasek, 2006: 71–73).

The critical question of why injury prevention has such a meagre impact in generating enthusiasm and channeling public interest still remains unanswered (Petridou *et al.*, 1995). Which strategy should be followed to obtain the greatest injury reduction from implementing injury prevention measures and whether this should target the community as a whole or certain high-risk population groups is currently being debated.

Community-based interventions

Community-based interventions refer to multicomponent interventions that generally combine individual and environmental change strategies across multiple settings aiming to prevent dysfunction and to promote well-being among population groups in a defined local community. In most cases, entire communities (e.g., neighborhood, city, county) are used as units of intervention. From the ethical point of view, it seems reasonable to offer prevention to all members of a community. Furthermore, community programs offer the opportunity to stimulate cultural changes. Such programs are, however, very expensive. Also, measuring the outcome of such interventions is difficult both in terms of the time period that is necessary to observe a significant change in injury rates and in terms of the number of cases required to attain a reasonable statistical power. Process measures may therefore be more appropriate for monitoring the effectiveness of community injury-prevention programs.

Targeting population groups at high risk for sustaining injuries may be a more feasible approach in terms of interventional costs as well as in measuring the outcome of such an initiative, as it has sufficient statistical power. Moreover, there is a great potential for injury reduction because of the higher exposure to the risk factor for injury. Identifying such population groups' use of reliable screening measures with an acceptable level of sensitivity and specificity is a prerequisite.

As a rule, injury prevention programs have no built-in evaluation components in their design, possibly due to the lack of data showing effectiveness and the intrinsic difficulty of detecting outcomes. Further methodological problems for measuring the outcomes relate to the appropriateness of random assignment and difficulties in finding suitable comparison sites. Consequently, it is extremely difficult to make recommendations for or against an injury

prevention measure when evidence of its effectiveness is still lacking. Where this evidence has been sought, however, it is not uncommon to see that the intervention may be unlikely to represent a cost-effective use of resources. For example, the effectiveness of a community-based smoke alarm give-away program was tested using data from a randomized controlled trial. This resulted in a 0.15 probability of being cost-effective, which is highly unlikely to represent a cost-effective use of resources. The Cambridge-Somerville Project, within the field of violence prevention, is another example of an ambitious randomized controlled trial to prevent juvenile delinquency, violence, and injury; in the end, it resulted in higher rates of crime, violence, and untimely death in the intervention group than in the control group.

The overall experience gained from community injury-prevention programs, however, has reached the conclusion that community participation and multidisciplinary collaboration are essential factors in solving local injury problems. The World Health Organization (WHO) Safe Community model is a prominent framework for injury prevention at the community level that uses multiple strategies and targets all age groups, environments, and situations. Similarly inspired national movements in other countries include the Canadian Safe Communities Foundation and the Beterem National Centre for Children's Health and Safety in Israel. In general, the findings of these programs show that the most successful interventions occurred in medium-sized Scandinavian communities, reveal the importance of social and cultural homogeneity of the participating intervention communities, and conclude that such programs may work better in cohesive, homogeneous, stable, and isolated communities.

Initiatives aiming at sharing views and exchanging information on injury prevention and improving reporting of nonfatal, non-hospital system-based events may be a good basis with actions coordinated across sectors. While economic evidence is growing, the specific costs and benefits of different strategies need to be calculated for different countries due to variable resource levels. Within a specific community, it may be more effective to target specific population groups, such as the safety needs of older people.

See also: Environmental and Occupational Epidemiology.

Citations

Brooks AJ, Sperry D, Riley B, and Girling KJ (2005) Improving performance in the management of severely injured patients in critical care. *Injury* 36: 310–316.
Centers for Diseases Control (2004) *Worker Health Chartbook 2004.* Cincinnati, OH: DHHS (NIOSH) Publications.
Champion HR, Copes WS, Sacco WJ, *et al.* (1990) A new characterization of injury severity. *Journal of Trauma* 30: 539–546.
Emergency Department Injury Surveillance System, data 1998–2001 and National Statistical Service of Greece, average number for

1998–2001 (data analyzed by CEREPRI, University of Athens). Greece: CEREPRI.

Gielen CA, Sleet AD, and DiClemente JR (2006) *Injury and Violence Prevention: Behavioral Science Theories Methods, and Applications*. San Francisco, CA: Josey Bass.

Girasek D (2006) Would society pay more attention to injuries if the injury control community paid more attention to risk communication science. *Injury Prevention* 12: 71–73.

Langley J and Brenner R (2004) What is an injury? *Injury Prevention* 10: 69–71.

Last JM (ed.) (2000) *A Dictionary of Epidemiology*, 4th edn. New York: Oxford University Press.

Petridou E (1995) Injury prevention: An uphill battle. *Injury Prevention* 1: 8.

Petridou E (2000) Childhood injuries in the European Union: Can epidemiology contribute to their control? *Acta Paediatrica* 89: 1244–1249.

Petridou E, Browne A, Lichter E, *et al.* (2002) What distinguishes unintentional injuries from injuries due to intimate partner violence: a study in Greek ambulatory care settings. *Injury Prevention* 8: 197–201.

Philippakis A, Hemenway D, Alexe DM, *et al.* (2004) A quantification of preventable unintentional childhood injury mortality in the United States. *Injury Prevention* 10: 79–82.

Pless B (2002) Taking risks with injury prevention. *Canadian Medical Association Journal* 167: 767–768.

Runyan WC (2003) Introduction: Back to the future – Revisiting Haddon's conceptualization of injury epidemiology and prevention. *Epidemiologic Reviews* 25: 60–64.

Sethi D, Watts S, Zwi A, Watson J, and McCarthy C (2004) Experience of domestic violence by women attending an inner city accident and emergency department. *Emergency Medicine Journal* 21: 180–184.

WHO Statistical Information System (WHOSIS) (2006) http://www.who.int/whosis/whostat2006YearsOfLifeLost.pdf (accessed 29 December 2006).

World Health Organization (2002) *World Report on Violence and Health*. Geneva: World Health Organization.

World Health Organization (2004) *World Report on Road Traffic Injury Prevention*. Geneva: World Health Organization.

Emergency Department Injury Surveillance System, data 1998–2001 and National Statistical Service of Greece, average number for 1998–2001 (data analyzed by CEREPRI, University of Athens). Greece: CEREPRI.

Laflamme L and Diderichsen F (2000) Social differences in traffic injury risks in childhood and youth – A literature review and a research agenda. *Injury Prevention* 6: 293–298.

Last JM (ed.) (2000) *A Dictionary of Epidemiology*, 4th edn. New York: Oxford University Press.

MacMahon B and Trichopoulos D (1996) *Epidemiology. Principle and Methods*. 2nd edn. Boston, MA: Little Brown and Company.

Murray CJ and Lopez AD (1997) Alternative projections of mortality and disability by cause 1990–2020: Global Burden of Disease Study. *Lancet* 349: 1498–1504.

National, Center for Injury Prevention and Control (2006) *CDC Injury Fact Book*. Atlanta, GA: Centers for Disease Control and Prevention.

Nilsen P (2004) What makes community-based injury prevention work? In search of evidence of effectiveness. *Injury Prevention* 10: 268–274.

Nilsen P, Hudson DS, Kullberg A, *et al.* (2004) Making sense of safety. *Injury Prevention* 10: 71–73.

Organization for Economic Cooperation, Development (OECD) (1998) *Safety of Vulnerable Road Users. Scientific Expert Group on the Safety of Vulnerable Road Users (RS7)*. Paris, France: OECD.

Robertson LS (1998) *Injury Epidemiology*. 2nd edn. New York: Oxford University Press.

Task Force on Burden of Injuries (BOI) of the EuropeanCommission, Working Party on Accidents and Injuries (WP-AI) (2005) Burden of Fatal Injuries in the European Union. Athens, Greece: CEREPRI. http://www.euroipn.org/cerepri (accessed November 2005).

Towner E (2005) Injury and inequalities: Bridging the gap. *International Journal of Injury Control and Safety Promotion* 12: 79–84.

Further Reading

Chishti P, Stone DH, Corcoran P, Williamson E, and Petridou E EUROSAVE Working Group (2003) Suicide mortality in the European Union. *The European Journal of Public Health* 13: 108–114.

Relevant Website

http://www.euroipn.org/stats_portal/ – Injury Statistics Portal within the Project Coordination and Administration of the European Injury Prevention Working Party on Accidents and Injuries Program.

Epidemiology of Tuberculosis

T H Holtz, Centers for Disease Control and Prevention, Atlanta, GA, USA

Published by Elsevier Inc.

Introduction

Tuberculosis has killed more persons in the history of the world than any other infectious disease and is currently the second most common infectious disease killer, claiming 1.6 million deaths per year (nearly 4400 per day) (World Health Organization, 2007). It is estimated that in the past two centuries, TB has accounted for approximately one billion deaths (Ryan, 1992). The discovery of deformities consistent with tuberculosis disease in skeletons suggest that the disease was common in Egypt at least 4000 years ago (Nerlich *et al.*, 1997). In 500 BC, Hippocrates described patients with 'consumptive disease,' a classic description that endures to this day, characterized by coughing bloody sputum, chest pain, and wasting. At the time, of course, there was no effective treatment and patients essentially withered away, consumed by their disease.

Tuberculosis grew in prevalence in Europe during the seventeenth century, as the growing population moved into larger cities, with concomitant crowded living conditions and poor sanitation and ventilation. By the first half of the nineteenth century, TB was responsible for one-quarter of all deaths on the continent as a result of industrialization and concentrated urban misery. As housing conditions improved toward the end of the nineteenth century, tuberculosis rates began to decline. However, as colonialism took Europeans to Africa and Asia, the disease accompanied the industrialization and urbanization processes in these regions. In India and China, TB rates reached epidemic levels at the turn of the twentieth century, though low population density limited the spread of TB in most of Africa. European immigration to the New World accompanied with early industrialization in Eastern urban centers brought high TB rates similar to the mainland European continent. Mortality rates similarly reflected epidemic proportions, with up to 600 deaths per 100 000 people (Stead et al., 1995).

TB declined in the industrialized world starting in the late nineteenth century aided by improvements in labor and housing conditions, and public health practices such as the advent of the Bacille Calmette–Guérin vaccine. It was not until widespread European immigration to South and sub-Saharan Africa at the turn of the twentieth century that TB became widespread there. The story was similar among the indigenous populations of what is now Alaska and Greenland, where TB took hold and ravaged the local population (with rates above 1000/100 000 persons) (Stead et al., 1995). In areas such as Indonesia and South East Asia, TB was introduced in the early twentieth century. It was not until the 1940s and the use of antibiotics – especially streptomycin and isoniazid – that the TB death rate began a steeper decline in Europe and North America (although the rate of decline in incidence did not change throughout that time). TB incidence rates in Western Europe and North America declined consistently through the twentieth century. In the late 1980s, however, a confluence of factors led to a reversal in the incidence rate in the United States (especially in New York City) (Frieden et al., 1995). This reversal was primarily due to the defunding of tuberculosis control programs, combined with a rise in HIV infection rates and outbreaks of multidrug-resistant tuberculosis (Binkin et al., 1999). Increasing economic inequality in the United States, with poverty, homelessness in urban settings, immigration from high-burden countries, and crowded housing also converged to cause a resurgence of TB.

A century ago, TB ravaged affluent and poor societies alike, although not equally. Today, however, rates of TB are telling indicators of a country's wealth or poverty status and particularly of resource disparities within societies. Therefore tuberculosis, and the distribution of drug-resistant TB, is not only a matter of the transmission of TB infection, it is also a reflection of global resource distribution (Kim et al., 2005). In much of sub-Saharan Africa where there are few resources, TB rates are highest. In countries where TB therapy was available but improperly prescribed, or where there were frequent drug shortages, rates of multidrug-resistant TB have risen. In areas where TB programs were defunded and political support for TB control waned, there were both increases in TB and multidrug-resistant TB. Understanding social inequalities is therefore central to understanding the persistence and re-emergence of TB. The unprecedented scale of the current TB epidemic and the human rights aspects of the problem demand effective and urgent action. The next section summarizes the epidemiology of the current TB epidemic in terms of morbidity, mortality, and economic burden.

Burden of TB Morbidity and Mortality

Case Notifications

Currently, approximately one-third of the world's population is infected with TB (World Health Organization, 2007). Among the 8.8 million estimated new cases, and 1.6 million estimated deaths, more than 95% are thought to occur in developing countries. This enormous disparity and imbalance of disease burden is due to the underfunding of public health services, the spread of HIV, and the emergence of drug-resistant tuberculosis. If tuberculosis control is not strengthened through improvements in both social conditions and health services, estimates are that approximately one billion people will be newly infected with the mycobacterium that causes TB, over 150 million people will develop TB disease, and 36 million people will die of TB between 2000 and 2020 (World Health Organization, 2002).

It is impossible to know the true incidence of TB, given that we do not know how many cases go undetected, which makes aggregate case notification data from countries very important. Case notification data reflect health service coverage and the efficiency of TB case-finding and reporting activities of a country's programs. In countries with effective TB control programs, case notifications can closely approximate the true incidence. Often, poor program performance results in underdetection and underreporting of cases. Therefore in most of the developing world notifications represent only a fraction of the true incident cases as large sectors of the population have no access to effective treatment. Despite limitations, case notifications under stable program conditions in most countries provide useful data on the trend of TB incidence and rates stratified by age, sex, and some risk characteristics. The World Health Organization uses case notifications and modeling methods to estimate the global TB disease burden.

In 2005, 199 countries (99.9% of the world's population) reported 5.1 million TB cases to WHO, of which 2.4 million of these were new sputum smear-positive cases. Of this total, 35% of these cases were diagnosed in the Southeast Asia region, 25% in the Western Pacific region, 23% in the African region, 4% in the American region, 5% in the Eastern Mediterranean region, and 7% in the European region (World Health Organization, 2007). **Figure 1** shows the TB notification rates from

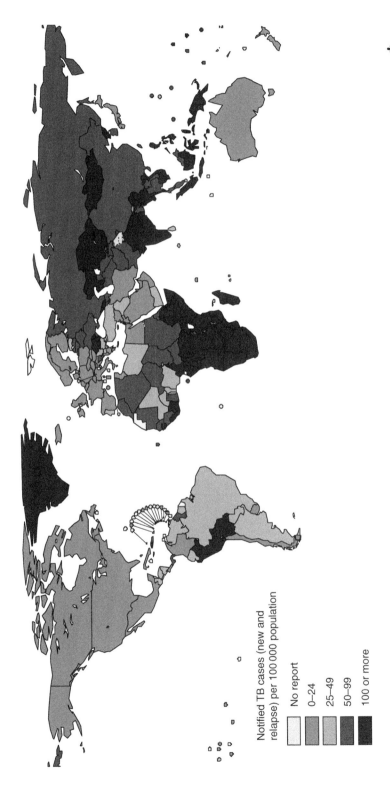

The boundaries and names shown and the designations used on this map do not imply the expression of any opinion whatsoever on the part of the World Health Organization concerning the legal status of any country, territory, city or area or of its authorities, or concerning the delimitation of its frontiers or boundaries. Dotted lines on maps represent approximate border lines for which there may not yet be full agreement.

Figure 1 Tuberculosis notification rates, 2005. From World Health Organization (2007) *Global Tuberculosis Control: Surveillance, Planning, Financing.* Geneva: World Health Organization.

2005. A total of 26.5 million new and relapse cases were notified by DOTS programs between 1995 and 2005. Case notifications have been steadily falling for at least the last two decades in Southeast Asia and Western Pacific regions, in Western and Central Europe, and North and Latin America. Case reports have been increasing in Eastern Europe (the former Soviet Union) since 1990, and in sub-Saharan Africa since the mid-1980s, although the rate of increase has slowed in the past few years (Dye, 2006). The resurgence of TB in Eastern Europe is due to economic decline, poor TB control, and a poor general health infrastructure. The elevated incidence of drug resistance in this region (sometimes over 10% of new cases have multidrug-resistant TB) is probably a byproduct of these forces and not a cause.

Estimated Incidence and Mortality

Global estimates of TB incidence are based on multiple inputs, including case notifications, such as population-based surveys of TB prevalence, vital registration data, and independent assessments of surveillance system quality (Dye, 2006). In 2007, WHO estimated that prevalence and death rates of TB had been falling for several years, peaking sometime between 2000 and 2005. By 2005 the incidence rate was stable or in decline in all six WHO regions, a measure of the success of global DOTS programs. However, WHO also estimated that the global incidence (absolute number of new cases per year) of

TB is growing at roughly 1% per year, due to the growing caseload in sub-Saharan Africa and countries of the former Soviet Union (Eastern Europe and Central Asia), and population growth (World Health Organization, 2007).

Worldwide, there were an estimated 8.8 million new cases of TB in 2005, with 3.9 million cases thought to be infectious (World Health Organization, 2007). The incidence and mortality rates vary widely by WHO region (**Table 1**). Developing countries show the brunt of the epidemic, precisely the places with fewer resources to combat the problem. It is estimated that 95% of the world's cases and 98% of the TB deaths occur in the developing world (Raviglione and Uplekar, 2006). **Figure 2** shows the estimated numbers of new TB cases charted by country. In 2005, almost 3 million new cases were diagnosed in South and Southeast Asia, which accounted for one-third of all cases worldwide. Nearly half of the world's cases that arise every year occur in Asia. While there were fewer cases in Africa (2.5 million), the incidence per capita is nearly twice that of Asia, with 343 cases per 100 000 population. Similarly, most deaths from TB occurred in Asia (807 000), but the highest mortality per capita was in Africa (74 per 100 000).

Twenty-two countries are labeled as high-burden countries and account for 80% of the world's case burden. The five countries with the highest burden of TB were India (1.8 million cases), China (1.3 million cases), Indonesia (533 000 cases), Nigeria (372 000 cases), and Bangladesh (322 000 cases). The American (North and South) and European regions (WHO designation) account

Table 1 Summary of tuberculosis estimates by WHO region, 2005

WHO region	AFR	AMR	EMR	EUR	SEAR	WPR	Global
Population in millions	738	890	541	882	1656	1752	6461
New cases of TB disease, all forms							
Number of incident cases (thousands)	2529	352	565	445	2993	1927	8811
Incidence rate (per 100 000)	343	39	104	50	181	110	136
HIV prevalence in new adult cases (%)	37	5.5	2.8	3.6	3.5	1.2	12
Attributable to HIV (thousands)	506	11	9.8	10.0	56	14	656
Attributable to HIV (%)	31	5.0	2.5	3.3	2.9	1.1	11
New sputum smear-positive cases of TB							
Number of incident cases (thousands)	1088	157	253	199	1339	866	3902
Prevalence rate SS + TB (per 100 000)	511	50	163	60	290	206	217
% Of incident cases HIV+	28	7.9	2.1	4.6	3.9	1.0	11
Deaths from TB disease							
Deaths from TB (thousands)	544	49	112	66	512	295	1577
Deaths from TB (per 100 000)	74	5.5	21	7.4	31	17	24
Deaths from TB in HIV+ adults (thousands)	208	3.7	4.8	3.0	26	5.5	251
% Of adult AIDS deaths due to TB	15	5.4	20	13	7.6	14	13
TB deaths attributable to HIV (%)	34	6.5	3.2	3.9	3.8	1.4	13

AFR, Africa; AMR, Americas; EMR, Eastern Mediterranean; EUR, Europe; SEAR, Southeast Asia; WPR, Western Pacific; TB, tuberculosis; SS+, sputum smear-positive, HIV+, HIV-positive; adult, 15–49 years old.
WHO African Region comprises sub-Saharan Africa and Algeria. The remaining North African countries are included in the WHO Eastern Mediterranean Region.
Data from World Health Organization (2007) *Global Tuberculosis Control: Surveillance, Planning, Financing.* Geneva: World Health Organization; Corbett EL, Watt CJ, Walker N, *et al.* (2003) The growing burden of tuberculosis: Global trends and interactions with the HIV epidemic. *Archives of Internal Medicine* 163: 1009–1021.

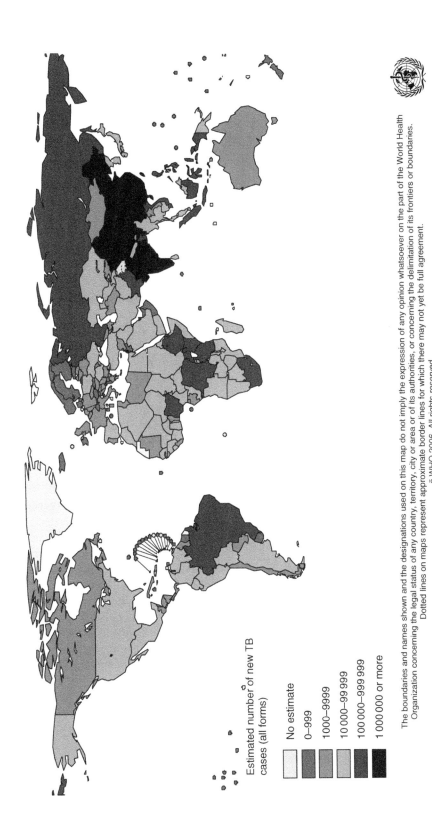

Figure 2 Estimated numbers of new TB cases, 2005. From World Health Organization (2007) *Global Tuberculosis Control: Surveillance, Planning, Financing.* Geneva: World Health Organization.

for 9% of the world's total TB burden. However, in North America and many European countries, more than 50% of the TB cases reported are among persons who were not born in those countries (foreign born). Among the 15 countries with the highest estimated TB incidence rates, 12 are in Africa. This is largely explained by the relatively high rates of HIV infection. Swaziland, Djibouti, Namibia, Lesotho, Botswana, Kenya, Zimbabwe, Zambia, and South Africa all have estimated incidence rates above 600 per 100 000 (World Health Organization, 2007).

In most locales, men have greater incidence rates of TB than women, although in many of these places women are more likely to have poor access to health facilities and diagnostic services. The observed difference in incidence between men and women is due to an observed epidemiologic difference in exposure to infection (in the workplace, poor housing conditions, other congregate settings) and susceptibility to development of disease. Where the transmission of the TB bacillus is stable or increasing, the incidence rate is highest in young adults as most cases result from recent infection or reinfection. As transmission falls, the caseload shifts to older adults, as a higher proportion of cases can be attributable to reactivation of latent infection (Dye, 2006). In the established market economies where rates of TB are low, indigenous persons with TB tend to be older. Immigrants in these countries from high incidence areas tend to be younger, although this depends on the maturity of the epidemic in the host country.

The ongoing global TB epidemic is of great concern for many reasons: (1) increasing global social and economic inequality, with a widening income gap between the rich and poor in various countries; (2) historical neglect of TB control programs; (3) changing global demographics (increasing world population and age structure); (4) worsening drug resistance in many areas; and (5) impact of the HIV pandemic (Maher et al., 2006).

TB/HIV

One of the primary causes of the resurgence in TB worldwide is the increase in HIV infection, even in rural areas. Among the 1.6 million estimated annual deaths, 195 000 are estimated to also be infected with HIV (World Health Organization, 2007). HIV is the strongest risk factor for persons infected with *Mycobacterium tuberculosis* to acquire TB disease – either drug-susceptible or drug-resistant TB – following infection. The HIV virus suppresses the body's immune system, which promotes progression of either recently acquired or latent tuberculosis infection to TB disease. Persons infected with HIV who become infected with *M. tuberculosis* have a very high risk of developing TB disease within 2 years. The HIV epidemic has therefore telescoped the TB epidemic of both susceptible and drug-resistant strains, shortening the time to

generate the epidemic from years to months (Maher et al., 2006). As a result, the global HIV epidemic has increased the burden of TB in many countries. Between 1990 and 1999, the incidence of TB in sub-Saharan Africa increased by over 250%, with an estimated one-third of all new TB cases occurring among people who were HIV-infected. This happened despite many countries having a well-functioning national TB control program. In areas of high tuberculosis prevalence, therefore, TB is one of the most common opportunistic infections. TB may also accelerate the course of HIV infection, increasing HIV viral load in some patients, and is thought to be the primary cause of death in up to 40% of those who are HIV infected (de Jong et al., 2004).

Table 1 shows estimates of TB taking into account interactions with HIV. In 2002, 11% of all new TB cases in adults aged 15–29 years were attributable to HIV infection (Corbett et al., 2003). Of the estimated global burden of 1.6 million deaths from TB, 13% were attributable to HIV. Again, sub-Saharan Africa bears the brunt of these colliding epidemics, with over 500 000 incident TB cases attributable to HIV and over 200 000 deaths from TB in HIV-infected individuals. WHO estimates that 11% of TB cases worldwide, and 31% in sub-Saharan Africa, were attributable to HIV infection in 2005 (Dye, 2006). **Figure 3** shows the estimate of TB/HIV co-infection rates by country.

The proportion of adults with TB who were infected with HIV varies greatly by region, from roughly 30% in Africa to less than 2% in the Western Pacific. In high TB burden countries such as China, Indonesia, Bangladesh, and Pakistan, HIV infection rates in TB cases have remained below 1%. Where HIV infection rates are high in the general population (generalized epidemic), they are generally also high in persons with TB. Estimates for high TB burden southern African countries such as South Africa, Botswana, Zimbabwe, and Zambia exceed 50%. HIV has probably had a smaller effect on the prevalence of TB than on the incidence of TB, as HIV significantly reduces the life expectancy of persons with TB, and in the general population as well (Dye, 2006). Due to HIV and TB mortality, life expectancy in many southern African countries has dropped below 45 years.

In some areas with both high TB and HIV prevalence, the symptoms of TB disease are often equated with HIV-positive status by lay people. Persons exhibiting TB symptoms are therefore often stigmatized as HIV-positive, which causes them to modify their social and health-seeking behavior, and ultimately hinders TB control efforts at a clinical level. The stigma surrounding both diseases promotes shame and silence, which further exacerbates the spread of both diseases. Approaching TB control with a human rights lens therefore becomes imperative (World Health Organization, 2001).

Although HIV has had a more profound impact on the epidemiology of TB worldwide than any other risk factor,

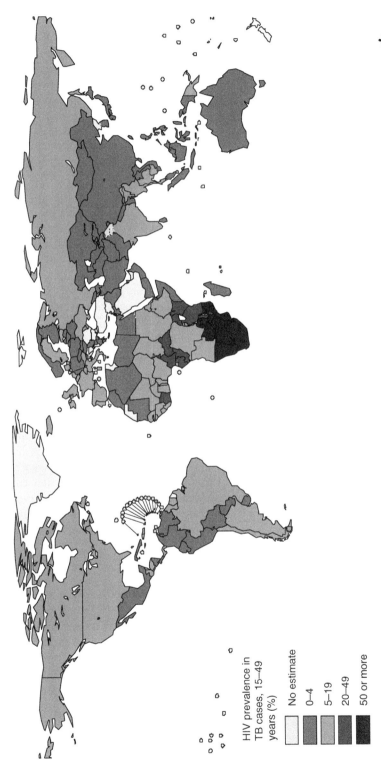

The boundaries and names shown and the designations used on this map do not imply the expression of any opinion whatsoever on the part of the World Health Organization concerning the legal status of any country, territory, city or area or of its authorities, or concerning the delimitation of its frontiers or boundaries. Dotted lines on maps represent approximate border lines for which there may not yet be full agreement.

Figure 3 Estimated HIV prevalence in new adult TB cases, 2005. From World Health Organization (2007) *Global Tuberculosis Control: Surveillance, Planning, Financing*. Geneva: World Health Organization.

HIV prevalence in TB cases, 15–49 years (%)

No estimate
0–4
5–19
20–49
50 or more

other important risk factors should not be ignored (Maher et al., 2006). More attention needs to be paid to the increased risk of developing TB from smoking, as well as from air pollution and other respiratory diseases. Chronic diseases such as diabetes also play a large role, as does the prevalence of undernutrition.

Drug-Resistant Tuberculosis

The emerging worldwide epidemic of drug-resistant tuberculosis is a byproduct of ineffective or poorly organized systems for TB control. It is therefore entirely a human-made problem. Modulation of gene expression, or dissemination of genes conferring drug resistance through transformation of stretches of DNA, do not occur in the TB bacteria as with other pathogens. Conversely, the natural selection of rare drug-resistant strains (for isoniazid–rifampin resistance, the mutation frequency is $1:10^{14}$) inside the human body occurs when inconsistent or interrupted treatment (health services and/or patient factors) is given, when the wrong drugs are prescribed for the wrong amount of time, when drugs of inferior quality are given, or when there is an interrupted supply of drugs. Strains are identified as MDR TB (multidrug-resistant TB) if they are resistant to at least isoniazid and rifampin, the two most important drug used to treat the disease. When susceptibility to these two core drugs is lost, more toxic and more expensive drugs must be used to treat the disease. While drug-susceptible TB is generally treatable, the regimen for MDR TB can take up to 2 years to complete and costs a TB program over 100 times more than treating a drug-susceptible case. Before the advent of a worldwide concerted effort to treat MDR TB, treatment success rates were 50% for new cases and 30% for retreatment cases in those who adhered to observed therapy instituted by a program (Espinal et al., 2000).

In 1994, the World Health Organization and International Union Against Tuberculosis and Lung Disease launched the Global Project on Antituberculosis Drug Resistance Surveillance. The project's goal is to measure the prevalence and monitor the trend of antituberculosis drug resistance worldwide using standardized methodology (World Health Organization, 2003). As of 2007, three reports have been published, with the further report due out in late 2007. Over 90 countries have contributed data to the reports, although there is a great deal of missing data from sub-Saharan Africa. According to the last report, the prevalence of MDR TB varies greatly by region. Tuberculosis patients in Eastern Europe and Central Asia are ten times more likely to have MDR TB than patients in the rest of the world. China, Ecuador, Peru, Israel, and South Africa also have problems with increasing MDR TB rates, with the latter country burdened by more than 6000 cases per year. The highest rates of MDR TB occur in Estonia, Kazakhstan,

Karakalpakstan (Uzbekistan), Tomsk Oblast in Russia, Lithuania, and Israel. Overall, MDR TB among isolates from new cases ranges from 0% to 14%, with a median of 1%. The median prevalence among previously treated cases was 7% (World Health Organization, 2005). Recent WHO modeling of the incidence of MDR TB estimated that 424 203 (95% CI 376 019–620 061) new cases occurred in 2004. China, India, and the Russian Federation accounted for 62% of the estimated global burden of MDR TB, roughly 261 362 cases (Zignol et al., 2006). **Figure 4** shows the countries or settings with the highest rates of MDR TB among new and previously treated cases of TB between 1999 and 2002.

In response to the MDR TB problem, WHO and partners formulated the DOTS-Plus Strategy in 1998, which provides for the treatment of patients with MDR TB using more effective second-line medications. Given the expense of these drugs, the Stop TB Partnership set up the Green Light Committee to allow access to concessionally priced second-line medications through a bulk-purchasing mechanism for those programs that could demonstrate an effective DOTS strategy. Beginning at five pilot projects, the DOTS-Plus strategy grew to include over 50 sites. Treatment success rates only approach 65–70% in the best of these programs (Leimane et al., 2005). International guidelines for the treatment of drug-resistant TB have been published (World Health Organization, 2006). The problem of default from therapy, however, continues to plague the treatment of MDR TB patients. DOTS-Plus and the treatment of MDR TB patients has now been rolled into the global WHO Stop TB Strategy.

In addition, HIV may also be contributing to increases in MDR TB prevalence among TB patients. HIV infection has been associated with many outbreaks of MDR TB (mainly due to a lack of infection control), as well as acquired rifamycin resistance. In the continent with the highest rates of HIV infection, the only country with trend data on anti-TB drug resistance is Botswana, a country with one of the highest TB incidence rates worldwide at approximately 600 TB cases per 100 000 population. Three national drug resistance surveys conducted from 1995 to 2002 reported statistically significant increases in resistance to any anti-TB drug, to isoniazid, and to streptomycin among new TB cases without a history of prior TB treatment (Nelson et al., 2005). The prevalence of MDR-TB among new cases increased from 0.2% to 0.8%, although this was not statistically significant. Given the challenges in Botswana and other sub-Saharan African countries, such as relatively high treatment default rates and uncontrolled use of second-line drugs for MDR TB, the possibility exists for further increases in MDR TB.

To make matters worse, extensively drug-resistant tuberculosis (XDR TB) was described in 2005–2006 following a joint survey by WHO and CDC (Centers for Disease Control and Prevention, 2006a). XDR TB is currently defined as MDR TB that is also resistant to any

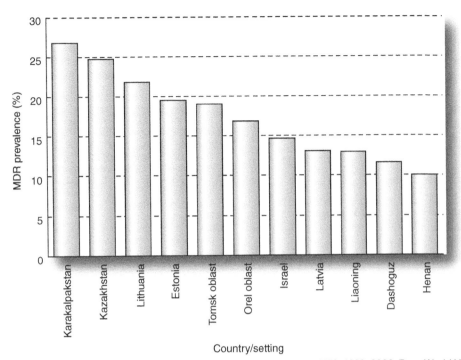

Figure 4 Countries/settings with combined MDR TB prevalence rates higher than 10%, 1999–2002. From World Health Organization (2005) Anti-tuberculosis Drug Resistance in the World: The WHO/IUATLD Global Project on Anti-Tuberculosis Drug Resistance Surveillance. Report No.3, Prevalence and Trends, WHO/HTM/TB/2004.343. Geneva: World Health Organization.

fluoroquinolone and one of the three second-line inject-able drugs (amikacin, kanamycin, or capreomycin) (Centers for Disease Control and Prevention, 2006b). The most recent reports have noted XDR TB in all areas of the world, but most commonly in Asia and Eastern Europe. The definition was created to put a name to a face of a problem that had been described by clinicians who reported encountering patients with difficult-to-treat highly resistant TB. Even the best estimates of successful treatment are that only 25–35% of XDR TB cases will be cured (Holtz *et al.*, 2005). In 2006, investigators from South Africa reported the occurrence of highly resistant TB in HIV-infected persons who were enrolled in antiretroviral treatment programs, but whose case-fatality was alarm-ingly high (98%) despite adequate response to drugs (Gandhi *et al.*, 2006). A large proportion of the cases had never had TB before, and several were health-care work-ers, raising the question about nosocomial spread and insufficient infection control practices in that region. The specter of virtually untreatable strains of TB being propagated throughout sub-Saharan Africa threatens to undo decades of TB control work in the region where TB is already on the rise.

Economic Burden of TB

Tuberculosis remains a prominent disease not only because of the number of people affected, or the human

rights concerns about the neglected global response despite its treatability, but also because it strikes down adults in the prime of their productive lives. More than 80% of the burden of TB, as measured by disability-adjusted life years lost, is due to premature death rather than illness or disability (World Health Organization, 2000). Tuberculosis therefore extracts an enormous eco-nomic burden on developing countries. These costs fall into two categories: (1) Direct costs to the health services and to the patient and patient's family and (2) indirect costs to society, community, and the patient's family through lost production (World Health Organization, 2000). Tuberculosis patients and their families pay the cost of TB through their suffering, pain, and grief. A protracted illness can also cause psychological and social stress and costs. There is a great deal of stigma that remains sur-rounding TB, as well as with TB/HIV, and many patients may be rejected by society, their job, or even their own family. In some societies, TB survivors are seen as unmar-riageable or unfit for work. Discrimination in the health sector and in society can lead to mental health stress and reduction in quality of life.

The largest indirect cost to the patient is lost income through debilitation and sickness. Most patients are too sick to work for 3–4 months during their illness, and up to 8–10 months if they have MDR TB, resulting in the loss of a significant portion of their annual income. If the patient dies, there is the further loss of 15–20 years of income depending on the age of the patient. The substantial nontreatment costs borne by patients and families of patients are often greater than the costs of treatment by the health sector. Households develop strategies for dealing with actual losses and potential losses. Selling assets is a common strategy, which is not advantageous in the long term for patients or families (Maher *et al.*, 2006). Reducing food intake, withholding school fees, or delaying marriages of children can all have important long-term consequences for families.

Conclusion

Tuberculosis is an age-old disease than continues to afflict the poor and disadvantaged populations around the globe with alarmingly high mortality rates. Due to poor attention to global TB control, the annual incidence of TB continues to rise at 1% per year, although recent gains have been made in fighting the disease where it kills the most people, such as in India and China. HIV and drug-resistant TB present challenges to the global public health community that will not be easily overcome. TB will continue to be with us for our lifetime. With the advent of more rapid diagnostic techniques and more effective drugs against drug-susceptible TB and drug-resistant TB, we will hopefully see an interruption in the transmission of TB and a reversal in the global incidence in the twenty-first century to correct the political, social, and public health missteps of the twentieth century.

Citations

Binkin N, Vernon AA, Simone PM, *et al.* (1999) Tuberculosis prevention and control activities in the United States: An overview of the organization of tuberculosis services. *International Journal of Tuberculosis and Lung Disease* 3(8): 663–674.

Centers for Disease Control and Prevention (2006a) Emergence of *Mycobacterium tuberculosis* with extensive resistance to second-line drugs – Worldwide, 2000–2004. *Morbid Mortal Weekly Report* 55(11): 301–305.

Centers for Disease Control and Prevention (2006b) Notice to readers: Revised definition of XDR-TB. *Morbid Mortal Weekly Report* 55(43): 1176.

Corbett EL, Watt CJ, Walker N, *et al.* (2003) The growing burden of tuberculosis: Global trends and interactions with the HIV epidemic. *Archives of Internal Medicine* 163: 1009–1021.

De Jong BC, Israelski DM, Corbett EL, and Small PM (2004) Clinical management of TB in the context of HIV infection. *Annual Review of Medicine* 55: 283–301.

Dye C (2006) Global epidemiology of tuberculosis. *Lancet* 367: 938–940.

Espinal MA, Kim SJ, Suarez PG, *et al.* (2000) Standard short-course chemotherapy for drug-resistant tuberculosis: Treatment outcomes in 6 countries. *Journal of the American Medical Association* 283(19): 2537–2545.

Frieden TR, Fujiwara PI, Washko RM, and Hamburg MA (1995) Tuberculosis in New York City – Turning the tide. *New England Journal of Medicine* 333(4): 229–233.

Gandhi NR, Moll A, Sturm AW, *et al.* (2006) Extensively drug-resistant tuberculosis as a cause of death in patients co-infected with tuberculosis and HIV in a rural area of South Africa. *Lancet* 368 (9547): 1554–1556.

Holtz TH, Riekstina V, Zarovska E, Laserson KF, Wells CD, and Leimane V (2005) XDR-TB: Extreme drug-resistance and treatment outcome under DOTS-Plus, Latvia, 2000–2002. *International Journal of Tuberculosis and Lung Disease* 9 (supplement 1): S258.

Kim JY, Shakow A, Mate K, Vanderwarker C, Gupta R, and Farmer P (2005) Limited good and limited vision: Multidrug-resistant tuberculosis and global health policy. *Social Science and Medicine* 61: 847–859.

Leimane V, Riekstina V, Holtz TH, *et al.* (2005) Clinical outcome of individualised treatment of multidrug-resistant tuberculosis in Latvia: A retrospective cohort study. *Lancet* 365: 318–326.

Maher D and Raviglione MC (2006) Tuberculosis – a WHO perspective. In: Schlossberg D (ed.) *Tuberculosis and Nontuberculous Mycobacterial Infections*, 5th edn., pp. 133–146. New York: McGraw-Hill Medical.

Nelson LJ, Talbot EA, Mwasekaga MJ, *et al.* (2005) Antituberculosis drug resistance and anonymous HIV surveillance in tuberculosis patients in Botswana, 2002. *Lancet* 366: 488–490.

Nerlich AG, Haas CJ, Zink A, Szeimies U, and Hagedorn HG (1997) Molecular evidence for tuberculosis in an ancient Egyptian mummy. *Lancet* 350: 1404.

Raviglione MC and Uplekar MW (2006) WHO's new stop TB strategy. *Lancet* 367: 952–955.

Ryan F (1992) *Tuberculosis: The Greatest Story Never Told.* Worcestershire, UK: Swift Publishers.

Stead WW, Eisenach KD, Cave MD, *et al.* (1995) When did *Mycobaterium tuberculosis* infection first occur in the New World? An important question with public health implications. *American Journal of Critical Care and Medicine* 151: 1267–1268.

World Health Organization (2000) *The Economic Impacts of Tuberculosis. The Stop TB Initiative 2000 Series,* (WHO/CDS/STB/2000.5) Geneva, Switzerland: World Health Organization.

World Health Organization (2001) *Guidelines for Social Mobilization: A Human Rights Approach to Tuberculosis,* WHO/CDS/STB/2001.9. Geneva, Switzerland: World Health Organization.

World Health Organization (2002) *Global tuberculosis control: Surveillance, planning, financing.* Geneva, Switzerland: World Health Organization.

World Health Organization (2003) *Guidelines for Surveillance of Drug Resistance in Tuberculosis,* WHO/CDS/CSR/RMD/2003.3. Geneva, Switzerland: World Health Organization.

World Health Organization (2005) Anti-tuberculosis Drug Resistance in the World: The WHO/IUATLD Global Project on Anti-Tuberculosis Drug Resistance Surveillance. Report No.3, Prevalence and Trends, WHO/HTM/TB/2004.343. Geneva, Switzerland: World Health Organization.

World Health Organization (2006) *Guidelines for the Programmatic Management of Drug-Resistant Tuberculosis.* WHO/HTM/TB/2006.361. Geneva, Switzerland: World Health Organization.

World Health Organization (2007) *Global Tuberculosis Control: Surveillance, Planning, Financing.* Geneva, Switzerland: World Health Organization.

Zignol M, Hosseini MS, Wright A, *et al.* (2006) Global incidence of multidrug-resistant tuberculosis. *Journal of Infectious Diseases* 194: 479–485.

Relevant Websites

http://www.who.int/tb/hiv/en/ – World Health Organization TB/HIV website.

http://www.who.int/tb/en/ – World Health Organization tuberculosis website.

http://www.who.int/tb/xdr/ – World Health Organization, XDR-TB: Extensively drug-resistant tuberculosis.

Epidemiology of HIV/AIDS and its Surveillance

R Choi and C Farquhar, University of Washington, Seattle, WA, USA

Introduction

During the last 25 years, human immunodeficiency virus (HIV) has claimed the lives of millions of men, women, and children across the globe and has developed into an international public health crisis. The HIV/AIDS (acquired immune deficiency syndrome) epidemic has spared few regions in the world and has been particularly devastating in sub-Saharan Africa, where more than 60% of all HIV-infected adults and 90% of HIV-infected infants reside (Joint United Nations Program on AIDS [UNAIDS]/World Health Organization [WHO], 2006). At the time of the first reports of AIDS cases among gay men in the United States during the early 1980s, it would have been difficult to envision such a calamitous outcome. Even after identification of the human immunodeficiency virus in 1983 and diagnosis of HIV infection among heterosexual men and women, infants and children, intravenous drug users, hemophiliacs, and recipients of other blood products, the enormity of the situation was not fully recognized. As a result, the global response to HIV was initially slow and in many parts of the world remains inadequate, despite in-depth knowledge of the salient risk factors for HIV transmission and improved surveillance data defining the nature of the epidemic.

Overall Prevalence of HIV

Despite significant advances in HIV prevention and treatment, HIV remains a disease without a cure and continues to threaten the social and economic stability of many developing nations. According to the *AIDS Epidemic Update 2006* by UNAIDS, an estimated 39.5 million (34.1–47.1) people worldwide were living with HIV in 2006 (**Figure 1**). Approximately 17.7 million (15.1–20.9) of HIV-infected were women, an increase of over 1 million between 2004 and 2006. In the same year, an estimated 4.3 million (3.6–6.6) became newly infected with HIV, and approximately 2.9 million (2.5–3.5) lost their lives to AIDS (**Figures 2** and **3**). HIV has infected over 65 million people and claimed over 25 million lives worldwide since 1981 (UNAIDS/WHO, 2006).

Distinctions between HIV Types 1 and 2

Two human immunodeficiency viruses have been identified and characterized in humans: HIV type 1 (HIV-1) and HIV type 2 (HIV-2). While HIV-1 and HIV-2 share the same modes of transmission, HIV-2 has a less efficient rate of transmission than HIV-1 (Kanki *et al.*, 1994). Studies conducted in Senegal estimated the HIV-2 transmission rate per sexual act with an infected partner to be 3.4- to 3.9-fold lower than that of HIV-1 (Gilbert *et al.*, 2003). Other studies conducted in The Gambia, Ivory Coast, and Senegal have demonstrated rates of mother-to-child HIV-2 transmission to be approximately 6- to 20-fold lower than those among women with HIV-1 infection (Andreasson *et al.*, 1993; Abbott *et al.*, 1994; Adjorlolo-Johnson *et al.*, 1994; O'Donovan *et al.*, 2000). Studies have also demonstrated that progression to AIDS is slower among individuals with HIV-2 compared to HIV-1, although the consequences of immunosuppression and the propensity for opportunistic infections remain similar at lower CD4 counts (Marlink *et al.*, 1994).

Another difference between HIV-1 and HIV-2 is in their antiretroviral susceptibility, which may be important in future delivery of antiretroviral therapy to Africa and management of the epidemic. The current antiretroviral therapy for HIV-1 includes various combinations of nucleotide or nucleoside reverse transcriptase inhibitors (NRTIs), nonnucleoside reverse transcriptase inhibitors (NNRTIs), and protease inhibitors (PIs). While NRTIs have been found to be as effective against HIV-2 as they are against HIV-1 *in vitro* (Mullins *et al.*, 2004), NNRTIs have been shown to be largely ineffective against HIV-2 *in vitro* (Witvrouw *et al.*, 1999). PIs have shown mixed effectiveness against HIV-2 (Pichova *et al.*, 1997).

Given lower rates of transmission and progression to disease with HIV-2, it is not surprising that HIV-1 is responsible for the majority of HIV infections and AIDS cases worldwide. HIV-2 is restricted to relatively small geographic areas and is the predominant HIV type in the West African countries of Guinea-Bissau, The Gambia, Cape Verde, and Senegal, where it was first described in 1985 (**Figure 4**) (Barin *et al.*, 1985). HIV-2 is also found in Portugal and former Portuguese colonies, such as Mozambique, Angola, southwestern India, and Brazil, although it is less prevalent in these regions than HIV-1 infection (Kanki, 1997).

While these differences between HIV-1 and HIV-2 promote a better understanding of HIV, it is clear that HIV-1 drives the HIV/AIDS epidemic globally, and HIV-1 will therefore be the focus of the remainder of this article.

HIV-1 Groups and Subtypes

The great genetic diversity of HIV is reflected in the many genotypes or clades that have been identified.

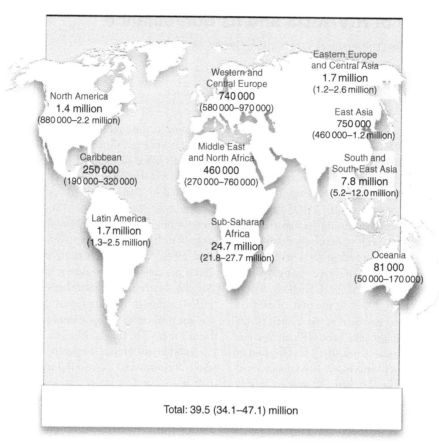

Figure 1 Adults and children estimated to be living with HIV in 2006. Reproduced with kind permission from UNAIDS/WHO (2007) *AIDS Epidemic Update 2006*. Geneva: UNAIDS/WHO.

Currently, HIV-1 genotypes are divided into Groups M, N, and O, with Group M being further subdivided into subtypes A to K because it is the most common. Groups N and O are limited to West Africa. Group O represents the outlier strains, while Group N represents 'new group' or non-O and non-M strains. Generally, intragenotype strain variation is less than 15%, while intergenotypic variation is 20–30% (Burke, 1997).

Subtypes A to K are defined by significant clustering across the genome and are often more prevalent in particular regions of the world (see **Figure 4**) (McCutchan, 2006). Of these subtypes, subtype C is currently the most common subtype worldwide, and is found in the eastern and southern parts of Africa and in India (McCutchan, 2000). Subtype B predominates in the United States and Europe, subtypes A and D are found in eastern parts of Africa, and subtype E in South-East Asia.

Several studies suggest that subtypes A to K differ in their primary mode of transmission, virulence, and infectivity. In Thailand, where subtypes B and E were both prevalent at the start of the epidemic, subtype E was initially the major subtype among female sex workers, while subtype B was associated with intravenous drug use (IDU) (Nelson *et al.*, 1993; Nopkesorn *et al.*, 1993).

However, subtype E subsequently became more common than subtype B among IDUs, indicating that mode of transmission may be less important than other biological or behavioral factors (Nopkesorn *et al.*, 1993). In Kenya, subtypes A, C, and D all circulate and individuals infected with HIV-1 subtype C have been found to have higher plasma RNA levels and lower CD4 counts compared to individuals with subtypes A or D (Neilson *et al.*, 1999). In Uganda and Kenya, HIV infection with subtype D has been associated with more rapid progression when compared to infection with subtype A (Kaleebu *et al.*, 2001; Baeten *et al.*, 2007). However, in Sweden, studies showed no differences among subtypes A, B, C, or D when examining clinical HIV disease progression (Alaeus *et al.*, 1999).

Individuals may also be coinfected with 2 strains of HIV-1 and these may be the same or different viral subtypes. Coinfection occurs when a person acquires two different viral strains simultaneously or when a chronically HIV-infected individual is reinfected with HIV-1, a phenomenon also known as super-infection. This has led to recombinant forms of HIV-1, which may in turn be transmitted and have the potential to become major strains within populations. For example, a recombinant form comprised of subtypes A and E is a

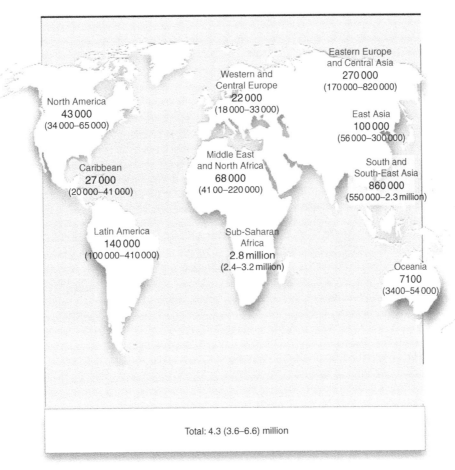

North America
43 000
(34 000–65 000)

Caribbean
27 000
(20 000–41 000)

Latin America
140 000
(100 000–410 000)

Western and
Central Europe
22 000
(18 000–33 000)

Middle East
and North Africa
68 000
(41 00–220 000)

Sub-Saharan
Africa
2.8 million
(2.4–3.2 million)

Eastern Europe
and Central Asia
270 000
(170 000–820 000)

East Asia
100 000
(56 000–300 000)

South and
South-East Asia
860 000
(550 000–2.3 million)

Oceania
7100
(3400–54 000)

Total: 4.3 (3.6–6.6) million

Figure 2   Estimated number of adults and children newly infected with HIV during 2006. Reproduced with kind permission from UNAIDS/WHO (2007) *AIDS Epidemic Update 2006.* Geneva: UNAIDS/WHO.

major circulating strain throughout South-East Asia and a recombinant strain of subtypes A and G is a major strain in West Africa. Recombinant strains will undoubtedly continue to emerge and challenge those involved in HIV vaccine development, surveillance efforts, and clinical care.

Modes of HIV Transmission: Rates and Risk Factors

Understanding the different modes of transmission and appreciating associated risk factors play an essential role in grasping the epidemiology of the HIV/AIDS epidemic. HIV may be transmitted via sexual intercourse (either male to female, female to male, or male to male), via IDU, vertically from mother to child, through transfusions of blood or other blood products, or via occupational exposure to HIV-infected bodily fluids.

Sexual Transmission

Sexual transmission accounts for the 75–85% of HIV infections worldwide and heterosexual intercourse accounts

for the vast majority of these transmission events (Royce *et al.*, 1997). The likely explanation for this is that heterosexual transmission predominates in those regions of sub-Saharan Africa with the highest HIV prevalence, rather than that heterosexual intercourse is a more efficient means of transmission. The average rate of infection for vaginal intercourse is estimated to be 0.0011 per contact and several studies suggest vaginal transmission from an infected male to an uninfected female is more efficient than when the female partner is HIV-infected (**Figure 5**) (Gray *et al.*, 2001). This is in comparison to significantly higher rates for unprotected anal sex, which is the most efficient mode of sexual transmission and has an average rate of infection of 0.0082 per contact (Vittinghoff *et al.*, 1999).

One of the most significant and well-established risk factors in sexual HIV-1 transmission is the quantity of HIV-1 in the blood of the infected partner. In a rural district of Uganda, one study demonstrated a significant dose–response relationship between increased HIV-1 RNA viral load in plasma and increased risk of transmission. For every $\log_{10}$ increment in the viral load, there was a 2.5-fold increase in HIV-1 transmission and no transmission occurred in this cohort when the infected partner

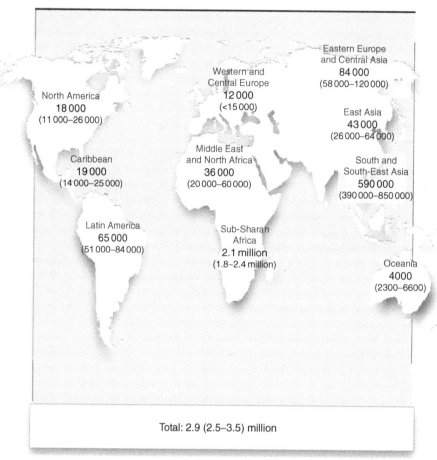

Figure 3 Estimated adult and child deaths from AIDS during 2006. Reproduced with kind permission from UNAIDS/WHO (2007) *AIDS Epidemic Update 2006*. Geneva: UNAIDS/WHO.

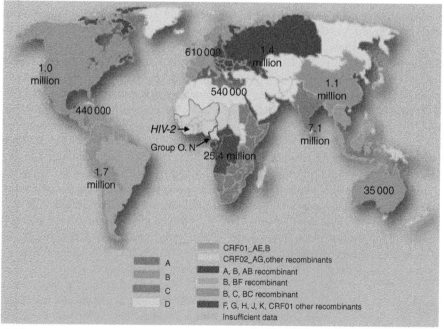

Figure 4 Global distribution of HIV-1 subtypes and HIV-2. Global epidemiology of HIV 78: s7–s12. Copyright 2006 Wiley & Sons, Inc. Reprinted with permission of Wiley-Liss, Inc., a subsidiary of John Wiley & Sons, Inc.

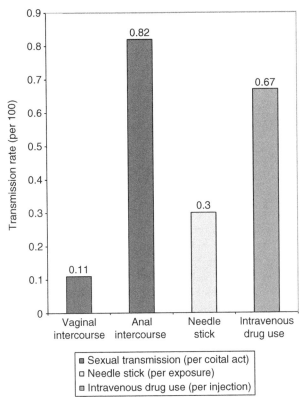

Figure 5 Rates for different modes of transmission.

had a plasma HIV-1 RNA level less than 1500 copies per milliliter (Quinn *et al.*, 2000).

The highest HIV-1 viral load occurs in the setting of end-stage AIDS and during primary HIV infection, making these periods of high transmission risk. The latter is a particular concern from a public health standpoint because when a person is first infected with HIV, he or she may not know his or her HIV status, and may unknowingly spread HIV at high rates. A study in Uganda demonstrated that the highest HIV transmission rates were within 2.5 months after seroconversion of the infected partner, which represents primary infection (0.0082 per coital act), and during the period 6–26 months before the death of the infected partner, which represents advanced AIDS (0.0028 per coital act). The average rates of HIV transmission were 0.0007 per coital act among chronically infected partners (Wawer *et al.*, 2005).

Genital shedding of HIV-1 may also increase HIV transmission risk and some have suggested that it may be a better predictor of HIV transmission than systemic HIV-1 viral load (Baeten and Overbaugh, 2003). A number of studies have reported strong correlation between plasma and genital tract HIV-1 levels; however, one published study has found a significant association between genital HIV shedding and increased transmission (Pedraza *et al.*, 1999).

Another factor that appears to increase risk of transmitting HIV, as well as risk of acquiring HIV in the exposed, uninfected partner, is the presence of sexually transmitted infections (STIs). STIs may facilitate HIV shedding in the genital tract, cause local recruitment of susceptible inflammatory cells, or disrupt genital mucosal surfaces. Increased risk of both HIV transmission and acquisition has been shown for both ulcerative and non-ulcerative STIs. Early studies identified syphilis as increasing risk of acquisition 3.1- to 12.8-fold (Otten *et al.*, 1994). A separate study found a fivefold increase in acquisition of HIV in the presence of genital ulcers, where 89% of the ulcers were chancroid (Cameron *et al.*, 1989). The ulcerative STI that has received the most attention recently has been herpes simplex virus type 2 (HSV-2). Two meta-analyses have demonstrated that having HSV-2 increases the risk of transmission approximately threefold (Freeman *et al.*, 2006) and increases risk of HSV-2 acquisition twofold (Wald, 2004). The association between HSV-2 infection and HIV systemically and in genital secretions has been firmly established in a recent trial in Burkina Faso which showed that HSV suppression therapy with valacyclovir significantly reduced genital and plasma HIV-1 RNA level in women who are coinfected with HSV-2 and HIV-1 (Nagot *et al.*, 2007). Randomized clinical trials (RCTs) testing the hypotheses that HSV-2 suppression will reduce risk of HIV transmission and acquisition are underway.

In terms of nonulcerative STIs, several studies have shown significantly increased risk in the acquisition of HIV in the presence of gonorrhea, chlamydia, trichomoniasis, and bacterial vaginosis (Plummer *et al.*, 1991; Laga *et al.*, 1993; Craib *et al.*, 1995; Sewankambo *et al.*, 1997; Taha *et al.*, 1998). These data and others led to four community-level RCTs conducted in Mwanza, Tanzania; Rakai, Uganda; Masaka, Uganda; and Manicaland, Zimbabwe to see the effect of STI treatment on HIV transmission. The study in Mwanza showed a 38% reduction in HIV incidence among those receiving the intervention to prevent STIs when compared with the nonintervention group (Grosskurth *et al.*, 1995); however, none of the other three studies was able to demonstrate a positive impact of STI treatment on HIV transmission (Wawer *et al.*, 1999; Kamali *et al.*, 2003). The main explanation for these discordant findings is that Mwanza represented a community that was in an early phase of the HIV epidemic, while the other three communities were in a more mature phase of the epidemic (Korenromp *et al.*, 2005). Therefore, new HIV epidemics characterized by high-risk behavior may benefit significantly more from interventions than HIV epidemics in a more mature phase.

Vaginal microbicides targeting STIs and HIV have also been evaluated for a protective effect against HIV transmission. Nonoxynol-9 has been studied in several RCTs, and to date, none has shown any benefit against HIV transmission (Kreiss *et al.*, 1992; Wilkinson *et al.*, 2002). In fact, some of these studies have demonstrated increased risk of HIV transmission among those women using the microbicide, probably secondary to increased genital inflammation and ulceration. Such risks are being closely monitored in ongoing RCTs examining other microbicides to determine their impact on HIV transmission.

Hormonal contraception is another potential risk factor for HIV acquisition that has been extensively studied. Hormonal contraception could increase a woman's susceptibility via hormonally induced changes in the vaginal mucosa or through associated cervical ectopy (Chao *et al.*, 1994; Daly *et al.*, 1994; Sinei *et al.*, 1996). However, recent studies, including a trial following 6109 women in Uganda, Zimbabwe, and Thailand, have not found an association between hormonal contraceptive use and HIV acquisition (Mati *et al.*, 1995; Morrison *et al.*, 2007; Myer *et al.*, 2007).

Increased transmission rates have also been associated with specific sexual practices and several partnership factors. The different modes of sexual intercourse differ in their efficiency of HIV transmission, with anal intercourse having the highest rates of transmission, followed by vaginal, and then oral sex (Royce *et al.*, 1997). In addition, traumatic sex (fisting, rape), sex while under the influence of alcohol or cocaine, sex during menses, sex during pregnancy, the use of vaginal desiccants, and the use of vaginal tightening agents have been associated with increased HIV transmission risk in several studies (Lazzarin *et al.*, 1991; Henin *et al.*, 1993; Seidlin *et al.*, 1993). Partnership factors that increase HIV transmission risk include high number of partners, high frequency of sexual contact, and concurrency. Concurrency is a partnership timing factor defined as being engaged in more than one sexual relationship at a single time point. In contrast, serial monogamy occurs when each partnership ends before the start of the next sexual relationship (Morris and Kretzschmar, 1997).

One important intervention to prevent HIV transmission is condom use. In several longitudinal studies, consistent condom use was 80–87% effective in preventing HIV transmission (Davis and Weller, 1999; Weller and Davis, 2002). Condom use is also associated with decreased transmission of gonorrhea, chlamydia, and HSV-2, all important HIV risk factors (Shafii *et al.*, 2004). Despite these compelling data, increasing condom use within at-risk populations has been a challenge. Several behavioral studies designed to reduce risky behavior and increase condom use have had no impact on HIV incidence (Hearst and Chen, 2004).

Strong data also support circumcision of adult men as a means to protect against HIV transmission. A number of observational studies have demonstrated a significant association between male circumcision and HIV transmission (Quinn *et al.*, 2000). These were recently validated in three large clinical trials, which randomized men to circumcision or no circumcision. One biological explanation is that keratinization of the glans when circumcised prevents tears and abrasions and decreases the presence of Langerhans cells and other HIV target cells (Quinn, 2006). The first RCT was completed in South Africa and showed 60% protection against HIV infection in the intention to treat analysis and 75% protection in the per protocol analysis (Auvert *et al.*, 2005). Two other concurrent RCTs in Kenya and Uganda were recently published and confirmed that male circumcision reduced HIV incidence in men with similar risk reduction as the RCT in South Africa (Bailey *et al.*, 2007; Gray *et al.*, 2007).

Transmission via Injection Drug Use (IDU)

HIV transmission from IDU accounts for 15–25% of HIV infection globally and approximately one-third of HIV infection outside sub-Saharan Africa. The rate of HIV transmission for IDU is 0.0067 per exposure (see **Figure 5**) (Kaplan and Heimer, 1992). The majority of HIV-infected intravenous drug users live in Southern China, East Asia, the Russian Federation, and the Middle East. In some regions, such as Eastern Europe and Central Asia, approximately 80% of incident HIV cases result from IDU (UNAIDS/WHO, 2006). As there are approximately 13 million intravenous drug users globally, and 8.8 million in Eastern Europe and Asia, HIV prevention efforts targeting IDU are essential in curbing the rapid spread of HIV in these regions.

The greatest risk factor for HIV transmission via IDU is the use of contaminated syringes, needles, and other paraphernalia. This is most often associated with the practice of sharing drug paraphernalia, which can occur for cultural, social, legal, or economic reasons. Sharing with multiple injection partners is an added risk factor. This can take place at sites where drugs are sold and injection equipment is made available for rental, such as in 'shooting galleries' (Marmor *et al.*, 1987). Practices that increase risk when sharing include backloading, frontloading, and booting. The first two occur when a drug solution is squirted from a donor syringe into another by removing the plunger (backloading) or needle (frontloading) from the receiving syringe. Booting is the practice of repeatedly drawing blood into the syringe and mixing it with drug.

In addition to drug practices, the type of drug may be important. The use of cocaine has shown higher risk of HIV transmission when compared to heroin (Anthony *et al.*, 1991), perhaps due to the need for more injection frequency and also the more frequent practice of booting in cocaine drug injection. Also, cocaine is associated with high-risk sexual practices.

Another risk factor that is intimately linked with IDU is commercial sex work (Astemborski *et al.*, 1994). Drug users often have to fund their habits by working as sex workers and drug-using commercial workers are less likely to use condoms than nonintravenous drug users.

HIV epidemics in China, Indonesia, Kazakhstan, Ukraine, Uzbekistan, and Vietnam are fueled by the overlap of commercial sex work and IDU (UNAIDS/WHO, 2006).

One way to decrease the risk of HIV transmission among intravenous drug users is through cessation of drug injection. Methadone or buprenorphine replacement has been associated with a decrease in risk of HIV infection among users as a result of decreases in drug use (Sullivan *et al.*, 2005). However, pharmacotherapy has overall been unsuccessful in complete cessation of IDU (Amato *et al.*, 2004). Other methods to decrease the risk of HIV include syringe and needle exchange programs. These programs offer clean syringes and needles in exchange for used injection equipment, with the goal of decreasing needle and syringe sharing. Several studies in the United States, the United Kingdom, and the Netherlands have shown them to be effective (Buning *et al.*, 1988; Donoghoe *et al.*, 1989; Watters *et al.*, 1994). Despite studies that show decreased needle sharing, there has been much controversy surrounding these programs due to concerns that the programs are condoning drug use and may increase the prevalence of drug use by making syringes and needles more available. These concerns have not been validated in other studies in the United States, Britain, France, Sweden, and the Netherlands, which showed no increase in the prevalence of drug use in the setting of needle exchange (Brickner *et al.*, 1989; Oliver *et al.*, 1994; Paone and Des Jarlais, 1994). An additional benefit of needle exchange programs is that they provide an opportunity for counselors to educate drug users about preventive interventions.

Mother-to-Child Transmission

Vertical transmission rates in many developing countries remain as high as 10–20% even though the likelihood an HIV-1-infected mother will transmit HIV-1 to her infant has been reduced to less than 1% in the United States and Europe. As a result, more than 500 000 infant HIV infections occur each year in sub-Saharan Africa and other resource-limited settings (UNAIDS/WHO, 2006). Differences in transmission rates may be attributed in part to poor access and uptake of HIV diagnostic testing and prevention interventions in those regions with the highest HIV prevalence among women of reproductive age. A number of other factors, including infant feeding practices, rates of coinfections, and breast pathology, also contribute.

HIV may be transmitted from mother to infant during pregnancy (*in utero*), during delivery (intrapartum), or through breast-feeding. In the absence of antiretroviral therapy, the overall transmission rate among non-breast-feeders is approximately 15–30% (**Figure 6**). Among non-breast-feeding women, approximately two-thirds of mother-to-child HIV-1 transmission events occur during delivery when the baby passes through the birth canal and is exposed to infected maternal blood and genital secretions. The remaining infant infections are attributable to *in utero* transmission.

In resource-limited settings, the majority of HIV-1-infected women breast-feed their infants due to lack of clean water or safe alternatives to breast milk, or due to stigma associated with not breast-feeding in regions where breast-feeding is the norm. Consequently, overall rates of transmission in the absence of antiretroviral prophylaxis increase to 30–45% (John and Kreiss, 1996) and several studies suggest that breast milk exposure accounts for one-third to one-half of these transmission events. Transmission during the *in utero* and intrapartum periods contributes the remainder of infections in proportions similar to those among non-breast-feeders (see **Figure 6**).

Valuable data on breast milk transmission rates were collected in a randomized clinical trial of breast-feeding versus formula feeding in Kenya where 16% of infants acquired HIV-1 via breast milk during the 2-year study period (Nduati *et al.*, 2000). The proportion of transmission events attributable to breast-feeding was 44%. A subsequent meta-analysis of nine cohorts of HIV-1-infected breast-feeding mothers found similar results, reporting that the proportion of infant infections attributable to breast-feeding after the first month postpartum was 24–42% (Coutsoudis *et al.*, 2004). Risk of breast milk transmission after the first month appears to remain relatively constant over time, with transmission events continuing to accumulate with longer duration of breast-feeding (Coutsoudis *et al.*, 2004). During this period, the risk of infant HIV-1 acquisition per liter of breast milk ingested is similar to the risk of an unprotected sex act among heterosexual adults (Richardson *et al.*, 2003).

High maternal plasma HIV-1 RNA load has been consistently associated with increased transmission and is considered the most important predictor of vertical transmission risk (Dickover *et al.*, 1996). Several studies have demonstrated that reduction of HIV-1 viral load with antiretroviral drugs decreases overall rates of transmission, and this has become the mainstay of global prevention efforts. HIV-1 viremia is highest in the setting of advanced disease and is usually associated with severe

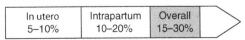

Breast-feeders

In utero 5–10%	Intrapartum 10–20%	Breast milk 10–20%	Overall 30–45%

Non-breast-feeders

In utero 5–10%	Intrapartum 10–20%	Overall 15–30%

Figure 6 Timing and absolute rates of vertical HIV-1 transmission.

immunosuppression. High HIV-1 levels also occur during acute HIV infection, a time when a woman may not realize she is at risk for transmitting HIV-1 to her child. This has been examined in one study of women acquiring HIV-1 postpartum which found that there was a twofold increased risk of transmitting HIV-1 via breast milk during acute HIV (Dunn and Newell, 1992).

In addition to HIV-1 viral load, several biological and behavioral factors contribute to increased transmission risk. Ascending bacterial infections that cause inflammation of the placenta, chorion, and amnion have been associated with increased *in utero* transmission in several observational studies (Taha and Gray, 2000). Sexually transmitted infections (STIs), such as syphilis and gonorrhea, are considered to increase risk of transmission via this mechanism (Mwapasa *et al.*, 2006), as well as chorioamnionitis resulting from infection with local vaginal or enteric flora. However, the role of chorioamnionitis was not confirmed in a randomized clinical trial of more than 2000 women comparing antibiotic treatment of ascending infections to placebo which found no difference in transmission events between the two arms (Taha *et al.*, 2006).

Other risk factors include infant gender and malarial infection of placental tissue, which has been inconsistently reported to increase mother-to-child HIV-1 transmission (Brentlinger *et al.*, 2006). Strong associations have been found between infant gender and *in utero* transmission in several cohorts (Galli *et al.*, 2005; Taha *et al.*, 2005; Biggar *et al.*, 2006). Female infants have a twofold increased risk of infection at birth when compared to male infants, perhaps because *in utero* mortality is higher for male HIV-1-infected infants than for females (Galli *et al.*, 2005; Taha *et al.*, 2005; Biggar *et al.*, 2006).

Risk factors influencing the intrapartum period include genital tract HIV-1 levels, genital ulcer disease, delivery complications, and breaks in the placental barrier that may cause maternal–fetal microtransfusions. Genital ulcer disease has been shown to increase mother-to-child HIV-1 transmission at least twofold, both in the presence and absence of antiretrovirals (John *et al.*, 2001; Chen *et al.*, 2005; Drake *et al.*, 2007). The majority of genital ulcers are caused by HSV-2, and in regions with high HIV-1 seroprevalence, HSV-2 seroprevalence is greater than 70% among women of reproductive age. Other risk factors for intrapartum transmission include prolonged duration of ruptured membranes and cervical or vaginal lacerations that occur during delivery. To restrict exposure to maternal HIV-1 in blood and mucosal secretions, cesarean section has been used effectively in many settings.

Two of the most important determinants of breast milk transmission risk are duration of breast-feeding and HIV-1 viral levels in breast milk. Introduction of food other than maternal milk may also exert an effect on HIV-1 transmission risk, potentially by compromising infant mucosal surfaces in the oropharynx and gut. Breast milk

viral load increases with increased plasma viremia and also as a result of local factors. These include breast inflammation resulting from mastitis, breast abscess, or other breast pathology, and inflammation within the breast milk compartment in the absence of clinical symptoms, which is known as subclincal mastitis (John *et al.*, 2001). Rates of subclinical mastitis are reported to be as high as 30% among HIV-1-infected breast-feeding women, and several studies have found it to be associated with increased HIV-1 levels in breast milk, as well as greater risk of infant HIV-1 acquisition (Willumsen *et al.*, 2003).

Transmission via Exposure to Blood Products

HIV transmission through blood transfusion and blood products has become rare after much progress in instituting careful screening and limiting the use of transfusions. Stringent screening of blood and blood products was a high priority at the start of the epidemic when it became known that transfusion with HIV-infected blood was an extremely efficient mode of transmission. In retrospective studies, approximately 90% of transfusion recipients were infected per single contaminated unit of blood (Donegan *et al.*, 1990), and 75–90% of recipients of Factor VIII concentrate acquired HIV (Caussy and Goedert, 1990).

In developed countries, blood product screening for HIV includes serologic and nucleic acid donor testing. In Canada, the estimated risk of HIV-infected donation being accepted was 1 per 7.8 million donations in the period from 2001 to 2005 (O'Brien *et al.*, 2007), and in the United States, the estimated risk of an HIV-infected donation being accepted was 1 per approximately 2.1 million donations in 2001 (Dodd *et al.*, 2002). While great strides have been made to improve the safety of the blood supply in many countries, antibody screening of blood donors is not universally done in many developing countries due to the lack of resources. In addition, some developing nations still rely on paid donors for their blood banks, and these paid donors have been shown to be at high risk for bloodborne infections (Volkow and Del Rio, 2005).

Occupational Exposure and HIV Transmission Risk

Health-care workers and laboratory personnel have a higher risk of HIV infection than individuals in other occupations. The average risk of HIV transmission is approximately 0.3% following percutaneous exposure to HIV-infected blood (see **Figure 5**) (Bell, 1997). Accidental percutaneous exposure carries the highest risk of subsequent infection and is the most important cause of occupational HIV transmission. Needlesticks are the most common cause of a percutaneous accident, and factors that increase transmission from a needlestick accident include deep puncture with a large-bore needle, larger quantity of blood, and exposure to blood from an HIV-infected individual with a high HIV viral load (Cox and Hodgson, 1988). Contaminated surgical instruments have also been associated with percutaneous injuries. Non-penetrating accidents that involve intact skin are far less risky. Retrospective data suggest that immediate initiation of effective antiretroviral drugs can decrease risk of acquiring HIV after an occupational exposure (Cardo *et al.*, 1997). Currently, recommended postexposure prophylaxis comprises a two- or three-drug antiretroviral regimen, depending on the nature and severity of the exposure (CDC, 2005).

Regional HIV Surveillance Data

The HIV epidemic has developed distinctly in different regions. Generalized epidemics occur when the general population HIV prevalence reaches 1% or more, and concentrated epidemics are described as an HIV prevalence of 5% or more in high-risk groups.

Sub-Saharan Africa: Overview

In 2006, HIV and AIDS continue to have a devastating effect on sub-Saharan Africa which is home to 24.7 million people living with HIV and 63% of all HIV-infected individuals in the world. Approximately 2.8 million people became newly infected in sub-Saharan Africa in 2006, and approximately 2.1 million people died from HIV in this same year. Women are more likely to be infected than men in this region, and 59% of all HIV-infected persons are estimated to be female (**Figure 7**) (UNAIDS/WHO, 2006).

Southern Africa

Within sub-Saharan Africa, Southern Africa has the highest burden of disease, accounting for 32% of HIV-infected individuals and 34% of AIDS deaths in the world. All countries of Southern Africa continue to increase in prevalence, except Zimbabwe, where HIV seroprevalence among adults has reduced to 20.1% from 22.1% in 2003. A decrease in HIV prevalence was reported in antenatal clinics in Zimbabwe from 30–32% in 2000 to 24% in 2004. Swaziland has the highest adult prevalence of HIV globally at 33.4%, and South Africa has the second greatest number of HIV-infected persons among all nations in the world after India. Across Southern Africa, the death rate from AIDS significantly increased in both men and women between 1997 and 2004, despite increased antiretroviral availability and use.

East Africa

Overall, HIV prevalence has been stabilizing or decreasing in this region of Africa. Kenya, Tanzania, and Rwanda have all shown a decline in prevalence over the last several years. In Kenya, adult HIV prevalence decreased from 10% in the late 1990s to approximately 6% in 2005 (Kenya Ministry of Health, 2005), and in Tanzania, adult HIV prevalence decreased from 8.1% to 6.5% between 1995 and 2004 (Somi *et al.*, 2006). There is concern that a similar trend may not continue in Uganda where there is a decrease in consistent condom use and increase in the number of men with more than one partner (Uganda Ministry of Health, 2006). In addition, there is concern that the growing number of intravenous drug users, especially in Kenya, Tanzania, and Zanzibar may significantly modify the course of the epidemic in these regions (Ndetei, 2004; Odek-Ogunde, 2004).

West and Central Africa

The epidemic has been less severe overall in West Africa compared to East and Southern Africa. There is declining HIV prevalence in Ghana, Cote d'Ivoire, and Burkina Faso; however, prevalence appears to be increasing in Mali (WHO, 2005). In Mali, the HIV seroprevalence using

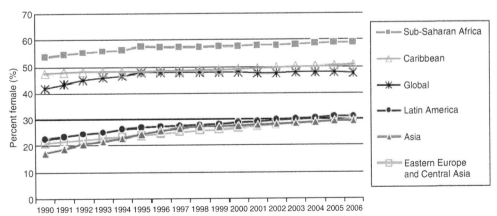

Figure 7   Percent of adults greater than 15 years of age living with HIV who are female, 1990–2006. Reproduced with kind permission from UNAIDS/WHO (2007) *AIDS Epidemic Update 2006*. Geneva: UNAIDS/WHO.

antenatal clinic data has increased from 3.3% in 2002 to 4.1% in 2005. In Nigeria, which is known to have the third largest number of HIV-infected persons in the world, as a result of its large population, HIV prevalence appears to have stabilized at approximately 4.4% in 2005.

Asia: Overview

In 2006, there were 8.6 million people infected with HIV in Asia. Of these, 960 000 people were newly HIV-infected in 2006, and approximately 630 000 people died from AIDS. Compared to countries in sub-Saharan Africa, seroprevalence in most Asian countries is lower; however, generalized epidemics are found in Thailand, Cambodia, and Myanmar.

South-East Asia

South-East Asian countries have the highest HIV prevalence in Asia due to the commercial sex industry, widespread IDU, and transmission among men who have sex with men (MSM) (**Figure 8**). While the epidemic appears to be stabilizing in Thailand, Cambodia, and Myanmar, in Vietnam the number of infected individuals has almost doubled in number between 2000 and 2005. Despite the overall stabilizing trend in Thailand, there is a growing concern that the epidemic is increasing within the general population. One-third of newly infected individuals in 2005 were married women. In Cambodia, the stabilizing trend may have been partly due to behavioral changes in the commercial sex work industry. Consistent condom use increased from 53% to 96% among brothel-based sex workers in the major cities of Cambodia (Gorbach *et al.*, 2006) and this was followed by a decline in the HIV prevalence among sex workers from 43% to 21% between 1995 and 2003 (National Center for HIV/AIDS, 2004).

China

Currently, there are 650 000 people living with HIV in China, and approximately 45% of these individuals are intravenous drug users (China Ministry of Health, 2006). The epidemic initially occurred in rural provinces along the major drug trafficking routes, and major outbreaks from HIV-1 commercial plasma donors worsened the epidemic (Wu *et al.*, 2001). Sexual transmission has further fueled the spread of HIV to urban areas in China, which from 1998 to 2005 experienced an exponential increase in new HIV cases (Wu *et al.*, 2007). New cases were estimated to climb from 3300 to 36 000 during this period, with a greater proportion due to sexual transmission in populations considered at lower risk. As a result, there is concern that the epidemic is now spreading from high-risk populations of intravenous drug users and commercial sex workers to the general population.

India

The second most populous nation, India, had approximately 5.7 million HIV-infected people in 2005, more than any other country in the world. Most of these reported HIV cases are concentrated in 6 of the 28 states of India where transmission is occurring through unprotected heterosexual intercourse. Among those infected, 38% are women and HIV prevalence among women from 206 antenatal clinics has declined from 1.7% in 2000 to 1.1% in 2004 (Kumar *et al.*, 2006). The epidemics in the northeast part of India are mainly due to IDU.

Eastern Europe and Central Asia

Currently, there are 1.7 million people living with HIV in Eastern Europe and Central Asia, where new cases of

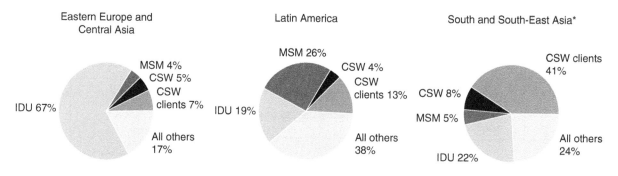

IDU: Injecting drug users
MSM: Men having sex with men
CSW: Commercial sex workers

* India was omitted from this analysis because the scale of its HIV epidemic (which is largely heterosexual) masks the extent to which other at-risk populations feature in the region's epidemics.

Figure 8   Proportions of HIV infections in different population groups by region, 2005. Reproduced with kind permission from UNAIDS/WHO (2007) *AIDS Epidemic Update 2006*. Geneva: UNAIDS/WHO.

HIV have grown significantly in the past decade and continue to increase. Ukraine and the Russian Federation comprise 90% of HIV infections of this region (EuroHIV, 2006), and approximately 80% of those infected in the Russian Federation are 15 to 30 years of age. The primary mode of transmission in this area is IDU, which makes up approximately 67% of cases in Eastern Europe and Central Asia (see **Figure 8**). However, the number of newly infected individuals through unprotected sex is also growing.

Latin America and the Caribbean

Approximately 250 000 people are living with HIV in the Caribbean. The epidemic was initially due to the commercial sex industry and eventually spread into the general population. In addition, 10% of those who are HIV-infected are MSM. The HIV infection rates have stabilized in the Caribbean, where Haiti and the Dominican Republic account for approximately 75% of HIV-infected cases.

In Latin America, the epidemic has stabilized overall with 1.7 million people living with HIV and approximately 140 000 new infections annually. The majority of the cases are due to unsafe IDU and MSM (see **Figure 8**), and more than 60% of HIV-infected persons reside in Argentina, Brazil, Colombia, and Mexico. There has been much international praise for the efforts of the Brazilian government for HIV prevention and treatment efforts during the last decade.

North America, Western, and Central Europe

In North America and Western and Central Europe, the number of living HIV-infected persons is 2.1 million, a number that continues to increase. The United States accounts for 1.2 million people living with HIV, which places it among the 10 countries in the world with the highest number living with HIV or AIDS. This is because individuals with HIV are living longer as a result of increased use of antiretroviral drugs in these parts of the world. In North America and Western and Central Europe, there were 65 000 new infections and approximately 30 000 deaths from AIDS in 2006.

The main populations at risk in the United States and Europe are MSM and intravenous drug users. However, women, African-Americans, and immigrants are increasingly affected by the HIV epidemic. The proportion of women newly infected with HIV increased from 15% before 1995 to 27% in 2004 in the United States, and between 2001 and 2004, half of all AIDS diagnoses were in African-Americans. In 2004, African-Americans had a significantly higher risk of HIV infection than among Whites in the United States,

7 times greater in men and 21 times greater in women. In Western and Central Europe, three-quarters of all heterosexually acquired HIV are among migrants and immigrants (EuroHIV, 2006).

Middle and North Africa

There are an estimated 450 000 people living with HIV, with 68 000 newly infected, in Middle and North Africa. The major modes of transmission are IDU, commercial sex, and sex among MSM. In this region, Sudan is the only nation with a generalized epidemic with a prevalence of 1.6%. Other nations in this region have poor surveillance, and therefore it may be difficult to understand fully the nature of the epidemic. Greater efforts are needed to improve surveillance and access to high-risk populations to control the HIV epidemic.

Oceania

In Oceania, an estimated 81 000 persons were infected with HIV and 7100 were newly infected in 2006. Three-quarters of the infected in this region reside in Papua New Guinea, where prevalence has increased to 1.8%. Risk factors for transmission in Papua New Guinea include inconsistent condom use, sex with commercial sex workers, high rates of concurrent sexual relationships, early sexual initiation, high rates of sexual violence against women, and high rates of STIs (Brouwer *et al.*, 1998; Bank, 2006). In Australia and New Zealand, transmission among MSM continues to drive the epidemic, accounting for 66% and 90% of all new HIV cases, respectively.

Citations

Abbott RC, NDour-Sarr A, Diouf A, *et al.* (1994) Risk factors for HIV-1 and HIV-2 infection in pregnant women in Dakar, Senegal. *Journal of Acquired Immune Deficiency Syndromes* 7: 711–717.

Adjorlolo-Johnson G, De Cock KM, Ekpini E, *et al.* (1994) Prospective comparison of mother-to-child transmission of HIV-1 and HIV-2 in Abidjan, Ivory Coast. *Journal of the American Medical Association* 272: 462–466.

Alaeus A, Lidman K, Bjorkman A, Giesecke J, and Albert J (1999) Similar rate of disease progression among individuals infected with HIV-1 genetic subtypes A-D. *AIDS* 13: 901–907.

Amato L, Minozzi S, Davoli M, Vecchi S, Ferri M, and Mayet S (2004) Psychosocial combined with agonist maintenance treatments versus agonist maintenance treatments alone for treatment of opioid dependence. *Cochrane Database of Systematic Reviews* 4, CD004147.

Andreasson PA, Dias F, Naucler A, Andersson S, and Biberfeld G (1993) A prospective study of vertical transmission of HIV-2 in Bissau, Guinea-Bissau. *AIDS* 7: 989–993.

Anthony JC, Vlahov D, Nelson KE, Cohn S, Astemborski J, and Solomon L (1991) New evidence on intravenous cocaine use and the risk of infection with human immunodeficiency virus type 1. *American Journal of Epidemiology* 134: 1175–1189.

Asian Development Bank (2006) www.adb.org/Documents/RRPs/PNG/39033-PNG-RRP.pdf (accessed April 2008).

Astemborski J, Vlahov D, Warren D, Solomon L, and Nelson KE (1994) The trading of sex for drugs or money and HIV seropositivity among female intravenous drug users. *American Journal of Public Health* 84: 382–387.

Auvert B, Taljaard D, Lagarde E, Sobngwi-Tambekou J, Sitta R, and Puren A (2005) Randomized, controlled intervention trial of male circumcision for reduction of HIV infection risk: The ANRS 1265 Trial. *Public Library of Science Medicine* 2: e298.

Baeten JM, Chohan B, Lavreys L, et al. (2007) HIV-1 Subtype D Infection Is Associated with Faster Disease Progression than Subtype A in Spite of Similar Plasma HIV-1 Loads. *Journal of Infectious Diseases* 195: 1177–1180.

Baeten JM and Overbaugh J (2003) Measuring the infectiousness of persons with HIV-1: opportunities for preventing sexual HIV-1 transmission. *Current HIV Research* 1: 69–86.

Bailey RC, Moses S, Parker CB, et al. (2007) Male circumcision for HIVprevention in young men in Kisumu, Kenya: a randomised controlled trial. *The Lancet* 369: 643–656.

Barin F, M'Boup S, Denis F, et al. (1985) Serological evidence for virus related to simian T-lymphotropic retrovirus III in residents of west Africa. *The Lancet* 2: 1387–1389.

Bell DM (1997) Occupational risk of human immunodeficiency virus infection in healthcare workers: an overview. *American Journal of Medicine* 102: 9–15.

Biggar RJ, Taha TE, Hoover DR, Yellin F, Kumwenda N, and Broadhead R (2006) Higher in utero and perinatal HIV infection risk in girls than boys. *Journal of Acquired Immune Deficiency Syndrome* 41: 509–513.

Brentlinger PE, Behrens CB, and Micek MA (2006) Challenges in the concurrent management of malaria and HIV in pregnancy in sub-Saharan Africa. *The Lancet Infectious Diseases* 6: 100–111.

Brickner PW, Torres RA, Barnes M, et al. (1989) Recommendations for control and prevention of human immunodeficiency virus (HIV) infection in intravenous drug users. *Annals of Internal Medicine* 110: 833–837.

Brouwer EC, Harris BM, and Tanaka S (1998) *Gender Analysis in Papua, New Guinea*. Washington, DC: World Bank.

Buning EC, van Brussel GH, and van Santen G (1988) Amsterdam's drug policy and its implications for controlling needle sharing. *NIDA Research Monographs* 80: 59–74.

Burke DS, McCutchan FE, and Francine E (1997) *Global Distribution of Human Immunodeficiency Virus-1 Clades*. Philadelphia, PA: Lippincott-Raven.

Cameron DW, Simonsen JN, D'Costa LJ, et al. (1989) Female to male transmission of human immunodeficiency virus type 1: risk factors for seroconversion in men. *The Lancet* 2: 403–407.

Cardo DM, Culver DH, Ciesielski CA, et al. (1997) A case-control study of HIV seroconversion in health care workers after percutaneous exposure. Centers for Disease Control and Prevention Needlestick Surveillance Group. *New England Journal of Medicine* 337: 1485–1490.

Caussy D and Goedert JJ (1990) The epidemiology of human immunodeficiency virus and acquired immunodeficiency syndrome. *Seminars in Oncology* 17: 244–250.

Center for Disease Control (2005) Updated U.S. Public Health Service Guidelines for the Management of Occupational Exposures to HIV and Recommendations for Postexposure Prophylaxis. *MMWR* 1–17.

Chao A, Bulterys M, Musanganire F, et al. (1994) Risk factors associated with prevalent HIV-1 infection among pregnant women in Rwanda. National University of Rwanda-Johns Hopkins University AIDS Research Team. *International Journal of Epidemiology* 23: 371–380.

Chen KT, Segu M, Lumey LH, et al. (2005) Genital herpes simplex virus infection and perinatal transmission of human immunodeficiency virus. *Obstetrics and Gynecology* 106: 1341–1348.

China Ministry of Health (MoH) (2006) 2005 update on the HIV/AIDS epidemic and response in China, ed. China MoH. UNAIDS Beijing, China: WHO.

Coutsoudis A, Dabis F, Fawzi W, et al. (2004) Late postnatal transmission of HIV-1 in breast-fed children: an individual patient data meta-analysis. *Journal of Infectious Diseases* 189: 2154–2166.

Cox J and Hodgson L (1988) Hepatitis B, AIDS and the neurological pin. *Medical Education* 22: 83.

Craib KJ, Meddings DR, Strathdee SA, et al. (1995) Rectal gonorrhoea as an independent risk factor for HIV infection in a cohort of homosexual men. *Genitourinary Medicine* 71: 150–154.

Daly CC, Helling-Giese GE, Mati JK, and Hunter DJ (1994) Contraceptive methods and the transmission of HIV: implications for family planning. *Genitourinary Medicine* 70: 110–117.

Davis KR and Weller SC (1999) The effectiveness of condoms in reducing heterosexual transmission of HIV. *Family Planning Perspectives* 31: 272–279.

Dickover RE, Garratty EM, Herman SA, et al. (1996) Identification of levels of maternal HIV-1 RNA associated with risk of perinatal transmission. Effect of maternal zidovudine treatment on viral load. *Journal of the American Medical Association* 275: 599–605.

Dodd RY, Notari EPt, and Stramer SL (2002) Current prevalence and incidence of infectious disease markers and estimated window-period risk in the American Red Cross blood donor population. *Transfusion* 42: 975–979.

Donegan E, Stuart M, Niland JC, et al. (1990) Infection with human immunodeficiency virus type 1 (HIV-1) among recipients of antibody-positive blood donations. *Annals of Internal Medicine* 113: 733–739.

Donoghoe MC, Stimson GV, Dolan K, and Alldritt L (1989) Changes in HIV risk behaviour in clients of syringe-exchange schemes in England and Scotland. *AIDS* 3: 267–272.

Drake AL, John-Stewart GC, Wald A, et al. (2007) Herpes simplex virus type 2 and risk of intrapartum human immunodeficiency virus transmission. *Obstetrics and Gynecology* 109: 403–409.

Dunn D and Newell ML (1992) Vertical transmission of HIV. *The Lancet* 339: 364–365.

EuroHIV (2006) *HIV/AIDS Surveillance in Europe: End-year Report 2005* vol. 73. Saint-Maurice: Institutde Veille Sanitaire.

Freeman EE, Weiss HA, Glynn JR, Cross PL, Whitworth JA, and Hayes RJ (2006) Herpes simplex virus 2 infection increases HIV acquisition in men and women: systematic review and meta-analysis of longitudinal studies. *AIDS* 20: 73–83.

Galli L, Puliti D, Chiappini E, et al. (2005) Lower mother-to-child HIV-1 transmission in boys is independent of type of delivery and antiretroviral prophylaxis: the Italian Register for HIV Infection in Children. *Journal of Acquired Immune Deficiency Syndrome* 40: 479–485.

Gilbert PB, McKeague IW, Eisen G, et al. (2003) Comparison of HIV-1 and HIV-2 infectivity from a prospective cohort study in Senegal. *Statistics in Medicine* 22: 573–593.

Gorbach PM, Sopheab H, Chhorvann C, Weiss RE, and Vun MC (2006) Changing behaviors and patterns among Cambodian sex workers: 1997–2003. *Journal of Acquired Immune Deficiency Syndrome* 42: 242–247.

Gray RH, Wawer MJ, Brookmeyer R, et al. (2001) Probability of HIV-1 transmission per coital act in monogamous, heterosexual, HIV-1 discordant couples in Rakai, Uganda. *The Lancet* 357: 1149–1153.

Gray RH, Kigozi G, Serwadda D, et al. (2007) Male circumcision for HIV prevention in men in Rakai, Uganda: a randomised trial. *The Lancet* 369: 657–666.

Grosskurth H, Mosha F, Todd J, et al. (1995) Impact of improved treatment of sexually transmitted diseases on HIV infection in rural Tanzania: randomised controlled trial. *The Lancet* 346: 530–536.

Hearst N and Chen S (2004) Condom promotion for AIDS prevention in the developing world: is it working? *Studies in Family Planning* 35: 39–47.

Henin Y, Mandelbrot L, Henrion R, Pradinaud R, Coulaud JP, and Montagnier L (1993) Virus excretion in the cervicovaginal secretions of pregnant and nonpregnant HIV-infected women. *Journal of Acquired Immune Deficiency Syndrome* 6: 72–75.

John GC and Kreiss J (1996) Mother-to-child transmission of human immunodeficiency virus type 1. *Epidemiologic Reviews* 18: 149–157.

John GC, Nduati RW, Mbori-Ngacha DA, et al. (2001) Correlates of mother-to-child human immunodeficiency virus type 1 (HIV-1) transmission: association with maternal plasma HIV-1 RNA load, genital HIV-1 DNA shedding, and breast infections. *Journal of Infectious Diseases* 183: 206–212.

Kaleebu P, Ross A, Morgan D, *et al.* (2001) Relationship between HIV-1 Env subtypes A and D and disease progression in a rural Ugandan cohort. *AIDS* 15: 293–299.

Kamali A, Quigley M, Nakiyingi J, *et al.* (2003) Syndromic management of sexually-transmitted infections and behaviour change interventions on transmission of HIV-1 in rural Uganda: a community randomised trial. *The Lancet* 361: 645–652.

Kanki P (1997) *Epidemiology and Natural History of Human Immunodeficiency Virus Type 2*. Philadelphia, PA: Lippincott-Raven.

Kanki PJ, Travers KU, S MB, *et al.* (1994) Slower heterosexual spread of HIV-2 than HIV-1. *The Lancet* 343: 943–946.

Kaplan EH and Heimer R (1992) A model-based estimate of HIV infectivity via needle sharing. *Journal of Acquired Immune Deficiency Syndrome* 5: 1116–1118.

Kenya Ministry of Health (MoH) (2005) AIDS in Kenya. 7th edn, ed. (NASCOP) NAaSCP Nairobi, Kenya: Ministry of Health Kenya.

Korenromp EL, White RG, Orroth KK, *et al.* (2005) Determinants of the impact of sexually transmitted infection treatment on prevention of HIV infection: a synthesis of evidence from the Mwanza, Rakai, and Masaka intervention trials. *Journal of Infectious Disease* 191 (supplement 1): S168–S178.

Kreiss J, Ngugi E, Holmes K, *et al.* (1992) Efficacy of nonoxynol 9 contraceptive sponge use in preventing heterosexual acquisition of HIV in Nairobi prostitutes. *Journal of the American Medical Association* 268: 477–482.

Kumar R, Jha P, Arora P, *et al.* (2006) Trends in HIV-1 in young adults in south India from 2000 to 2004: a prevalence study. *The Lancet* 367: 1164–1172.

Laga M, Manoka A, Kivuvu M, *et al.* (1993) Non-ulcerative sexually transmitted diseases as risk factors for HIV-1 transmission in women: results from a cohort study. *AIDS* 7: 95–102.

Lazzarin A, Saracco A, Musicco M, and Nicolosi A (1991) Man-to-woman sexual transmission of the human immunodeficiency virus. Risk factors related to sexual behavior, man's infectiousness, and woman's susceptibility. Italian Study Group on HIV Heterosexual Transmission. *Archives of Internal Medicine* 151: 2411–2416.

Marlink R, Kanki P, Thior I, *et al.* (1994) Reduced rate of disease development after HIV-2 infection as compared to HIV-1. *Science* 265: 1587–1590.

Marmor M, DesJarlais DC, Cohen H, *et al.* (1987) Risk factors for infection with human immunodeficiency virus among intravenous drug abusers in New York City. *AIDS* 1: 39–44.

Mati JK, Hunter DJ, Maggwa BN, and Tukei PM (1995) Contraceptive use and the risk of HIV infection in Nairobi, Kenya. *International Journal of Gynaecology and Obstetrics* 48: 61–67.

McCutchan FE (2000) Understanding the genetic diversity of HIV-1. *AIDS* 14(supplement 3): S31–S44.

McCutchan FE (2006) Global epidemiology of HIV. *Journal of Medical Virology* 78(supplement 1): S7–S12.

Morris M and Kretzschmar M (1997) Concurrent partnerships and the spread of HIV. *AIDS* 11: 641–648.

Morrison CS, Richardson BA, Mmiro F, *et al.* (2007) Hormonal contraception and the risk of HIV acquisition. *AIDS* 21: 85–95.

Mullins C, Eisen G, Popper S, *et al.* (2004) Highly active antiretroviral therapy and viral response in HIV type 2 infection. *Clinical Infectious Diseases* 38: 1771–1779.

Mwapasa V, Rogerson SJ, Kwiek JJ, *et al.* (2006) Maternal syphilis infection is associated with increased risk of mother-to-child transmission of HIV in Malawi. *AIDS* 20: 1869–1877.

Myer L, Denny L, Wright TC, and Kuhn L (2007) Prospective study of hormonal contraception and women's risk of HIV infection in South Africa. *International Journal of Epidemiology* 36: 166–174.

Nagot N, Ouedraogo A, Foulongne V, *et al.* (2007) Reduction of HIV-1 RNA levels with therapy to suppress herpes simplex virus. *New England Journal of Medicine* 356: 790–799.

National Center for HIV/AIDS Dermatology and STDs (2004) *HIV Sentinel Surveillance (HSS) in Cambodia, 2003*. Phnom Penh, Camodia: National Center for HIV/AIDS Dermatology and STDs.

Ndetei D (2004) Study on the assessment of the linkages between drug abuse, injecting drug abuse and HIV/AIDS in Kenya: a rapid situation assessment 2004. Nairobi, Kenya: United Nations Office on Drugs and Crime.

Nduati R, John G, Mbori-Ngacha D, *et al.* (2000) Effect of breastfeeding and formula feeding on transmission of HIV-1: a randomized clinical trial. *Journal of the American Medical Association* 283: 1167–1174.

Neilson JR, John GC, Carr JK, *et al.* (1999) Subtypes of human immunodeficiency virus type 1 and disease stage among women in Nairobi, Kenya. *Journal of Virology* 73: 4393–4403.

Nelson KE, Celentano DD, Suprasert S, *et al.* (1993) Risk factors for HIV infection among young adult men in northern Thailand. *Journal of the American Medical Association* 270: 955–960.

Nopkesorn T, Mastro TD, Sangkharomya S, *et al.* (1993) HIV-1 infection in young men in northern Thailand. *AIDS* 7: 1233–1239.

O'Brien SF, Yi QL, Fan W, Scalia V, Kleinman SH, and Vamvakas EC (2007) Current incidence and estimated residual risk of transfusion-transmitted infections in donations made to Canadian Blood Services. *Transfusion* 47: 316–325.

O'Donovan D, Ariyoshi K, Milligan P, *et al.* (2000) Maternal plasma viral RNA levels determine marked differences in mother-to-child transmission rates of HIV-1 and HIV-2 in The Gambia. MRC/Gambia Government/University College London Medical School working group on mother-child transmission of HIV. *AIDS* 14: 441–448.

Odek-Ogunde M (2004) World Health Organization phase II drug injecting study: behavioural and seroprevalence (HIV, HBV, HCV) survey among injecting drug users in Nairobi. Nairobi, Kenya: WHO.

Oliver KMS, Friedman S, Maynrd H, *et al.* (1994) *Behavioral and Community Impact of the Portland Syringe Exchange Program*. Washington, DC: National Academy Press.

Otten MW Jr, Zaidi AA, Peterman TA, Rolfs RT, and Witte JJ (1994) High rate of HIV seroconversion among patients attending urban sexually transmitted disease clinics. *AIDS* 8: 549–553.

Paone D, Des Jarlais DC, *et al.* (1994) *New York City Syringe Exchange: An Overview*. Washington, DC: National Academy Press.

Pedraza MA, del Romero J, and Roldan F (1999) Heterosexual transmission of HIV-1 is associated with high plasma viral load levels and a positive viral isolation in the infected partner. *Journal of Acquired Immune Deficiency Syndrome* 21: 120–125.

Pichova I, Weber J, Litera J, *et al.* (1997) Peptide inhibitors of HIV-1 and HIV-2 proteases: a comparative study. *Leukemia* 11(supplement 3): 120–122.

Plummer FA, Simonsen JN, Cameron DW, *et al.* (1991) Cofactors in male-female sexual transmission of human immunodeficiency virus type 1. *Journal of Infectious Diseases* 163: 233–239.

Quinn TC (2006) Male circumcision as a preventive measure limiting HIV transmission. *Retrovirology* 3(supplement 1): S109.

Quinn TC, Wawer MJ, Sewankambo N, *et al.* (2000) Viral load and heterosexual transmission of human immunodeficiency virus type 1. Rakai Project Study Group. *New England Journal of Medicine* 342: 921–929.

Richardson BA, John-Stewart GC, Hughes JP, *et al.* (2003) Breast-milk infectivity in human immunodeficiency virus type 1-infected mothers. *Journal of Infectious Disease* 187: 736–740.

Royce RA, Sena A, Cates W Jr., and Cohen MS (1997) Sexual transmission of HIV. *New England Journal of Medicine* 336: 1072–1078.

Seidlin M, Vogler M, Lee E, Lee YS, and Dubin N (1993) Heterosexual transmission of HIV in a cohort of couples in New York City. *AIDS* 7: 1247–1254.

Sewankambo N, Gray RH, Wawer MJ, *et al.* (1997) HIV-1 infection associated with abnormal vaginal flora morphology and bacterial vaginosis. *The Lancet* 350: 546–550.

Shafii T, Stovel K, Davis R, and Holmes K (2004) Is condom use habit forming?: Condom use at sexual debut and subsequent condom use. *Sexually Transmitted Diseases* 31: 366–372.

Sinei SK, Fortney JA, Kigondu CS, *et al.* (1996) Contraceptive use and HIV infection in Kenyan family planning clinic attenders. *International Journal of STD and AIDS* 7: 65–70.

Somi GR, Matee MI, Swai RO, *et al.* (2006) Estimating and projecting HIV prevalence and AIDS deaths in Tanzania using antenatal surveillance data. *BMC Public Health* 6: 120.

Sullivan LE, Metzger DS, Fudala PJ, and Fiellin DA (2005) Decreasing international HIV transmission: the role of expanding access to opioid agonist therapies for injection drug users. *Addiction* 100: 150–158.

Taha TE, Brown ER, Hoffman IF, *et al.* (2006) A phase III clinical trial of antibiotics to reduce chorioamnionitis-related perinatal HIV-1 transmission. *AIDS* 20: 1313–1321.

Taha TE and Gray RH (2000) Genital tract infections and perinatal transmission of HIV. *Annals of the New York Academy of Science* 918: 84–98.

Taha TE, Hoover DR, Dallabetta GA, *et al.* (1998) Bacterial vaginosis and disturbances of vaginal flora: association with increased acquisition of HIV. *AIDS* 12: 1699–1706.

Taha TE, Nour S, Kumwenda NI, *et al.* (2005) Gender differences in perinatal HIV acquisition among African infants. *Pediatrics* 115: e167–e172.

Uganda Ministry of Health (MoH) (2006) Uganda HIV/AIDS Sero-behavioural Survey 2004/2005, Ministry of Health and ORC Macro, ed. Calverton, MD: Ministry of Health and ORC Macro.

UNAIDS/WHO (2006) *AIDS Epidemic Update 2006.* Geneva, Switzerland: UNAIDS/WHO.

Vittinghoff E, Douglas J, Judson F, McKirnan D, MacQueen K, and Buchbinder SP (1999) Per-contact risk of human immunodeficiency virus transmission between male sexual partners. *American Journal of Epidemiology* 150: 306–311.

Volkow P and Del Rio C (2005) Paid donation and plasma trade: unrecognized forces that drive the AIDS epidemic in developing countries. *International Journal of STD and AIDS* 16: 5–8.

Wald A (2004) Synergistic interactions between herpes simplex virus type-2 and human immunodeficiency virus epidemics. *Herpes* 11: 70–76.

Watters JK, Estilo MJ, Clark GL, and Lorvick J (1994) Syringe and needle exchange as HIV/AIDS prevention for injection drug users. *Journal of the American Medical Association* 271: 115–120.

Wawer MJ, Gray RH, Sewankambo NK, *et al.* (2005) Rates of HIV-1 transmission per coital act, by stage of HIV-1 infection, in Rakai, Uganda. *Journal of Infectious Disease* 191: 1403–1409.

Wawer MJ, Sewankambo NK, Serwadda D, *et al.* (1999) Control of sexually transmitted diseases for AIDS prevention in Uganda: a randomised community trial. Rakai Project Study Group. *The Lancet* 353: 525–535.

Weller S and Davis K (2002) Condom effectiveness in reducing heterosexual HIV transmission. *Cochrane Database Systemic Reviews* 3, CD003255.

WHO (2005) HIV/AIDS epidemiological surveillance report for the WHO African region-2005 update. Harare, Zimbabwe: WHO Regional Office for Africa.

Wilkinson D, Tholandi M, Ramjee G, and Rutherford GW (2002) Nonoxynol-9 spermicide for prevention of vaginally acquired HIV and other sexually transmitted infections: systematic review and meta-analysis of randomised controlled trials including more than 5000 women. *The Lancet Infectious Diseases* 2: 613–617.

Willumsen JF, Filteau SM, Coutsoudis A, *et al.* (2003) Breastmilk RNA viral load in HIV-infected South African women: effects of subclinical mastitis and infant feeding. *AIDS* 17: 407–414.

Witvrouw M, Pannecouque C, VanLaethem K, Desmyter J, DeClercq E, and Vandamme AM (1999) Activity of non-nucleoside reverse transcriptase inhibitors against HIV-2 and SIV. *AIDS* 13: 1477–1483.

Wu Z, Rou K, and Detels R (2001) Prevalence of HIV infection among former commercial plasma donors in rural eastern China. *Health Policy Plan* 16: 41–46.

Wu Z, Sullivan SG, Wang Y, Rotheram-Borus MJ, and Detels R (2007) Evolution of China's response to HIV/AIDS. *The Lancet* 369: 679–690.

Relevant Websites

http://www.aidsinfo.nih.gov – AIDSinfo, HIV/AIDS Treatment Information, Department of Human and Health Services Guidelines.

http://www.cdc.gov – Centers for Disease Control and Prevention (CDC).

http://www.hivma.org/Content.aspx?id=1922 – HIV Medicine Association (HIVMA) Practice Guidelines.

http://www.unaids.org – Joint United Nations Programme on HIV/AIDS (UNAIDS).

http://www.iasusa.org/pub/arv_2006.pdf – *Treatment for Adult HIV Infection: 2006 Recommendations of the International AIDS Society – USA Panel.*

Epidemiology of Influenza

P V Targonski, Mayo Clinic and University of Minnesota, Rochester, MN, USA
G A Poland, Mayo Clinic, Rochester, MN, USA

Introduction

Influenza, or 'flu,' is an acute, seasonally occurring respiratory illness that has a global reach and is thought to have been described by Hippocrates in 412 BC in his *Of the Epidemics.* The name 'influenza' came about in the Middle Ages as a derivation of the Latin *coeli influenza,* which referred to the belief that the illness was the result of celestial influences. Later it was attributed to exposure to the cold. The English used influenza to describe a European outbreak in the mid-1700s, but European and other geographic outbreaks had clearly occurred prior to that time (Potter, 2001). An example of the global reach of this illness was observed in CE 1580, when it spread from Asia to Africa and Europe and then to America.

History of Viral Isolation and Viral Characteristics

Influenza illness in humans is, of course, not caused by astrological influences or evil humors but rather by influenzavirus A and influenzavirus B – both single-stranded RNA viruses from the virus family Orthomyxoviridae (Wright and Webster, 2001). Influenzavirus C can cause infection in children, but the magnitude of clinically relevant infection rates from influenza C overall is relatively insignificant when compared with influenza A and B (**Table 1**). Richard Pfeiffer isolated *Haemophilus influenzae* in 1892, and it was commonly accepted that this organism caused influenza because it was frequently found in the throats of influenza victims from the Russian flu (1889–1890) and Spanish flu (1918–1919) outbreaks. It has since been recognized that this organism reflected a bacterial super-infection. In the 1920s, Richard Shope demonstrated that a swine form of influenza could be transmitted to pigs through bronchial secretions of infected animals, and he proposed a virus as an etiologic agent for influenza illness. Subsequently, Smith, Andrewes, and Laidlaw isolated influenza virus from human influenza patients in 1933. Although this article focuses on influenza in humans, viral influenza can occur in birds, swine, horses, dogs, and other animals.

The classification of influenza into A, B, and C types is based on antigenic differences in nuclear material. Influenza A in particular exhibits a variety of subtypes based on differences in viral surface antigens: hemagglutinin (H) and neuraminidase (N). Varying combinations of H and N antigens make up the observed subtypes of influenza A (for example, H1N1 or H3N2). There are 16 recognized H antigens, 3 of which are usually associated with infections in humans (H1, H2, and H3), and 9 recognized N antigens, 2 of which are usually associated with infections in humans (N1 and N2). Antibody against one influenza virus type or subtype confers limited or no protection against another type or subtype of influenza (Smith *et al.*, 2006). Furthermore, antibody to one antigenic variant of influenza virus might not completely protect against a new antigenic variant of the same type or subtype.

Influenza strains are identified through surveillance by organizations such as the National Institute of Infectious Diseases (Japan), the National Institute for Medical Research (United Kingdom), the Centers for Disease Control and Prevention (CDC; United States), and globally by the U.S. Department of Defense and the World Health Organization (WHO). Any new strains are conventionally designated on the basis of virus type, the geographic area

from which the strain was identified, the strain number, and the year of identification, as well as the H and N antigen subtypes (see **Figure 1**).

For influenza viruses, the H and N antigens change over time, usually the result of point mutations in specific gene segments of the influenza A virus – so-called antigenic drift (**Figure 2**). Antigenic drift is a manifestation of natural selection pressures as host populations develop full or partial immunity to the virus, and drift can occur in influenza B and C as well (CDC, 2007). Antigenic drift can result in epidemic influenza, or influenza that results in cases and/or mortality in excess of expected amounts on a local, regional, or national level. Of course, recognition of epidemics requires a standard definition of 'normal' or 'expected' levels of disease, as well as surveillance. As an example, the CDC monitors influenza occurrence and mortality in the United States, and the severity of an influenza season is determined by excess pneumonia- and influenza-related deaths. The CDC also maintains influenza-related mortality surveillance through the 122 Cities Mortality Reporting System, which obtains weekly overall death data and influenza/pneumonia death data from 122 U.S. cities and metropolitan areas. An epidemic of influenza mortality is defined as 1.645 standard deviations above the expected seasonal baseline, which is established from the previous 5 years of influenza and pneumonia mortality data.

In addition to antigenic drift, which is an ongoing process generally resulting in minor antigenic changes in the influenza A virus, periodic 'antigenic shift' (**Figure 3**) can also be observed at varying time intervals. This process can result in major changes in the H and N surface antigens and the emergence of a new influenza A virus to which human populations have little or essentially no immunity. This shift is thought to occur predominantly through reassortment, or gene segment exchange, between human and avian influenza viruses. This reassortment may be facilitated by hosts such as swine, which are

Table 1 Influenza types and characteristics

Type A	Moderate to severe illness
	All age groups
	Humans and other animals
Type B	Milder disease
	Primarily affects children
	Humans only
Type C	Rarely reported in humans
	No epidemics

Centers for Disease Control and Prevention (2007) Influenza. In: Atkinson W, Hamborsky J, McIntyre L, and Wolfe S (eds). *Epidemiology and Prevention of Vaccine-Preventable Diseases.* 10th edn, pp. 235–256. Washington, DC: Public Health Foundation. The textbook Vaccines, edited by Plotkin, Orenstein, and Offit, 5th edition, 2008.

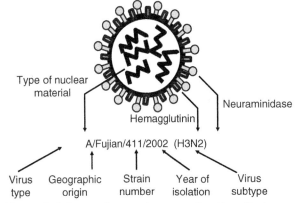

Figure 1 Influenza virus naming convention. From Centers for Disease Control and Prevention (2007) Influenza. In: Atkinson W, Hamborsky J, McIntyre L, and Wolfe S (eds). *Epidemiology and Prevention of Vaccine-Preventable Diseases.* 10th edn, pp. 235–256. Washington, DC: Public Health Foundation.

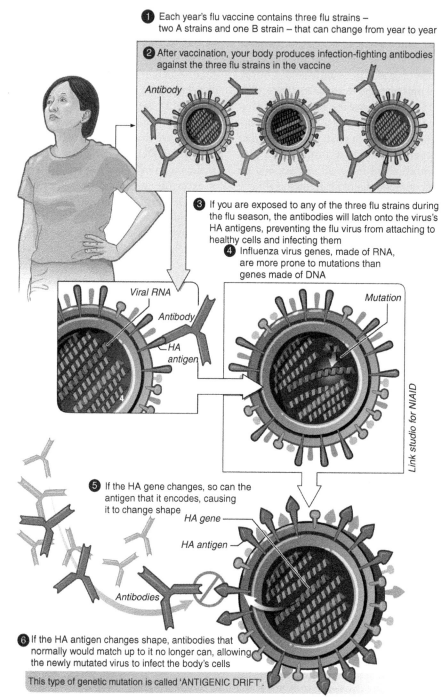

① Each year's flu vaccine contains three flu strains – two A strains and one B strain – that can change from year to year

② After vaccination, your body produces infection-fighting antibodies against the three flu strains in the vaccine

Antibody

③ If you are exposed to any of the three flu strains during the flu season, the antibodies will latch onto the virus's HA antigens, preventing the flu virus from attaching to healthy cells and infecting them

④ Influenza virus genes, made of RNA, are more prone to mutations than genes made of DNA

Viral RNA

Antibody

HA antigen

Mutation

Link studio for NIAID

⑤ If the HA gene changes, so can the antigen that it encodes, causing it to change shape

HA gene

HA antigen

Antibodies

⑥ If the HA antigen changes shape, antibodies that normally would match up to it no longer can, allowing the newly mutated virus to infect the body's cells

This type of genetic mutation is called 'ANTIGENIC DRIFT'.

Figure 2 Antigenic drift. From http://www3.niaid.nih.gov/NR/rdonlyres/A68ECEB4-8292-499B-B33F-FAEEDBAC7BBC/O/AntigenicDrift_HiRes.jpg.

susceptible to infection by both avian and human influenza viruses, thus creating a 'mixing pot' for reassortment when concurrent infection occurs. Since in humans, antibody against specific influenza virus types and subtypes in general offers little to no protection against other influenza types or subtypes, new influenza A viruses occurring through antigenic shift can lead to influenza pandemics, or a global disease outbreak.

Pandemic Influenza

Pandemics require a new virus causing infection in humans and sustained human-to-human transmission of that virus. An average of three pandemics per century have occurred since the 1600s, usually at 10- to 50-year intervals. In the twentieth century, pandemics occurred in 1918–1919 (Spanish flu), 1957 (Asian flu), and 1968

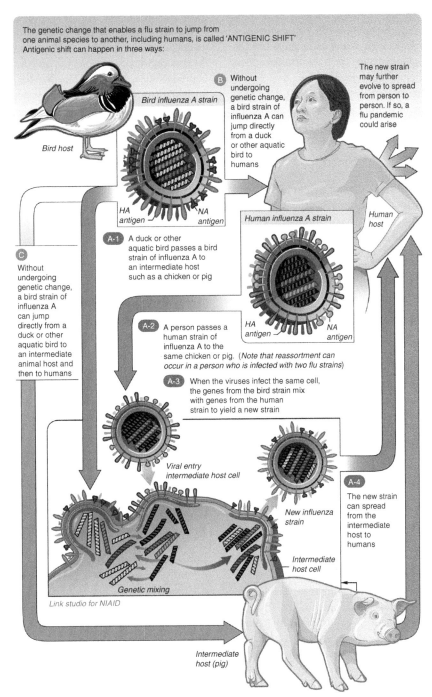

The genetic change that enables a flu strain to jump from one animal species to another, including humans, is called 'ANTIGENIC SHIFT'. Antigenic shift can happen in three ways:

Bird host

Bird influenza A strain

HA antigen   *NA antigen*

B Without undergoing genetic change, a bird strain of influenza A can jump directly from a duck or other aquatic bird to humans

The new strain may further evolve to spread from person to person. If so, a flu pandemic could arise

Human host

A-1 A duck or other aquatic bird passes a bird strain of influenza A to an intermediate host such as a chicken or pig

Human influenza A strain

HA antigen   *NA antigen*

C Without undergoing genetic change, a bird strain of influenza A can jump directly from a duck or other aquatic bird to an intermediate animal host and then to humans

A-2 A person passes a human strain of influenza A to the same chicken or pig. (*Note that reassortment can occur in a person who is infected with two flu strains*)

A-3 When the viruses infect the same cell, the genes from the bird strain mix with genes from the human strain to yield a new strain

Viral entry intermediate host cell

New influenza strain

A-4 The new strain can spread from the intermediate host to humans

Intermediate host cell

Genetic mixing

Link studio for NIAID

Intermediate host (pig)

Figure 3 Antigenic shift. From http://www3.niaid.nih.gov/NR/rdonlyres/30377A8B-747F-480A-832E-O2ABE091B3C/O/AntigenicShift_HiRes.jpg/.

(Hong Kong flu). Mortality from the Asian flu and the Hong Kong flu was estimated at 700 000–1 million deaths and 1–2 million deaths, respectively – large and frightening numbers. The Spanish flu epidemic of 1918–1919, however, wreaked human, social, and economic impact like no scourge previously recorded in human history, including the Black Death of the Middle Ages. It has been estimated that up to 20% of the world's population developed influenza during the Spanish flu pandemic, and up to 100 million people died worldwide. Furthermore, many of the dead were young, healthy individuals. The Spanish flu virus was an avian H1N1 subtype of influenza A that may have crossed the species barrier from birds to humans without an intermediary host such as swine. The Asian flu was caused by an avian H2N2 influenza A strain, and the Hong Kong flu was caused by an H3N2 strain that was a reassortment of human and avian viruses as well. Given the tremendous adverse public health consequences of an influenza pandemic, as well as the time since the last global pandemic, heightened awareness and preparedness for an influenza pandemic are warranted.

The WHO has articulated the phases of an influenza pandemic alert as part of a larger preparedness and action plan (WHO, 2005c), from the interpandemic period (phase 1), in which the threat to humans from pandemic influenza is thought to be low, through an actual influenza pandemic (phase 6), in which sustained human-to-human transmission occurs (**Table 2**). Currently, the WHO and national public health agencies across the globe are closely monitoring the H5N1 avian influenza viruses that have led to 307 recognized human infections and 186 deaths as of 24 May 2007, resulting in the designation of a global phase 3 pandemic alert.

Signs and Symptoms of Influenza Infection

One of the difficulties in pinpointing influenza as a cause of illness throughout history is the relatively nonspecific nature of influenza symptoms and signs. Illness is characterized by acute onset of fever, with headache, myalgias, fatigue, sore throat, cough, nasal congestion, rhinorrhea, and less commonly nausea, vomiting, and diarrhea (more frequently seen in children). Symptoms last 2–7 days from onset, although cough and fatigue may persist for more-prolonged periods, and severe bouts of illness can lead to prostration, secondary respiratory bacterial infections, hospitalization, and death. The primary mode of spread is through airborne respiratory droplets, although direct contact with virally contaminated materials can also lead to infection. The incubation period is 1–3 days, and the period of communicability is from up to a day before through 5–7 days following development of clinical symptoms, and perhaps longer in children: up to 10 days following development of clinical symptoms (Stohr, 2004).

Recent reviews examined the value of medical history and physical examination findings in the outpatient diagnosis of influenza infection, and neither study found that individual signs or symptoms were high yield for identifying or excluding a diagnosis. Symptom complexes, which combine the presence or absence of specific signs and symptoms suggestive of influenza, can be used to refine diagnostic possibilities as well as to monitor for influenza disease regionally, nationally, and internationally. In the United States, the CDC utilizes a Sentinel Providers Surveillance Network of approximately 1200 health-care providers, who report age-group-specific numbers of total patient visits as well as visits to monitor occurrence of 'influenza-like illness' (ILI), which is defined as the symptom complex of fever (temperature $\geq 100\,°F$, or $37.8\,°C$) and a cough and/or a sore throat in the absence of a known cause other than influenza. The concept and definition of ILI are also frequently used in clinical trials and other research studies evaluating the effectiveness of influenza prevention or treatment regimens.

Epidemiology: Disease Distribution and Surveillance

Although influenza activity in humans occurs year-round in tropical climates such as southeast Asia and equatorial Africa, influenza is more commonly associated with seasonal epidemics that occur annually in the temperate regions of the northern and southern hemispheres. In the United States, the first infections in which virus is isolated are usually seen in early- to mid-October, and influenza-positive infections continue to be observed through May. In the 2005–2006 U.S. season, influenza A H3N2 was most commonly seen overall, but as the season progressed, influenza B was more frequently isolated from respiratory specimens. While this has been the most common strain predominance and temporal pattern in the United States for some years, influenza B viruses have tended to be more commonly reported in Europe, and influenza A (H1N1) and influenza B viruses predominated in Asia in 2005 and 2006.

During influenza seasons, between 5% and 15% of the total population in affected countries may develop respiratory infections. As the leading cause of health-care encounters for acute respiratory tract infections in the United States, influenza is associated with 20 000–40 000 deaths, up to 300 000 hospitalizations, and countless sick days and episodes in which individuals are temporarily unable to attend to their normal life activities every year.

Table 2   World Health Organization phases of pandemic alert

1	Interpandemic phase	Low risk of human cases
2	New virus in animals, no human cases	Higher risk of human cases
3	Pandemic alert	No or very limited human-to-human transmission
4	New virus causes human virus	Evidence of increased human-to-human transmission
5		Evidence of significant human-to-human transmission
6	Pandemic	Efficient and sustained human-to-human transmission

Adapted from http://www.who.int/csr/disease/avian_influenza/phase/en/index.html

Globally, annual influenza is thought to cause between 3 million and 5 million cases of severe illness and between 250 000 and 500 000 deaths in the world's population annually (WHO, 2003).

Young children, those with chronic diseases, and older people are disproportionately at risk for illness and death from influenza. Annual global influenza attack rates in children are higher than in all adults (20–30% vs. 5–10%, respectively), although mortality rates in adults increase with age and comorbidity. In the United States, more than 90% of influenza and pneumonia deaths that occur during influenza epidemic periods are among persons age 65 or older. This predominance of excess mortality in the older population tends to reflect the experience of developed countries, although less is known regarding the descriptive epidemiology of influenza in the developing world. Morbidity and mortality from influenza are likely to be severely underestimated in the tropics and subtropics.

Global Surveillance

The WHO Global Influenza Program has four major foci aimed at addressing influenza control globally: Provide influenza surveillance, promote global and national pandemic preparedness, provide standards for influenza surveillance and control, and provide leadership toward mitigating the health and economic burden of influenza in the world.

The WHO Global Influenza Surveillance Network consists of 121 influenza centers in 93 countries (**Figure 4**). The centers obtain respiratory samples from patients with ILI and submit specimens to four international WHO Collaborating Centers for isolation and identification of influenza strains. The Surveillance Network has been collecting information on circulating influenza strains and documenting trends in influenza infection since 1948, and extending coverage to all countries would provide more-accurate data on circulating strains, emerging new strains, and disease trends that can inform resource allocation toward optimal prevention and control of global influenza.

Influenza Control

Influenza control is principally achieved through the use of vaccination to prevent the development and transmission of illness. However, influenza vaccination is not universally available on a global level; 90% of the world's influenza vaccine production capacity is centered in North American and European countries, which represent only 10% of the world's population. Nor is influenza vaccine optimally utilized in developed countries: The United States has not met national objectives for vaccination rates to eligible individuals, including those involved in the provision of health care to the population in general (USDHAS, 2000). Significant health disparities also exist

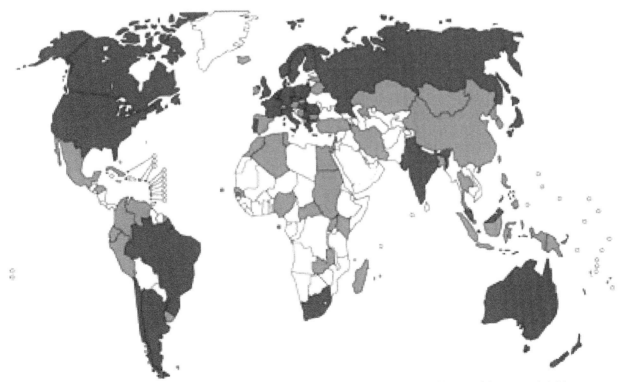

Figure 4 Geographic distribution of National Influenza Centers, 2007. White, no laboratory; blue, one laboratory; dark blue, more than one laboratory. From http://www.who.int/csr/disease/avian_influenza/centres/en/index.html.

for vaccine receipt among different racial and socioeconomic groups (O'Malley, 2006).

As with other infectious diseases, education of local populations and health-care providers regarding basic personal hygiene, such as hand washing, avoidance of mucus contamination, and control of coughs and sneezes, can contribute to improved influenza control. Maintenance of adequate barrier protections and supplies to maintain adequate hygiene during periods of increased clinic or hospital use associated with influenza outbreaks may serve to dampen nosocomial transmission as well. In hospitals, where patients may be at increased risk for severe complications of influenza, restricting visitors with respiratory illness or elective procedures has been proposed in the literature. Isolation of cases is difficult because of delays in presentation that may coincide with the period of communicability and because of delays in diagnosis, even where rapid laboratory testing exists. Rapid diagnostic testing for influenza A and B can now take as little as 30 min with commercially available kits processed by trained laboratory personnel. In general, these tests are 90–95% specific and 70–75% sensitive when compared with routine influenza culture as a gold standard.

While quarantine is not routinely applied to influenza cases, the WHO is vigorously promoting pandemic preparedness, including case investigation and treatment, prevention of the spread of disease in the community, maintenance of essential services, and planning for recovery (WHO, 2005a). The next pandemic is not a matter of if, but of when.

Antivirals

In addition to prevention and control of influenza through the use of vaccines and general hygiene measures, two classes of antiviral agents exist for prevention and treatment of influenza infections: adamantanes and neuraminidase inhibitors (NIs) (Moscona, 2005). The adamantanes include amantadine and rimantadine, both of which have activity only against influenza A, not influenza B. Furthermore, viral resistance to the adamantanes was observed to increase dramatically over the past 3 years, from 1.9% in 2004 to 91% of isolates tested through 12 January 2006 by the CDC. On January 14, 2006, the CDC issued a health alert recommending the use of amantadine or rimantadine in the 2005–2006 season for prevention or treatment of influenza in the United States. This recommendation has carried forward to the 2006–2007 influenza season. The CDC currently recommends against the use of amantadine or rimantadine for prevention or treatment of influenza in the United States.

The NIs include oseltamivir and zanamivir, and these agents are active against both influenza A and influenza B. Oseltamivir is approved for treatment and prevention in persons 1 year old and older, and Zanamivir is approved

for treatment in persons 7 years old and older and prevention in persons 5 years old and older. While resistance to the adamantanes has led to recommendations against their use, all influenza isolates tested for drug resistance by the CDC in the 2005–2006 season remained susceptible to the NIs. Thus, these agents are the antivirals of choice for influenza prevention and treatment.

For treatment of influenza, the NIs should be started within 2 days of the onset of illness – clearly a challenge in practice, given the often nonspecific early symptoms of influenza as well as the highly variable time among patient populations between onset of symptoms and presentation to medical attention. Nonetheless, if started within the recommended time frame, duration of uncomplicated illness can be decreased by approximately 1–2 days in otherwise healthy individuals. There may be a similar benefit in high-risk individuals as well. Treatment with the NIs should last 5 days.

For prevention of influenza, vaccination remains the preferred method to minimize or avoid morbidity and mortality. Both NIs may be used for contact postexposure or community prophylaxis (zanamivir was approved for prevention of influenza in the United States in 2006). Efficacy for protection against laboratory-diagnosed influenza is approximately 80%. These agents may be used in vaccinated individuals, and in settings such as nursing homes experiencing influenza outbreaks, NIs may confer added protective benefit. In addition, the NIs may have wider application when strain mismatch occurs between vaccine and circulating influenza virus.

Vaccines

Using data obtained through the WHO Global Influenza Surveillance Network and laboratory analysis of circulating influenza strains by the WHO Collaborating Centres, the WHO twice annually convenes a panel of international influenza experts to make recommendations for the composition of influenza vaccine for the northern hemisphere (February) and southern hemisphere (September). These recommendations are published in the WHO's *Weekly Epidemiological Record* and influence the production of more than 250 million influenza vaccine doses annually. A WHO Global Immunization and Vision Strategy has been created to serve as a template for national vaccination strategies, with the ultimate goal of extending vaccination to all eligible persons (WHO, 2005). The introduction of new vaccines and vaccine technologies is a key component of the WHO's vision.

Inactivated trivalent influenza viral vaccine (TIV), targeted at inducing systemic rather than local immunity, has been licensed in the United States since the late 1950s and has been recommended routinely since 1963. TIVs are safe and are highly purified, containing only noninfectious, inactivated viruses that cannot cause influenza. Composed of whole virus or purified subunit antigens of the N and H viral surface glycoproteins, antibodies to inactivated virus in vaccines can neutralize viral replication, but when administered intramuscularly they may not induce adequate mucosal responses that minimize the risk of infection. As previously noted, the WHO and national agencies such as the Food and Drug Administration in the United States recommend the composition of annual TIV. The standard approach is to include two vaccine virus strains that mirror the predominant circulating influenza A virus or viruses with an influenza B vaccine virus strain (hence, trivalent). Protection conferred by the vaccine has been shown to correlate directly with the immune response elicited in the recipient. However, the strength of this association is not as clear in older vaccinees, and inactivated vaccines are predominantly effective only against viral strains that have similar H and N antigens. When the viruses chosen for the vaccine resemble those of the circulating epidemic strains, vaccine efficacy for prevention of hospitalization and death approaches 70–90% among healthy young adults. Gross and colleagues, in a meta-analysis conducted in the mid-1990s, found that the pooled estimates of TIV efficacy for 20 cohort studies in the older population were as follows: 56% for preventing respiratory illness, 53% for preventing pneumonia, 48% for preventing hospitalization, and 68% for preventing death (Gross et al., 1995).

Live attenuated, cold-adapted vaccines against influenza have been explored for more than three decades, and a live attenuated intranasal vaccine (LAIV) was licensed and has been available since the 2003–2004 influenza season in the United States (Flumist; MedImmune Vaccines). Overall, however, few countries recommend or use live attenuated influenza vaccines, and they are not recommended by the WHO for influenza prevention because of cold-chain and cost considerations. However, the vaccine is safe and highly efficacious. Limited availability, complexities in large-scale production, and vaccine storage and handling issues likely influence this recommendation. Administered intranasally as a large-particle aerosol to the upper respiratory epithelium, the vaccine is targeted at inducing an IgA response to the influenza virus. Although inactivated vaccines administered intramuscularly frequently produce higher titers of serum antibody to influenza virus, LAIV intranasally induces higher levels of secretory and local antibody. One of the argued benefits of the LAIV is that the mucosal immune response to the live attenuated vaccine virus may more closely resemble a naturally occurring immune response than the response that is produced by inactivated vaccines. However, the true mechanism of protection remains incompletely understood.

Like TIV, LAIV contains vaccine virus strains (or the antigenic equivalent) that are recommended annually and is administered annually to eligible individuals. Unlike TIV, LAIV uses live virus, and vaccine receipt could result in mild influenza-like illness associated with infection by an influenza vaccine virus. Some recipients shed detectable virus in nasal secretions for a short duration after vaccination. However, there has been only one report of a placebo recipient acquiring an attenuated viral strain from a LAIV recipient, and no other published studies to date have reported such transmission from vaccinated to unvaccinated persons. Although the attenuated vaccine strains theoretically could recombine with a wild-type variant and cause the potential for illness or a novel viral pandemic, more than 30 years of study have shown that the vaccine virus is genotypically stable, and the hypothetical reassortments have not been identified among any of the clinical trial participants to date.

LAIV has been targeted to children and young to middle-aged adults in the United States. Prevention of influenza among children likely holds benefit for other age and at-risk groups as well, as time lags in age-specific morbidity and mortality suggest that children may represent a primary vector for viral transmission in communities. As such, intensive efforts focused on vaccination of children (and protection of children through vaccination of contacts) may provide the added benefit of decreased morbidity and mortality among the older population.

Vaccine Strategies

The scaling of strategies to undertake and improve influenza vaccine receipt rates is highly dependent on the underlying health-care infrastructure and cultural and social factors that influence the decision to give and receive vaccine. In the absence of integrated and comprehensive outpatient and hospital-based patient medical record systems and registries, which most of the world does not possess, the best approach is to take the vaccine to eligible populations and remove as many barriers to vaccine receipt as possible. Patient and provider education regarding the cost–benefit of vaccine receipt, as well as the potential health consequences of acquiring influenza infection at the individual and community level, are important foundations of improved vaccination coverage. Immunizing individuals in a variety of settings can improve coverage as well; not only hospitals and health or health-related service clinics but also home health visits, long-term care facilities, group homes, and even community centers, places of religious worship when appropriate, schools, and places of employment could be considered.

One effective strategy for improving vaccination coverage rates when vaccine is routinely available is simply recommending vaccination to patients when appropriate. A health-care provider's recommendation is among the strongest determinants for inducing adult patients to receive vaccinations. Recommending and offering influenza vaccination consistently throughout the influenza season, rather than predominantly or only in the weeks preceding the influenza season or at the onset of influenza activity, presents another opportunity. System-based opportunities to improve vaccination coverage exist as well. Both immunization registries and recall and reminder systems can be effective in improving vaccination coverage in primary care clinics with sufficient administrative support to maintain accurate records-based systems.

Many studies have shown standing orders to be a valuable system approach to vaccine delivery, and computer-based standing orders have demonstrated utility as well. In the hospital setting, physicians with the highest volume of pneumonia care in their hospital practices may actually do significantly worse (35–40%) in completing vaccine provision to their hospitalized patients than do their colleagues treating lower pneumonia volumes, further supporting the rationale for taking vaccine delivery out of physicians' hands and utilizing standing orders. Additional information on standing order templates and other programs to improve vaccination rates, including client education, drop-in clinics, recall and reminder, performance feedback, and other programs may be found at the CDC National Immunization Program website (www.cdc.gov/vaccines/recs/remider-sys.htm, June 2007).

Future Directions

Events in the past decade leading to the current phase 3 pandemic alert regarding human infection by the H5N1 avian influenza virus are dictating much of the recent energy and efforts concentrating on influenza pandemic preparedness, and appropriately so. Given the relatively long period of 40 years since the last influenza pandemic, many people are concerned that the next pandemic is on the immediate horizon and that H5N1 may be it. This threat is complicated by inadequate supplies of antiviral agents and increasing drug resistance to commonly used antivirals against influenza. Recognition by the WHO and other public health agencies of the need for better, less expensive, and more easily and rapidly produced, stored, and handled influenza vaccine to allow more complete worldwide coverage in the event of an influenza pandemic is both timely and necessary. Unfortunately, this need also highlights, not only the immense global disparities in vaccine availability and delivery, but also the tremendous international racial and socioeconomic disparities in public health and medical infrastructure. While emerging technologies and the wave of knowledge associated with the Human Genome Project may help us solve many theoretical problems in the control and prevention of influenza, we must also solve the practical problems adversely affecting health equity and health promotion in order to optimize the public health and wellness of our global community.

See also: Global Burden of Disease; Surveillance of Disease.

Citations

Centers for Disease Control and Prevention (2007) Influenza. In: Atkinson W, Hamborsky J, McIntyre L, and Wolfe S (eds) *Epidemiology and Prevention of Vaccine-Preventable Diseases,* 10th edn. 10th edn, pp. 235–256. Washington, DC: Public Health Foundation.

Gross PA, Hermogenes AW, Sacks HS, *et al.* (1995) The efficacy of influenza vaccine in older persons: A meta-analysis and review of the literature. *Annals of Internal Medicine* 123: 518–527.

Moscona A (2005) Neuraminidase inhibitors for influenza. *New England Journal of Medicine* 353: 1363–1373.

National Center for Immunization and Respiratory Disease, Centers for Disease Control and Prevention (2007) Recommendations and Guidelines, Reminder Systems and Strategies for Increasing Vaccination Rates. http://www.cdc.gov/vaccines/recs/reminder-sys/htm (accessed May 2007).

O'Malley AS and Forrest CB (2006) Immunization disparities in older Americans: Determinants and future research needs. *American Journal of Preventive Medicine* 31: 50–158.

Potter CW (2001) A history of influenza. *Journal of Applied Microbiology* 91: 572–579.

Smith NM, Bresee JS, Shay DK, Uyeki TM, Cox NJ, and Strikas RA (2006) Prevention and control of influenza: Recommendations of the Advisory Committee on Immunization Practices. *MMWR. Morbidity and Mortality Weekly Report* 55(RR10): 1–42.

Stohr K (2004) Influenza. In: Heymann DL (ed.) *Control of Communicable Disease in Man,* 18th edn, pp. 307–312. Washington, DC: American Public Health Association.

U.S. Department of Health and Human Services (2000) *Healthy People 2010 Immunization Goals.* Washington, DC: U.S. Government Printing Office.

World Health Organization (2005a) *Checklist for Influenza Pandemic Preparedness Planning.* Geneva, Switzerland: World Health Organization. Document WHO/CDS/CSR/GIP 2005.4.

World Health Organization (2005b) *Draft Global Immunization Strategy (WHA 58.15, agenda item 13.8).* Geneva, Switzerland: World Health Organization.

World Health Organization (2005c) *Global Influenza Preparedness Plan: The Role of WHO and recommendations for National Measures Before and During Pandemics.* Geneva, Switzerland: World Health Organization. Document WHO/CDS/CSR/GIP/2005.5.

World Health Organization (n.d.) *Influenza.* http://www.who.int/mediacentre/factsheets/2003/fs211/en/ (accessed 28 October 2007).

Wright PF and Webster RG (2001) Orthomyxoviruses. In: Knipe DM, Howley PM, Griffin DE, *et al.* (eds.) *Fields Virology.* 4th edn., pp. 1534–1579. Philadelphia, PA: Lippincott Williams & Wilkins.

Further Reading

Barry JM (2004) *The Great Influenza: The Story of the Deadliest Pandemic in History.* New York: Viking.

Call SA, Vollenweider MA, Hornung CA, Simel DL, and McKinney WP (2005) Does this patient have influenza? *Journal of the American Medical Association* 293: 987–997.

Couch RB (1981) Summary of medical literature. Review of effectiveness of inactivated influenza virus vaccine. In: *Office of Technology Assessment (ed.) Cost-Effectiveness of Influenza Vaccination,* pp. 43–45. Washington, DC: Office of Technology Assessmentt.

Lewis PA and Shope RE (1931) Swine influenza II: A hemophilic bacillus from the respiratory tract of infected swine. *Journal of Experimental Medicine* 54: 361–371.

Poland GA, Jacobson RM, and Targonski PV (2007) Avian and pandemic influenza: An overview. *Vaccine* 25: 3057–3061.

Reichert TA, Sugaya N, Fedson DS, *et al.* (2001) The Japanese experience with vaccinating schoolchildren against influenza. *New England Journal of Medicine* 344: 889–896.

Shope RE (1931) Swine influenza I: Experimental transmission and pathology. *Journal of Experimental Medicine* 54: 349–359.

Shope RE (1931) Swine Influenza III: Filtration experiments and etiology. *Journal of Experimental Medicine* 54: 373–385.

Smith W, Andrewes CH, and Laidlaw PP (1933) A virus obtained from influenza patients. *Lancet* 2: 66–74.

Targonski PV and Poland G (2003) Adult Immunizations. In: Land R and Hensrud D (eds.) *Clinical Preventive Medicine*, pp. 573–589. Chicago, IL: American Medical Association.

Taubenberger JK, Reid AH, Lourens RM, Wang R, Jin G, and Fanning TG (2005) Characterization of the 1918 influenza virus polymerase genes. *Nature* 437: 889–893.

Relevant Websites

http://www.cdc.gov/flu/ – Centers for Disease Control and Prevention, Seasonal Flu.

http://www.cdc.gov/nip/home-hcp.htm – Centers for Disease Control and Prevention, Vaccines & Immunizations.

http://www.pandemicflu.gov/ – U.S. Department of Health and Human Services Pandemic Flu Home page.

http://www.who.int/csr/disease/influenza/en/ – World Health Organization Epidemic and Pandemic Alert Response page.

http://gamapserver.who.int/GlobalAtlas/home.asp – World Health Organization Global Atlas of Infectious Disease.

http://www.who.int/topics/influenza/en/ – World Health Organization Influenza page.

SECTION 4
DEMOGRAPHY

Demography, Epidemiology and Public Health

O S Miettinen, McGill University, Montreal, QC, Canada

The Classical Outlook

The disciplines of demography, epidemiology, and public health all are concerned with human populations, with epidemiology dependent on demography and public health dependent on both demography and epidemiology.

Demography addresses human populations as populations *per se*, that is, their sizes and structures – distributions by such fundamental, 'demographic' person-characteristics as age and gender – and the dynamics influencing these – such demographic factors as rates of birth ('nativity' rates), rates of death ('mortality' rates), and patterns of migration.

These demographic concerns about populations are ones of knowing and understanding, for whatever societal purposes – raising armies, raising taxes, and so forth – in addition to those of epidemiology and public health.

Epidemiology addresses human populations, demographically characterized, in respect to their 'health,' meaning the frequency of particular types of ill-health – illness (Miettinen and Flegel, 2003b) – in them. The frequency of, or the 'morbidity' from, a particular illness is quantified in terms of a rate of its occurrence (Miettinen and Flegel, 2003f).

If the illness phenomenon at issue is of the form of a state (of notable duration), the rate is one of 'prevalence,' expressing the proportion of individuals in the (sub)population at issue that are afflicted by the illness at a particular time (Miettinen and Flegel, 2003f).

If, on the other hand, the illness phenomenon is an event (of no notable duration), the rate is one of incidence (Miettinen and Flegel, 2003f). This can be, again, of the proportion type, as in the 'secondary attack rate' expressing the proportion of the 'contacts' of a person with a communicable disease that contract this disease, or in the rate of subsequent gastroenteritis among participants in a communal supper. Alternatively, an incidence rate is of the form of incidence density: the number of cases occurring, or diagnosed, in a given amount of population-time, in 10 000 person-years, for example.

If, in a population's course over time, a rate of a given time is unusually high, it is said to signify the presence of an epidemic, while the level of occurrence that is usual for the population is referred to as the endemic rate.

The epidemiological concern about (the level of) morbidity from a particular illness ultimately is its control, meaning reduction of the rate through population-level measures aimed at prevention of cases of the illness.

To this end, epidemiological inputs guide, for one, population-level health education concerning preventive interventions – generally changes of behavior – that the population's individual members might adopt.

The epidemiological inputs may also guide decisions about community-level interventions, whether regulatory or of the form of service.

This practice of epidemiology can be, and is, also thought of as community medicine, which is characterized by the client of a doctor being a population, in contrast to the individual clients in clinical medicine.

In community medicine, just as in clinical medicine, the doctor is a professional in the etymological meaning of 'doctor': teacher, specifically one who is capable of getting to know, beyond what is possible for a layperson, about the client's health, and who on the basis of this knowing – gnosis (dia-, etio-, pro-) (Miettinen and Flegel, 2003d) – teaches the client (or the client's representative(s)) about the client's own health (Miettinen and Flegel, 2003e).

Actually intervening on the course of the client's health is by no means common, much less inherent, in an epidemiologist's practice, just as it isn't in a clinician's practice (Miettinen and Flegel, 2003e).

The knowledge base of epidemiological practice/community medicine, like that of clinical medicine, increasingly derives from research and science.

Epidemiological research, in its service to community-level preventive medicine, typically addresses causation – etiology/etiogenesis (Miettinen and Flegel, 2003c) – of illness. Focusing on whatever (potential) cause, the research addresses the extent to which this cause increases the incidence of particular illnesses among people exposed to the cause. The causal rate ratio for a particular illness, then, implies the proportion of its incidence that is due to this cause among people exposed to this cause. This general 'etiologic fraction' among the exposed, when coupled with the *ad hoc* proportion of cases of the illness arising from the exposed subpopulation, implies the proportional reduction in the cared-for population's overall incidence that would result from complete removal of the cause (Miettinen, 1974).

Eminent in research of this type has been study of cigarette smoking in the etiology of lung cancer. While the risk of this disease is strongly dependent on the particulars of that smoking, the research has shown the incidence density typically to be about tenfold relative to that of nonsmokers. This implies an etiologic fraction of

$(10 - 1)/10 = 0.90$ for a population of cigarette smokers; and if, in the cared-for population, 85% of lung cancer cases have been determined to arise from among cigarette smokers, then the proportion of the overall lung cancer incidence that is due to cigarette smoking can be taken to be $0.90 \times 0.85 = 77\%$ – and this means that disappearance of cigarette smoking in the cared-for population would, in time, reduce lung cancer incidence by 77% (or so).

When the preventive measure is not removal of a cause but the introduction of a novel means to enhance resistance to the cause, epidemiological research takes the form of an experimental introduction of that intervention, generally in a comparative trial.

Very notable among epidemiological preventive-intervention trials have been those on vaccinations against infectious diseases, including the polio vaccination trials half a century ago and those concerning cervical cancer most recently. But there have been such trials on other types of preventive intervention as well, dietary supplementation with antioxidants for the prevention of cancer, for example.

Epidemiology, whether as the practice of community medicine or as the research (under whatever science) that produces the scientific knowledge base for this practice, no longer constitutes a single, coherent discipline. Instead, it now is the aggregate of differentiated subdisciplines – 'specialties' – of epidemiologic/community medicine practice or of their associated research disciplines (Miettinen, 2004). There is communicable disease epidemiology, cancer epidemiology, nutritional epidemiology, community psychiatry, and so on. And besides, in modern textbooks of 'epidemiology,' the term generally refers to theory – concepts and principles – of epidemiological research.

Public health, as a term, commonly refers to the 'health' of people at large, meaning their collective level of ill health/illness (Miettinen and Flegel, 2003a, 2003b) – their morbidity – in some particular respect(s). It is in this meaning that one speaks, for example, of the public health impact of the aggregate of a particular type of preventive practice in clinical medicine. Public health in this meaning – of the 'public's' health – is quite informal a concept, generally with no associated concern for express quantification of the level(s) of morbidity *per se* or of effects on the level(s).

Epidemiology in the meaning of (the disciplines of) community medicine is an approximation to the concept of public health as one of health care, specifically the classical health-care concept of public health. 'Public' in this disciplinary term refers to a community/population of people as being the client of the health care; and it also can be taken to refer to the fact that community health care, different from clinical health care, inherently is publicly – societally – financed (Miettinen and Flegel, 2003a). The meaning of 'health' in this is that of health care, but expressly more inclusive than that of 'medicine.'

In today's terminology, health care is medicine only insofar as it is provided by a physician (Miettinen and Flegel, 2003a), a graduate of a 'medical' school, while public health professionals commonly are not physicians. They include public health nurses, sanitary engineers, food hygienists, occupational safety experts, radiation protection experts, public health educators, and others.

While the conceptual distinction between public health and clinical medicine thus has been very sharp, there nevertheless has been quite an interdependence between these two. Looking at this from the vantage of public health – in which actions most broadly fall in the categories of education, regulation, and service – its education may be aimed at promoting the use of clinical services (in usual clinical settings) – diagnostic, as in screening for a cancer, or interventive, as in the management of hypertension or diabetes. Public health regulations, while commonly directed to extramedical matters – sanitary, environmental, and so on – are also directed to clinical medicine, as in removing a dangerous medication from the clinical formulary or requiring reporting of (select) communicable disease diagnoses. A public health service to the cared-for population generally is para-clinical in the meaning that it is individual-oriented but extrinsic to the general system of clinical care, as in providing, in settings outside the usual clinical ones, sterile needles for drug addicts or vaccinations in the context of an epidemic.

Current Extensions

Epidemiological research addressing the etiology/etiogenesis of an illness, while up to now principally serving community etiognosis, and clinical etiognosis besides, is now being refined in such a way that individuals in the community, and clinical clients also, can be given individualized information on the magnitude of the effects of a preventive intervention, effects specific to particular points in prospective time. Thus, future epidemiological research on the cigarette smoking etiology of lung cancer, or re-analyses of data from past studies on this, will provide for estimating, for an individual of a particular age, smoking history, and so forth, the probability with which stopping smoking now would have the consequence of preventing the emergence of symptomatic lung cancer in the next ten years, the next 20 years, and so on. Similarly, epidemiological research on the causation of death from a cancer by not having been screened for it (by not having thus provided for its early treatment) will provide for setting period-specific prognostic probabilities, also specific to a person's risk profile, of preventing death from the cancer by prospective screening (its associated early treatment) initiated now and regularly repeated.

This novelty in the theory and practice of etiologic/etiognostic research will secondarily imply a corresponding innovation in intervention-prognostic research, epidemiologically in preventive trials for community medicine – for individualized intervention decisions in it, following community-level health education – and, by analogy, for clinical medicine also. Thus, intervention trials, whether preventive or therapeutic, will produce empirical probability functions of the type sketched above as arising from etiologic studies. And a byproduct will be descriptive-prognostic functions – of person characteristics and prospective time – conditional on the choice of intervention.

In this way, epidemiologists' advanced etiologic research for community medicine, providing individualized inputs to decisions about preventive interventions, will become the paradigm for studies on clinical interventions, randomized trials in particular (Miettinen, 2004), while up to now the latter have commonly been held to be paradigmatic for the former.

Epidemiologists' descriptive research on the prevalence of an illness, concerning the prevalence as a joint function (descriptive) of various person-characteristics, already is being brought, as a novelty, to clinical research. The context is the development of the scientific knowledge base for that which is pivotal in clinical medicine: diagnostic probability-setting for a given illness in the differential-diagnostic set, given the set of available facts on a set of diagnostic indicators, the diagnostic profile of the case, that is. Correct diagnosis of a particular illness, given the diagnostic profile, is characterized by the correct probability with which that illness is taken to be present; and this probability in turn is defined/determined by the prevalence of that illness in instances of the profile in general (Miettinen, 2001), given that the profile is formulated in generally meaningful terms. Diagnostic research, still incipient only, thus concerns diagnostic prevalence functions – joint functions of the diagnostic indicators involved in the diagnostic profile, specific to particular domains of client presentation (chief complaint together with a broad range of age, say) (Miettinen, 2001).

As the requisite knowledge base of clinical medicine – in its gnosis (dia-, etio-, pro-) – is about probabilities in the meaning of proportions (relative frequencies), and as these are based on rates of prevalence or incidence, clinical research of the quintessentially 'applied' (instrumentalist) variety has a distinctly epidemiological flavor. And indeed, research for clinical gnosis, and application of the resulting knowledge also, now is commonly spoken of as being 'clinical epidemiology.' This term, however, can be said to be a contradiction in terms, as epidemiology really is, as both research and practice, a matter of community medicine, the essence of which sharply contrasts with that of clinical medicine (Miettinen, 2004).

Public health in most modern countries has recently changed dramatically, not so much as a matter of progress within its classical domain as of domain expansion, of what it encompasses as its health-care concerns. By far

the biggest innovation in public health in most modern countries in the second half of the twentieth century was the introduction of national health insurance, bringing clinical health care into the public domain, though initially only as a matter of public financing (Miettinen and Flegel, 2003a). At present, in countries with this vastly expanded realm of public health, the principal concerns of a minister of health are quality assurance and cost containment – overwhelmingly in clinical health care.

Quality assurance in health care presupposes definitions of good, normative health care in various components of it. Beyond this, it requires monitoring of health-care actions with a view to their classifications on their respective scales of quality; but ultimately it is a matter of administrative actions aimed at curtailing substandard practices in health care.

This has substantially broadened the range of epidemiological activity in public health practice (Miettinen, 2004). In classical epidemiology, sample surveys were confined to the context of 'community diagnoses' as a matter of assessing the rates of prevalence of particular illnesses (Morris, 1955), supplemented by surveys to assess distributions of particular risk factors for the development of particular illnesses with a view to preventive interventions. Now the principal need for epidemiological surveys in public health practice is in the quality monitoring of clinical health care. As for meeting this need, however, a limiting factor still is the very incomplete development of norms of clinical health care (Liberati et al., 1989).

Correspondingly, the principal challenge in modern public health is the need to develop national standards for clinical health care, and especially to thus define the clinical health care that is subject to societal financing, the associated challenge being to design the national system(s) of the delivery of clinical health care with a view to efficiency and its consequent cost containment.

See also: Clinical Epidemiology; Concepts of Health and Disease.

Citations

Liberati A, Chatziandreou E, and Miettinen OS (1989) Health care research: What is it about? *Quality Assurance in Health Care* 1: 249–257.

Miettinen OS (1974) Proportion of disease caused or prevented by a given exposure, trait or intervention. *American Journal of Epidemiology* 99: 325–332.

Miettinen OS (2001) The modern scientific physician: 3. Scientific diagnosis. *Canadian Medical Association Journal* 165: 910–911.

Miettinen OS (2004) Epidemiology: *Quo vadis? European Journal of Epidemiology* 19: 713–718.

Miettinen OS and Flegel KM (2003a) Elementary concepts of medicine: II. Health, health fields, public health. *Journal of Evaluation in Clinical Practice* 9: 311–313.

Miettinen OS and Flegel KM (2003b) Elementary concepts of medicine: III. Illness: Somatic anomaly with ... *Journal of Evaluation in Clinical Practice* 9: 315–317.

Miettinen OS and Flegel KM (2003c) Elementary concepts of medicine: VI. Genesis of illness: Pathogenesis, aetiogenesis. *Journal of Evaluation in Clinical Practice* 9: 325–327.

Miettinen OS and Flegel KM (2003d) Elementary concepts of medicine: VIII. Knowing about a client's health: Gnosis. *Journal of Evaluation in Clinical Practice* 9: 333–335.

Miettinen OS and Flegel KM (2003e) Elementary concepts of medicine: IX. Acting on gnosis: Doctoring, intervening. *Journal of Evaluation in Clinical Practice* 9: 337–339.

Miettinen OS and Flegel KM (2003f) Elementary concepts of medicine: XI. Illness in a community: Morbidity. *Journal of Evaluation in Clinical Practice* 9: 345–348.

Morris JN (1955) The uses of epidemiology. *British Medical Journal* 2: 395–401.

Population Growth

S Haddock and E Leahy, Population Action International, Washington, DC, USA
R Engelman, Worldwatch Institute, Washington, DC, USA

Dynamics of Population Growth

In the last half-century, population growth has proceeded at a rate unprecedented in the history of the planet. The human population took hundreds of thousands of years to grow to 2.5 billion people in 1950. Then, within the time span of just 50 years, the world's population more than doubled to exceed six billion people. Most of this growth has occurred in developing countries where advances in public health have contributed to lower mortality at all ages. Until recently, death rates fell faster than birthrates, resulting in rapid population growth.

While growth rates have fallen from their all-time high, human numbers are still increasing. The world population is growing by about 1.2% a year, down from a peak of roughly 2% in the late 1960s. However, even at this lower growth rate, the world's population still experiences a net increase of about 76 million people each year; many more than the 50 million or so added annually in the 1950s when the term population explosion first gained currency.

Population Projections

World population could reach anywhere between 7.7 billion and 10.6 billion by the mid-21st century, based on the 2004 United Nations (UN) projections, depending mostly on future birthrates (UN, 2007). A population projection is a conditional forecast based on assumptions about current and future fertility, mortality, and migration. **Figure 1** shows the UN's high, medium, and low projections for 2300. The variances between these three projections stem from differences in projected fertility; that is, the average number of children a woman has in the study population. In the high projection, global fertility averages around 2.6 children per woman. In the medium, it averages about 2.1 children per woman. The lowest fertility projection assumes an average of about 1.6 children per woman. Most users of these projections tend to cite the medium projection as the most likely. It is important, however, to be aware of the low and high projections as a kind of outer bounds of demographic possibility.

Recent UN projections are lower than most previous projections for the same period, reflecting earlier-than-expected declines in family size in some countries. Yet even under the UN's slow-growth scenario, the population would continue to grow for at least four more

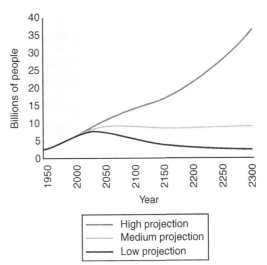

Figure 1 Population projections (high, medium and low to 2300). The United Nations high, medium, and low population projections are based on assumptions about current and future fertility, mortality, and migration. Data from United Nations Population Division (2004) *World Population to 2300*. New York, United Nations Population Division.

decades, to about 7.8 billion people, before declining gradually. Under the UN's high-growth scenario, the world population would exceed 35 billion late in the 23rd century and continue growing rapidly. The long-term medium projection suggests that the population would peak just above 9.1 billion around 2075, then drift downward to around 8.5 billion before growing again late in the 23rd century.

However, there is no certainty in projecting future population trends. All population projections are based on fairly rigid assumptions and therefore cannot provide completely reliable guides to the world's demographic future.

The Demographic Transition

The transformation of a population that is characterized by high birth and death rates to one in which people tend to live longer lives and raise smaller families is called the demographic transition. This transition typically shifts population age structure from one dominated by children and young adults up to age 29 to one dominated by middle-aged and older adults age 40 and above. About one-third of the world's countries, including most of Europe, Russia, Japan, and the United States, have effectively completed this transition. These 65 or so countries contain half of the world's population.

In **Figure 2(a)** and **2(b)**, two population pyramids geometrically display age structures: The proportion of people per age group, relative to the population as a whole. Afghanistan is an example of a country in the early phase of the demographic transition. Such countries typically have age structures composed predominantly of young adults and children (commonly called a youth bulge). As countries advance into the late phase of transition, as shown by the population age structure of South Korea, the proportion of children begins to decrease, but a youth bulge persists for a decade or two, moving upward into the older age cohorts.

Fertility Rates

Improvements in the education of girls and the overall status of women, together with increased access to contraceptive methods, have played important roles in advancing the demographic transition and reducing the global average fertility rate from 4.9 children in the first half of the 1960s. Nevertheless, the world's average fertility rate is currently 2.7 children, considerably higher than the level of fertility that would ultimately stabilize the growth of most populations (UN, 2005). This level, called replacement fertility, represents the number of children a couple needs to have in order to replace themselves in the population. The values for replacement fertility are surprisingly diverse and vary by

country, reflecting mostly differential rates of survival of children to their own reproductive ages. Replacement fertility rates range today from a low of 2.04 for Réunion Island to a high of 3.35 in Swaziland (Engelman and Reahy, 2006).

In nearly all developing countries, the average number of childbirths per woman has decreased in recent decades. While a number of factors have contributed to this revolution in childbearing, improved access to modern contraceptive methods has played a key role, in most of sub-Saharan Africa, in many countries of the Middle East, and in parts of South Asia. Growing at rates of 2.5–3.5% annually, these countries could double in size in 20 to 30 years. Almost all industrialized countries now have an average family size of fewer than two children and are growing relatively slowly, or even declining in population. In some eastern and southern European countries, women have an average of 1.2 or 1.3 children. These nations comprise less than 5% of the world's population, however, and thus have little influence on overall global trends (**Figure 3**).

Population Aging

Due to low fertility rates in some developed countries, concerns are emerging about population aging and the possibility of population decline. Population aging is defined as a rising average age within a population and is an inevitable result of longer life expectancies and lower birthrates. In many societies, population aging is a positive social and environmental development, but its potential persistence to extreme average ages is worrisome to governments concerned with the funding of social security programs and general economic growth. However, like population growth itself, population aging cannot continue indefinitely and will eventually end, even in stabilized populations.

Population decline is occurring in some industrialized countries. European population growth, which fueled immigration to the Americas for three centuries, has ended and begun to reverse course, despite significant streams of migration from developing countries. If low fertility rates persist, the populations of Germany, Italy, Russia, and Spain could shrink by 5–10% by 2025-an average reduction of 0.5% per year. In East Asia, the populations of Japan, China, and South Korea are likely to peak and begin a gradual decline in size before the middle of the 21st century. However, major declines outside Europe and East Asia are unlikely for decades.

Factors That Influence Population Growth
Contraceptive Prevalence

Demographers attribute much of the recent decline in global fertility to improved access to and use of family

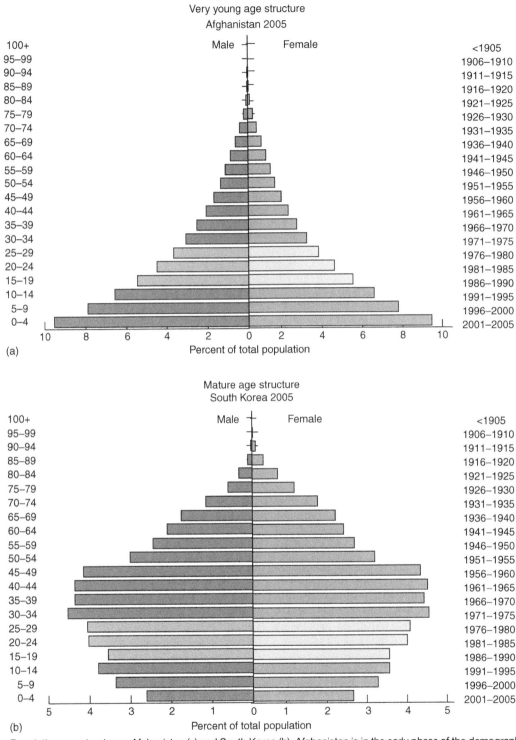

Figure 2 Population age structures: Afghanistan (a) and South Korea (b). Afghanistan is in the early phase of the demographic transition, with a large youth bulge. South Korea, which is in the late phase of transition, has a decreasing proportion of youth. Data from United Nations Population Division (2005) *World Population Prospects: The 2004 Revision*. New York: United Nations Population Division.

planning information and methods. More than half of all married women in developing countries now use family planning, compared to 10% in the 1960s. Across the developing world, use of modern methods of contraception ranges from less than 8% of married women in Western and Central Africa to 65% in South America. The highest contraceptive prevalence rate in the world is in Northern Europe, where 75% of married women are currently using a modern method of family planning (**Figure 4**) (UN, 2004).

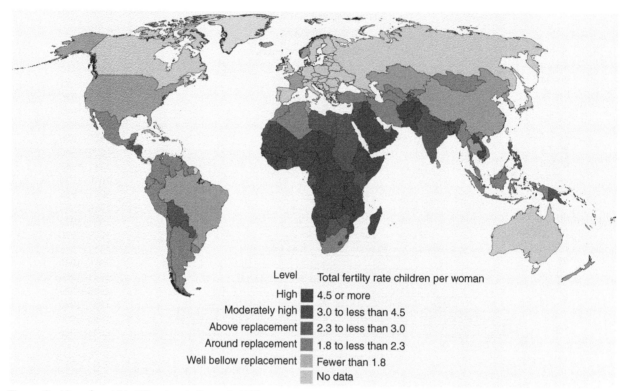

Figure 3 Map of world fertility rates. In the early 1970s, women in almost every developing country were estimated to have, on average, more than four children during their lives. In the three decades that followed, a revolution in childbearing spread across the world. Yet progress along the demographic transition has been uneven and lags in several regions. Data from United Nations Population Division (2005) *World Population Prospects: The 2004 Revision*. New York: United Nations Population Division.

Despite these gains in availability, contraceptive services are still difficult to obtain, unaffordable, or of poor quality in many countries. Approximately 201 million married women worldwide who would prefer to delay or avoid having another child are not using modern methods of contraception (Alan Guttmaches Institute and UNFPA, 2003). Unmet need is highest in sub-Saharan Africa, where 46% of women at risk of unintended pregnancy are not using any contraceptive, presumably reflecting lack of access or other barriers. Meanwhile, in developing countries, the number of women in their childbearing years is increasing by about 22 million women a year. For fertility rates to continue their global decline, family planning services will have to expand rapidly to keep up with both population growth and rising demand.

Mortality from HIV/AIDS and Other Infectious Diseases

Like no other disease, AIDS debilitates and kills people in their most productive years. Ninety percent of HIV-associated fatalities occur among people of working age, who leave behind large numbers of orphans – currently 11 million in sub-Saharan Africa

alone – with few means of supporting themselves. A projected 10–18% of the working-age population will be lost in the next 5 years in nine central and southern African countries, primarily due to AIDS-related illnesses (Cincotta *et al.*, 2003).

High rates of AIDS mortality lead to a bottle-shaped population age structure, with very high proportions of young people and many fewer older adults. As birth rates remain high while people of reproductive age die from AIDS-related causes, the share of young dependants to each working-age adult rises dramatically. Without significant advances in HIV prevention or in access to life-saving drugs in poor countries, AIDS-related mortality rates could increase significantly. UN population projections suggest that some countries will experience lower population growth rates from AIDS, but high fertility rates mean that population size in these countries is likely to still increase significantly (**Figure 5**).

Population growth also threatens global health through increased vulnerability to other infectious diseases. A growing population size living in and moving to and from densely populated areas creates expanded opportunities for disease to spread and intensify. At the country and community levels, governments often lack the resources to improve sanitation and public health services

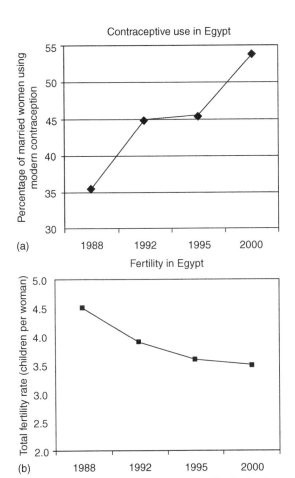

(a)

(b)

Figure 4 Contraceptive prevalence and fertility decline in Egypt. These figures illustrate the negative correlation between contraceptive use and total fertility rates that occurred over a 12-year period in Egypt. As an additional 20% of married women began using modern contraception between 1988 and 2000 (a), the country's total fertility rate (b) decreased from 4.5 to 3.5 children per woman. El-Zanaty F and Way A (2001) *Egypt Demographic and Health Survey 2000.* Calverton, MD: Ministry of Health and Population (Egypt), National Population Council and ORC Macro.

at the same rate that populations are increasing. At the household level, evidence from demographic surveys suggests that children born after several siblings tend to receive fewer immunizations and less medical attention than children born earlier or in smaller families (Rutstein, 2005). The cumulative effect of all these influences is a greater risk of disease with higher birthrates and rapid population growth.

Gender Equity

When women are able to determine the size of their families, fertility rates are generally lower than in settings where women's status is poor. In particular, there is a strong correlation between female school enrollment rates and fertility trends. In most countries, girls who are educated, especially those who attend secondary school, are more likely to delay marriage and childbearing. Women with some secondary education commonly have between two and four fewer children than those who have never been to school (Conly, 1998).

Early childbearing often limits educational and employment opportunities for women. When women have an education, their children tend to be healthier; in India, a baby born to a woman who has attended primary school is twice as likely to survive as one born to a mother with no education. By delaying marriage and childbearing, educating girls also helps lengthen the span between generations and slow the momentum driving future population growth.

Migration

The movement of people from one country to another – emigration in the case of those who leave their native country and immigration to describe the increase in a country's foreign-born population – continues to increase in both scale and frequency. International migration has doubled in the past 25 years, with about 200 million people – 3% of the world's population – today living in a country different from the one in which they were born. Approximately 60% of international migrants have chosen to live in developed countries, but migration within developing countries remains significant. Asia has three times as many international migrants as any other region of the developing world.

Although there are many reasons for increases in migration, the dramatic population growth of the past few decades has been a primary impetus. This has led, with a 15- to 20-year time lag, to the rapid growth of the world's labor force, especially among the young adults who make up the age group most likely to migrate. Tens of millions of people are added to the labor force each year, and the search for decent jobs is the leading reason people migrate. In addition deteriorating environmental conditions related to population growth – water and food shortages, for example, or human-induced climate change – can also spur large movements of population across international borders. Lower rates of population growth can help ease the pressures to migrate and improve the underlying conditions that force many people to seek a better life elsewhere.

Government Policies

Throughout history, government regulations on fertility – either by promoting or restricting childbirth – have directly affected population dynamics. Authoritarian regimes have pursued pro-natalist policies to increase the size of a population for militaristic, nationalist, and/or economic reasons. A few countries, including the world's most populous – China and India – have placed direct and indirect

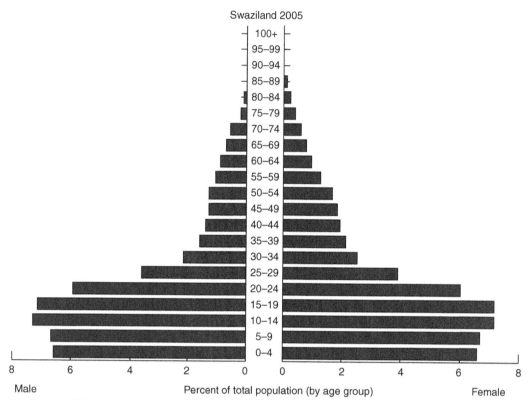

Figure 5 The Impact of HIV/AIDS on population age structure in Swaziland. The age structure of Swaziland's population in 2005 shows the decimating impact of the HIV/AIDS pandemic. As the disease leads to high mortality rates among working-age adults, high fertility rates create a youthful population. Data from United Nations Population Division (2005) *World Population Prospects: The 2004 Revision*. New York: United Nations Population Division.

regulations on their citizens' fertility as a means of reducing population growth.

All state regulation of fertility, whether pro-natalist or intended to slow population growth, has been strongly criticized by human rights advocates. The importance of individual freedom of choice concerning fertility and reproductive health was outlined and agreed upon by 19 countries in 1994 at the International Conference on Population and Development.

Worldwide, more than one-fifth of all pregnancies are terminated annually. The prevalence of abortion is one indication of the high level of unintended pregnancy worldwide. Political disagreements over the highly contentious issue of abortion have in recent years hampered the funding of population and reproductive health programs in both the United States and in many developing countries.

As in the case of abortion, government policy related to international migration cannot really be called population policy, since in no cases is it expressly designed to remedy perceived deficiencies in national population trends. Nonetheless, government policies on migration and the process itself do influence the pace and distribution of population change, and it remains possible that some countries with especially low fertility may design

future migration policies specifically to slow either the aging or the decline of their populations, or both.

Impacts of Population Growth

Health

High fertility rates can have an adverse effect on the health of women and children, especially in developing countries that lack a health infrastructure. Every year, an estimated 529 000 women die in pregnancy or childbirth (WHO, 2004), and for every woman who dies as many as 30 others suffer chronic illness or disability (Ashford 2002). Moreover, every year more than 46 million women resort to an induced abortion; 18 million do so in unsafe circumstances. Each year, approximately 68 000 women die from unsafe abortions and tens of thousands more suffer serious complications leading to chronic infection, pain and infertility (WHO, 2005).

Pregnancy-related deaths overall account for one-quarter to one-half of deaths to women of childbearing age. For both physiological and social reasons, pregnancy is the leading cause of death for young women aged 15–19 worldwide, with complications of childbirth and unsafe abortion being the major factors (WHO, 2004).

Furthermore, each year 3.3 million babies are stillborn, more than 4 million die within 28 days of birth, and another 6.6 million children die before age 5 (UN, 2005).

The timing of births has an impact on child health. When a pregnant woman has not had time to fully recover from a previous birth, the new baby is often born underweight or premature, develops too slowly, and has an increased risk of dying in infancy or contracting infectious diseases during childhood (Rustein, 2005). Research shows that children born less than 2 years after the previous birth are about 2.5 times as likely to die before age 5 than children who are born 3–5 years apart (Setty-Venugopal and Upadhyay, 2002).

Chronic hunger, which affects an estimated 852 million undernourished people worldwide, is another critical health issue that is directly linked to population growth. The number of chronically hungry people in developing countries increased by nearly 4 million per year in the latter part of the 1990s. Globally, the number of food emergencies each year has doubled over the past two decades, totaling more than 30 per year. Africa has the highest number and proportion of countries facing food emergencies. The average number of food emergencies in Africa has almost tripled since the 1980s, and one-third of the population of sub-Saharan Africa is undernourished. A 1996 study by the Food and Agriculture Organization estimated that Africa's food supply would need to quadruple by 2050 just to meet people's basic caloric needs under even the lowest, and most optimistic, population growth projections (Food and Agriculture Organization, 2004).

Poverty

Improving reproductive health care, including family planning, can have economic benefits. The expanded provision of family planning services was responsible for as much as a 43% reduction in fertility between 1965 and 1990 in developing countries; falling fertility rates, in turn, have been associated with an average 8% decrease in the incidence of poverty in low-income countries. Countries with poverty rates above 10% have fertility rates that are double those in richer countries (Leete and Schoch, 2003).

Lowering fertility rates through access to family planning information and contraceptive supplies has both macro- and microeconomic benefits. Just as national governments are able to spend more per capita on social welfare when population growth slows, parents can invest more in health and education costs for each child if they have fewer children. Couples who have smaller families are often able to have women work outside the home and to save more of their income, thus increasing the national labor supply, investment, and growth.

Economists credit declining fertility over the past four decades as one contributor to sustained economic growth among the East Asian Tiger countries, which include South Korea, Taiwan, Thailand, Singapore, Indonesia, Malaysia, and Hong Kong. Research indicates that shifts to smaller family size and slower rates of population growth in the region helped create an educated workforce, expand the pool of household and government savings, raise wages, and dramatically increase investments in manufacturing technology (Williamson and Higgins, 1997; Williamson, 2001). A shift to smaller families produced three important demographic changes: Slower growth in the number of school-age children, a lower ratio of dependants to working-age adults (dependency ratio), and a reduced rate of labor force growth. As fertility declined, household and government investments per child increased sharply, as did household savings, while governments reduced public expenditures. Domestic savings rose to displace foreign funds as the leading source of private sector investment and countries that had been major foreign aid recipients emerged to become a significant part of industrialized countries' export market. Although this model of fertility decline and economic growth has not yet been replicated in other regions of the world, the East Asian experience demonstrates how important a smaller average family size can be to economic development.

Natural Resources

Greater numbers of people and higher per capita resource consumption worldwide are multiplying humanity's impacts on the environment and natural resources. While population is hardly the only force applying pressure to the environment, the challenges of sustainability and conservation become harder to address as the number of people continues to increase. Currently, more than 1.3 billion people live in areas that conservationists consider the richest in nonhuman species and the most threatened by human activities. While these areas comprise about 12% of the planet's land surface, they hold nearly 20% of its human population. The population in these biodiversity hotspots is growing at a collective rate of 1.8% annually, compared to the world population's annual growth rate of 1.3% (Engelman, 2004). Human pressure on renewable freshwater, cropland, forests, fisheries, and the atmosphere is unprecedented and continually increasing.

Changes in ecosystems (natural systems of living things interacting with the nonliving environment) can greatly impact human prosperity, security, and public health. Food supply, fresh water, clean air, and a stable climate all depend upon healthy ecosystems. Human-induced or human-accelerated disturbances to ecosystems can increase the risk of acquiring infectious diseases, either directly or through the impact made to biodiversity. For example, air and water pollution are linked to increases in asthma and other respiratory problems, as well as cancer and heart disease. The emergence of Lyme disease in the United States is thought to be associated with habitat loss and diminished biodiversity. Many experts believe that climate change is also contributing to a rise of infectious disease worldwide, as warmer temperatures bring pathogens to new geographical areas (Epstein *et al.*, 2003).

Currently, more than 745 million people face water stress or scarcity (Engelman, 2004). Much of the fresh water now used in water-scarce regions originates from aquifers that are not being refreshed by the natural water cycle. In most of the countries where water shortage is severe and worsening, high rates of population growth exacerbate the declining availability of renewable fresh water. Cultivated land is at similar levels of critical scarcity in many countries. Despite the Green Revolution and other technological advances, agriculture experts continue to debate how long crop yields will keep up with population growth. The food that feeds future generations will be grown mostly on today's cropland, which must remain fertile to keep food production secure. Easing world hunger would be even more difficult if population growth resembles demographers' higher projections.

Likewise, future declines in the per capita availability of forests, especially in developing countries, are likely to pose major challenges for both conservation and for the provision of food, fuel, and shelter necessary for human well-being. Based on the United Nations' medium population projection and current deforestation trends, by 2025 the number of people living in forest-scarce countries could swell to 3.2 billion in 54 countries (Engelman, 2004). Most of the world's original forests have been lost to the expansion of human activities.

In 2002, per capita emissions of CO_2 continued a 3-year upward climb that appeared unaffected by the global economic jolt from the September 2001 terrorist attacks on the United States. In the 1999–2002 period, population growth and increasing per capita fossil-fuel consumption joined forces on an equal basis to boost global CO_2 emissions rapidly. With about 4.7% of the world's population, the United States accounted for almost 23% of all emissions from fossil-fuel combustion and cement manufacture, by far the largest CO_2 contributor among nations. (China, with more than four times the U.S. population, is number two.) Emissions remained grossly inequitable, with one-fifth of the world's population accounting for 62% of all emissions in 2002, while another — and much poorer — fifth accounted for 2%. Population growth and the corresponding increase in global CO_2 emissions are of crucial importance to scientists and policy makers concerned with the potential effects of global climate change.

Conflict and Security

During the last three decades of the twentieth century, the demographic transition was correlated with continuous declines in the vulnerability of countries to civil conflicts, including ethnic wars, insurgencies, and terrorism. Progress through the demographic transition gives countries a more mature and less volatile age structure, slower workforce growth, and a more slowly growing school-age population. It reduces urban growth and gives countries additional time to expand infrastructure, meet the demand for public services, and conserve dwindling natural resources. Countries in the early and middle phases of demographic transition have cumulatively been significantly more vulnerable to civil conflict than late-transition countries.

The likelihood of civil conflict steadily decreased for high-risk countries as they experienced overall declines in birth and death rates. From the 1970s to the 1990s, a decline in a country's annual birth rate of ten births per 1000 people corresponded to a decrease of approximately 10% in the likelihood of an outbreak of civil conflict.

The demographic factors most closely associated with the likelihood of a new outbreak of civil conflict during the 1990s were a high proportion of young adults ages 15–29 years and a rapid rate of urban population growth. When coupled with a large youth bulge, countries with a very low availability of cropland and/or renewable fresh water, plus a rapid rate of urban population growth, had a roughly 40% probability of experiencing an outbreak of civil conflict in the 1990s. Migration and differential rates of population growth among ethnic groups competing for political and economic power have also played important roles in political destabilization.

Over the past 40 years, the demographic transition has been progressing impressively in nearly all of the world's regions. Most of the world's countries are moving toward a distinctive range of population structures that make civil conflict less likely. Yet this progress through the demographic transition is not universal. Continuing declines in birth rates and increases in life expectancy in the poorest and worst-governed countries will be required.

Conclusion

In summary, the world is demographically complex, diverse, and divided in ways that have no precedent in human history. No one can say with confidence how problematic this diversity is or how humanity's demographic future will unfold. However, it is certain that given the linkages between world population growth and disease and mortality, environmental resources, gender equity, and civil conflict, demography will play a major role in the future of global public health.

See also: Demography, Epidemiology and Public Health; Demography of Aging; Epidemiology of HIV/AIDS and its Surveillance; Genetic Epidemiology; Populations at Special Health Risk: Migrants; Trends in Human Fertility.

Citations

The Alan Guttmacher Institute (1999) *Induced Abortion Worldwide.* New York: The Alan Guttmacher Institute.

The Alan Guttmacher Institute and UNFPA (2003) *Adding it up: The Benefits of Investing in Sexual and Reproductive Health Care.* New York: AGI and UNFPA.

Ashford L (2002) *Hidden Suffering: Disabilities from Pregnancy and Childbirth in Less Developed Countries.* Washington, DC: Population Reference Bureau.

Conly S (1998) *Educating Girls: Gender Gaps and Gains.* Washington, DC: Population Action International.

El-Zanaty F and Way A (2001) *Egypt Demographic and Health Survey 2000.* Calverton, MD: Ministry of Health and Population (Egypt), National Population Council and ORC Macro.

Engelman R (with Anastasion D) (2004) *Methodology. People in the Balance: Update 2004.* http://www.populationaction.org/ resources/publications/peopleinthebalance/downloads/ AcknowlAndMethodo.pdf.

Engelman R and Leahy E (2006) *How Many Children Does It Take to Replace Their Parents? Variation in Replacement Fertility as an Indicator of Child Survival and Gender Status.* Paper presented at the Population Association of America annual conference Los Angeles, 30 March–1 April.

Epstein PR, Chivian E, and Frith K (2003) Emerging diseases threaten conservation. *Environmental Health Perspectives.* 111(10): A506–A507.

Food Agriculture Organization (2004) *The State of Food Insecurity in the World 2004.* Rome: FAO.

Global Commission on International Migration (2005) *Migration in an Interconnected World: New Directions for Action.* Geneva, Switzerland: GCIM.

Joint United Nations Programme on HIV/AIDS (2005) *AIDS Epidemic Update: December 2005.* Geneva, Switzerland: UNAIDS.

Leete R and Schoch M (2003) Population and poverty: Satisfying unmet need as the route to sustainable development. *Population and Poverty: Achieving Equity, Equality and Sustainability* 8: 9–38.

Rutstein S (2005) Effects of preceding birth intervals on neonatal, infant and under-five years mortality and nutritional status in developing countries: Evidence from the Demographic and Health Surveys. *International Journal of Gynecology and Obstetrics* 89 (supplement 1): s7–s24.

Setty-Venugopal V and Upadhyay UD (2002) *Three to Five Saves Lives. Population Reports. L13: 2.* Baltimore, MD: Johns Hopkins University.

UNFPA. State of World Population (2004) *Reproductive Health and Family Planning.* http://www.infpa.org/swp/2004/english/ch6/ page3.html (accessed February 2006).

United Nations Children's Fund (2005) *State of the World's Children 2005.* New York: UNICEF.

United Nations Population Division (2004) *World Population to 2300.* New York, United Nations Population Division.

United Nations Population Division, Department of Economic and Social Affairs (2004) *World Contraceptive Use 2003.* New York: United Nations.

United Nations, Department of Economic and Social Affairs, Statistics Division (2005) *Word Population Prospects: The 2004 Revision.* New York: United Nations.

United Nations Population Division (2005) *World Population Prospects: The 2004 Revision.* New York: United Nations Population Division.

United Nations Population Division (2007) *World Population Prospects: The 2006 Revision.* New York: United Nations Population Division.

Williamson JG and Higgins M (1997) The accumulation and demography connection in East Asia. *Proceedings of the Conference on Population and the East Asian Miracle.* Honolulu, Hawaii: East-West Center.

Williamson JG (2001) Demographic change, growth, and inequality. In: Birdsall N, Kelley AC, and Sinding SW (eds.) *Population Matters: Demographic Change, Economic Growth, and Poverty in the Developing World,* pp. 107–136. Oxford,UK: Oxford University Press.

World Health Organization (2004) *Maternal Mortality in 2000: Estimates Developed by WHO, UNICEF and UNFPA.* Geneva, Switzerland: WHO.

World Health Organization (2005) *The World Health Report 2005: Make Every Mother and Child Count.* Geneva, Switzerland: WHO.

Further Reading

Ashford L (1995) *New Perspectives on Population: Lessons from Cairo.* Washington, DC: Population Reference Bureau.

Birdsall N, Kelley A, and Sinding S (eds.) (2001) *Population Matters: Demographic Change, Economic Growth, and Poverty in the Developing World.* New York: Oxford University Press.

Bongaarts J (1994) Population policy options in the developing world. *Science* 263: 771–776.

Chivian E (ed.) (2002) *Biodiversity: Its Importance to Human Health: Interim Executive Summary.* Cambridge, MA: Center for Health and the Global Environment Harvard Medical School.

Cincotta R, Wisnewski J, and Engelman R (2000) Human population in the biodiversity hotspots. *Nature* 404: 990–992.

Coale A and Hoover E (1958) *Population Growth and Economic Development in Low-Income Countries.* Princeton, NJ: Princeton University Press.

Cohen JE (1995) *How Many People Can the Earth Support?* New York: Norton.

Engelman R and LeRoy P (1993) *Sustaining Water: Population and the Future of Renewable Water Supplies.* Washington, DC: Population Action International.

Food and Agriculture Organization (1996) *Food Requirements and Population Growth.* World Summit Background Document No. 4. Rome: FAO.

Livi-Bacci M (1992) *Concise History of World Population.* Cambridge, MA: Blackwell Publishers.

Lutz W, O'Neill B, and Scherbov S (2003) Europe's population at a turning point. *Science* 299: 1991–1992.

Mason A (ed.) (2002) *Population Change and Economic Development in East Asia: Challenges Met, Opportunities Seized.* Stanford, CA: Stanford University Press.

National Research Council (1986) *Population Growth and Economic Development: Policy Questions.* Washington, DC: National Academy of Science Press.

Robey B, Rutstein S, and Morris L (1993) The fertility decline in developing countries. *Scientific American* 269: 60–67.

Smil V (1991) Population growth and nitrogen: An exploration of a critical existential link. *Population and Development Review* 17: 569–601.

United Nations (1994) *Programme of Action Adopted at the International Conference on Population and Development.* New York: United Nations.

Relevant Websites

http://www.measuredhs.com – Demographic and Health Surveys.
http://www.popact.org – Population Action International.
http://www.un.org/esa/population/unpop.htm – United Nations Population Division.
http://www.who.int – World Health Organization.

Trends in Human Fertility

J G Cleland, Centre for Population Studies, London School of Hygiene and Tropical Medicine, London, UK

Introduction

The number of children born per woman and the timing of births are directly relevant to public health and health services in many ways. The level of childbearing, for instance, determines the demand for obstetric and child health services and has a direct effect on the maternal mortality rate. The age pattern of childbearing influences the incidence of obstetric complications, because pregnancies in the early teenage years and at ages over 35 years pose an increased risk to the mother. Fecundity also declines after age 35, and thus postponement of births will increase the need for assisted reproduction. The spacing of births has important health implications; conceptions occurring within 24 months of a previous live birth are at elevated risk of fetal death, prematurity, low birth weight for gestational age, and infant mortality. Unintended pregnancies may result in induced abortion, which in many countries is restricted and unsafe.

Fertility also affects public health indirectly through socioeconomic pathways. Birth rates are the crucial determinant of population growth (or decline) and the age structure of populations, and both factors have profound socioeconomic implications. Countries growing at 2% per year or more (implying a doubling in population size every 36 years or less), because mortality has declined but fertility remains high, face greater difficulties in escaping from poverty and illiteracy than other countries, mainly because nearly half the population is aged under 15 years, thus placing a heavy dependency burden on the adult population. When fertility falls, an era of several decades follows when the labor force is proportionately large, the dependency burden is atypically low, and prospects for making rapid socioeconomic progress are especially bright. This era is inevitably followed by a return to a high-dependency burden because of an increase in the elderly population, which poses a strain on governments' health and welfare budgets.

The sequence is well illustrated by the case of the Republic of Korea (**Figure 1**). By 1960, mortality had already declined but fertility remained high at about six births per woman, and the population was growing at 2.8% per year. At that time, 42% of the total population was aged under 15 years but only 3% were aged 65 or more. In the next 40 years, fertility fell sharply and by 2000 the number of births per woman was about 1.4 and the growth rate had abated to 0.6% per year. Between 1960 and 2000 the number of working-age adults (15–64 years)

per 100 dependants rose from 120 to 250. Between 2000 and 2040 it is projected that the proportion of Korea's population aged 65 or more will rise from 7.4% to 30.5% and the ratio of workers to dependants will have fallen from 250 to 137 per 100 dependants. All industrialized countries now face similar problems of population aging.

In the absence of any constraints, it is estimated that the average number of births per woman would be about 15. In all societies, fertility is held well below this biological maximum by a blend of four main factors: restrictions on sexual intercourse, typically operating through marriage systems; lactation that inhibits ovulation; contraception; and induced abortion. The highest fertility recorded for a national population was 8.7 births per woman in Yemen between 1970 and 1985. In premodern societies, fertility was typically in the range of four to six births.

Between 1950 and 2005, the global fertility rate halved from about five to 2.5 births. Under conditions of moderate to low mortality, a little over two births per woman is required to bring about long-term stabilization of population size. Thus, the world as a whole may be approaching the end of an era of sustained growth, from 1 billion in 1830 to 6.5 billion in 2005 and a projected total of 9.2 billion in 2050 (United Nations, 2006). However, these global figures mask huge differences between regions and countries. The level of childbearing in most industrialized countries has fallen well below the two-child mark and therefore these countries face the possibility of population decline, combined with population aging. Conversely, many of the poorest countries in the world still retain buoyant fertility levels and can expect substantial increases in population size. In this article, fertility trends since 1950 will be described and the underlying causes and implications discussed.

Trends in Industrialized Countries

In most of Europe and in North America, fertility decline started in the late 19th century (well before the development of modern contraceptives) and birth rates fell to low levels in the Great Depression of the 1930s, giving rise to concerns about population decline. These concerns were short-lived because, following the end of World War II, fertility rose in most industrialized countries and in some it continued to rise throughout the 1950s (**Figure 2**). This postwar baby boom was most pronounced in the United States, where fertility climbed from 2.9 births in 1946

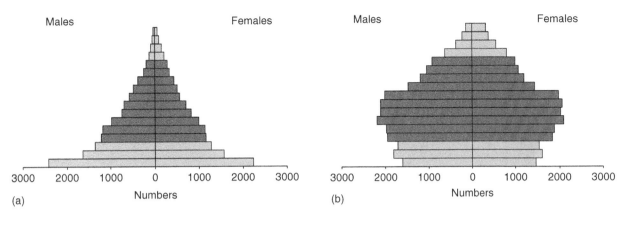

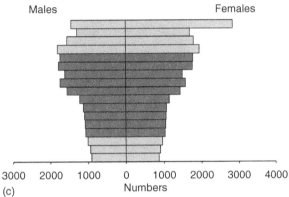

Figure 1 Age structure in Republic of Korea: 1960 (a), 2000 (b), and 2040 (c) (projected). Population aged 15–64 years is darkly shaded. Source: UN Department of Economic and Social Affairs, Population Division (2007) *World Population Prospects: The 2006 Revision.* New York: United Nations.

to peak at 3.7 births in 1957. Japan is the clearest exception: This country experienced a dramatic decline from 4.5 births in 1947 to 2.0 births a decade later, partly in response to a shift from pro- to antinatalist policies and liberalization of abortion laws.

The mid-1960s marked the start of a second and unforeseen phase of fertility decline. By 1980, fertility in most (developed) countries had fallen below the replacement level of two births. In 2005, childbearing was below 1.5 births in Italy, Spain, Germany, Austria, the Russian Federation, and much of Eastern Europe, and also in the economically advanced East Asian states and territories (Japan, Hong Kong, Singapore, Taiwan, Republic of Korea). Some of this decline can be attributed to increased efficiency in the prevention of unintended births. The advent of oral contraception in the 1960s represented a decisive break of the sex–reproduction nexus. Access to legal abortion was also made easier in many countries. In 2000, about 20% of known pregnancies were legally terminated in France, Norway, Denmark, Italy, the United Kingdom, and Sweden. This percentage exceeded 40% in many countries of the former Soviet bloc and the Russian Federation itself (United Nations, 2005). In the United States, the fraction of births reported by women as

unwanted fell from 20% in the early 1960s to 7% by the late 1970s, and the same trend no doubt occurred in many industrialized countries, though is less well documented.

However, most commentators have sought explanations in more fundamental changes than improved birth control. The fertility decline in many industrialized countries has been accompanied and partly propelled by postponement of marriage and parenthood, rises in cohabitation, nonmarital births, and divorce, increased acceptance of diverse sexual lifestyles, and a growing independence of women. These interwoven features, dubbed the 'second demographic transition,' represent an appreciable departure from marriage and parenthood as the central pillars of adult life. The key underlying cause is identified by some as the changing roles of women in society, together with the sluggish adaptation of men to this emancipation, for instance, by reluctance to shoulder a more equal share of the burden of housekeeping and childrearing. The shift away from marriage and motherhood has been called 'the revenge of women on men.' Paradoxically, however, the level of childbearing is lowest in countries where women's labor force participation is also very low: Japan, Greece, Italy, and Spain. It is also of note that these same countries have low proportions of nonmarital births.

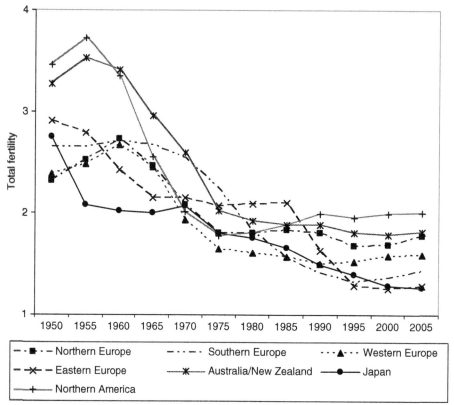

Figure 2 Fertility trends, 1950–2005: selected industrialized regions and countries. Source: UN Department of Economic and Social Affairs, Population Division (2007) *World Population Prospects: The 2006 Revision*. New York: United Nations.

Other experts, such as Ronald Lesthaeghe and Dirk van de Kaa, have sought an explanation in the development of broader 'postmodern' values of individualism, secularism, and the desire for self-fulfillment. Compelling region-specific explanations abound. For instance, the turbulence and insecurity caused by the break-up of the Soviet bloc coincides with the period of sharpest decline in these countries. Given the economic, social, and cultural diversity of the very-low-fertility countries, it seems unlikely that there is a single underlying cause.

A sustained fertility rate of 1.5 births implies a halving of population size approximately every 65 years. While this prospect of population shrinkage is welcomed by some environmental groups, it is regarded with alarm by many European and Asian governments. International migration on a sufficient scale to offset low birth rates and prevent population decline does not appear to be politically feasible. Hence, the main policy responses have been aimed at stimulating reproduction and have included generous maternity/paternity allowances (Sweden), child allowances that increase with parity (France), and cash payments at birth (Australia, Italy). Many other countries have shunned explicit pronatalist policies but have attempted to make family building and work more compatible, for instance, by better provision of infant care centers. None of these policies can claim long-term

effectiveness at raising birth rates, and the demographic futures of industrialized countries is uncertain (Gauthier, 1996). While most experts foresee the continuation of very low fertility, the United Nations envisages a slight but steady increase over the next 40 years. One factor favoring an increase concerns postponement of births, which depresses period rates but may not affect the number of children that women have over their life course. Sooner or later, the trend toward delayed childbearing must end and, when this happens, period fertility rates will increase, typically by an average of 0.2–0.4 births per woman (Lutz *et al.*, 2003). It is also true that a two-child family remains a widespread aspiration despite downward shifts in some countries (Goldstein *et al.*, 2003).

Trends in Developing Regions

In Asia, Latin America, and to a lesser extent Africa, life expectancy increased sharply while birth rates remained high in the two decades following World War II. The resulting acceleration of rates of population growth rang alarm bells because of evidence that socioeconomic progress would be jeopardized. Key U.S. leaders, such as President Lyndon Johnson and Robert MacNamara, president of the World Bank, became convinced of the need to reduce birth rates through the promotion of family planning. In 1969, the United Nations Fund for Population Activities (now the United Nations Population Fund – UNFPA) was created, with the shrewd choice of a Filipino Roman Catholic as its first executive director. Knowledge, attitude, and practice (KAP) surveys indicated the existence of favorable attitudes toward smaller family sizes and contraception in many poor countries. Pilot programs in Taiwan and the Republic of Korea showed that a ready demand existed for modern contraception, specifically the intrauterine device. Thus, the stage was set for a novel form of social engineering, the reduction of fertility through government-sponsored family planning programs. The number of developing countries with official policies to support family planning rose from two in 1960 to 115 by 1996.

Between 1950 and 2005, fertility in both Asia and Latin America fell from a little under six births per woman to about 2.5 births (**Figure 3**). The main exceptions are Afghanistan, the Lao People's Democratic Republic and Pakistan in Asia, and Guatemala, Bolivia, and Paraguay in Latin America. In the Arab states of North Africa, the corresponding decline was from 6.8 births to 3.2 births. Only in sub-Saharan Africa does fertility remain high at 5.5 births.

The relative influence of family planning promotion and socioeconomic development (in particular, increased life expectancy and education, which raise the number of surviving children and the costs of rearing them) on fertility trends is hotly contested. In most Latin American countries, the role of state intervention has been minor. Governments in this region were hesitant to promote

birth control partly because of the influence of the Roman Catholic church, and early efforts to popularize contraception were spearheaded by nongovernmental organizations with the prime objective of reducing illegal and unsafe abortions. The imprint of government actions can be more clearly discerned in Asia, notably in China, Bangladesh, and Indonesia. In China, programs to reduce population growth started in 1972 and, in the next seven years, fertility fell sharply – but not sufficiently, in the opinion of government planners. In 1979, the one-child policy was enacted and enforced rigorously in urban areas, where fertility fell quickly to one child. In rural areas, however, there was entrenched resistance and in the 1980s policy implementation in many provinces was relaxed to permit two children, particularly if the first born was a daughter (Gu *et al.*, 2007). China's fertility is currently estimated to be 1.7 births per woman. Because of the vast size of China's population, government policies in this country have made a major contribution to global stabilization but the price has also been high: denial of reproductive freedom, sex-selective abortion, abandonment of daughters, and instances of female infanticide.

In Bangladesh, one of the poorest and least literate countries in Asia, governments, faced with a highly visible population problem, had little choice but to address it as a top priority. Starting in 1975, a comprehensive family planning service was created, accompanied by incessant publicity through the mass media and other channels. Between 1975 and the 2000, fertility halved from six to three births per woman – a vivid demonstration that poverty and illiteracy are not incompatible with small families.

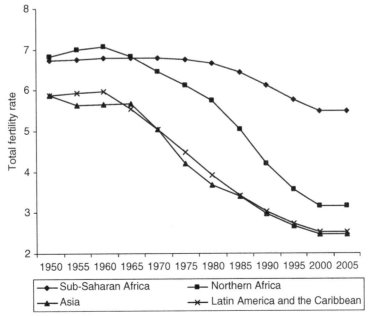

Figure 3 Fertility trends, 1950–2005: Selected developing regions. Source: UN Department of Economic and Social Affairs, Population Division (2007) *World Population Prospects: The 2006 Revision*. New York: United Nations.

The demographic histories of the Philippines and Indonesia also demonstrate that high educational levels and reasonably high status of women, factors thought to be particularly conducive to low fertility, do not always have this effect. In 1960, the Philippines was one of the wealthiest countries of Southeast Asia. The level of adult literacy was 72%, compared with only 39% in Indonesia. Income per head was almost double the Indonesian level at that time, life expectancy was 10 years longer, and infant mortality correspondingly lower. It came as no surprise, therefore, that fertility decline started earlier in the Philippines than in Indonesia. However, since the mid-1970s, the pace of decline has been much greater in Indonesia; the level of fertility in 2000–05 was estimated to be 2.5 births, one birth lower than in the Philippines.

The explanation for this unexpected outcome lies well beyond the realm of statistical evidence, but almost certainly involves the intertwined factors of religion and government policy. The Indonesian government skillfully evaded the potential danger of opposition from Islamic leaders by eschewing abortion and contraceptive sterilization. It mounted a very forceful family planning program, with considerable community pressure on couples to adopt birth control (Warwick, 1986). In the Philippines, no compact between church and state was reached, and Roman Catholic leaders remain strongly and openly opposed to modern birth control. This opposition has both inhibited the evolution of comprehensive family planning services and no doubt influenced the climate in which reproductive decisions are taken.

The persistence of rather high fertility in the Philippines is made even more surprising in view of the relatively high status of women in that country. Educational levels for women are exceptionally high, as is labor force participation. However, the example of the Philippines suggests that the status of women – if defined in terms of participation in public life, including paid employment – is not such an important precondition for sustained fertility decline as so often claimed. Indeed, it is probably more a consequence of decline than a cause.

Though fertility in sub-Saharan Africa remains high on average, the subregion is demographically diverse. In the Republic of South Africa and Zimbabwe (then Rhodesia), vigorous family planning promotion started before the advent of majority rule and fertility in both countries, and in Botswana is now at a relatively low level. HIV epidemics in southern Africa are especially severe and thus falling fertility has been accompanied by rapidly rising mortality. These countries face an exceptionally abrupt end to an era of population growth.

In eastern Africa, fertility decline has started in most countries, but most markedly in Kenya. In that country, a vigorous family planning effort was initiated in the early 1980s and, in the next 15 years, fertility fell from nearly eight to 4.8 births. Unexpectedly, the rate then plateaued, one likely reason being that funds and energy were diverted

from family planning to HIV/AIDS. Between 1988 and 2003, the proportion of contraceptive users relying on government services dropped from 68% to 53% and the percentage of births reported by mothers as unwanted rose from 11% to 21% (Westoff and Cross, 2006). Both trends imply a deterioration of government services. In 2002, the United Nations projected Kenya's population in 2050 at 44 million. In 2004, this projection was raised to 83 million, mainly in response to the fertility stall but also to a reduction in expected AIDS-related mortality.

This sequence of events in Kenya may be an extreme example of a more pervasive trend throughout much of the region. Rather than gathering pace in the past 15 years, the trend toward lower fertility has faltered. In west and central Africa, fertility typically remains close to six births per woman, contraceptive use prevalence among married women remains below 10%, and desired family sizes are still high. The United Nations projects that fertility in sub-Saharan Africa will decline steadily to reach 2.5 births by midcentury. Even if this projection is accurate, Africa's population is set to rise from 0.77 billion in 2005 to 1.76 billion in 2050. Most countries will double in population size in the next 40 or so years, and some will triple in size.

Is the persistence of high fertility throughout much of sub-Saharan Africa simply a reflection of low socioeconomic development or of distinctive features of culture and social organization that set the region apart from Asia and Latin America? Certainly, standards of living for many Africans worsened in the 1990s, but equally high levels of poverty and illiteracy did not stifle fertility transition in Asia, as trends in Bangladesh and Nepal since the 1980s show. It is also true that countless surveys reveal that Africans attach a higher value to large families than citizens elsewhere. According to Caldwell, the explanation for this pronatalism lies in the subordination of the nuclear family to the lineage. For lineage leaders, the patriarchs, high fertility is advantageous because it enhances their prestige, power, and patronage. Thus, they see children as sources of wealth rather than as drains on emotional and financial resources. A related explanation stems from the multiplicity of ethnic and linguistic groups in Africa, with the inevitable tension and conflict over resources that this diversity implies. A buoyant birth rate and numerical strength may well have conferred advantage in these circumstances, thus engendering strongly pronatalist values.

Since the most recent International Conference on Population and Development in Cairo, in 1994, policies to reduce population growth through family planning promotion have fallen from fashion and been replaced by a broader agenda of women's reproductive health and rights. The topic of population has been marginalized in key reports on development and was omitted from the Millennium Development Goals. International funding for family planning has fallen. This neglect may prove to be mistaken. **Figure 4** shows a display of the 76 poorest

	Low (<10%)	Medium (10%–19%)	High (20%+)
High (5.0 or more)		Mozambique [5.52] Nigeria [5.85] Niger [7.45] Nicaragua [8.00]	Senegal [5.22] Kenya [5.00] Togo [5.37] Cote d'Ivoire [5.06] Zambia [5.65] Madagascar [5.28] Ethiopia [5.78] Tanzania [5.66] Rwanda [6.01] Guinea [5.84] Yemen [6.02] Benin [5.87] Malawi [6.03] Chad [6.54] Burkina Faso [6.36] Somalia [6.43] Sierra Leone [6.50] Angola [6.75] Mali [6.70] Burundi [6.80] D R Congo [6.70] Afghanistan [7.50] Uganda [6.75]
Medium (3.0–4.99)	Egypt [3.17]	Sri Lanka [3.02] India [3.11] Bangladesh [3.22] Paraguay [3.48] Jordan [3.53] Philippines [3.54] Zimbabwe [3.56] Hounduras [3.72]	Syria [3.48] Laos [3.59] Cambodia [3.64] Nepal [3.68] Tajikistan [3.81] Bolivia [3.96] Pakistan [3.99] Haiti [4.00] Papua New Guinea [4.32] Ghana [4.59] Guatemala [4.60] Sudan [4.82] Iraq [4.86] Cameroon [4.92]
Low (1.0–2.9)	Romania [1.29] Cuba [1.63] China [1.70] Thailand [1.83] Korea, Dem Rep [1.92] Kazakhstan [2.01] Vietnam [2.32] Indonesia [2.38] Brazil [2.35] Colombia [2.47]	Ukraine [1.15] Belarus [1.24] Azerbaijan [1.67] Tunisia [2.04] Kyrgyz Republic [2.50] Morocco [2.52] Algeria [2.53] Peru [2.70] Uzbekistan [2.74] Ecuador [2.82] El Salvador [2.88] Dominican Republic [2.95]	Bulgaria [1.26] Serbia [1.75] Myanmar [2.25]

Total fertility (births per woman) 2000–2005

Unmet need for family planning

Figure 4 Classification of low-income countries by fertility rate (2000–05) and unmet need for family planning. Figures in parentheses show the fertility rate.

countries with a current population of 5 million or more, by fertility rate (2000–05) and by the level of unmet need for family planning – defined as the percent of married women who want no child for at least 2 years but are using no method of contraception. Over one-third of these countries, mostly in Africa, still have high fertility of five births or more per woman, and the vast majority of these countries also have a high unmet need for family planning. In a further 25 countries, fertility is in the range of three to five births, well above replacement level.

Conclusions

For millennia, the human population grew at a miniscule rate because moderate fertility was matched by high, albeit fluctuating, mortality. The scientific and technological revolution of the past 200 years broke this demographic balance and gave rise to an unprecedented surge in human numbers. The past 50 years has seen a necessary and welcome return toward balance; fertility has fallen in most countries, and world population may stabilize in the latter half of this century. Thus, the prospect of the Malthusian nightmare of famine and warfare, so prominently proclaimed in the 1960s by Paul Ehrlich and others, has receded.

No consensus on the ideal level of fertility exists, but a range of 1.7 to 2.3 births per woman has much to recommend it, as it implies modest growth or decline. As shown in this article, the world is still far away from such a benign outcome. Fertility rates in many industrialized countries have plunged well below 1.7 while many poor countries have rates well above 2.3. Indeed, the fertility of nations has rarely been so diverse. Our demographic future is still uncertain. Will birth rates in Africa fall as fast and pervasively as in Asia and Latin America, and will fertility edge steadily up in countries such as Japan and Italy? What happens in Africa is partly a matter of political priorities because a large body of successful experience at reducing fertility has accumulated. Policies to raise fertility do not have a successful track record, and so trends in low-fertility countries are particularly difficult to predict.

Citations

Gauthier AN (1996) *The State and the Family: A Comparative Analysis of Family Policies in Industrialised Countries*. Oxford, UK: Clarendon Press.

Goldstein J, Lutz W, and Testa MR (2003) The emergence of sub-replacement family size ideals in Europe. *Population Research and Policy Review* 22(5–6): 479–496.

Gu B, Wang F, Guo Z, and Zhang E (2007) China's local and national fertility policies at the end of the twentieth century. *Population and Development Review* 33: 129–147.

Lutz W, O'Neill BC, and Scherbov S (2003) Europe's population at a turning point. *Science* 299: 1991–1992.

United Nations (2005) *The New Demographic Regime: Population Challenges and Policy Responses*. Geneva, Switzerland: Economic Commission for Europe and United Nations Population Fund.

United Nations (2006) *World Population Prospects: The 2006 Revision*. New York: Department of Social and Economic Affairs, Population Division.

Warwick DP (1986) The Indonesian family planning program: Government influence and client choice. *Population and Development Review* 12: 453–490.

Westoff C and Cross A (2006) *The Stall in the Fertility Transition in Kenya*. Demographic and Health Surveys Analytical Study No. 9. Calverton, MD: ORC Macro.

Further Reading

Caldwell JC and Caldwell P (1987) The cultural context of high fertility in sub-Saharan Africa. *Population and Development Review* 13: 409–437.

Caldwell JC and Schidlmayr T (2003) Explanation of the fertility crisis in modern societies: A search for commonalities. *Population Studies* 57: 241–264.

Cleland J, Bernstein S, Ezeh A, Faundes A, and Innis J (2006) Family planning: The unfinished agenda. *Lancet* 368: 1810–1827.

Davis K, Bernstam MS, and Ricardo-Campbell R (eds.) (1986) Below-replacement fertility in industrial societies: Causes, consequences, policies. *Population and Development Review*, 12 (supplement).

Guzmán JM, Singh S, Rodríguez G, and Pantelides EA (eds.) (1996) *The Fertility Transition in Latin America*. Oxford, UK: Clarendon Press.

Kirk D (2000) The demographic transition. *Population Studies* 50: 361–388.

Leete R and Alam I (eds.) (1993) *The Revolution in Asian Fertility: Dimensions, Causes and Implications*. Oxford, UK: Clarendon Press.

Lesthaeghe R and Meekers D (1986) Value changes and the dimension of familism in the European community. *European Journal of Population* 2: 225–268.

van de Kaa DJ (2001) Post modern fertility preferences: From changing value orientation to new behavior. In: Bulatao RA and Casterline JB (eds.) Global Fertility Transition. *Population and Development Review*, pp. 290–331.

Relevant Websites

http://www.populationaction.org – Population Action International.

http://www.prb.org – Population Reference Bureau.

http://www.un.org/esa/population/unpop.htm – United Nations Department of Economic and Social Affairs, Population Division.

http://unstats.un.org/unsd/demographic/default.htm – United Nations Statistics Division.

Life Expectancy Measurements

D M J Naimark, University of Toronto, Toronto, Ontario, Canada

Introduction

Life expectancy (LE) is one of the key issues in clinical medicine. It is of interest to individual patients and their medical practitioners as well as to policy makers when trying to understand the impact of a given health program on the longevity of members of the general population. Estimation of the gains in LE associated with medical interventions that are considered to be effective some-times seem small. For example, there is little doubt that cigarette smoking has the potential to shorten life because it causes cancer. One would think, therefore, that smoking cessation should be associated with a significant increase in LE. However, the gain for 35-year-old women is only 8 months (Tsevat, 1991; Wright, 1998). To a lay person and to many health professionals, this increase hardly seems worth the considerable effort required by smokers in order to stop smoking. In fact, this particular magnitude of LE gain can be shown to be quite significant.

The objectives of this article are to explore the mean-ing of LE and gains or losses thereof, to understand those factors inherent in a disease state or in a health interven-tion that determine the magnitude of a change in LE, and to illustrate some methods for estimating LE values from empirical data. In this chapter, the LE associated with a closed cohort is considered, that is a group of individuals that is gathered together at some inception point and then followed over time. Dynamic cohorts, of interest to demo-graphers, in which new individuals are added to the group as time passes, by birth for example, are not within the scope of the current discussion.

Definition of Life Expectancy

Average Life Span

In the ideal case, LE is a straightforward concept. It is equal to the average life span of a cohort of individuals who are observed after an inception time point. Some examples of cohorts include the members of an arm of a randomized clinical trial (RCT), a particular exposure group in a prospective, observational study, and a hypo-thetical cohort in a Markov decision model. Examples of inception points include birth, the onset or diagnosis of a disease, the initiation of treatment, or the first cycle of a Markov process (see 'Life Expectancy as the Output of a Markov Process').

From a theoretical perspective, calculating the LE for a cohort involves observing it until all of the members have died, summing the total amount of time, e.g., the life-months, that the cohort accrued and then dividing by the number of individuals in the cohort at the inception point. A graphic illustration of this is shown in **Figure 1**. The life spans, in months, since the inception of the cohort is shown for a group of ten individuals. If the total number of life-months experienced by the members of the cohort was 130, then the life expectancy of the cohort is equal to 130 life-months/10 lives = 13.0 months. Note that LE is always an average: Some individuals may live more and some may live less than the average. Given an individual with the same characteristics, placed in the same environment, and at the same point in his or her life history as the members of the cohort were at the inception point, one would expect him or her to live 13 months, on average.

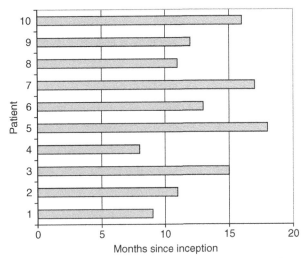

Figure 1 Life expectancy as the sum of the life spans of members of a cohort divided by the number of individuals in the cohort.

Equivalent Way of Thinking about LE

An alternative way to conceptualize the calculation of LE is not to think of horizontal life spans of members of the cohort as shown in **Figure 1**, but rather to think of verti-cal cohort membership as shown in **Figure 2**. The number of individuals remaining in the cohort each month after the inception point is plotted as a series of vertical bars. As members of the cohort die, the vertical bars shrink in size.

The members of the cohort who survive the first month each add 1 life-month to the cumulative total of the cohort. One can see that the number of life-months accrued by the members of the cohort during the first month after the inception is equal to the area of the rectangle above month 1 in **Figure 2**. The width of the rectangle is equal to 1 month and its height is equal to the number of indivi-duals who survived for at least 1 month. The total number of life-months experienced by the cohort is therefore the sum of the areas of the rectangles. If that sum happened to be 8236 life-months, and there were 684 individuals in the cohort at the inception, then the LE of the cohort would be $8236/684 = 12.04$ months.

Area Under a Survival Curve

The process of calculating LE by adding up the areas of the rectangles as shown in **Figure 2** and then dividing by the number of individuals in the cohort at inception can be represented symbolically as:

$$L \approx \frac{vn_1 \cdot \Delta_1 + n_2 \cdot \Delta_2 + \ldots + n_m \cdot \Delta_m}{n_0} \quad [1]$$

where n_0 is the number of individuals in the cohort at time zero, n_i, is the number left in the cohort after the ith interval, which is the same as the height of the ith rectangle ($i\varepsilon[1,m]$), and Δ_i is the width of the ith interval.

In this case, $\Delta_1 = \Delta_2 = \ldots = \Delta_m = 1$ month. The area of the rectangle associated with the ith interval is the product of its width and its height, $n_i \Delta_i$, and the sum of those products equals the total number of life-months accrued by the cohort. Distributing the denominator through the terms in the numerator yields:

$$L \approx \frac{v n_1}{n_0} \cdot \Delta_1 + \frac{v n_2}{n_0} \cdot \Delta_2 + \ldots + \frac{v n_m}{n_0} \cdot \Delta_m \qquad [2]$$

Since n_i/n_0 is the proportion of individuals, or the probability of an individual surviving the ith interval, the equation for LE can be rewritten as:

$$L \approx P_1 \cdot \Delta_1 + P_2 \cdot \Delta_2 + \ldots + P_m \cdot \Delta_m \qquad [3]$$

As shown in **Figure 3**, if, instead of representing the absolute number of individuals remaining in the cohort at a given time, the proportion surviving or the probability

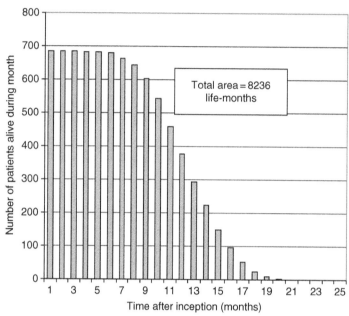

Figure 2 An alternative way to conceive of life expectancy: The sum of the areas representing the number of cohort members remaining alive at each month after inception divided by the number of people initially in the cohort.

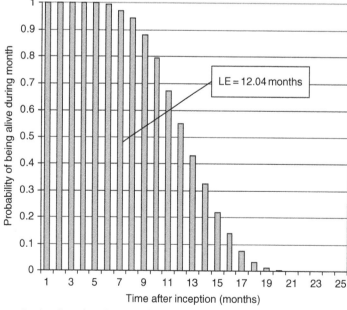

Figure 3 Life expectancy can also be viewed as the sum of the areas of rectangles representing the probability of remaining alive at each month after inception.

of survival is plotted as a function of time since inception, then the LE of the cohort is equal to the area of the rectangles themselves rather than the area of rectangles divided by the number of individuals at inception.

As shown in **Figure 4**, if LE is calculated as the area of the rectangles in a discrete, survival probability graph, whether the probability of survival for a given month is calculated at the end (**Figure 4(a)**) or the beginning (**Figure 4(b)**) of each interval will produce significantly

different answers for the LE estimate. In the figure, the ideal survival curve is shown as a smooth line. The ideal curve represents the more likely scenario that deaths in the cohort occur randomly throughout the interval, rather than at discrete times as has been assumed thus far. **Figure 4(a)** shows the results of using a discrete process to account for deaths at the end of the interval. In that case, the resulting LE estimate will underestimate the ideal value. Conversely, as shown in **Figure 4(b)**, the LE estimate

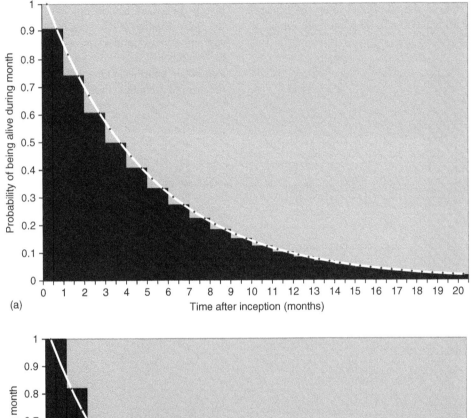

(a)

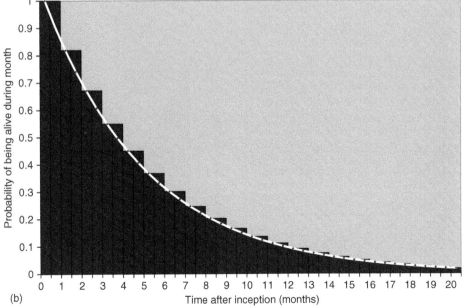

(b)

Figure 4 The sum of the areas of rectangles representing the probability of survival differs if the heights correspond to points on the ideal curve (the white line) at the beginning or end of each month. (a) The rectangles are arranged so that they represent points on the ideal curve at the end of each interval and LE is underestimated. (b) Conversely, the rectangles are arranged to represent the height of the ideal curve at the beginning of each month and LE is overestimated.

derived from accounting for survival at the beginning of the interval will overestimate the ideal value.

The error introduced will be significant if the size of the interval is a substantial fraction of the time horizon of the cohort. The horizon can be thought of as the number of intervals where the remaining fraction of the cohort is above some minimal value. As shown in **Figure 5**, as the width of the intervals decreases, and their number increases, then the LE calculated as the sum of rectangular areas approaches the ideal value. In the case shown in the figure, membership in the cohort is counted at the beginning of each interval. Thus, as the number of intervals increases, the LE estimate decreases toward the ideal value. Finally, in the limit:

$$L = \lim_{\substack{n \to \infty \\ \Delta \to 0}} \sum_{i=1}^{n} P_i \cdot \Delta_i = \int_0^{\infty} S(t)dt \qquad [4]$$

In other words, LE can be understood to be equivalent to the area under a smooth survival function, S(t). The latter statement is true regardless of the shape of the curve.

Figure 6 demonstrates a cumulative survival curve. With each interval, the number of life-months generated by the members of the cohort during the current interval is added to the cumulative total for all of the prior intervals. The height of each rectangle represents the current value of the cumulative total. As shown in the figure, the cumulative total approaches a certain value asymptotically. This value is equivalent to the areas of the rectangles, i.e., approximately the LE, of the noncumulative survival curve. Just as the approximation of life expectancy in the noncumulative case improves when the size of the intervals decreases and their number increases, the asymptotic value obtained from a cumulative survival plot approaches the ideal when it is in the form of a smooth curve.

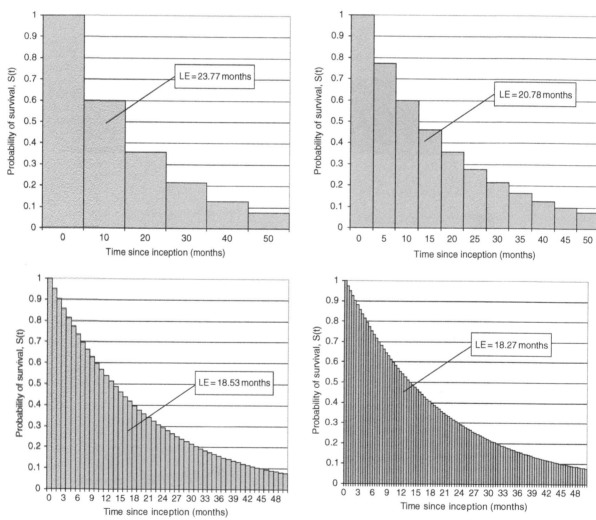

Figure 5 The LE estimate when taken as the areas of probability rectangles approaches the true value as the number of rectangles increases and their width decreases. In this case, since the heights of the rectangles correspond to probabilities at the beginning of each interval, and thus overestimate the true LE, as the number of rectangles increases the LE estimate decreases toward the true value.

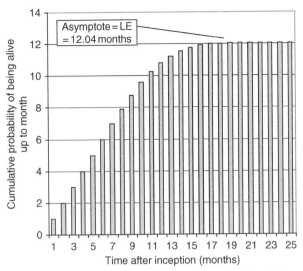

Figure 6 A cumulative probability plot approaches the LE asymptotically.

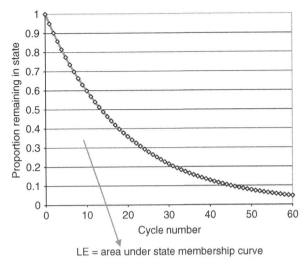

LE = area under state membership curve

Figure 7 The area underneath the state membership graph for the well state in a two-state Markov process is equivalent to the survival curve for a real cohort. Both represent LEs.

Life Expectancy as the Output of a Markov Process

A Markov process is a method of simulating the behavior of a cohort of individuals with a particular health scenario. The simulation traces the distribution of the hypothetical cohort among a set of mutually exclusive health states over time. The passage of time is represented by a cycle counter. Each cycle consists of a set of steps: (1) Transitioning hypothetical individuals from one state to another via a set of probability rules; (2) determining the new distribution of the cohort among the health states; and then (3) awarding each hypothetical individual an increment of life equivalent to the length of the cycle. At the end of each cycle, the total number of life-months experienced by the cohort is added to a cumulative total.

Time in a Markov process is represented by the product of the cycle length (in units of days, months, or years) and the number of cycles that have elapsed since the initiation of the process. A Markov model should have one or more absorbing states into which hypothetical individuals may enter but from which they cannot leave and which does not award life increments. Eventually when the proportion of the cohort that has not been absorbed reaches a preset minimum, the Markov process terminates. The total accumulated life increments for the cohort approaches a final value asymptotically. This latter value, when divided by the size of the hypothetical cohort, is the output of the Markov process.

One can appreciate that the procedure of calculating the accumulating life increments of a hypothetical cohort in a Markov process is equivalent to the procedure of calculating the LE of a real cohort of individuals using a cumulative survival plot. Also, it is easy to see, therefore, that the output of a Markov process is a LE. **Figure 7** shows a state membership graph in which the proportion of a hypothetical cohort remaining in the alive health state of a two-state Markov process is plotted as a function of cycle number. The other state, dead, represents the absorbing state for the process. The state membership plot is equivalent to a survival curve for the alive state. The area underneath the graph represents the contribution of life increments from members of the cohort who have spent time in that state to the cumulative total for the entire cohort.

Quality-Adjusted LE

Figure 8 shows a state membership graph for a slightly more complicated Markov process. In this case, there is a well state, an intermediary sick state and an absorbing dead state. The unadjusted LE for the Markov process is equal to the sum of the areas under the well and sick curves. However, a common practice is to assign a relative value, known as an incremental utility, to each state. For example, if an incremental utility of 0.6 is assigned to the sick state, it implies that a cycle spent in that state is only worth 60% of a cycle spent in the well state. Formal systems for eliciting judgments about the relative value of health states exist. If the area underneath each state membership curve is multiplied by its associated incremental utility, then the sum of those products is known as a quality-adjusted LE.

Event-Free LE

Until this point, the event of interest has been the death of members of the cohort. However, the concept of LE can be extended to any irreversible outcome. An example of this is

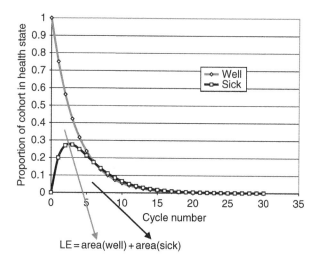

$$LE = area(well) + area(sick)$$

$$QALE = area(well)*Uwell + area(sick)*Usick$$

Figure 8 The sum of the areas under the well and sick states of a three-state Markov process after being multiplied by their respective incremental utilities yields the quality-adjusted LE for the hypothetical cohort.

the freedom from first cancer recurrence. A cohort of patients who have experienced an initial remission of their cancer would exist in this state until the first recurrence happens. Since they can never again be said to have not experienced a first recurrence, the transition out of the freedom-from-first-recurrence health state is irreversible. The area under a plot of the proportion of individuals free of first recurrence would give the event-free LE of that cohort.

Gains in LE

The discussion to this point has focused on the LE of a single cohort. However, clinicians are often interested in the relative difference between two alternative strategies. Given that the LE of a cohort is equivalent to the area under its survival curve. It follows that the gain in LE, ΔLE, associated with membership in one cohort relative to another is equal to the area between their respective survival curves, as is shown in **Figure 9**.

Determinants of the Magnitude of Gains in LE

The gain in LE associated with adopting one health strategy over another is equal to the area between their respective survival curves. Therefore, the magnitude of gains in LE is determined by the two factors that alter the area between survival curves: (1) The vertical or horizontal separation of the curves, and (2) the slope of the curves.

As shown in **Figure 10**, the vertical separation of two survival curves at some time point is equivalent to the absolute difference in survival between the two strategies, which is the same as the absolute risk reduction (ARR)

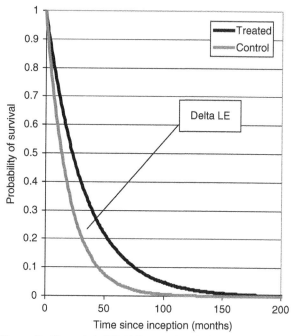

Figure 9 The gain in LE, ΔLE, associated with one health strategy versus another represents the area between their survival curves.

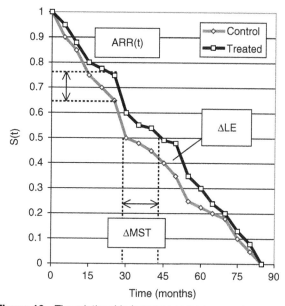

Figure 10 The relationship between some commonly employed measures of treatment effect. The absolute risk reduction at some time t, ARR(t), is the vertical separation of the curves at t, the change in median survival time, ΔMST, is the horizontal separation of the curves at a survival probability of 0.5. ΔLE represents the area between the survival curves that integrates the ARR at all times, t, and the change in survival time at all survival probabilities.

at that time. The horizontal separation of the curves at a survival probability of 0.5 is equivalent to the difference in median survival time between the two strategies.

In the case of curves representing a control group and an intervention group, the separation of the curves, vertical or horizontal, is determined by the absolute efficacy of the intervention and the proportion of people in the cohort who will benefit from it. For example, the benefit from vaccination against a rare but lethal infectious disease is distributed unevenly in the cohort of vaccinated individuals. The vaccine produces a very large gain in LE in those who would have ultimately contracted the disease but has zero effect in those who would not. The gain in LE for the former group is very large but since they represent only a small fraction of the cohort, and since the majority of the cohort experience zero gain, the LE gain for the cohort overall is quite small. For example, in the smoking cessation example mentioned in the introduction, the gain of 8 months represents the population-wide gain for all 35-year-old women regardless of their smoking history. When the gain is recomputed for the 35-year-old female smokers who are actually at risk, its value is a more impressive 2.8 years (Tsevat, 1991; Wright, 1998).

The other determinant of the magnitude of a gain in LE is the slope of the survival curves. For any given ARR at a fixed time (or change in median survival time), the steeper the decline in the control (baseline) group curve, the lower the gain in LE associated with adopting an intervention (see **Figure 11**). One approach to help put gains into perspective would be to report both the absolute gain in LE and the proportion or percentage that the gain represents of the LE in the control group. For example, in the smoking cessation example mentioned in the introduction, the ΔLE was 8 months on a baseline LE of 542 months, which represents a gain of 1.5%. In a cohort at much higher

risk, with a baseline LE of 24 months, the same absolute gain in LE would represent a 33% increase.

Wright *et al.* (1998) have suggested using baseline risk in a qualitative sense as a criterion for categorizing the gains associated with medical interventions. Their goal was to help readers of studies that report gains in LE to put the results into the correct context and thereby determine if the gain is significant. They have proposed that gains of 1 month or more should be considered for preventative strategies in populations at average risk – for example, a decade of biennial mammography for women aged 50 produced a gain of 0.8 months. Prevention strategies aimed at populations with elevated risk yielded gains that were typically about 1 year. For example, reduction of diastolic blood pressure from an initial value between 90 and 94 mmHg to a value less than 88 mmHg in 35-year-old hypertensive patients yielded a gain of 13 months for men and 11 months for women. The authors found that gains associated with the treatment of established disease varied with the severity of the disease but rarely exceeded 1 year.

Perceptual Difficulties

One of the reasons that gains in LE may seem to be small is a misconception regarding their meaning. As we have seen, a gain (or loss) of LE represents the area between two survival curves. However, readers often make the mistake of thinking that gains in LE come as additional time tacked onto the end of a fixed life span. For example, a 20-year-old female smoker, anticipating a LE of an additional 60 years, might think that a LE gain of 8 months means that he or she will live to be 80.67 years rather than 80 years if she were to stop smoking.

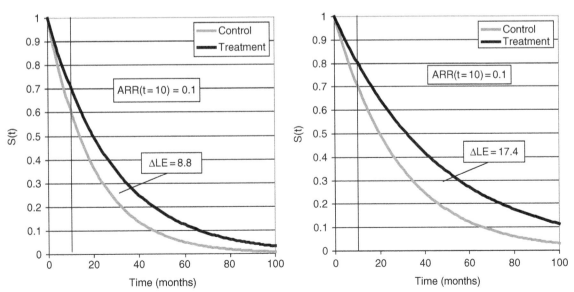

Figure 11 The same absolute risk reduction (ARR) at 10 years can produce different ΔLE values depending on the slope of the curves – the steeper the curves, the lower the resulting ΔLE.

Such a gain seems small to her because of the process of discounting. The latter concept refers to the fact that benefits we receive in the future are less valuable to us in present terms than benefits we receive immediately. For example, imagine a 20-year-old individual being told that he or she will lose 1 year of life due to smoking: In the first case, the individual will die immediately instead of living until age 21 and in the second case, he or she will live only until age 80 instead of 81. Most people would consider the former scenario to represent a much more significant loss even though the numerical change in life span is identical. This implies that we value life in the near-term more than life in the future. Thus, if it was true that LE gains merely represent extensions of life span in the distant future, then they would have little value to us in the present because of the process of discounting. In reality, the fact that gains in LE are equivalent to the separation of survival curves means that the benefit starts to occur as soon as the two curves start to separate.

Estimation of LE from Empirical Sources

In contrast to the simplicity of the calculation of LE in an ideal and theoretical sense wherein one follows a complete cohort of individuals until all have died, estimation of LE using commonly available data is not so straightforward. The difficulty lies in the fact that cohorts are rarely followed until all of its members have died. Censoring and incomplete observation requires some degree of extrapolation when estimating LE. Extrapolation can be achieved with parametric and nonparametric approaches.

Closed-Form, Parametric LE Estimation

The goal of the closed-form parametric approach is to produce an expression of LE that is relatively simple and that can be evaluated with a hand-held calculator (i.e., that does not need numerical approximation using a computer simulation).

The exponential survival function
The simplest closed-form approach is to assume a survival model in which the hazard remains constant – the exponential model – which has the following form:

$$S(t) = \exp(-\mu t) \qquad [5]$$

where μ is a constant value. LE, as has been shown above, is equal to the area under the survival function:

$$L = \int_0^\infty S(t)dt \qquad [6]$$

Evaluating the integral yields $L = 1/\mu$.

From the data for a group in a RCT or a prospective observational study, one can obtain the estimated proportion of deaths, P(t), during the observation interval, *t*. The latter estimate may be derived from a Kaplan-Meier estimate. Alternatively, P(t) may represent the raw proportion of events observed in the cohort under observation at the median observation time, *t*. The estimate of the survival function is therefore:

$$\hat{S}(t) = 1 - \hat{P}(t) \qquad [7]$$

Using this estimate of the survival function at *t*, an estimate of the LE of the cohort can be obtained:

$$\hat{\mu} = -\ln\left[\hat{S}(t)\right]/t \qquad [8]$$

$$\hat{L} = v1/\hat{\mu} = -t/\ln\left[\hat{S}(t)\right] \qquad [9]$$

Caution is required when using this approach since Kuntz and Weinstein (1995) have shown that LE estimates generated in this way are statistically biased. In other words, since the LE estimate is a nonlinear function of the survival function estimate, the expected value of the LE estimate is not equal to the true LE value.

Using a Taylor series expansion, they show that:

$$\in(\hat{L}) = \in\left(\frac{v-t}{\ln\left[\hat{S}(t)\right]}\right) = \left(\frac{v-t}{\ln[S(t)]}\right)$$
$$- \frac{vt\sigma^2(t)[2 + \ln[S(t)]]}{2S(t)^2[\ln[S(t)]]^3} \qquad [10]$$

In other words, the expected value of the LE estimate can be decomposed into the true value (the first term on the right-hand side) and a bias term (the second term on the right-hand side). The magnitude of the bias is a function of *t*, $\sigma^2(t)$, representing the variance of the survival function estimate, and the true survival function value S(t).

Kuntz and Weinstein point out that the bias term is zero when $\ln[S(t)] = -2$ and S(t) is, therefore, approximately 0.135. When S(t) is greater than 0.135, the bias tends to be positive and vice versa. The variance of the survival function estimate depends both on the sample size and on the percentage of censoring within the study on which the estimate was based. Through simulation, they show that the magnitude of the bias increases as the sample size on which P(t) is based decreases, the observation interval shortens and as μ decreases. The bias also increases with a higher percentage of censoring. In order to mitigate against this bias in practice, they recommend the use of larger studies with a low percentage of censoring and choosing the observation interval *t* such that estimate of S(t) is as close to 0.135 as possible.

The DEALE
Beck *et al.* (1982a, 1982b) have proposed an extension to the use of the exponential model called the DEALE, or declining exponential approximation of life expectancy, in which the hazard is broken into two components, an age, sex, and

race specific hazard, μ_{ASR}, due to causes of death other than the disease in question (i.e., natural causes), and a constant disease-specific hazard, μ_D. In the DEALE approach and in all of the subsequent methods described in this section, it is assumed that a table of life expectancies, L, is available for each age in the general population. These estimates may be averaged over race and sex, i.e., L_a, or else stratified by the latter demographic features, i.e., L_{asr}.

For example, in order to calculate the LE with the DEALE methodology for the intervention group in a RCT, one first obtains an estimate of the probability of disease-specific mortality for the cohort over some time, P(t), and estimates the disease-specific hazard, μ_D, as described in eqns [7] and [8]. Next, one obtains the age, sex, and race-adjusted LE from published demographic tables for the general population, L_{asr}. The particular value to take from the table is the one for people whose age, sex, and race most closely corresponds to the characteristics of the intervention group. The hazard due to natural causes, μ_{ASR}, is therefore equal to $1/L_{asr}$. According to the DEALE, one assumes that both the disease-specific and natural hazards remain constant over time. Therefore, LE with disease, L_D is estimated by:

$$\hat{L}_D = \frac{1}{\hat{\mu}_D + \mu_{ASR}} \qquad [11]$$

The Gompertz mortality function

Although the DEALE is attractive because of its simplicity, it can lead to inaccurate estimates of LE because, in reality, the hazard due to natural causes is not constant. The function that most closely approximates the mortality observed in the general population, the Gompertz function (named after its discoverer, Benjamin Gompertz) has the form:

$$\mu_{ASR}(t) = k \cdot \exp(a \cdot t) \qquad [12]$$

The hazard associated with natural causes increases with time: It doubles approximately every eight and one-third years. Assuming that the hazard from natural causes remains constant, as in the DEALE method, results in a risk of death that is too high for younger and too low for older individuals. This can be seen in the original description of the DEALE method by Beck *et al.* where they compared LE estimates with the latter method and with a Gompertz-based approach: Underestimation by the DEALE was most pronounced for younger individuals.

A logical extension of the Gompertz hazard function, the Makeham-Gompertz function, is formed by the addition of a constant disease-specific hazard to the Gompertz hazard:

$$\mu(t) = \mu_D + k \cdot \exp(a \cdot t) \qquad [13]$$

However, there is no closed-form expression for LE that incorporates the latter hazard function.

Extensions to the DEALE

Keeler *et al.* (1992) have proposed a set of alternatives to the DEALE that satisfy the closed-form requirement and provide a better approximation to Gompertz-based LE.

The first of these has $\mu_{ASR}(t) = bt$. In other words, the natural hazard increases with time, just not exponentially. They show that the corresponding survival function is:

$$S(t) = \exp\left(-\frac{vbt^2}{2}\right) \qquad [14]$$

LE without disease, L_{asr}, is the area under the latter survival function:

$$L_{asr} = \int_0^\infty \exp\left(-\frac{vbt^2}{2}\right) dt \qquad [15]$$

This expression for LE without disease is a variation of the error function,

$$\mathrm{erf}(x) = \frac{v2}{\sqrt{\pi}} \int_0^x e^{-t^2} dt \qquad [16]$$

and so Keeler *et al.* call this approach the ERror Function Approximation to Life Expectancy or the ERFALE. As in the case of LE estimation with the DEALE, the first step in the ERFALE method, and in all of the techniques suggested by Keeler *et al.*, is to obtain an estimate of the LE without the disease in question, L_{asr}, from a demographic table that corresponds most closely to the age, sex, and race distribution of the cohort of interest. In order to calculate the LE with disease, one needs to develop an expression for the hazard parameter, b, in terms of L_{asr}.

Note that the probability density of a normal variable (x) is:

$$\phi(x) = \frac{v1}{\sigma\sqrt{2\pi}} \exp\left[\frac{-(x-\mu)^2}{2\sigma^2}\right] \qquad [17]$$

Let $x = t$, $\mu = 0$ and $\sigma^2 = (1/b)$ then

$$\phi(t) = \sqrt{\frac{vb}{2\pi}} \exp\left[\frac{v - bt^2}{2}\right] \qquad [18]$$

The probability mass function is therefore:

$$\Phi(t) = \sqrt{\frac{vb}{2\pi}} \int_{-\infty}^t \exp\left[\frac{v - bt^2}{2}\right] dt \qquad [19]$$

Because the latter is a probability mass function, it follows that

$$1 = \Phi(\infty) = \sqrt{\frac{vb}{2\pi}} \int_{-\infty}^\infty \exp\left[-\frac{vbt^2}{2}\right] dt \qquad [20]$$

and therefore, since the cumulative normal probability mass function is symmetrical

$$\frac{v1}{2} = \sqrt{\frac{vb}{2\pi}} \int_0^\infty \exp\left[-\frac{vbt^2}{2}\right] dt \qquad [21]$$

substituting eqn [15]

$$\frac{v1}{2} = \sqrt{\frac{vb}{2\pi}} \cdot L_{asr} \qquad [22]$$

and therefore

$$b = \frac{v\pi}{2(L_{asr})^2} \qquad [23]$$

$$\text{Let } \hat{y} = \frac{v\hat{\mu}_D}{\sqrt{b}}$$

then Keeler *et al.* have shown that

$$\hat{L}_D = \frac{v\hat{y} \cdot \Phi(-\hat{y})}{\hat{\mu}_D \phi(\hat{y})} \qquad [24]$$

which can be approximated by

$$\hat{L}_D = \frac{v1}{\hat{\mu}_D}\left(1 - \frac{v1}{\hat{y}^2} + \frac{v3}{\hat{y}^4}\right) \qquad [25]$$

Another alternative to the DEALE is the delayed DEALE in which the LE, L_{asr}, for a person without disease but with the same age, sex, and race as the cohort is divided into two time periods: An initial period, kL_{asr}, in which the hazard is 0 followed by a second period $(1-K)$ L_{asr} in which the hazard function is $1/[(1-K) L_{asr}]$. LE for a patient with disease is estimated by:

$$\hat{L}_D = \frac{v1}{\hat{\mu}_D}\left[1 - \frac{v\exp(-\hat{\mu}_D K L_{asr})}{1 + \hat{\mu}_D(1 - K)L_{asr}}\right] \qquad [26]$$

Finally, the mixed DEALE is a model where a proportion, p, of a healthy population lives exactly L_{asr} more years and the remainder, $(1-p)$ follow the DEALE. In this case, the LE for patients with disease is estimated by:

$$\hat{L}_D = p \cdot \left[\frac{v1 - \exp(-\hat{\mu}_D L_{asr})}{\hat{\mu}_D}\right] + (1 - p) \cdot \left[\frac{v1}{\hat{\mu}_D + \frac{1}{L_{asr}}}\right] \qquad [27]$$

Keeler *et al.* found that the best values for the fractions *k* and *p* were 0.5 and 0.75, respectively. Using a variety of values for L_{asr} and μ_D, they found that the estimates for LE with disease using the DEALE approximation consistently underestimates the Gompertz-based LE, while the ERFALE, delayed DEALE, and mixed DEALE had variable results but tended to overestimate Gompertz.

The GAME Approximation

One of the issues with the latter extensions to the DEALE is that they require natural hazard functions to assume piecemeal, nonsmooth, forms, and they also assume that the disease-specific hazard remains constant with time. Van Den Hout (2004) has proposed a closed-form approach that addresses these concerns for the situation in which the disease-specific hazard function declines with time in a smooth, monotonic, and concave-upward fashion. Natural hazards are modeled with a GAmma distribution and disease-specific hazards with Mixed Exponential distributions hence the name of the approach: GAME.

In this model, the remaining life span of a healthy individual at a given age *a*, T_a, has a gamma distribution:

$T_a \sim$ Gamma (k_a, θ_a). From the fundamental characteristics of gamma probability distributions, the expected value of T_a, $E(T_a)$, which is the LE, L_a, is equal to $k_a\theta_a$. The variance of T_a, $var(T_a)$, is equal to $k_a\theta_a^2$. For convenience, Van Den Hout reparameterized the distribution using the squared coefficient of variation, $s_a = var(T_a)/E^2(T_a) = k_a\theta_a^2/k_a^2\theta_a^2 = 1/k_a$. Thus the reparameterized gamma distribution for T_a is Gamma$(1/s_a, s_a L_a)$. In order to derive a survival function for healthy individuals at various ages, it is necessary to have values of s_a for each age. While values of $L_a = E(T_a)$, the LE for the general population at each age, are readily available, information on the variance of T_a at each age is not. Van Den Hout therefore describes an iterative method for deriving the variance values from a table of life expectancies:

$$P_a = \frac{L_a - \frac{1}{2}}{L_{a+1} + \frac{1}{2}} \qquad [28]$$

where p_a is the probability of a healthy individual at age *a* surviving for at least 1 more year. Then Van den Hout shows that

$$var(T_a) = E(T_a^2) - E^2(T_a)$$
$$= p_a \cdot \left(var(T_{a+1}) + (1 + L_{a+1})^2\right)$$
$$+ (1 - p_a) \cdot (1/3) - L_a^2 \qquad [29]$$

Thus, the production of the table of variances for T_a by age requires one to start at the oldest age and work iteratively toward younger ages. How to specify the value of $var(T_{a+1})$ for the oldest age group in the table is not mentioned by Van Den Hout, but presumably this would be arbitrarily set to zero. With both the tables of life expectancies and variances in hand, then for a healthy individual at age *a*:

$$s_a = v var(T_a)/E^2(T_a) = v var(T_a)/L_a^2 \qquad [30]$$

The survival function, $S_0(t)$ for a healthy person at age *a* is 1-CDFgamma$(1/s_a, s_a L_a)$, i.e., one minus the cumulative distribution function for a gamma probability distribution with shape parameter $1/s_a$ and scale parameter $s_a L_a$. Note that:

$$CDFgamma(t; k, \theta) = \frac{v\gamma(k, t/\theta)}{\Gamma(k)} \qquad [31]$$

so

$$S_0(t; a) = 1 - \frac{v\gamma(1/s_a, t/s_a L_a)}{\Gamma(1/s_a)} \qquad [32]$$

also note that

$$\gamma(1/s_a, t/s_a L_a) + \Gamma(1/s_a, t/s_a L_a) = \Gamma(1/s_a)$$

where $\gamma(a,b)$ is the lower incomplete gamma function, $\Gamma(a,b)$ is the upper incomplete gamma function, and $\Gamma(a)$ is the complete gamma function (note that the gamma function is not the same as the gamma probability distribution).

Therefore

$$S_0(t; a) = 1 - \frac{v\Gamma(1/s_a) - \Gamma(1/s_a, t/s_a L_a)}{\Gamma(1/s_a)} \qquad [33]$$

If $1/s_a$ is an integer then $\Gamma(1/s_a) = ((1/s_a) - 1)!$ and

$$\Gamma(1/s_a, t/s_a L_a) = ((1/s_a) - 1)! \cdot \exp(-t/s_a L_a) \cdot \sum_{j=0}^{(1/s_a)-1} t^j/j!$$

Thus

$$S_0(t; a) = 1 - \left\{ \frac{((1/s_a) - 1)! - ((1/s_a) - 1)! \cdot \exp\left(\frac{-t}{s_a L_a}\right) \cdot \sum_{j=0}^{(1/s_a)-1} \frac{t^j}{j!}}{((1/s_a) - 1)!} \right\}$$

and

$$S_0(t; a) = \exp(-t/s_a L_a) \cdot \sum_{j=0}^{(1/s_a)-1} t^j/j! \qquad [34]$$

The exponential distribution is a special case of the gamma distribution, gamma(k, θ), where $k = 1$ and $\theta = 1/\mu$. Recall that under the reparameterization, $s_a = 1/k_a$ and $\theta_a = s_a L_a$, therefore, $s_a = 1/s_a = 1$ and $-t/s_a L_a = -t\mu_a$. Thus, the survival function shown in eqn [34] simplifies to: $S_0(t; a) = \exp(-t\mu_a)$.

Excess hazard due to disease is modeled by a mixture of exponential distributions. This allows the effect of disease to be heterogeneous among different groups of patients:

$$S_D(t) = \sum_{i=1}^{n} \pi_i \cdot \exp(-\mu_i t) \qquad [35]$$

where $\pi_1 + \pi_2 + \ldots + \pi_n = 1$ represents the proportion of the diseased cohort that belongs to each group. Note that the overall hazard starts as a composite of the hazards in the n groups but decreases toward that in the group with the smallest hazard as time passes and the members of the higher risk groups make up a smaller proportion of the survivors.

Van Den Hout describes two methods for estimating the π_i and μ_i parameters from observed survival curves for the disease. In the first method, one assumes that there are two groups, one of which has no excess mortality. From the observed disease-specific survival curve, one picks an arbitrary time, x and another time halfway between 0 and x, then:

$$\hat{\pi}_1 = \frac{v(1 - \hat{S}_D(x/2))^2}{(1 - \hat{S}_D(x/2)) - (\hat{S}_D(x/2) - \hat{S}_D(x))}, \hat{\pi}_2 = 1 - \hat{\pi}_1$$

$$\hat{\mu}_1 = \frac{2}{x} \ln\left(\frac{v1 - \hat{S}_D(x/2)}{\hat{S}_D(x/2) - \hat{S}_D(x)}\right), \hat{\mu}_2 = 0 \qquad [36]$$

In the second method, the parameters for any arbitrary number of groups can be found using a spreadsheet with a

optimization procedure by minimizing an error function. The method is described in detail in the paper by Van Den Hout and in a worked example in a spreadsheet that is available on his website (Van Den Hout, 2004).

Finally, the survival functions for healthy and diseased individuals are assumed to be independent and therefore the overall survival function is their product. The GAME estimate of LE is then the area under the combined survival curve for individuals at age a:

$$L_d(a) = \int_0^\infty S_D(t) \cdot S_0(t; a) dt \qquad [37]$$

Using a complex derivation, Van Den Hout shows that the combined LE estimate for a patient at age 'a' is:

$$L_d(a) = \sum_{i=1}^{n} \frac{\pi_i}{\mu_i} \left\{ 1 - \left(\frac{v1}{1 + \mu_i(s_a L_a)}\right)^{1/s_a} \right\} \qquad [38]$$

Note that if a particular disease group has no excess mortality, then the expression above involves division by zero. In that case, the summand for that group should be replaced with $\pi_i L_a$.

Van Den Hout validated the GAME approach using LE tables for Dutch women with ages from 0 to 100 years and with a range of constant disease-specific hazards, μ, from 0 to 1. The GAME and DEALE methods were compared to a gold standard model:

$$L_d(a) = [p_a p_d \cdot (1 + L_d(a + 1)] + [(1 - p_a p_d) \cdot (1/2)] \qquad [39]$$

where p_d is equal to $\exp(-\mu)$. Once again, LE estimates for the gold standard are computed starting with the oldest age and working backward. The DEALE underestimated the gold standard LE to a much greater degree (a maximum of 10 years) than did the GAME approach (a maximum of 2 months). However, a better validation might have been achieved if the two methods were compared to a LE estimate produced with a Markov process (see the section titled 'Parametric LE estimation using Markov processes' below) implementing a Gompertz-Makeham hazard.

For validation of the GAME method in a scenario where disease-specific hazard decreases with time, survival curves and LE estimates for both the DEALE and GAME approaches were calculated for breast cancer survival data from the National Cancer Institute. The GAME method more closely approximated the observed data.

Conclusions Regarding the Closed-Form Approaches

The advantage of the closed-form approaches is that, despite the complex derivation for some of them, they all result in formulae that are relatively easy to implement with a hand-held calculator or a spreadsheet. There are, however, a few unresolved issues. First, the clinical studies that one might hope to use for LE estimation are often heterogeneous. This complicates the choice of the particular L_{asr} value to use in the estimation formulae. Furthermore, in order to use these methods – except for the GAME approach – one must make the assumption that the disease-specific hazard estimated from the clinical data is constant across age, sex, race, and other factors. The GAME method has the advantage that a single observed survival curve from a heterogeneous diseased population can be decomposed into a set of subgroups, each with its own constant disease-specific hazard rate. Alternatively, if one has the luxury of having disease-specific mortality data for the subgroups of a cohort then the other methods could be used to estimate an LE for each in turn. Indeed, Benbassat *et al.* (1993) showed that substantially different LE results were obtained for cancer patients if cancer-specific hazard was modeled to be constant, a function of age at diagnosis, or a function of both age at diagnosis and time since diagnosis.

Second, the natural hazards computed from LE tables for the general population represent the composite risk from all causes of death including the disease of interest. Thus methods that combine natural hazards in the general population and disease-specific hazards are actually counting the effect of the disease twice. For rare causes of death, this issue is negligible, but for studies of mortality due to cardiovascular disease, common cancers, and diabetes, the error would be expected to be more substantial.

Parametric LE Estimation Using Markov Processes

If one is willing to forego a closed-form approach and engage in numerical approximation, then discrete, Markov process-based calculation of LE has advantages. A two-state (alive and dead) Markov process can be set up and allowed to run until the proportion of the theoretical cohort left in the alive state reaches some negligible value. The resulting output of the Markov process is the LE estimate (see 'Life Expectancy as the Output of a Markov Process'). Note that commonly used decision-analytic software accounts for alive state membership in discrete Markov processes at the end of each time increment or cycle and therefore underestimates the true LE value. This is particularly true when the Markov process is coarse – i.e., when the length of each cycle is a significant proportion of the time horizon (see above). This can be remedied by shortening the cycle length and by adding a value equivalent to a half-cycle length to the LE estimate produced by the Markov process. As an example of the Markov-based approach, Tsevat *et al.* (1991) used a more complex Markov model to estimate the gain in

LE associated with population-wide cardiovascular risk-reduction strategies.

Because the Markov process is discrete, the incorporation of annual age-, sex-, and race-specific natural hazards becomes straightforward. It is also straightforward to incorporate disease hazards that have either a multiplicative or an additive effect on natural hazards.

For example, a feature of the DEALE method and its extensions is the assumption that the disease-specific and natural hazards are additive. Kuntz and Weinstein (1995) have used a Markov-based approach to examine the differences in calculated LE values when additive and multiplicative models are used. The effect of these different disease-specific effects on the calculated gain in LE associated with treatment was also examined.

They use a step function to represent survival without disease:

$$S_0(t) = \exp\left(-\sum_{i=1}^{t} \mu_{ASR}(i)\right) \qquad [40]$$

where $\mu_{ASR}(i)$ is the age-, sex-, and race-specific annual hazard rate for the general population in the ith year after some arbitrary starting age. Then LE at the starting age without disease is:

$$L_{asr} = \frac{1}{2} + \sum_{t=1}^{n} S_0(t) \qquad [41]$$

where n is chosen so that $S_0(n)$ is negligible. Equation [41] is representative of a two-state Markov process that is allowed to run for n cycles.

Under the model where hazard due to disease is additive:

$$S_D(t) = \exp\left(-\sum_{i=1}^{t} (\mu_{ASR}(i) + \mu_D)\right) \qquad [42]$$

and the survival function for a cohort of diseased individuals who are treated is:

$$S_R(t) = \exp\left(-\sum_{i=1}^{t} (\mu_{ASR}(i) + \mu_D \lambda_a)\right) \qquad [43]$$

where λ_a has the value 0 for a perfectly effective treatment and the value 1 for a completely ineffective one. LEs for diseased individuals with and without treatment were computed using Markov processes, as represented in eqn [41], by replacing $S_0(t)$ with estimates of $S_D(t)$ and $S_R(t)$. Estimates for μ_D and λ_a were obtained by using RCT data and rearranging eqns [42] and [43], respectively:

$$\hat{\mu}_D = \frac{v - \ln[\hat{S}_D(t)]}{t} - \frac{v\sum_{i=1}^{t} \mu_{ASR}(i)}{t} \qquad [44]$$

and

$$\hat{\gamma}_a = \frac{v - \ln[\hat{S}_R(t)] - \sum_{i=1}^{t} \mu_{ASR}(i)}{t_{\hat{\mu}D}} \qquad [45]$$

Under the model where hazard due to disease is multiplicative:

$$S_D(t) = \exp\left(-\sum_{i=1}^{t}(\mu_{ASR}(i) \cdot \beta_D)\right) \qquad [46]$$

and the survival function for a cohort of diseased individuals who are treated is:

$$S_R(t) = \exp\left(-\sum_{i=1}^{t}(\mu_{ASR}(i) \cdot \beta_D \lambda_m)\right) \qquad [47]$$

where λ_m has the value '$1/\beta_D$' for a perfectly effective treatment and the value 1 for a completely ineffective one. Estimates for β_D and λ_m were obtained by using RCT data and rearranging eqns [46] and [47], respectively:

$$\hat{\beta}_D = \frac{\ln[\hat{S}_D(t)]}{\ln[S_0(t)]} \qquad [48]$$

and

$$\hat{\gamma}_m = \frac{\ln[\hat{S}_R(t)]}{\ln[S_0(t)] \cdot \hat{\beta}_D} \qquad [49]$$

Kuntz *et al.* derived these parameter estimates for three large RCTs comparing medical and surgical therapy for coronary artery disease. In general, the multiplicative model produced lower LE estimates and smaller gains in LE for surgery over medical therapy than did the additive model. The difference in ΔLE between the two approaches ranged from 0.42 to 0.98 years for LE estimates that averaged 21.3 and 14.1 years, respectively, across treatment arms and types of disease-specific effect.

When the parameter estimates derived from patients as old as the enrollees in the cardiovascular RCTs were extrapolated to other ages, predictable behavior of the ΔLE occurred. Under the additive model, the gain in LE associated with surgery declined monotonically with age and was always lower for men. Kuntz *et al.* show that this is due to the fact that, in the additive model, constant disease-specific hazard has a smaller relative magnitude (and therefore treatment is less efficacious in absolute terms) as age increases. Furthermore, since men have a larger burden of death from natural causes at any given age, if disease-specific hazard is the same for men and women, then men have a smaller relative effect of disease-specific hazard and therefore less absolute benefit from treatment.

In the multiplicative case, the ΔLE rises with age and then falls. Men have larger ΔLE values at younger ages and then lower values at older ages compared to women. Kuntz *et al.* show that this effect is due to the fact that two factors are in tension: While the relative magnitude of a multiplicative disease effect remains constant, its absolute size increases. Thus treatment efficacy increases with age,

while at the same time the LE and therefore the number of years over which the treatment can have an effect decreases with age. For young people who have large LEs, the higher natural hazard experienced by men produces a larger absolute treatment effect compared to women. For older people, shorter LEs become the limiting factor so that women, who have longer LEs than men, experience a larger treatment effect.

These effects are artifacts and result from extrapolation of LE estimates from RCT data to other age groups. Kuntz and Weinstein recommend that, wherever possible, parameter estimates for the disease-specific effects should be obtained from RCTs that break survival estimates down by age. Furthermore, the relative proportion of disease-specific to natural deaths across age groups can give a clue as to which model, additive or multiplicative, is operating. If disease-specific deaths fall as a proportion of total mortality in older patients, then an additive effect is likely. Conversely, if the proportion of disease-specific deaths remains constant with age, then a multiplicative model should be used.

Nonparametric LE Estimation

It is possible to estimate LE from clinical studies that report Kaplan-Meier (KM) survival curves without resorting to estimating parameters. One must be cautious because a curve derived from heavily censored data is likely to be biased unless the censoring is purely random. Furthermore, the estimated cumulative survival probability of the right-hand tail of the KM curve tends to be unstable because it is based on the data from fewer patients. Also, a true LE estimate cannot be made unless the KM curve extends down to zero probability of survival. Otherwise, the method described below will provide an estimate of the number of life-months accrued by the cohort during the period of observation. In that case, a true LE estimate will require an extrapolation of the KM curve.

In order to produce a LE estimate, one must have access to the life table upon which the Kaplan-Meier curve was based. Suppose that there are n observed subjects, and that the ith subject has an associated observation time, t_i, and an estimated cumulative survival probability, $S(t_i)$, at that time. Estimates of the number of life units associated with the ith individual and the LE are:

$$\hat{l}_i = \begin{cases} t_i, i = 1 \\ S(t_{i-1}) \cdot (t_i - t_{i-1}), i > 1 \end{cases}$$

$$\hat{L}_D = \sum_{i=1}^{n} \hat{l}_i \qquad [50]$$

LE estimates are also possible to derive from Cox regression models if one has access to the original data. The Cox proportional hazard model is:

$$S(t, \vec{X}) = \exp\left[-H(t, \vec{X})\right]$$

$$H(t, \vec{X}) = H_0(t) \cdot \exp(\beta_1 X_1 + \beta_2 X_2 + \ldots + \beta_p X_p) \qquad [51]$$

Statistical software is readily available for estimating the beta coefficients of a Cox model for right-censored, time-to-event data. If the statistical program reports a value of the survival function for each case in the data set, then it is possible to arrange these estimates and observation times into a table, order them in an ascending fashion by observation time and apply eqn [50] in order to calculate a LE estimate for the cohort.

However, one may wish to calculate the LE of a person with particular values for the X variables or the ΔLE associated with a change in the value of one or more of them. In that case, an estimate of the baseline hazard function, $H_0(t)$, is required. Unfortunately, $H_0(t)$ is not often reported by statistical programs. However, in the course of estimating the Cox model, if the statistical package offers the option of calculating a log-minus-log (lml) and x-beta statistic for each case in the data set, then it is possible to reconstruct the estimated baseline hazard function. Rearranging eqn [51] for the ith case in the data set yields:

$$\hat{H}_0(t_i) = \exp\left\{\left[\ln(-\ln(s(t_i, \vec{X}_i)))\right] - \hat{\beta} \cdot \vec{X}_i\right\}$$

$$\hat{H}_0(t_i) = \exp(\text{lml}_i - \text{xbeta}_i) \qquad [52]$$

Here, lml_i represents the log of the minus log of the estimated survival function for the ith case at t_i and xbeta_i represents the linear combination of the estimated Cox regression coefficients with the ith case's particular vector of values for the predictor variables, $\mathbf{X}i$. One calculates an estimate of the baseline hazard function value for each case in the data set. These values, when ordered by t_i, can then be used as a lookup table which is set up for interpolation. Then

$$\widehat{L}_D \approx \sum_{j=1}^{T} \exp\left[-_0(j) - \exp(\hat{\beta} \cdot \vec{X}_{new})\right] \qquad [53]$$

where the LE value is estimated over T units of time, such that the value of the summand at T is negligible, $H_0(j)$ is the interpolated value of the baseline hazard function obtained from the lookup table and $\mathbf{X}_{new}$ is the new vector of values for the predictor variables. In order to calculate the effect on LE of a difference in one or more of the predictor variables, eqn [53] can be implemented twice using the different values of the vector $\mathbf{X}_{new}$ and subtracting the resulting L_D estimates. An expression for the variance of the LE estimate using this method has not been developed, nor has the magnitude of the bias in the estimate of the baseline hazard function been determined. As discussed in 'Closed-form, Parametric LE Estimation' above, this bias may exist because $H_0(j)$ is a nonlinear

function of the survival estimate. As for nonparametric LE estimation from KM curves, this method will only provide true LE estimates if the survival function extends down to a value close to zero. Otherwise the method provides the number of life-months (or years) accrued by a cohort – or the difference in life-months between two cohorts – during the observation time.

Conclusion

Life expectancy can be understood to be equal to the area under a survival curve regardless of its shape. A gain in life expectancy associated with adopting one health strategy over another (or of being in one exposure group versus another) is the area between the respective survival curves. In order to put a given gain into proper perspective, it is necessary to understand the baseline risk in the control group and the proportion of people who are likely to benefit from the intervention. It is certainly a misconception to view gains in life expectancy as increments of time tacked onto the end of a fixed life span. Life expectancy can be estimated from empirical data by a variety of methods that each have strengths and weaknesses.

See also: Clinical Epidemiology; Longevity in Specific Populations; Methods of Measuring and Valuing Health.

Citations

Beck JR, Kassirer JP, and Pauker SG (1982a) A convenient approximation of life expectancy (the DEALE): 1. Validation of the method. *American Journal of Medicine* 73: 883–888.

Beck JR, Pauker SG, Gottlieb JE, Klein K, and Kassirer JP (1982b) A convenient approximation of life expectancy (the DEALE): 2. Use in medical decision making. *American Journal of Medicine* 73: 889–897.

Benbassat J, Zajicek G, Van Oortmarssen GJ, Ben-Dov I, and Eckman MH (1993) Inaccuracies in estimates of life expectancies of patients with bronchial cancer in clinical decision making. *Medical Decision Making* 13: 237–244.

Keeler E and Bell R (1992) New DEALES: Other approximations of life expectancy. *Medical Decision Making* 12: 307–311.

Kuntz KM and Weinstein MC (1995) Life expectancy biases in clinical decision making. *Medical Decision Making* 15: 158–169.

Tsevat J, Weinstein MC, Williams LW, *et al.* (1991) Expected gains in life expectancy from various coronary heart disease risk factor modifications. *Circulation* 83: 1194–1201.

Van Den Hout WB (2004) The GAME estimate of reduced life expectancy. *Medical Decision Making* 24: 80–88.

Van Den Hout WB (2004) *The GAME Estimate of Reduced Life Expectancy: Worked-out Example.* https://www.lumc.nl/2050/research/home_hout.htm (accessed November 2007).

Wright JC and Weinstein MC (1998) Gains in life expectancy from medical interventions–standardizing data on outcomes. *New England Journal of Medicine* 339: 380–386.

Further Reading

Cox DR (1972) Regression models and life tables. *Journal of the Royal Statistical Society B* 34: 187–220.

Gompertz B (1825) On the nature of the function expressive of the law of human mortality. *Philosophical Transcripts of the Royal Society (London)* 115: 513–585.

Kaplan EL and Meier P (1958) Nonparametric estimation from incomplete observations. *Journal of the American Statistical Association* 53: 457–481.

Laupacis A, Sackett DL, and Roberts RS (1988) An assessment of clinically useful measures of the consequences of treatment. *New England Journal of Medicine* 318: 1728–1733.

Naglie G, Krahn M, Naimark D, Redelmeier DA, and Detsky AS (1997) Primer on medical decision analysis. Part 3. Estimating probabilities and utilities. *Medical Decision Making* 17: 136–141.

Naimark D, Naglie G, and Detsky AS (1994) The meaning of life expectancy: What is a clinically significant gain? *Journal of General International Medicine* 9: 702–707.

Naimark D, Krahn M, Naglie G, Redelmeier DA, and Detsky AS (1997) Primer on medical decision analysis. Part 5. Working with Markov processes. *Medical Decision Making* 17: 152–159.

Olshansky SJ, Carnes BA, and Cassel C (1990) In search of Methuselah: Estimating the upper limits to human longevity. *Science* 250: 634–640.

Sonnenberg FA and Beck JR (1993) Markov models in medical decision making: A practical guide. *Medical Decision Making* 13: 322–338.

Tsai SP, Lee ES, and Hardy RJ (1978) The effect of a reduction in leading causes of death: Potential gains in life expectancy. *American Journal of Public Health* 68: 966–971.

Active Life Expectancy

K G Manton, Duke University, Durham, NC, USA

Glossary

Active life expectancy The proportion of total life expectancy expected to be lived without chronic disability.

Cox regression A procedure to analyze the effects of covariates of hazard functions assuming only that the hazard functions are proportional.

Fokker-Planck equation A matrix equation describing how the means and variances of J variables change over time due to (1) dynamics and (2) diffusion.

Fuzzy sets Methods for partial classification of individual cases into two or more categories.

GoM A multivariate analytic procedure in which persons are assigned intensity scores on a set of K dimensions represented by the data.

Logistic regression A regression model in which the dependent variable is a nonlinear (i.e., logistic) function of the probability of an event occurring.

Markov models Transition models based on the assumption that the change in state from t to $t+1$ is based only on the person's state at t (and not earlier states as $t-1$).

Principal components A multivariate procedure used to identify the K dimensions representing the J variables in a second-order moments matrix.

Sullivan method A commonly used strategy for studying active life expectancy by using life table functions calculated from vital statistics mortality data and data on the age-specific prevalence of chronic disability from nationally representative survey data.

Introduction

Active life expectancy (ALE) is a useful, and increasingly used, concept for measuring the combined health, functional, and longevity status of relatively long-lived national populations. It has recently received emphasis as a public health measure for cross-national comparisons of the health of economically developed countries by, for example, the World Health Organization (Robine and Michel, 2004). This was, in part, because health policy analysts became concerned that life expectancy in developed countries might continue to increase, not primarily because of improved health, but rather due to increasingly expensive medical interventions that possibly were increasing the length of life spent in disabled life states at later ages with poor quality of health and impaired function.

This concern emerged most strongly in the United States in the early 1980s because actuaries at the Social Security Administration (SSA) had failed to anticipate the renewed acceleration of the increase in overall life expectancy in the United States starting in 1969 after significant declines in male life expectancy due to increased cardio-vascular disease mortality rates had been observed from 1954 to 1968. This was because the SSA actuarial fore-casting models were based on extrapolations of prior long-term (e.g., 10-year) cause-specific national mortality trends. Thus, when U.S. male mortality started to increase in 1954 due to increased circulatory disease risks, a trend that continued to 1968, their cause-specific mortality projections in the early 1970s, based primarily on that 14-year period of adverse male mortality experience, suggested that life expectancy would not increase further in the United States as a result of having reached what some demographic researchers believed was the biological upper bound to human life expectancy (Myers, 1981). This occurred despite U.S. female's life expectancy continuing to increase over the same period.

In 1982, sufficient new positive U.S. male mortality experience (e.g., from 1969 to 1980) had accumulated to suggest, in contrast to the prior SSA projections, that continuing future reductions in adult male morta-lity would be likely and, therefore, future increases in life expectancy. As a consequence, it became necessary to consider how to change the normal retirement age (then 65) for the income-support component of the U.S. Social Security program to preserve the long-term (75-year) fiscal integrity of the SSA trust fund. Although the evidence on U.S. life expectancy increases after 1968 was strong and consistent, there did not exist sufficient data on the direction and magnitude of the longitudinal correlation of disability and morbidity trends with those life expectancy increases to confidently determine the quality of life and level of functioning in the increasing number of years expected to be lived at ever more advanced ages (e.g., at ages 65 and above) (Feldman, 1983).

This concern was supported by a number of public health researchers who argued that it was the intrinsic nature of modern industrial society (e.g., due to social stress and environmental pollution) to increase the prevalence of chronic diseases. They viewed modern industrial society as incapable of mounting effective public health responses to chronic disease pandemics or to modulate the effects of those chronic health problems on functioning at later ages (e.g., Kramer, 1980; Gruenberg, 1977). These pessimistic arguments, however, were also based on insufficient longi-tudinal national morbidity and health data and thus were speculative. For example, many examples were taken from the mental health arena, where disease definition and diag-nosis are often difficult and ambiguous. One set of argu-ments was based on the increased survival of persons with certain genetic disorders to reproductive age because of medical advances (e.g., the improved surgical repair of cardiac anomalies in persons afflicted with Down's syn-drome (Greunberg, 1977)). This, it was argued, would serve to increase the future prevalence of these genetic syndromes and their health and functional sequelae.

In contrast, other authors (e.g., Fries, 1980) suggested that by appropriately targeting preventative measures (e.g., exercise and nutrition programs) to the general elderly population – and rehabilitation services to the disabled elderly – the period of life expected to be spent without chronic disability could increase faster than total life expec-tancy. This beneficial state of population health dynamics was called "morbidity compression" (Fries, 1980). Fries, however, continued to assume that the upper bound for life expectancy was biologically fixed. Manton (1989) argued, in his dynamic equilibrium model, that the cor-relation of disability-free and total life expectancy was not genetically fixed but modifiable through appropriate public health policy supported by biomedical research intended to improve clinical and rehabilitative interven-tions in disablement processes and chronic morbidity at late ages. Recent analyses (Manton *et al.*, 2006b) tend to support the dynamic equilibrium model in that active life expectancy continues to increase faster than overall life expectancy.

A different, but equally optimistic, argument suggested that modern societies had indeed evolved in ways that would better support the genetic constitution of humans by modifying many social, environmental, and medical conditions. This complex dynamic situation, labeled by Professor Robert Fogel of the University of Chicago "techno-physiological" evolution, reflects both improve-ment in nutrition and environmental quality (e.g., water treatment), which, by increasing body size and strength, led to increased economic productivity and reduced health problems through rapid modification of technol-ogy and environmental quality. In such conditions, health improvements occurred far more rapidly than they could have if changes were solely dependent on genetic selection operating over multiple biological generations.

Fogel's formulations were, fortunately, empirically veri-fiable by using data on the health of Union army soldiers both at enlistment in the Civil War (the Gould sample) and later, when Civil War veterans applied for pensions from 1900 to 1910. The health of Union army veterans could be compared, for example, with veterans of World War II as assessed in national health surveys such as the National Health Interview Surveys (NHIS) and the National Health Nutrition and Examination Survey (NHANES) in the late 1980s and early 1990s. It was found that many chronic diseases (e.g., CVD) and chronic disability declined 6% over prevalence per decade in most of the twentieth century.

Associated with these trends, body mass index (BMI) increased as life expectancy increased. Fogel argued that increases in BMI reflected better health as a result of improved nutrition and water quality and reductions in caloric expenditures directed to fighting acute and chronic effects of infectious diseases. The rate of improve-ment in health and functioning, in multiple analyses of the

National Long Term Care Surveys for 1982 to 2004, was observed to accelerate starting in 1982 – results confirmed both in other national surveys (e.g., the Medicare Current Beneficiary Survey (MCBS), the Health and Retirement Survey (HRS), and the NHIS) and in Medicare expenditure and service use files longitudinally linked to the 49 000 sample persons from the six National Long Term Care Surveys (NLTCS).

In contrast, recent increases in BMI were argued by Lakdawalla and others (2005) to represent a potential health risk for the future U.S. elderly population by causing increases in disability prevalence (e.g., as early as 2012 to 2015), although the most recent available data (i.e., the 2004 NLTCS; Manton et al., 2006a) do not yet show such adverse health effects. Indeed, recent analyses of the relation of BMI to mortality and morbidity by Flegal and other researchers at the U.S. Center for Disease Control suggested prior estimates of the health and mortality effects of elevated BMI had been overestimated because of a failure to use recent data reflecting large improvements in the medical management of such obesity-related risk factors as hypertension, hypercholesterolemia, and elevated blood glucose. Rand researchers, in a comprehensive report to the CMS actuaries, also did not find a significant relation of elevated BMI to Medicare expenditures to at least 2030.

Since it was argued that there were insufficient data on disability and morbidity in 1980 to evaluate the longitudinal correlation of age trends in the prevalence of disability and longevity, it was decided in 1982 by Congress and the Greenspan Commission to conservatively increase the SSA normal retirement age by only two years (from age 65 to 67) starting in 2000, with the increase to be phased in gradually by 2020. No corresponding changes were proposed for the Medicare entitlement age, which was left at age 65. A number of European countries and Japan have begun to consider similar changes. In Britain, an increase in the normal retirement age to 67, with a further increase to age 69 in 2050, is being considered. It has been suggested that pension benefits in Japan be restricted to a fixed proportion of the total population. To maintain pension coverage for 17% of the Japanese population would require, with current Japanese mortality, increasing the normal retirement age to 73.2 years.

It is thus of interest that recent U.S. Bureau of Labor Statistics projections of labor force participation rates at ages 65+ from 2004 to 2014 suggest there will be significant future increases in the economic activity of the U.S. elderly population. A number of economists suggest that increased labor force activity in the United States at later ages may be stimulated by the transition from defined-benefit pension programs to joint individual-enterprise savings pension programs such as 401(k) systems (defined contribution pensions), in which benefits continue to increase as long as one continues to work and pay into the system.

Active Life Expectancy: Definition and Operationalization

To quantify the population health consequences of improved survival, Sullivan (1971) argued that survival curves estimated from U.S. vital statistics data could be paired with age-specific disability or disease prevalence data provided by national health surveys to calculate the average amount of time that one could expect to live in a healthy state in a national population; i.e., active life expectancy, or ALE. This quantity could be compared to total life expectancy, with changes in the ratio of those two quantities being a sensitive measure of population health dynamics and the rate of creation of human capital at later ages. The calculation of ALE over time on a cross-sectional basis (the Sullivan methodology) is illustrated in **Figure 1**, where we present total age-specific survival and survival without disability observed for 1935, 1999, and projected to 2080 (Manton et al., 2006b). In all of our ALE computations, U.S. longitudinal data will be used.

The survival curves in **Figure 1** are based upon longitudinal data from the 1982 to 1999 NLTCS that were used to make survival and age-specific chronic disability prevalence estimates (Manton and Gu, 2001) from historical data on the Civil War veterans analyzed by Fogel and Costa, and from official U.S. life tables. Future projections of ALE were made from these curves using an assumption of a 1.7% per annum decline in the prevalence of chronic disability (Singer and Manton, 1998; Manton et al., 2006b). In **Figure 1**, the dotted lines are survival curves. The solid lines are age-specific disability prevalence rates among survivors to each age.

Figure 1 suggests that there is a considerable increase in ALE over time, both absolutely and proportionally (morbidity compression), above age 65. The increases in ALE above age 85 are, interestingly, relatively even greater than those found at age 65. In Manton et al. (2006b), the relatively faster rate of ALE increase, especially at age 85+ when long-term care (LTC) use is most prevalent, suggested that the projected rapid growth of both Medicare and Medicaid expenditures to 2080 (i.e., to reach 24% of total GDP) might be significantly dampened if the observed trend (1982 to 2004; Manton et al., 2006a) toward the reduction of chronic disability prevalence were to continue at the rate of roughly 1.5% per annum (Singer and Manton, 1998). This would have to occur even with the projected large increases in survival at advanced ages; e.g., almost 15% of persons alive at age 65 are expected to survive to age 100 in 2080.

These ALE calculations (Sullivan, 1971), based on the sequential comparison over time of national life tables and disease and disability age-specific prevalence rate cross-sections, are also important because they help illustrate (1) potential changes in human capital in the U.S. aging population due to the effects of compression of morbidity

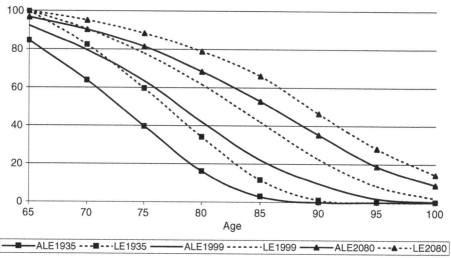

Figure 1   Survival curves for 1935, 1999, and 2080. Source: United Nations (2007), 'World population prospects: The 2006 Revision', http://esa.un.org/unpp/.

and (2) how recent public health, education, and clinical innovations and the future benefits of current investments in biomedical research may help drive future changes in ALE and human capital at later ages.

The latter point is crucial to the debate about the rate of growth of U.S. health expenditures and the future size, relative to GDP, of the Medicare and Medicaid programs. Specifically, if appropriately targeted acute and post-acute care medical expenditures operate to increase the proportion of life after age 65 that can be expected to be lived in potentially socially or economically productive states, then increases in Medicare expenditures may be beneficial to human capital creation and maintenance, and thereby further stimulate economic growth and increase GDP. If GDP can be significantly increased due to such targeted investments in health care, then the proportion of GDP spent on expenditures on health care in the future may grow relatively less rapidly than in current Medicare Trust Fund and Medicaid projections.

One issue for continuing debate is the sources of the declines in disability at later ages. Cutler and colleagues, analyzing the 1982 to 1999 NLTCS, suggest that a large proportion of recently observed declines in chronic disability at later ages may be due to improved medical management of circulatory diseases (see 'Further Reading'). The importance of medical innovations in reducing chronic disability also has been suggested by a number of other economists. Behavioral changes such as reductions in male smoking rates and increased educational attainment at later ages have undoubtedly contributed to the observed declines in chronic disability – as have changes in Medicare reimbursement policy (e.g., the Balanced Budget Act of 1997), which mandated the use of prospective payment for skilled nursing facilities.

One of the crucial issues in the construction and interpretation of ALE estimates is how disability is to be measured. For example, one approach is to assess whether a person has difficulty performing activities of daily living (ADLs) (Katz *et al.*, 1963) or instrumental activities of daily living (IADLs). It is generally agreed that the disability measured should be chronic in nature (expected to last 90+ days) and involve physical, sensory, and cognitive components. Other analysts have used panels of experts to subjectively weight the functional impact of specific impairments. Some suggest that objective physical performance tests should be employed, such as the Nagi items. Others would like to include clinical measures, although practical concerns may apply when attempting to do so in in-person home visits in a large nationally representative survey.

In general, the wide range of possible disability measures available suggests the need for objective multivariate statistical procedures to identify the smaller number of core disability dimensions represented by the measures – each of which may be relatively crude and subject to error. Although individual measures of ADLs and IADLs may be crude, their ability – taken as a group – to predict both service use (e.g., Medicare expenditures) and mortality is quite high, so ADLs are frequently used in policy studies, legislation, and in service use eligibility criteria (e.g., by HIPPA based on the Health Insurance Portability and Accountability Act (HIPAA) in setting LTC standards; for example, impairment in two or three ADLs requiring personal assistance as a trigger to receive LTC insurance benefits). The fact that disability is multidimensional and dynamic suggests that a single ALE index (e.g., defined as the threshold of the sum of ADLs), although conceptually useful, is probably too crude for effective economic and actuarial Medicare and Medicaid policy studies. For realistic use in economic and health policy analysis, the disabled portion of total life expectancy should be broken down into several subtypes, or be continuously graded on several qualitatively distinct dimensions, using disability scores rigorously constructed in a multivariate procedure.

For example, in an economy dominated by information technology, physical impairments may be less important than cognitive impairment for many socially and economically important activities. This is in part due to the ability to at least partially compensate for physical impairments by the appropriate construction of physical space (i.e., office buildings and private residences), the creation of physical aides, and, in the future, even re-engineering of various body parts (e.g., currently, the intraocular lens replacement for cataracts, knee and hip replacements).

In addition, Fogel and other economists have recently argued that, in a modern industrial economy, the relative rate of short-term expenditures on health care perhaps should increase as a proportion of total GDP as expenditures made on, say, electronics and other consumer goods become saturated and as disposable income increases. Fogel suggests that if the short-term elasticity of health-care expenditures is 1.6%, then the relative share of GDP spent on health care could increase to roughly 20% without adverse national economic consequences; that is, we will make relatively more expenditures on preserving human health as our ability to saturate consumer demands (e.g., for televisions) and to manufacture highly durable electronics and robust machinery (e.g., automobiles with smart chips to monitor their internal state for efficient, prophylactic maintenance) increases. Other economists have projected that in the United States up to 30% of GDP could be spent on health care by 2050.

Thus, as durable goods have increased in longevity and durability, it is reasonable to argue that equivalent or greater expenditures need to be made on maintaining and improving human capital by increasing human longevity and durability (health and functioning). An analogue of this capital maintenance process in humans is to improve early diagnosis of disease and to monitor and improve individual health states (e.g., use of indwelling insulin reservoirs to better maintain blood glucose homeostasis as evaluated in real time by a microchip blood glucose sensor; indwelling cardiac defibrillators; and, recently, use of left ventricular cardiac assist devices).

Cross-National Implications of ALE/LE Ratio Differences

ALE/LE ratio calculations have importance not only for the U.S. economy but also in making economic comparisons cross-nationally for economically advanced countries. Japan is currently the most rapidly aging population in modern industrial nations. The Japanese fertility rate is already so low (1.3 overall; 1.1 in Tokyo) that Japan will soon begin to experience a rapid contraction in population size (from a peak of 127 million persons in 2006 to

between 110 to 100 million persons by 2050), as may the Russian Federation population and several other European (e.g. Italy) and Eastern European (e.g. Latvia) nation states.

This aging-population health dynamic provides the double burden on future economic growth and technological innovation that large proportions of the national population in developed countries will be retired (under current labor and tax law and economic conventions) and that growing proportions of this elderly population will be extremely elderly (e.g., aged 85+ and 95+) and thus require significant LTC – consequently promoting rapid growth of LTC service industries and requiring large amounts of human capital – but, without significant biomedical research, perhaps not adding significant value to the productivity (measured in terms of improved health) of LTC. This will be true if LTC continues to be defined primarily as a labor-intensive residential warehouse service function for what has been previously assumed to be an economically non-productive very elderly population with little capacity for rehabilitation (e.g., the hypothetical consequences of Baumol's disease in a labor-intense service industry).

Such negative conceptions of the ability of LTC to change population health conditions are beginning to be successfully challenged – at least in the United States. As originally conceived, post-World War II nursing home care was viewed primarily as a residential, not a true medical, service option. Concerns were often expressed about the quality of medical care received in nursing homes – especially for patients whose care was primarily funded by state Medicaid programs. The Balanced Budget Act of 1997 imposed a prospective payment formula for Medicare-reimbursed skilled nursing facilities (RUGS-III – or Resource Utilization Groups Version III) that required fixed amounts (in minutes) of rehabilitation services be provided for skilled nursing facility (SNF) residents with specific morbidity and disability case mixes. The net effect of this policy was that discharge rates from acute care hospitals to SNFs were reduced by 15% and discharges from SNFs increased – without a corresponding increase in the U.S. community-resident severely disabled population. Under the Medicare reimbursement formulas, per capita payments (inflation-adjusted) were found in the 1982 to 2004 NLTCS to have increased over time for severely disabled persons and to have declined for nondisabled persons (Manton et al., 2006a). This illustrates that it is possible to increase productivity on a national level (here measured by the expenditures necessary to achieve a unit of disability reduction), even in LTC facilities for elderly residents, if efficient provision of existing rehabilitation services is emphasized. This may increase the rate at which patients can be returned to independent living and has been further promoted by the recent emphasis (in part due to the Olmstead court decision in 1999) on Home- and

Community-based waivers for LTC within the U.S. Medicaid program.

The problem is that few other economically developed countries have been as successful as the United States in redefining the LTC system and in intervening in the health and function of the elderly and oldest-old population. China will shortly face this problem (i.e., rapid growth in the demand for LTC) but, with past government-mandated restrictions on fertility rates, without the human capital historically available in China from traditional family sources to help solve it. The World Bank has determined that if life expectancy and health in Russia do not increase to the levels observed in the rest of Europe, the Russian human capital situation may serve to severely depress its future rate of economic expansion – GDP growth – despite its economically dominant position in terms of natural resources.

The effects of these recent morbidity and disability trends are enhanced by recent economic, demographic, and epidemiological conditions and fertility rates in different countries – but in very different ways. In the United States, the post-World War II baby boom cohorts of 1946 to 1964 were both preceded by a birth dearth due to the Great Depression and World War II – and then again followed by a birth dearth. Part of the recent reductions in fertility in the United States (and Canada) is due to the increasing participation of females in higher education, professional careers, and the labor force, with a consequent delaying of first births until later ages. In China, human resource problems may result due to population aging because of the one-child, one-family policy enhanced by the current Chinese pattern for LTC delivery based heavily on the extended family.

In the United States, the outline of a preferred public health and health-care systems approach, by intervening directly in the health and functional consequences of the individual's aging processes to expand the proportion of the total life span that can be expected to be spent in an active and economically productive state, is only beginning to be consciously elaborated as part of a federal policy initiative to help maintain U.S. global economic competitiveness (Manton *et al.*, 2007). Such a plan necessarily involves significant investment in biomedical research, so disability rate declines can, in the future, occur at very advanced ages (e.g., above age 95), where the prevalence of chronic disability and loss of social independence is currently the highest. It also requires retraining and other human capital enhancement activities, as envisioned in the Lisbon Agenda.

The fact that the decline in U.S. chronic disability prevalence rates has averaged 1.5% per annum from 1982 to 2004, and the per annum rate has continued its acceleration of decline to 2004 to 2.2% per annum 1999 to 2004 (Manton *et al.*, 2006a), suggests that this strategy is functioning well in the United States in dealing with the

projected large increases in Medicare and Medicaid expenditures expected to be initiated starting in 2010 with the passing of age 65 by the initial post-World War II baby boom cohorts. By 2080, the combination of Medicare and Medicaid is currently projected to consume 24% of GDP – compared to only 7% for Social Security. One set of projections by Manton *et al.* (2007), based on modifications of the economic growth models of Romer, Hall and Jones, and Jones and Williams, suggests that increased investment in biomedical and other research might reduce the proportion of GDP consumed by Medicare and Medicaid to 12% (i.e., a reduction by half from the 24% projected to be consumed in 2080). This reduction would be achieved by (1) stimulating the rate of GDP growth by better maintenance of human capital and (2) slowing of the rate of growth of health-care costs by the lagged effect of increased Medicare expenditures in improving health. The latter argument holds if the period projected to be spent chronically disabled by individuals increases more slowly than the rate of increase in total life expectancy – as has been observed by Manton *et al.* (2006a, 2006b) using the 1982 to 2004 NLTCS.

Longitudinal Methods for Calculating Active Life Expectancy

The type of cross-sectional ALE calculation that has been most often used is due to Sullivan (1971).

This calculation has great utility as a summary index of one important facet of the quality of life and human capital dynamics in a national population. It can be compared over a sequence of points in time to examine aggregate longitudinal health changes. Such aggregate increases in health and function, however, are less useful in attempting to identify how changes in functioning occur in individuals over time or the specific factors that are associated with, and which may cause, improvements in function at late ages. Such factors, if identified, could be applied at the population level to promote continuing declines in chronic disability and disease prevalence. This analytic effort requires considerably more longitudinal data (i.e., the tracking of individual health and disability changes), in which the measurement characteristics of the interview instrument and the survey sample design are preserved over a lengthy enough period to make meaningful estimates of ALE changes for specific elderly birth cohorts. It is also necessary that covariates that may affect the emergence of chronic disability (e.g., education, nutrition, exercise, health care, BMI) be longitudinally measured in those same surveys.

One nationally representative U.S. survey series with the appropriate longitudinal sample design and measurement characteristics to track such changes in disability and disability risk factors is the six 1982 to 2004 NLTCS.

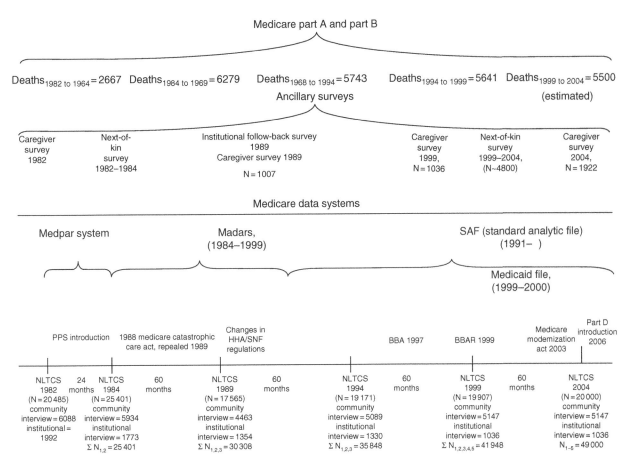

Figure 2 Observation plan, time frame, and sample sizes. World Bank Moscow Office, Economic Unit (2006), Russian Economic Report No.12, p. 20 (http://ns.worldbank.org.ru/files/rer/RER_12_eng.pdf).

The temporal sampling and interview structure of the six surveys is briefly summarized in **Figure 2**.

In addition to the six NLTCS survey waves (1982, 1984, 1989, 1994, 1999, 2004), there is also continuous (daily) information from Medicare administrative service use and expenditure records for individuals linked to the NLTCS survey records – currently for the period 1982 to 2005. A crucial aspect of the NLTCS for estimating longitudinal changes is that response rates were high (~95% from 1982 to 1999), so that there is relatively little chance for response bias to affect disability trend estimates. In 2004, to deal with an overall drop in the response rate to roughly 91%, data from longitudinal Medicare files, available for all persons in the sample, were used to adjust for health-related response bias in disability transition rate estimates (Manton *et al.*, 2006a). These adjustments, based on the ratio of Medicare Part A expenditure estimates for nondisabled persons to the Medicare Part A estimates for disabled persons, were retrospectively applied to nonresponders in all NLTCS waves so that a set of longitudinal weights consistently adjusted for nonresponse over all NLTCS 1982 to 2004 was generated (Manton *et al.*, 2006a).

Given that one has data on changes in an individual's functional status over time, as in the NLTCS, the question arises as to how best to estimate disability state transition parameters between surveys. This requires consideration of the types of disability transition rates one attempts to estimate and the rates of disability change in various age and demographic groups. There are several possible methodological approaches to estimate the necessary disability transition rates for calculating such longitudinal ALE measures.

One model that could be used is the standard discrete time Markov model. This model is relatively crude when assessed in terms of the types of disability changes one can estimate and what covariates might be included due to conventional sample size limitations (e.g., in the NLTCS, $N \sim 20\,000$ persons per wave). The model also assumes that there is no higher-order time dependency – the Markov condition – and that disability is a homogeneous and discrete measure.

Regression models can also be used to estimate disability transition rates when the sample size is insufficient to support stratification on all relevant control variables. One type of regression model, due to Cox, does not require estimating the time dependence of hazard rates, but only that, conditional on covariate values, the unobserved time-dependent hazard rates are proportional over time. This is an empirically testable assumption that may not hold for long periods of observation – especially if the force of mortality selection on the population systematically varies over disability status. Other regression models employ logistic functions of the probability of discrete transitions to ensure that the estimated probabilities fall within the range 0 to 1. In these models, there can be difficulties in trying to compare population estimates over time as temporal experience is accumulated; that is, mathematically updating transition rates with incremental adjustments for new experience collected over different periods of time can be difficult due to certain inconvenient parametric properties of logistic distributions. In all of these models, the dependent variable is a discrete change in functional status and not a continuous disability score.

An alternate approach is to use a large number of measures of functional impairment to calculate, in a multivariate procedure, convex (bounded to the range 0 to 1) continuous scores for multiple dimensions of disability. In using a principal component or factor analytic type of measurement model to calculate such disability scores, one is restricted by the assumption that the scores have a multivariate normal distribution; that is, information on moments higher than order two is lost.

An alternate method of calculating chronic disability indices involves using grade of membership (GoM) procedures (e.g., see Manton *et al.*, 1991, 1992, 1993, 1994) in which cases are assigned by using scores to 'fuzzy' sets, that is, persons are generally not in one homogeneous category but share properties of two, or more, fuzzy states. The model does not require the assumption of multivariate normality (i.e., they deal with more general distributions with informative moments of order three or higher). Furthermore, in GoM procedures, the K scores are estimated so that they sum to 1 for each person and are non-negative. This is equivalent to assuming disability changes occur in a convexly constrained multidimensional space and that the health trait scores for an individual vary between 0 and 1 for each of the K health and functional status dimensions.

In engineering studies, in which fuzzy set methods and computer algorithms are routinely used to study the dynamic control of complex nonlinear stochastic processes, such a measurement modeling step might be referred to as 'state fuzzification,' with the dynamics of the process studied in the more parsimonious, lower-dimension, less noisy fuzzy-state variable space. Importantly, after the fuzzy disabilities, state space process (with diffusion) is modeled, the new (forecast) distribution of the original disability measures can be extracted by reversing the measurement process to 'de-fuzzify' the distribution to get the new updated disability measure distribution.

Use of fuzzy set process models to model disabling processes has two other advantages. First, because the parameters of a continuous state stochastic process are being modeled, it is possible to calculate optimal solutions under certain marginal resource, or control variable, constraints. Second, because an individual's state is described as a continuous mixture of K health and functional dimensions, the measure precisely quantifies the health-determined functional capacity of the population under study.

Computing multivariate convex scores (i.e., bounded by 0 to 1) in GoM is an important modeling difference, compared to the calculations of DALYs and QALYs (disability-adjusted and quality-adjusted life years, respectively) and their application to planning for maximizing health and functioning in a population under resource constraints. In the latter two procedures, health status is also scaled over a 0 to 1 range on a single dimension; for example, death has a quality-of-life value of 0 and perfect health of 1. This is done to force decisions under a Game Theoretic model with a fixed payoff; that is, a zero sum game with finite, fixed resources.

In reality, the operation of the health-care process may serve, over time, to increase economic resources to further improve future health; that is, a positive feed forward mechanism. In GoM, persons are evaluated on multiple dimensions so that there is not a fixed unidimensional choice of an optimal state; that is, exchanges might be made between different types and levels of impairment. For example, if one dimension reflects primarily physical dysfunction, and another cognitive dysfunction, there might be very different payoffs for optimizing on one dimension versus another. It is also possible that synergistic (health-enhancing), as well as antagonistic, interactions may emerge in the stochastic nonlinear process. Also, it is possible that the timing and sequencing of specific interventions may be crucial to the disabling dynamics.

Stated differently, using the GoM-characterized multidimensional state of active life expectancy, the primary optimization criteria (e.g., using the scores in a quadratic optimization problem) could be an objectively identified set of health states where the status on different health dimensions for specific persons can be improved. This arises because this model views increased investment in health expenditures as a way to increase human capital productivity as a strategy for stimulating economic growth. It is arguable that this occurred during techno-physiological evolution as discussed by Fogel and Costa; that is, the work capacity and productivity of each person might increase over time as nutrition improved and body size and work capacity grew. Arguments by Flynn and others suggest such enhancements may have also occurred in cognitive skills (i.e., I.Q. increased) – again, possibly due to improved nutrition, better education and health, and smaller family size. Under these conditions, it would be erroneous to assess health on one dimension with a maximum value of one. This is made clear in evaluations of human capital, in which skill level, training, and socioeconomic factors have to be considered in adding quality dimensions to human capital calculations.

Empirical Example of Longitudinal Active-Life-Expectancy Calculations

As a first step in our example, the GoM measurement model was applied to 27 ADL, IADL, Nagi performance scores, and vision measures made in each of the six NLTCS for the period 1982 to 2004. That analysis showed that the 27 disability measures could be described by six types of disability profiles/dimensions found in community residents and a seventh discrete institutional residence disability category. With these seven disability scores, and the sample weights for individuals, it was possible to calculate a matrix of age-specific population disability transition parameters and age- and disability-dependent quadratic mortality functions estimated conditionally on the temporally current disability score values determined by the stochastic disability transition matrix. With disability dynamic equations and a disability-specific hazard function, life expectancy and ALE can be calculated conditionally upon the GoM disability scores by using generalizations of the well-known Fokker-Planck equations (Manton et al., 1993). In addition, the disability scores can themselves be made functions of medical conditions and other possibly exogenous factors that may affect individual disability trajectories over age/time. For example, stroke may operate to decrement both the physical and cognitive functions of an individual. This is one way to bring exogenous (control) variable information into calculations of endogenous changes of disability scores between NLTCS waves and to make projections of scores conditional on assumptions about trends in exogenous factors (i.e., either as observed or as may be generated by targeted interventions in control variables; Manton et al., 1993, 1994).

It was found (**Table 1**) that life expectancy estimates calculated using NLTCS data and exact times of death from linked Medicare files were quite close to those calculated by Social Security actuaries (SSA, Actuarial Study No. 116). This confirms that the NLTCS sample is representative of the survival experience of the entire U.S. elderly population, a property not always found in national health survey samples. This is illustrated in **Table 1**.

At age 65, the SSA cohort and NLTCS life expectancy values are quite close (i.e., 0.41 years higher in the NLTCS than for the SSA for males and 0.29 years lower

Table 1 Life expectancy for aged 65+ in 1982–2004 NLTCS

		Estimations from SSA life tables (LT)	
Age	GoM model	Period	Cohort (birth year 1917)
Male			
65	15.32	14.23	14.91
67	14.08	13.21	13.74
72	11.23	10.80	11.02
77	8.70	8.48	8.55
82	6.56	6.34	6.37
87	4.91	4.58	4.62
Female			
65	18.61	18.48	18.90
67	17.20	17.16	17.02
72	13.83	14.02	13.99
77	10.76	10.85	10.83
82	8.09	7.98	8.05
87	5.94	5.71	5.76

than in SSA female cohort). The difference is, in part, due to comparing the cross-sectional experience in the NLTCS with the experience of the single year of age cohort born in 1917.

In addition, longitudinal life tables showing the time/age dependence of both survival and disability changes may be calculated from the NLTCS. The disability dynamic dependent life table is presented for males and females in **Table 2**.

Table 2 was actually calculated as a complete (single year of age) table but, because of space considerations, we presented in the table only every fifth year of age up to 95 (where estimates begin to vary significantly due to small counts). The columns to the right represent the proportion of life expectancy at that age that is expected to be lived in each of the seven disability states. The overall life expectancy is a continuously weighted mixture of life tables for each of the seven disability types. That is, there exists a separate life table for PT1 (persons with no functional impairment) for all persons exactly like that pure type; that is, $g_1 = 1$. The life expectancy for this first type will be higher than the weighted average for the total, mixed population. Likewise, the life table for frail persons (i.e., $g_6 = 1$) will have a much lower life expectancy than the total (mixed) population.

The first pure type (PT1) in **Table 2** represents people with no chronic disability or physical limitations. The second and third types have partial limitations only in performing specific physical tasks. Pure type four is IADL-impaired; PT5 and PT6 represent persons with ADL dependency and with increasing levels of IADL impairment. The sixth type is frail; that is, highly ADL- and IADL-impaired. The seventh pure type represents respondents in institutional/nursing home residence. Such persons have significant functional limitations (e.g., 4.8 ADLs impaired on average) similar to the frail population; that is, PT6.

Table 2   Life tables with male and female cross-sectional disability covariates for 1982 to 2004 NLTCS

Age	L_x	E_x	PT 1	PT 2	PT 3	PT 4	PT 5	PT 6	PT 7
Male									
65	100 000	15.32	0.91	0.05	0.01	0.01	0.02	0.00	0.00
			0.28	0.10	0.06	0.06	0.08	0.07	0.00
75	69 652	9.67	0.88	0.03	0.01	0.01	0.02	0.02	0.02
			0.33	0.07	0.09	0.10	0.09	0.14	0.15
85	30 754	5.51	0.78	0.04	0.02	0.02	0.04	0.04	0.06
			0.42	0.09	0.10	0.14	0.12	0.18	0.24
95	4606	3.30	0.71	0.06	0.01	0.03	0.05	0.03	0.10
			0.45	0.10	0.09	0.16	0.14	0.18	0.30
Female									
65	100 000	18.61	0.92	0.02	0.02	0.01	0.02	0.01	0.00
			0.27	0.11	0.09	0.07	0.12	0.11	0.06
75	79 761	11.95	0.84	0.04	0.02	0.01	0.03	0.02	0.04
			0.37	0.13	0.11	0.10	0.16	0.15	0.19
85	46 235	6.73	0.66	0.05	0.03	0.03	0.07	0.05	0.12
			0.47	0.15	0.13	0.16	0.23	0.21	0.32
95	10 816	3.74	0.52	0.04	0.03	0.04	0.08	0.07	0.22
			0.50	0.15	0.13	0.18	0.24	0.26	0.42

Source: World Bank Moscow Office, Economic Unit (2006) Russian Economic Report No. 12, p. 21 (http://ns.worldbank.org.ru/files/rer/RER_12_eng.pdf).

In **Table 2**, L_x and e_x have standard demographic interpretations; for example, that 30.8% of the male population with a mixed disability distribution survives from age 65 to 85, with life expectancy declining from 15.3 years at age 65 to 5.5 years at age 85. The first disability dimension represents persons free of disability. The value in parentheses is the standard deviation of the disability score estimate. Since the space is convexly constrained, the standard deviation of 0.28 for PT1 at age 65 suggests the distribution of nondisabled persons is concentrated in the interior of the K-dimensional disability state space. The mean value of 0.78 (standard deviation of 0.42) for the nondisabled PT1 at age 85 indicates the burden of disability is much higher past age 85, with 16% of the male population living in the community in impaired states (i.e., 8% in highly impaired states 5 and 6) and 6% of males resident in nursing homes.

In the bottom panel of **Table 2** is the corresponding abbreviated life table for females. Life expectancy is higher for females (18.6 years at age 65; 6.7 years at age 85) as is the age-specific prevalence of chronic disability at later ages; for example, 34% of females are impaired at age 85 compared to 22% of males.

Although the life tables are the end product of the ALE analysis done cross-sectionally (Sullivan, 1971), certain intermediate transition parameters are of interest if one wishes to examine the individual biological mechanisms, and their control parameters, by which total and active life expectancy are generated over time in cohorts of individuals. One set of intermediate estimates are the parameters describing the change in the disability scores over time and the dependency of those transition parameters on factors (e.g., disease or disability risk factors

such as smoking, diabetes, or obesity) that are potentially controllable by specific interventions. The second set of intermediate coefficients describes the risk of death specific to disability state at a specific time and age. These two sets of coefficients interact over time to determine the life expectancy and risk factor distribution in the disability-dependent life tables previously described.

In **Table 3**, we present the matrix of disability-state transition coefficients calculated at ages 65 to 67 and ages 85 to 87. In the first row of the top panel (disability changes from age 65 to 67; or two-year transitions), 94% of the nondisabled male (and female) population (the first disability dimension or PT1) at age 65 remains nondisabled at age 67. The diagonal of the matrix represents the two-year persistence of persons in each of the seven disability states. For example, whereas males in the second pure type have little disability, though with some moderate physical performance limitations, after two years, only 34% of males remain in this type, while 33% of the type become nondisabled (i.e., move to PT1), and 26% become more severely disabled (with a transition to PT4 to PT7). PT3 to PT6 have only modest persistence, though at ages 65 to 67 there is a significant likelihood of returning to a less disabled state. Only the group of severely disabled persons resident in institutions has a high persistence and tends to remain in institutions.

At age 85 to 87, the disability changes for males (**Table 3**) show a persistence in disabled states that tends to be higher than at age 65 to 67 except for the nondisabled state (PT1). The return to the nondisabled state for females (column 1) is lower than at age 65, whereas the moderately disabled show a greater likelihood of their disability's worsening. The transitions for

Table 3 Disability state two year transitions between profiles for age 65 and 85

	Profiles for age 67						
Age 65	PT 1	PT 2	PT 3	PT 4	PT 5	PT 6	PT 7
Male							
PT 1	0.94	0.02	0.01	0.01	0.01	0.01	0.00
PT 2	0.33	0.34	0.06	0.05	0.10	0.09	0.02
PT 3	0.37	0.14	0.19	0.06	0.08	0.10	0.06
PT 4	0.27	0.15	0.09	0.21	0.13	0.12	0.03
PT 5	0.26	0.15	0.07	0.07	0.32	0.09	0.05
PT 6	0.23	0.11	0.07	0.06	0.09	0.38	0.06
PT 7	0.06	0.03	0.03	0.02	0.04	0.04	0.78
Female							
PT 1	0.94	0.01	0.01	0.01	0.01	0.01	0.00
PT 2	0.35	0.32	0.10	0.04	0.10	0.07	0.01
PT 3	0.29	0.12	0.29	0.05	0.11	0.11	0.02
PT 4	0.34	0.12	0.10	0.15	0.12	0.12	0.04
PT 5	0.28	0.10	0.11	0.05	0.32	0.12	0.02
PT 6	0.19	0.06	0.13	0.06	0.14	0.36	0.05
PT 7	0.19	0.03	0.03	0.02	0.02	0.03	0.67

	Profiles for age 87						
Age 85	PT 1	PT 2	PT 3	PT 4	PT 5	PT 6	PT 7
Male							
PT 1	0.87	0.02	0.01	0.01	0.03	0.03	0.03
PT 2	0.18	0.50	0.05	0.05	0.10	0.08	0.04
PT 3	0.18	0.10	0.41	0.07	0.10	0.10	0.05
PT 4	0.17	0.07	0.06	0.46	0.07	0.10	0.07
PT 5	0.20	0.07	0.05	0.04	0.50	0.08	0.05
PT 6	0.16	0.05	0.03	0.04	0.06	0.58	0.07
PT 7	0.17	0.01	0.01	0.02	0.02	0.02	0.76
Female							
PT 1	0.81	0.02	0.02	0.02	0.04	0.03	0.06
PT 2	0.16	0.45	0.06	0.06	0.10	0.09	0.09
PT 3	0.17	0.08	0.40	0.05	0.10	0.10	0.10
PT 4	0.17	0.07	0.05	0.43	0.08	0.09	0.11
PT 5	0.16	0.06	0.05	0.04	0.55	0.07	0.08
PT 6	0.15	0.04	0.04	0.04	0.05	0.57	0.11
PT 7	0.10	0.02	0.01	0.01	0.02	0.03	0.80

Source: World Bank Moscow Office, Economic Unit (2006) Russian Economic Report No. 12, p. 20 (http://ns.worldbank.org.ru/files/rer/RER_12_eng.pdf).

Table 4 Hazard matrix B at age 65 (proportion of deaths in one year) in NLTCS 1982–2004

	PT 1	PT 2	PT 3	PT 4	PT 5	PT 6	PT 7
Male							
PT 1	0.04	0.06	0.07	0.07	0.07	0.09	0.08
PT 2		0.08	0.09	0.10	0.09	0.12	0.11
PT 3			0.11	0.12	0.11	0.15	0.13
PT 4				0.13	0.11	0.16	0.14
PT 5					0.11	0.14	0.13
PT 6						0.20	0.18
PT 7							0.16
Female							
PT 1	0.03	0.04	0.04	0.06	0.05	0.08	0.07
PT 2		0.04	0.05	0.07	0.06	0.08	0.08
PT 3			0.06	0.08	0.07	0.10	0.09
PT 4				0.11	0.10	0.14	0.12
PT 5					0.08	0.12	0.11
PT 6						0.17	0.16
PT 7							0.14

Source: Economic and Social Commission for Asia and the Pacific, United Nations (2005) Economic and Social Survey of Asia and the Pacific 2005, United Nations publication Sales No. E.05.11.F.10, ISBN: 91-1-120420-8, http://www.unescap.org/pdd/publications/survey2005/9_Survey05_Ch-III.pdf.

Table 5 The difference of senescence process (θ) on disability covariate model and Gompertz model

		NLTCS 1982–2004 Age 65 and over	
		Female	Male
Disability covariate dynamics	θ (%)	6.96	6.54
	χ^2	7816	2890
	Ex (year) at age 65	18.61	15.32
Gompertz Function	θ (%)	9.62	8.62
	(SE)	(0.39)	(0.20)
θ difference between two models (%)		−2.66	−2.08
z value		−4.9	−7.4

Source: Economic and Social Commission for Asia and the Pacific, United Nations (2005) Economic and Social Survey of Asia and the Pacific 2005, United Nations publication Sales No. E.05.11.F.10, ISBN: 91-1-120420-8, http://www.unescap.org/pdd/publications/survey2005/9_Survey05_Ch-III.pdf.

females show patterns similar to those of males, though with a higher retention in institutional residence. As a consequence, one way to view the transition matrix is as a web of transition paths between the two 'anchor' states of the convex disability space; i.e., PT1 for persons nondisabled and PT7 for persons wholly disabled in institutions. The intermediate states in the web connecting the two end points appear to be snapshots of the qualitative intermediate state changes that evolve at that age. A completely dynamic picture of changes would require attaching time parameters (waiting times) to the intermediate states.

Interacting with these transitions is the risk of death for age-specific disability states. This is illustrated for both males and females in **Table 4**.

The hazard coefficients in **Table 4** show that at age 65 there is a small survival advantage for females for most pure types and pure type interactions (i.e., persons whose disability status is described by a mixture of two, or more, disability dimensions). That means, for a given disability profile, that female mortality at age 65 will be lower than for males. Those coefficients are, however, dependent on age, as shown in **Table 5**. Because the θ (rate of aging parameter) for females is larger than for males, female mortality rates in specific disability states tend to increase more rapidly with age.

In **Table 5**, we show the age-dependence of the male and female mortality functions, both without adjustments for the seven disability types and with adjustments for those disability types (scores).

The increase of mortality, specific to disability, is faster for females than for males (i.e., the θ value is larger for females), indicating that a crossover will be expressed in male/female mortality trajectories at later ages. This is consistent with studies of gender differences in mortality and of disability trajectories.

Discussion

Active life expectancy is a useful measure of the amount of healthy, socially independent life expectancy existing in a particular national population. It has often been examined (e.g., Robine and Michel, 2004) by comparing, over time, cross-sectional life tables of the type proposed by Sullivan (1971) (see Manton *et al.*, 2006b). It is now widely accepted as a basic measure of the quality of health in a country by WHO – especially in highly developed countries.

If, however, those measures are to be useful for studying how to intervene in the disablement/mortality processes determining active life expectancy, then longitudinal data on the functioning and survival of individuals must be available, and those data must be analyzed longitudinally; that is, to explicitly identify the interactions of age-specific disability and mortality over time in well-defined groups (e.g., birth cohorts). This requires either special longitudinal health surveys or long-term population registries of health events and mortality.

We presented a stochastic fuzzy state model of these disability dynamics and their interaction with mortality that will allow more detailed study of the biological mechanisms that generate and sustain chronic disability of different types. This will permit better estimation of the temporal parameters of disability processes – even at very advanced ages. Indeed, because longitudinal estimates of ALE require both age-specific estimates of disability dynamics and age and disability-specific mortality, additional component parameters of the process are estimated that can be examined to help better understand sources of change in the processes.

With improved parameter estimates it will be possible to (1) better quantitatively forecast change in ALE and (2) better simulate the effects of specific interventions. Thus, although true longitudinal analysis of ALE process is more complex and has greater data requirements, it is also intrinsically more informative and can be used to assess a broader range of issues, and in greater depth, than can the Sullivan-type cross-sectional estimates. Furthermore, by using an explicit stochastic model of disability dynamics, more formal analysis of resource allocation models can be conducted. The formal analyses will better (more naturally and with fewer assumptions)

describe population health and functional changes over time. This may lead ultimately to more effective and better-targeted strategies to improve ALE/LE ratios at late ages and thus to increase the human capital present at late ages in developed nations.

Citations

Feldman JJ (1983) Work ability of the aged under conditions of improving mortality. *Milbank Memorial Fund Quarterly* 61(3): 430–444.

Fries J (1980) Aging, natural death, and the compression of morbidity. *New England Journal of Medicine* 303: 130–135.

Gruenberg EM (1977) The failure of success. *Milbank Memorial Fund Quarterly* 55(1): 3–24.

Katz S, Ford A, Moskowitz R, Jackson B, and Jaffe M (1963) Studies of illness of the aged: the index of ADL, a standardized measure of biological and physical function. *Journal of the American Medical Association* 185: 914–919.

Kramer M (1980) The rising pandemic of mental disorders and associated chronic diseases and disabilities. *Acta Psychiatrica Scandinavica* 285: 382–397.

Lakdawalla DN, Goldman DP, and Shang B (2005) The health and cost consequences of obesity among the future elderly. *Health Affairs* 26: W5-R30–W5-R41.

Manton KG (1989) Epidemiological, demographic, and social correlates of disability among the elderly. *Milbank Quarterly* 67(Part 1 Suppl. 2): 13–58.

Manton KG, Stallard E, and Liu K (1993) Forecasts of active life expectancy: Policy and fiscal implications. *Journals of Gerontology* 48 (Special No): 11–26.

Manton K, Woodbury M, and Tolley HD (1994) *Statistical Applications Using Fuzzy Sets*. New York: Wiley Interscience.

Manton KG and Gu XL (2001) Changes in the prevalence of chronic disability in the U.S. black and non-black population above age 65 from 1982 to 1999. *Proceedings of the National Academy of Sciences, USA* 98(11): 6354–6359.

Manton KG, Gu XL, and Lamb VL (2006a) Change in chronic disability from 1982 to 2004/2005 as measured by long-term changes in function and health in the U.S. elderly population. *Proceedings of the National Academy of Sciences USA* 103(48): 18374–18379.

Manton KG, Gu XL, and Lamb VL (2006b) Long-term trends in life expectancy and active life expectancy in the United States. *Population and Development Review* 32(1): 81–105.

Manton KG, Lowrimore G, Ullian A, XiLiang G, and Tolley HD (2007) Labor force participation and human capital increases in an aging population and implications for U.S. research investment. *Proceedings of the National Academy of Science* 104(26): 10802–10807.

Myers GC (1981) Future age projections and society. In: Gilmore A (ed.) *Aging: A Challenge to Science and Social Policy*, pp. 248–260. Oxford, UK: Oxford University Press.

Robine JM and Michel JP (2004) Looking forward to a general theory on population aging. *Journals of Gerontology Series A-Biological Sciences and Medical Sciences* 59(6): 590–597.

Singer B and Manton KG (1998) The effects of health changes on projections of health service needs for the elderly population of the United States. *Proceedings of the National Academy of Science* 95: 15618–15622.

Sullivan DF (1971) A single index of mortality and morbidity. *HSMHA Health Reports* 86: 347–354.

Further Reading

Cutler D, Landrum M, and Stewart K (2006) Intensive medical care and cardiovascular disease disability reductions. *NBER Working Paper No. 12184* May 2006.

Fogel R (2004) *The Escape from Hunger and Premature Death, 1700–2100: Europe, America, and the Third World*. Cambridge studies in population, economy and society in past time. London: Cambridge University Press.

Fogel R and Costa D (1997) A theory of technophysio evolution, with some implications for forecasting population, health care costs, and pension costs. *Demography* 34(1): 49–66.

Freedman V, Martin L, and Schoeni R (2002) Recent trends in disability and functioning among older adults in the United States: A systematic review. *Journal of the American Medical Association* 288(24): 3137–3146.

Freedman VA, Crimmins E, Schoeni RF, *et al.* (2004) Resolving inconsistencies in old-age disability trends: Report from a technical working group. *Demography* 41(3): 417–441.

Manton KG and Stallard E (1988) *Chronic Disease Risk Modelling: Measurement and Evaluation of the Risks of Chronic Disease Processes*. London: Charles Griffin Limited. Griffin Series of the Biomathematics of Diseases.

Manton KG, Stallard E, and Woodbury MA (1991) A multivariate event history model based upon fuzzy states: Estimation from longitudinal surveys with informative nonresponse. *Journal of Official Statistics* 7(3): 261–293.

Manton KG, Stallard E, and Singer BH (1992) Projecting the future size and health status of the U.S. elderly population. *International Journal of Forecasting* 8: 433–458.

Manton KG and Gu XL (2005) Disability declines and trends in Medicare expenditures. *Ageing Horizons* 2: 25–34.

Manton KG, Gu XL, and Ukraintseva SV (2005) Declining prevalence of dementia in the U.S. elderly population. *Advances in Gerontology* 16: 30–37.

Schoeni R, Freedman V, and Wallace R (2001) Persistent, consistent, widespread, and robust? Another look at recent trends in old-age disability. *Journals of Gerontology Series B-Psychological Sciences & Social Sciences* 56(4): S206–S218.

Stallard E and Yee RK (2000) Noninsured home and community-based long-term care incidence and continuance tables. *Actuarial Report Issued by the Long-Term Care Experience Committee*. Schaumberg, IL: Society of Actuaries.

Walston J (2004) Frailty – the search for underlying causes. *Science of Aging Knowledge Environment* 4: pe4.

Demography of Aging

K C Land, Duke University, Durham, NC, USA
V L Lamb, North Carolina Central University, Durham, NC, USA

Introduction

Demography, the scientific study of population, is concerned with distributions of vital rates in populations, sources of variations in these rates or population dynamics, demographic consequences of changes in the structures of populations over time, and population forecasting. Age is an important indicator in demography because it is a critical part of the structure of populations, and it directly affects basic demographic processes of fertility (births), mortality (deaths), and migration. Demography of aging is a subfield of demography that focuses on the older members of a population as well as the processes and consequences of population aging. Research in the demography of aging examines a number of topics, including the state and status of the older population, changes in the numbers, proportionate size, and composition of the older population, demographic forces of fertility, mortality, and migration that bring about these changes, and effects of these changes on the social, economic, health, and personal well-being of the elderly (Myers, 1990).

Demographic and Epidemiologic Transitions

There has been a long-standing interest within the social sciences and epidemiology in determining the historical sequence and major stages of important socioeconomic and epidemiological transformations. This has been especially true in the field of demography, in which the notion of a demographic transition became embedded in the field to describe fairly universal patterns of declining mortality levels and subsequent declines in fertility, with accompanying characteristic changes in population growth rates and population structure.

Epidemiologic transition theory focuses upon changes in the complex patterns of disease and mortality associated with the demographic transition (Omran, 1971). The intent of the theory was to direct focus on the shifts in disease patterns and causes of mortality, and the resulting impacts upon life expectation and population growth. According to the theory, as nations modernized in the twentieth century, they improved their social, economic, and health conditions. Part of the modernization process is the replacement of life conditions that previously were conducive to the spread of infectious and parasitic diseases by more sanitary conditions, improved medical technology, and better lifestyles. This reduces the population's risk of dying from infectious diseases. Those saved from dying from such diseases survive into middle and older ages where they face the elevated risk of dying from chronic and degenerative diseases. Since such diseases tend to kill at much older ages than infectious diseases, this transition in causes of death is characterized generally by a redistribution of deaths from younger to older ages.

Omran's original statement of epidemiologic transition theory focused on population-level consequences of the modernization of societies and identified three stages of epidemiologic transition: The age of pestilence and famine, the age of receding pandemics, and the age of degenerative and man-made diseases. The major premise of the theory assumes mortality to be the fundamental factor in population dynamics.

The twentieth century was a period of reductions in mortality rates. The rapid declines in overall mortality in more developed countries slowed in the 1960s to a fairly stagnant trend. However, a decade later the declines resumed, particularly at older ages. The result was unprecedented increases in life expectancy during the twentieth century. The mortality declines and subsequent increases in life expectancy were due to reductions in the prevalence of chronic and degenerative diseases, contrary to Omran's theory.

A number of researchers suggested that the epidemiologic transition framework be extended to include a fourth stage. Several factors – including a pronounced shift in the age structure toward older ages, advances in medical technology, and public health measures that favored the old over the young, federal health-care programs that favored the elderly and poor, and reductions in risk factors on a population scale – are responsible for this new era in human epidemiologic history.

Olshansky and Ault (1986) argued that the timing and magnitude of this mortality transition was significant and distinct enough to qualify as a fourth stage of epidemiologic transition, which they termed the age of delayed degenerative diseases. This fourth stage is characterized, first, by rapidly declining age-specific death rates that are concentrated mostly in advanced ages and that occur at nearly the same pace for males and females. Second, the age distribution of deaths from degenerative and chronic conditions shifts progressively toward older ages. Third, relatively rapid improvements in survival across the life course and life expectancy are concentrated among the population at advanced ages. The result is that the expectation of life at birth has risen rapidly in recent years to the upper end of the seventh decade of life, and, among some populations in the developed world, to more than eight decades. In the United States, life expectancy increased from 47.3 years in 1900 to 76.9 years in 2000, as shown in **Figure 1**, and Japan's life expectancy increased from 44 to 80.7 years during that same period.

Population Aging

Population aging refers to changes in the age composition of a population such that there is an increase in the

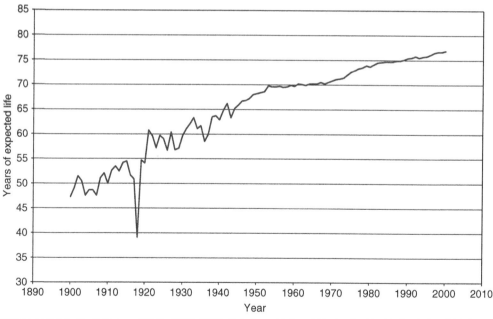

Figure 1   Average U.S. Life Expectancy at Birth, 1900–2000. Data from National Center for Health Statistics (1996) *Vital Statistics of the United States, 1991, Vol. II, Mortality Part A*. Washington DC: Public Health Service; (1900–1991); Hoyert DL, Arias E, Smith BL, Murphy SL, and Kochanek KD (2001) *Deaths: Final Data for 1999. National Vital Statistics Reports; Vol. 49 No. 8*. Hyattsville MD: National Center for Health Statistics (1992–1999); Minino AM, Arias E, Kochanek KD, Murphy SL, and Smith BL (2002) *Deaths: Final Data for 2000. National Vital Statistics Reports, Vol. 50, No. 15*. Hyattsville MD: National Center for Health Statistics (2000).

proportion of older persons. Demographers use age/sex pyramids to illustrate the distribution of populations across all age groups. **Figure 2** presents age/sex pyramids for 2000 and projected 2025 and 2050 for Brazil and Italy. Each bar represents the percent of total population in 5-year age groups for males (left) and females (right). In 2000, Brazil has a large portion of the population in the younger ages. By 2025 and 2050, the proportion of the younger population has decreased dramatically, and the proportion in the oldest group, 85 years and older, has increased dramatically. In contrast, in 2000

Italy's young population already constitutes a smaller portion of the total population. By 2050, persons under the age of 20 will constitute only 16.5% of the total Italian population, whereas those 60 and older will make up almost 40%.

Epidemiologic transition theory highlights how changes in the causes of mortality, from infectious and parasitic diseases to chronic and degenerative diseases, result in longer life expectation for populations. Thus, the changing process of mortality is one factor affecting population aging. A second important factor is changes

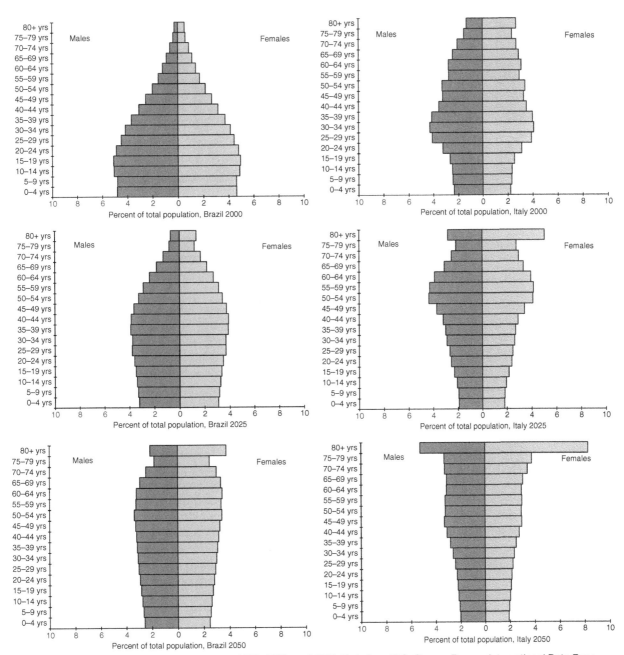

Figure 2 Age/sex pyramids for Brazil and Italy, 2000, 2025, and 2050. Data from U.S. Census Bureau, International Data Base.

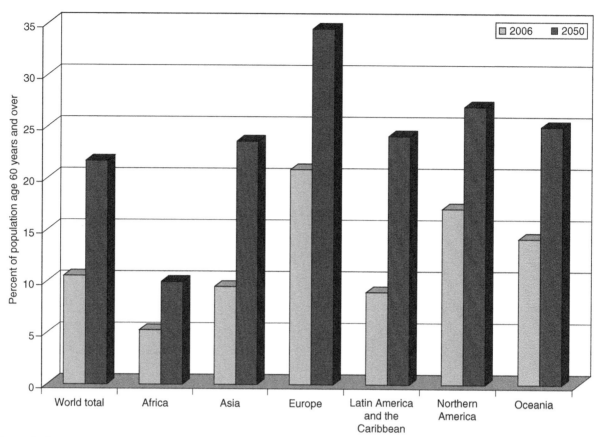

Figure 3 Percent of population age 60 and over by region, 2006–2050. United Nations (2002) *World population ageing: 1950–2050.* New York: United Nations. http://www.un.org/esa/population/publications/worldageing19502050/ (accessed October 2007).

in the rates of fertility or births. The changing age/sex structure of Brazil is due, in part, to reductions in the average number of children born per female. Italy is among the more developed countries that already have low birth rates in 2000, as represented by the small proportion of the population in the younger age groups.

A third factor affecting population aging is migration; however, the effect of migration on population aging is not as influential as that of changes in trends in population mortality and fertility. Patterns of migration into and out of nations can affect the age structure of populations. Immigrants tend to be younger, and first-generation immigrants tend to follow marriage and fertility patterns typical of their original country. Thus, a large flow of immigrants into a country can potentially shift the age structure to younger ages. A country that experiences significant out-migration may also shift to an older population structure if those migrating out are young adults and their children.

All regions of the world are experiencing population aging, although the rates of increase differ across regions, as shown in **Figure 3**. Europe is the oldest region, with 21%

of its population aged 60 years and over in 2006, and the rate is expected to rise to 34% in 2050. The youngest region is Africa, with only 5% of the population over the age of 60 in 2006, which will double to 10% in 2050. The proportion of older persons in both Asia and Latin America and the Caribbean regions are expected to increase from 9% to 24% between 2006 and 2050, due to both reductions in rates of fertility and increases in life expectancy.

A United Nations report, *World Population Aging: 1950–2050* (2002), set forth four important conclusions regarding the trend of population aging. First, population aging is unprecedented in the history of humanity. By 2050, it is predicted the worldwide number of persons aged 60 years and older will be larger than the number of persons aged 15 years and under. Second, population aging is a global phenomenon that affects persons of all ages in all nations. Third, population aging has serious implications for economic, political, social, and other areas of human life. Fourth, population aging is enduring. The trend will continue through the twenty-first century, and it is unlikely any nation will return to younger populations of the past.

Health, Disability, and Active Life Expectancy

As countries progress through the later stages of the epidemiologic transition, the traditional indicators of population health based on death rates alone are expected to change very little. Therefore, the incidence, prevalence, and duration of chronic conditions, and the disabling effects of chronic and degenerative conditions are increasingly important concerns in the examination of population health.

The epidemiologic transition theory has been extended to include a disability transition framework that focuses on changes in the causes and levels of disability and the distribution of disablement within different segments of the population (Myers *et al.*, 2003). In the early stages of the epidemiologic transition, the causes of disability will be infectious and parasitic diseases, and thus, the rate of new cases (incidence) will be high, particularly in the younger ages. As the cause of death changes to chronic and degenerative diseases, the total rate of disability cases (prevalence) will increase, and be compressed at older ages.

With the increase in life expectancy at older ages at the end of the twentieth century, some forecasts indicated that the result would be an increase in the proportion of older persons with serious health and disability problems, which would make large demands on the health-care system. Others predicted that there would be a postponement of serious chronic diseases and disabilities until the very end of life, resulting in a compression of morbidity (Fries, 1980). A third scenario is that the serious effects of chronic diseases would be lessened, and therefore there would not be large increases in the prevalence of more serious disabilities.

Much of the analysis of the relation between mortality and disability has been carried out using estimates of active or healthy life expectancy, which can elucidate the relation between disability and mortality quantitatively. Active life expectancy (ALE) refers to the proportion or years of total life expectancy that will be spent in a healthy or nondisabled state. In many ALE studies, disability is based on sample survey reports of difficulties or problems in performing activities of daily living (ADLs), which are personal care activities, such as eating, dressing, bathing, grooming, or getting in and out of a bed or chair. Persons are defined as disabled if they report having problems performing at least one ADL function. The age-specific disability rate is calculated to reflect the percentage of persons who are disabled in designated age intervals (e.g., 60–64, 65–69, 70–74). Population life tables, which estimate total years of life expectancy, are partitioned to estimate years of disabled and active (or healthy) life expectancy.

International studies of ALE in the 1980s were inconsistent in that some studies showed fluctuations with little to no improvement in health, whereas other studies documented modest disability declines. Research in the more developed nations at the end of the twentieth century has shown declines in the rates of disabilities, particularly severe disabilities, which have resulted in longer years of ALE. Regarding gender differences, studies have indicated that females have longer years of life expectancy and males tend to have a higher proportion of ALE. Part of the gender differences in total and active life expectancy is due to differences in the types of illnesses experienced in old age. Women have higher rates of disabling and degenerative diseases, such as arthritis, and men have higher rates of lethal acute conditions, such as heart attacks and stroke. Differences in social, economic, and lifestyle/behavioral experiences over the life course are factors that are linked with gender differences in morbidity and mortality in old age.

A question is whether disability declines will continue into the future. Combining results of early to mid to late-twentieth-century U.S. disability trends, Manton *et al.* (2006) calculated active and total life expectancy estimates from 1935 to 1999 and, using modest projected disability rate changes, made active life expectancy forecasts to 2080. The forecasts showed significant long-term improvements in the ratio of active to total life expectancy at age 65, with larger rates of improvement in the ratio at ages 85+, as shown in **Figure 4**.

The Elderly as a Subpopulation

The demography of aging also examines the characteristics and needs of the elderly as a subpopulation, often based on survey or vital statistics data. A society's older population is a very diverse and heterogeneous group. As populations move through the epidemiologic transition, the age structure within the older population also changes. In more developed countries, the fastest growing age group is the oldest old, or persons aged 85 years and older. The mortality changes have also affected the proportion of women and minorities in older ages.

With the rapidly changing structure and diversity of the older population, many demographers have studied the social and economic implications of population aging. Such studies have focused on a number of important concerns, including patterns of social and economic support across generations within families; factors associated with the process of retirement and exiting from the work force; changes in the socioeconomic status of elderly cohorts; patterns and types of migration at older ages; national pension, medical, and social programs to support the elderly; and changing patterns of health and disability, health-seeking behaviors, and sources of long-term care.

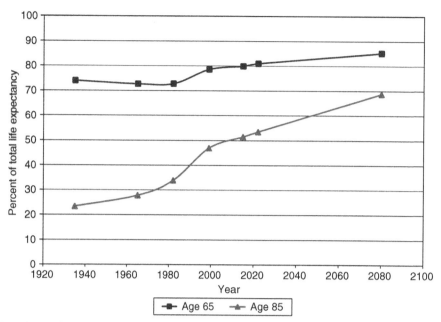

Figure 4 Proportion of total life expectancy to be spent in good health at ages 65 and 85, United States, 1935–2080. Source: Data from Table 1 in Manton KG, Gu X, and Lamb VL (2006) Long-term trends in life expectancy and active life expectancy. *Population and Development Review* 32: 81–106.

See also: Active Life Expectancy; Longevity in Specific Populations.

Citations

Fries JF (1980) Aging, natural death, and the compression of morbidity. *New England Journal of Medicine* 61: 130–135.

Hoyert DL, Arias E, Smith BL, Murphy SL, and Kochanek KD (2001) *Deaths: Final Data for 1999. National Vital Statistics Reports; Vol. 49 No. 8.* Hyattsville, MD: National Center for Health Statistics.

Manton KG, Gu X, and Lamb VL (2006) Long-term trends in life expectancy and active life expectancy. *Population and Development Review* 32: 81–106.

Minino AM, Arias E, Kochanek KD, Murphy SL, and Smith BL (2002) *Deaths: Final Data for 2000. National Vital Statistics Reports, Vol. 50, No. 15.* Hyattsville, MD: National Center for Health Statistics.

Myers GC (1990) Demography of aging. In: Binstock RH and George LK (eds.) *Handbook of Aging and the Social Sciences,* 3rd edn., pp. 19–44. New York: Academic Press.

Myers GC, Lamb VL, and Agree EM (2003) Patterns of disability change associated with the epidemiologic transition. In: Robine J-M, Jagger C, Mathers CD, Crimmins EM and Suzman RM (eds.) *Determining Health Expectancies,* pp. 59–74. West Sussex, UK: John Wiley & Sons Ltd.

National Center for Health Statistics (1996) *Vital Statistics of the United States, 1991, Vol. II, Mortality Part A.* Washington, DC: Public Health Service.

Olshansky SJ and Ault AB (1986) The fourth stage of the epidemiological transition: The age of delayed degenerative diseases. *Milbank Memorial Fund Quarterly* 64: 355–391.

Omran AR (1971) The epidemiologic transition: A theory of the epidemiology of population change. *Milbank Memorial Fund Quarterly* 49: 509–538.

United Nations (2002) *World population ageing: 1950–2050.* New York: United Nations. http://www.un.org/esa/population/publications/worldageing19502050/ (accessed October 2007).

Further Reading

Hanuschek EA and Maritato NL (eds.) (1996) *Assessing Knowledge of Retirement Behavior.* Washington, DC: National Academy Press.

Kinsella K and Phillips DR (2005) Global aging: The challenge of success. *Population Bulletin* 60: 1–40.

Martin LG and Preston SH (eds.) (1994) *Demography of Aging.* Washington, DC: National Academy Press.

Martin LG and Soldo BJ (eds.) (1997) *Racial and Ethnic Differences in the Health of Older Americans.* Washington, DC: National Academy Press.

National Research Council (2001) *Preparing for an Aging World: The Case for Cross-National Research.* Washington, DC: National Academy Press.

National Research Council (2004) *Understanding Racial and Ethnic Differences in Health in Late Life.* Washington, DC: National Academy Press.

Robine J-M, Jagger C, Mathers CD, Crimmins EM and Suzman RM (eds.) (2003) *Determining Health Expectancies.* West Sussex, UK: John Wiley & Sons Ltd.

Wachter KW and Finch CE (eds.) (1997) *Between Zeus and the Salmon: The Biodemography of Longevity.* Washington, DC: National Academy Press.

Longevity in Specific Populations

T T Samaras, Reventropy Associates, San Diego, CA, USA

Introduction

Human longevity can be defined in three ways. The first and most common approach is average life expectancy for a particular age; the second is age-specific all-cause mortality rate (deaths/100 000 people/year), which is the inverse of longevity. A third but unconventional definition deals with the percentage of centenarians in a population, which indirectly reflects the longevity of the adult population. Note that the maximum life span (MLS) of humans appears to be fixed at approximately 120 years. Unlike life expectancy, which has increased substantially since ancient Rome, MLS has not changed over thousands of years. The following material reviews the longevity of various populations.

Factors Affecting Longevity

It is well established that environment is a key factor affecting the longevity of individuals and entire populations. This includes socioeconomic status (SES), the quality of medical care, educational facilities, and exposure to various diseases. Nutrition also has a critical role because malnutrition can cause susceptibility to infections and premature death (Samaras, 2006, 2007). While many populations suffer from food deprivation, many developing and developed populations experience excessive food intake, and obesity is now a worldwide health problem leading to reduced longevity (Elrick et al., 2002). In view of the increasing weight trend, the body mass index (BMI) has become an important guideline for predicting mortality and longevity. Generally, a BMI (weight/height^2) of 19 to 23 kg/m^2 with good nutrition predicts greater longevity.

Other factors that affect longevity are heredity; stress levels; traumatic events; regular physical activity; toxins in the environment, food, and water; and exposure to disease-producing bacteria, viruses, and parasites. Although climate may play a role in longevity, long-living people are found in semitropical, cold, and temperate climates. The same is true for sea level and mountainous elevations. However, longevity appears to favor relatively small populations, such as Andorra (~80 000) and Sweden (~9 million) as shown in **Table 1**.

Worldwide Variations in Life Expectancy

Life expectancy is the average age at death for a particular population group. Note that life expectancies are also determined for each age group, usually in 10-year increments.

Life expectancies are available for 225 populations ranging from China to the tiny sovereign states of Andorra and San Marino. As shown in **Table 1**, life expectancies at birth for males and females combined range from 33.23 years for Swaziland to 83.52 years for Andorra (Central Intelligence Agency, 2007).

Consistent with findings that a good environment and SES promote longevity, most of the longest living populations are found in highly developed populations with superior sanitation, education, and health care. The worst life expectancies are found in Africa with its lower economic development and very high rate of mortality from HIV/AIDS infection. The top ten populations in terms of descending life expectancy (83.52 to 80.59 years) are Andorra, Macao, Japan, Singapore, San Marino, Hong Kong, Sweden, Australia, Switzerland, and France. (Rankings shift from year to year but most of these states stay in the top ten or close to it.)

The low life expectancy of developing populations does not mean that elderly people are absent from developing populations. Since poor countries tend to have much higher infant death rates, this situation lowers the average life expectancy. In addition, early deaths of

Table 1 Life expectancies for various populations (estimated 2007)

Rank	Population (both sexes)	Life expectancy at birth in years
1	Andorra	83.52
2	Macao	82.27
3	Japan	82.02
4	Singapore	81.80
4	San Marino	81.80
6	Hong Kong	81.68
7	Sweden	80.63
8	Australia	80.62
8	Switzerland	80.62
10	France	80.59
12	Iceland	80.43
20	Norway	79.67
28	Netherlands	79.11
32	Germany	78.95
47	Denmark	77.96
103	China	72.88
145	India	64.59
184	Kenya	55.31
222	Swaziland	33.23

children and young adults due to malnutrition, trauma, and infections reduce the average life expectancy. However, if early death is avoided, adults often reach advanced ages (Walker, 1974; Samaras, 2007).

A common misconception in comparing today's life expectancy to that of earlier times, such as the 1900s, is the belief that individuals can expect to live 25–30 years longer. However, if we look at the life expectancy of elderly people, the picture is quite different; e.g., 60-year-old white males lived 6.6 years longer in 2004 vs 1900, and 80-year-olds lived 3 years longer.

Gender and Life Expectancy

Females commonly have greater longevity compared to men throughout their lives. Exceptions exist, such as in Martinique and Afghanistan. However, there is a substantial difference of less than 2 to more than 10 years in longevity between the sexes, depending on the populations involved. Generally, the greatest differences are found in developed populations. Several reasons for gender differences in longevity have been proposed, such as hormonal protection, more robust physiology, better health-care habits, and lower rates of high-risk activities. These factors no doubt have an impact, but animal and human research indicates that differences in body size may play a major role (Samaras, et al., 2002; Samaras, 2007). For example, one study reported that the average height for males in 21 European nations was 7.7% taller than females, and males had an 8.0% lower life expectancy (Samaras et al., 2003a). Another study by Miller, based on about 1700 men and women in Ohio, found that when men and women of the same height were compared, there was essentially no difference in average life span (Samaras, 1996). Rollo also found that when he compared male and female mice of the same body weight, the usual difference in average life span disappeared (Samaras, 2007). Brown-Borg and Bartke also reported that dwarf male mice lived substantially longer than normal-size female siblings (Samaras, 2007).

Centenarians

Centenarians are another population of interest. Gerontologists have studied people who live to be 100 or more years in an attempt to define the qualities or conditions that characterize centenarians as a special population. They have identified a variety of positive attributes, such as not smoking, small body size, diet, regular exercise, avoidance of stress, good environment, family connectedness, avoidance of worry, and a positive attitude toward life.

The greatest concentration of centenarians has been found in Okinawa, Japan, with 340–400/million, Bulgaria with 199/million, and Sardinia with 136/million. The Okinawans have been studied for many years and

researchers have attributed their longevity to good nutrition and low caloric intake. Okinawan children in the recent past consumed about 40% fewer calories than children in mainland Japan (Samaras, 1996). Other factors were a simple life and life-long physical activity.

It should be noted that centenarians tend to be relatively short and light. This could be an artifact due to the trend toward greater height and body size during the last 150–200 years. In addition, people tend to shrink with age due to postural changes and compression of the discs in the spine, although shorter people shrink less than taller ones. However, the Okinawan male and female centenarians are quite short, averaging 148.3 cm and 138.6 cm respectively. After accounting for shrinkage and secular growth, these are still small people; for example, males equal to or exceeding 100 years were over 10 cm shorter than elderly men averaging 73 years of age (Chan et al., 1997). In addition, Paolisso et al. (1995) found Italian male centenarians averaged 162 cm and were 15 cm shorter than elderly men averaging 77.6 years. Note that shorter female centenarians normally outnumber taller males by a factor of three or four.

Longevity and Body Height

If we look at the countries with the greatest life expectancies, developed countries lead the world. Based on this fact, it would appear that the tallest and heaviest (and sometimes the fattest) populations in the world live the longest. However, a number of factors contradict this hypothesis. In fact, if the top six populations in terms of life expectancy are examined for height, it appears that most of them are relatively short. For example, the populations of Andorra (mostly Catalans and Spaniards), Macao (mostly Chinese), San Marino (similar to Italians), Singapore (mostly Chinese), Hong Kong (mostly Chinese), and Japan are shorter than the populations of northern Europe. In contrast, although Sweden ranks 7th from the top, other equally tall populations, such as Iceland, Norway, the Netherlands, Germany, and Denmark, average 29th from the top ranking (vs 3.3 for the top six populations). Note that the Dutch are the tallest people in the world and rank 28th in longevity.

The negative impact of excess weight on longevity is widely accepted in the medical community (Samaras, 2006, 2007). However, the role of height is controversial, and the following material will highlight conflicting findings on longevity based on height differences among several populations.

Studies Showing Taller People Have Greater Longevity

A review of life expectancy data shows that the tallest countries (and most developed) have on average the greatest longevity. Although not as great as the six top-ranking populations, Western and southern Europe, Australia, Canada, New Zealand, the UK, and the United States have substantially longer life expectancies compared to shorter nations in the Middle East, most of Asia, South America, and Africa. Approximately 40 studies found taller people have lower all-cause or cardiovascular disease mortality (CVD) (Samaras et al., 2003a). Since CVD is a major factor in reducing longevity, it indirectly supports the hypothesis that taller people live longer.

Waaler (1983) conducted a study of 176 574 deceased Norwegians and found that taller people had about a 15% lower mortality compared to shorter ones. However, at advanced ages, tall males experienced higher mortality. This study did not adjust findings for smoking, birth defects, accelerated growth, childhood illness, or SES. However, a more recent study from South Korea evaluated 386 627 middle-aged males and found all-cause mortality dropped 6% for a 10 cm increase in height when adjusted for SES and other factors (Song et al., 2003). However, no height trend was found for coronary heart disease (CHD).

Studies Showing Shorter People Have Greater Longevity

Data supporting the greater longevity of shorter people is at least as impressive as the findings showing taller people live longer. For example, a California study involved 1 million deaths of various ethnic groups and found tall people have over 100% higher all-cause mortality compared to short people, i.e., whites and blacks had over twice the all-cause mortality of the Chinese and Japanese. Latinos and South Asians, who were slightly taller than the Chinese, had similar mortality rates (Samaras, 2007). A similar pattern was found for CHD.

Another study involving 1.3 million Spanish military recruits tracked them for 70 years into their 80s and 90s and found a strong negative correlation ($r = -0.58$) between height and survival age (Samaras, 2007). The findings were based on measured conscription heights and deaths from national census data.

Insurance studies involving 4.5 million men and women reported that all-cause mortality increased with increasing height for middle-aged women and men (~30% for the tallest men) (Samaras et al., 2003a). In addition, several longevity studies of athletes in Finland and the United States revealed that shorter athletes lived longer than taller ones. The loss of life with increasing height averaged about 0.52 year/cm (Samaras, 2007).

Shorter people throughout the world have been found to have superior longevity or reduced chronic disease. These findings are summarized in **Figure 1**. Note that the lower left hand rectangle only lists four sample populations for low CHD. Many others exist, including Solomon Islanders, Congo Pygmies, Vietnamese, Papua New Guinea inhabitants, the Chinese and the Japanese.

Based on a review of 300 studies by Gunnell et al., shorter people also have lower cancer mortality (Samaras, 2007).

Potential Confounders in Height Studies

There are a number of explanations for the conflicts between studies showing positive or negative relations between longevity and body height. As mentioned before, longevity is a function of many factors and conditions, and height is only one factor, probably representing roughly 10–20% of the total impact. For example, SES for all major phases of life has an important bearing on longevity independent of height. In addition, since people in higher SES are generally taller, the benefits due to SES can offset the negative effects of increased body height. Another confounder is BMI because taller people tend to have higher BMIs when of similar proportions as shorter people (Samaras, 2007). However, most epidemiological studies use the same BMI to evaluate the mortality of tall and short people. This process results in comparing taller, leaner people against shorter, stockier people. Since leaner people tend to have a lower mortality, this bias can favor taller people (Samaras, 2007).

Other confounders involve prenatal and postnatal care and early growth patterns. In recent years, it has been found that catch up or accelerated growth in height and weight promotes obesity and chronic disease in adulthood (Samaras et al., 2003b; Samaras, 2007). Since low-birth-weight children generally become shorter adults compared to their normal-weight peers, their increased mortality is interpreted to result from their shorter height or lower SES rather than to accelerated growth and related health problems caused by excess weight (Samaras, 2007). Another potential problem is congenital or early childhood illness that results in shorter adult height and poorer health.

Animal Findings

There is strong evidence that larger animal species live longer than small ones. The obvious example includes a comparison between a mouse and an elephant. This advantage is mainly due to lower metabolic rate and evolutionary changes that resulted in greater cell replication potential and improved free radical defenses and DNA repair mechanisms. However, since the 1930s, robust findings indicate that within a species, smaller size promotes greater longevity. Rollo (Samaras, 1996, 2007) evaluated hundreds of longevity studies involving mice and rats and found a highly significant and substantial inverse relationship between body size and longevity. In addition, Miller and Austad (2006) reported that small dogs had greater longevity than medium and large ones. The most recent study on dogs found that there was a substantial

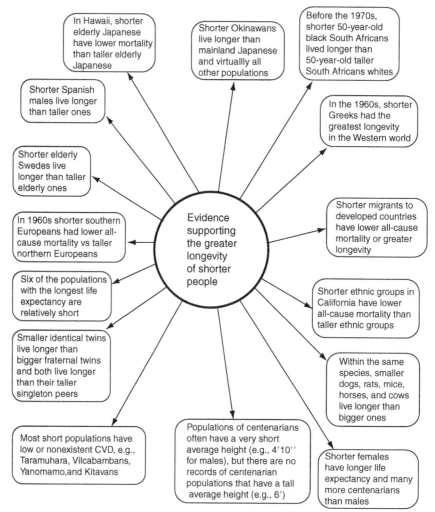

Figure 1 Partial summary of evidence supporting greater longevity of shorter, lighter people.

negative correlation between height and survival (Greer et al., 2007). For a wide height range of 15–94 cm, they found $r = -0.603$, $p < 0.05$. For a weight range of 0.9–89 kg, $r = -0.679$, $p < 0.05$.

Biological Factors and Mechanisms That Affect Longevity

If tallness is a real advantage for promoting longevity, what are the mechanisms that promote this feature? Certainly, recent human history shows a relation between improved education and economic status and increased height. However, this condition is environmentally driven rather than related to biological factors, although biological factors favoring taller height include lower heart and resting metabolic rates. Another beneficial factor is avoiding low birth weight (<2500 g). Since taller

people are less likely to have been low-birth-weight infants, this reflects better maternal nutrition and SES as long as birth weight does not exceed 4000 g (macrosomic). In contrast to taller people, shorter people have a larger number of biological advantages if their proportions and life-long SES are the same as taller people (see **Table 2**).

Conclusion

The preceding findings indicate that when tall people remain thin and experience the benefits of high SES, they can attain improved longevity compared to shorter people in disadvantaged populations. However, it appears that shorter, lighter bodies within the framework of positive environments and good nutrition have a number of inherent biological advantages.

Since height has a moderate impact on longevity, short and tall people can benefit from following

Table 2 Summary of biological mechanisms that may increase the longevity of shorter people

Biological factor	Description
Larger organs in proportion to body weight	Except for the heart and lungs, shorter people have relatively larger organs, which provide greater functional capacity. In addition, maximum oxygen uptake per kilogram is substantially higher
Greater cell duplication potential	Greater cell proliferation potential because fewer cell doublings are needed to attain adult height and weight. (A tall person may have 100 trillion cells compared to 60 trillion for a short person.) Note that many cells cannot reproduce after 50–100 replications according to the Hayflick limit
Lower need for cell replication	Lower demands for lifetime replacement of defective cells due to fewer cells in the body
Lower DNA damage	Much lower DNA damage, e.g., one study found an 85% higher rate of DNA damage in people who were 18% taller (Samaras, 2007: chapter 7).
Reduced toxin exposure	Lower food and water needs reduce exposure to toxins, parasites, bacteria, and viruses
Lower CVD risk	Lower blood pressure and lower left ventricular mass or hypertrophy reduce risk of CVD. Lower rates of atrial fibrillation. (However, shorter people in developed countries have more strokes)
Lower cancer risk	Lower risk of cancer due to fewer body cells and lower surface area (Samaras and Elrick, 2005)
Lower insulin and glucose levels	Lower insulin, insulin-like growth factor-1, and glucose levels increase longevity (chapters 6–8, Samaras, 2007)
Lower risk of obesity	In general, taller people were heavier babies and heavier infants tend to have increased risk of obesity (Samaras and Elrick, 2005: chapter 7; Samaras, 2006)
Lower risk of injury or death	Lower risk of hip fractures and injury or death in motor car accidents (Samaras, 2007: chapter 4)

well-established health practices. These include (1) maintenance of low BMIs (19–23), (2) consumption of diets high in vegetables, whole grains, and fruits and low in saturated fat, trans fats, and salt, (3) regular exercise, (4) adequate sleep, (5) avoiding exposure to harmful bacteria, viruses, and toxins, (6) management of stress, (7) maintenance of social networks, and (8) total avoidance of smoking and limited use of alcohol (Samaras, 2006, 2007).

See also: Active Life Expectancy; Demography of Aging.

Citations

Central Intelligence Agency (2007) World Factbook. http://www.cia.gov/library/publications/the-world-factbook (accessed October 2007).

Chan Y-C, Suzuki M, and Yamamoto S (1997) Dietary, anthropometric, hematological and biochemical assessment of the nutritional status of centenarians and elderly people in Okinawa, Japan. *Journal of American College of Nutrition* 16: 229–235.

Elrick H, Samaras TT, and Demas A (2002) Missing links in the obesity epidemic. *Nutrition Research* 22: 1101–1123.

Greer KA, Canterberry SC, and Murphy KE (2007) Statistical analysis regarding the effects of height and weight on life span of the domestic dog. *Research in Veterinary Science* 82: 208–214.

Miller RA and Austad SN (2006) Growth and aging: Why do big dogs die young? In: Masoro EJ and Austad SN (eds.) *Handbook of the Biology of Aging*, 6th edn., pp. 512–529. Burlington, MA: Academic Press.

Paolisso G, Gambardella A, Balbi V, Ammendola S, and D'Amore A (1995) Body composition, body fat distribution, and resting metabolic rate in healthy centenarians. *American Journal of Clinical Nutrition* 62: 746–750.

Samaras TT (1996) How body height and weight affect our performance, longevity and survival. *Journal of the Washington Academy of Sciences* 84: 131–156.

Samaras TT (2006) Nutrition, obesity, growth and longevity. In: Starks TP (ed.) *Trends in Nutrition Research*, pp. 1–40. New York: Nova Science Publishers.

Samaras T (ed.) (2007) Chapters 2, 5, 7–9. In: *Human Body Size and the Laws of Scaling. Physiological, Performance, Growth, Longevity and Ecological Ramifications.* New York: Nova Science Publishers.

Samaras T and Elrick H (2005) An alternative hypothesis to the obesity epidemic: Obesity is due to increased maternal size, birth size, growth rate, and height. *Medical Hypotheses* 65: 676–682.

Samaras TT, Storms LH, and Elrick H (2002) Longevity, mortality and body weight. *Ageing Research Reviews* 1: 673–691.

Samaras TT, Elrick H, and Storms LH (2003a) Is height related to longevity? *Life Sciences* 72: 1781–1802.

Samaras TT, Elrick H, and Storms LH (2003b) Birthweight, rapid growth, cancer, and longevity: A review. *Journal of the National Medical Association* 95: 1170–1183.

Song Y-M, Davey Smith G, and Sung J (2003) Adult height and cause-specific mortality: A large prospective study of South Korean men. *American Journal of Epidemiology* 158: 479–485.

Walker ARP (1974) Survival rate at middle age in developing and Western populations. *Postgraduate Medical Journal* 50: 29–32.

Waaler HT (1983) Height, weight and mortality – the Norwegian experience. *Acta Medica Scandinavica Supplement* 679: 1–51.

Further Reading

Samaras TT, Elrick H, and Storms LH (2004) Is short height really a risk factor for coronary heart disease and stroke mortality? A review. *Medical Science Monitor* 10: RA63–76.

Relevant Websites

http://www.okicent.org/cent.html – Centenarians.
http://www.ssc.wisc.edu/cdha/ – Center for Demographics of Health and Aging.
http://www.geri.duke.edu/china_study/ – Chinese Longitudinal Healthy Longevity Survey (CLHLS).
http://www.un.org/NewLinks/older/99/older.htm – Demographics of Older Persons.

http://longevity2.stanford.edu/GlobalAging.html – Global Aging Program-Stanford Center on Longevity.
http://www.shortsupport.org/Research/samaras.html – Longevity of Short and Tall People.
http://longevity-science.org/ – Longevity Research.
https://www.cia.gov/library/publications/the-world-factbook/rankorder/2102rank.html – World Life Expectancy Ranking.

Populations at Special Health Risk: Migrants

O Razum, University of Bielefeld, Bielefeld, Germany
F Samkange-Zeeb, Institute of Medical Biometry, Epidemiology and Informatics, Mainz, Germany

Definition of Migrants, Demography, and Types of Migration

Definition of Migrant

Migrants are individuals who move from one country or place of residence to settle in another. The move can be either across an international border or within a state, and it can be temporary or permanent. People migrate for economic reasons or to join their relatives; others are refugees, displaced persons, or uprooted people. Voluntary migrants are those who have made their own decision to migrate; the decision could, however, have been brought about due to economic or other pressures. Forced migrants are people who have to move because of external factors such as individual persecution, general conflict, or natural disasters (Braunschweig and Carballo, 2001; IOM, 2005). Any such classification remains theoretical, however. Often, push-and-pull effects are at work simultaneously; whether the migration is permanent may only be decided in the future, or the decision may be revised. **Table 1** provides an overview of population groups covered by the term migrant.

For health reporting and epidemiological purposes, foreign-born persons or holders of foreign passports are categorized as migrants. This underestimates the profound heterogeneity of foreign-born populations: they may be migrant workers, refugees, asylum seekers, or students. Their history and legal status, in turn, affects health determinants and outcomes. The offspring of immigrants may face similar problems but often do not appear in routine migration statistics because they are not foreign-born. Different regulations make comparisons of the health status of migrants between neighboring countries difficult.

Number of Migrants Globally and Sex Distribution

The number of international migrants worldwide has been increasing steadily over the last decades and is expected to continue doing so. In 1960, there were 76 million international migrants globally (IOM, 2005). By 2000, this number had reached an estimated 175 million, meaning that 1 out of every 35 persons in the world was an international migrant (**Table 2**). The total number was predicted to rise up to between 185 and 192 million by early 2005 and to reach 230 million by 2050 (IOM, 2005).

The proportion of women migrants went up from 47% in 1970 to 49% in 2000, and is higher in developed than in developing regions (**Table 2**). It is usually easier for men than for women to migrate legally: Efforts to recruit labor

Table 1   Population groups covered by the term migrant

Voluntary migrants
Labor migrants
Temporary contract workers
Foreign students
Family reunification
Spouses from country of origin
Migrants returning to county of origin (permanent; 'pendulum migration')
Ethnic or religious groups (e.g., ethnic German 'Aussiedler' from former Soviet Union states to Germany; Jews to Israel)
Undocumented ('irregular') migrants
Forced migrants
Refugees, asylum seekers
Internally displaced persons (not always counted as refugees/migrants)
Environmental migrants
Trafficked persons

Table 2   Numbers of international migrants in the world and by major region, including proportion of females among the international migrants, 1970 to 2000

Major region	Number of international migrants (in millions)				Percentage of females	
	1970	1980	1990	2000	1970	2000
World	81.5	99.8	154.0	174.9	47.2	48.6
Africa	9.9	14.1	16.2	16.3	42.7	46.7
Asia[a]	28.1	32.3	41.8	43.8	46.6	43.3
Latin America and the Caribbean	5.8	6.1	7.0	5.9	46.8	50.2
Northern America	13.0	18.1	27.6	40.8	51.1	50.3
Oceania	3.0	3.8	4.8	5.8	46.5	50.5
Europe[b]	18.7	22.2	26.3	32.8	48.0	51.0
Former USSR	3.1	3.3	30.3	29.5	48.0	52.1

[a]Excluding Armenia, Azerbaijan, Georgia, Kazakhstan, Kyrgyzstan, Tajikistan, Turkmenistan, and Uzbekistan.
[b]Excluding Belarus, Estonia, Latvia, the Republic of Moldova, the Russian Federation, and Ukraine.
Source: UN Trends in Total Migrant Stock: The 2003 Revision, In: IOM 2005.

frequently focus on employment in construction and agriculture, which tends to be male-dominated.

Changing Motives for Migration

People have been moving from one place to another, internally and across borders, throughout human history. Contemporary movement, however, differs significantly from that of past times. Continued economic disparities within nations – between rural and urban areas, regions or states, and among nations – have always played an important role in furthering internal and international migration. Today's migration patterns and the environment in which people migrate are defined by economic and humanitarian crises. In addition, modern communication and transportation, as well as the opening up of borders between countries and regions, have made it possible for people to travel farther, faster, and more easily than ever before. Migration has become a global issue, with all states of the world now functioning as either points of origin, transit, or destination, and, at times, all three at once (UNFPA/IMP, 2004; IOM, 2005). In 2000, the United States was the country with the largest number of international migrants with 35 million people, equivalent to 20% of world migrant stock. Regionally, Asia (excluding Armenia, Azerbaijan, Georgia, Kazakhstan, Kyrgyzstan, Tajikistan, Turkmenistan, and Uzbekistan) had the largest number: 43.8 million, or 25% of world migrant stock (IOM, 2005).

Traditional countries of immigration such as Australia, Canada, and the United States continue to be attractive destinations for international migrant workers. However, recently there have been significant shifts in labor migration. In the 1980s, for example, economic development in Japan and in East and Southeast Asia offered alternative destinations for migrant workers from economically less well-off countries in the region (IOM, 2005). In sub-Saharan Africa, the political liberalization of the Republic of South Africa in the 1990s and the continued deterioration in the economies of many neighboring countries led to a marked increase in migrant flows from the region into that country (Gushulak and MacPherson, 2004).

Internal migration, although often voluntary or economically based, can also be involuntary due to environmental degradation, natural disaster, human rights abuse, or political upheaval and armed conflict. Currently, 25 million persons in more than 50 countries are internally displaced due to conflict. While they remain within the borders of their own country, they are often without access to basic services such as health care and education, and beyond the reach of international aid organizations (UNFPA/IMP, 2004).

Migration: A Challenge to Individuals and Societies

Migration offers opportunities and is associated with risks – for individual migrants and their families, for the societies from which migrants originate, and for the receiving countries. Many countries are not well prepared and lack policies needed to make migration a healthy and socially productive process. This has public health implications for the people who move, for the families they have left behind, and for the communities they come in contact with during transition or in the host countries (Carballo and Nerukar, 2001).

Migration and Health

Under normal circumstances migration in itself should not pose a risk to health. However, the conditions surrounding the migration process can increase vulnerability for ill health. Some of the health risks are related to the conditions before departure, to travel conditions, and to the arrival or transit stage. The reasons why the movement is taking place – whether the individual can control them or not (voluntary or forced migration), the mode of movement, as well as the regulations and level of acceptance in the receiving country – all play a role in determining the health of migrants (Braunschweig and Carballo, 2001; IOM, 2004). These factors are examined later.

Exposures in Country of Origin

Persons fleeing persecution, leaving areas with high disease prevalence or limited access to health care, are likely to have different health profiles from those voluntarily emigrating from countries where health services are optimal and disease prevalence is low. A considerable number of migrants come from developing countries where infectious diseases such as tuberculosis (TB) and HIV/AIDS contribute significantly to morbidity. Persons originating from such a country and migrating to a developed country have, at the time of arrival, a higher risk of suffering from these diseases than persons of the same age in the general population of the country of destination (Cookson *et al.*, 1998; Carballo and Nerukar, 2001; Razum and Twardella, 2002; Gushulak and MacPherson, 2004; IOM, 2004). The problem is compounded by poor living conditions and the barriers to accessing preventive and curative health care that migrants often face (see following section titled 'Access to health services').

Between 1995 and 2000, the incidence of TB cases in Denmark increased steadily and the proportion of foreign-born persons among all cases rose from 18% in 1986 to 60% in 1996. Approximately 40% of all TB infections in England and Wales are occurring in immigrants from the Indian subcontinent. The incidence of TB in the Netherlands rose by 45% between 1987 and 1995, with more than half of the new cases being reported among immigrants. In Germany and France, migrants are three to six times more likely to be diagnosed with TB than nonmigrants. The risk of HIV/AIDS among migrants in many EU countries reflects the global epidemiologic pattern of the disease. For example, migrants of African origin residing in Sweden have a higher HIV/AIDS incidence than Swedish nationals. A similar pattern can be observed in Germany, where the number of HIV-infected persons among migrants is rising (Carballo and Nerukar, 2001; Robert Koch-Institut, 2005a, 2005b).

Exposures in the country of origin can also be to the benefit of migrants. Lifestyle factors such as diet, tobacco, and alcohol consumption are often more favorable for health in developing than in developed countries. With regard to smoking, the proportion of smokers in lower-income countries might be higher, but the amount consumed per person will often be substantially lower than in the high-income countries. Besides lung cancer, the incidence of breast cancer and colon cancer also tends to be lower. Studies show that migrants 'take along' their low risk for some chronic diseases and keep this advantage for many years, depending on the adopted lifestyle in the host country and the lag time of the disease in question. The risk of diseases, such as stomach cancer and stroke that are associated with poor hygienic and living conditions in childhood, tends to be higher, however (Razum and Twardella, 2002).

Patterns of Mobility (Regular Versus Irregular)

Movement as such can constitute a considerable and immediate health risk if it involves fleeing, forceful displacement, or illegal crossing of borders. Planned migration, in which the necessary travel documents have been organized beforehand and entry requirements are met, will be safer than a journey taken clandestinely or under duress.

Health risks of irregular migration

In June 2000, an attempt by 54 Chinese would-be immigrants to enter the United Kingdom in a sealed truck designed to carry fruit ended in their death by suffocation. Thousands of people are taking similar risks on a daily basis, with many of them losing their lives in the process. The death toll at sea among Africans and Albanians trying to enter Europe through Spain and Italy, respectively, is giving rise to international concern (Carballo and Nerukar, 2001).

The International Organization for Migration (IOM) reports that the number of irregular migrants is increasing. Precise figures are not available, but IOM estimates that one-third to one-half of migrants to developed countries travel without documents or with false ones, which is said to constitute an increase of 20% over the past 10 years (UNFPA/IMP, 2004). Correspondingly, the number of migrants in an irregular situation (which includes persons who enter legally but whose legal status has expired) within a country is difficult to estimate. Irregular migration does not necessarily involve traffickers; however, trafficking and smuggling of humans have become major criminal enterprises, often involving exploitation and abuse. Women and children are more vulnerable than men (Carballo and Nerukar, 2001; UNFPA/IMP, 2004).

Healthy Migrant Effect

It has frequently been observed that migrants have a lower mortality (and occasionally also morbidity) compared to the majority population of the host country, in spite of being socioeconomically disadvantaged. This phenomenon is known as 'healthy migrant effect.' Attempts to explain it have focused on a selection or self-selection of particularly healthy individuals into migration and on the differentials in risk of chronic diseases (e.g., cardiovascular disease) between populations. Hence, people migrating from countries with low mortality from coronary heart disease (CHD) to countries with high cardiovascular disease (CVD) mortality, initially experience a mortality advantage. Examples for such a scenario are the migration from southern to northern Europe and from Latin American countries to the United States. Due to the long lag periods in chronic disease, such mortality advantages may persist for years or even decades after migration (see following paragraph). Ultimately, as was shown in the Nihosan study of Japanese men migrating to Hawaii and San Francisco, mortality rates converge with those of the majority population. There is considerable evidence that initially advantageous cause-specific mortality rates of immigrants may turn into a mortality disadvantage when socioeconomic conditions are unfavorable and access to health care is difficult.

Exposures in Country of Immigration

By migrating to industrialized countries, migrants from lower-income countries benefit from environmental and public health measures that prevent the epidemic spread of infectious diseases, and from better access to biomedical care that provide a cure for many conditions (Razum and Twardella, 2002; Razum and Geiger, 2003). Changes in lifestyle (diet, tobacco, alcohol) can quickly lead to unfavorable changes in risk factor profiles for cardiovascular disease, lung and colon cancer, and other noncommunicable diseases. Due to long lag periods, disease and death rates may show appreciable increases only after decades of exposure. This potentially positive situation becomes problematic when public health policies of the host countries only target the general population but elude migrants.

Migrants are exposed to an excess risk of contracting infectious diseases even in high-income countries. For example, many migrant workers travel without their spouses or partners and might resort to unsafe sexual practices, thereby risking the contraction of sexually transmitted diseases (STDs). In Belgium and Sweden, the number of STD cases among foreign-born men is higher than that of men born in the two countries (Carballo and Nerukar, 2001).

Social Class

Social class is a strong determining factor for health. Migrants, upon the time of arrival, frequently become part of the lower social stratum of the host country. They then are exposed to similar risk factors, and face similar health risks, as the lower social class within the general population, such as a high smoking prevalence and poor working as well as housing conditions.

Housing can both determine the health of people, as well as indicate the quality of life they enjoy and are allowed to enjoy. Many migrants arrive with little money and usually have temporary official status that does not allow them to 'invest' in good-quality housing. Often this is further reinforced by social barriers. Newcomers from abroad (or rural areas in the case of rural to urban migration) tend to move to low-income areas of towns and cities where they are exposed to crowding, substandard housing, and poor sanitation (WHO, 2003). The situation is more problematic for seasonal workers.

In an agricultural site in southern Spain, 85% of the workers were living in crowded temporary structures. These were situated in close proximity to greenhouses and warehouses where pesticides were used and stored. In Portugal, more than three-quarters of migrant shantytowns had no running water, toilet facilities, electricity, or refuse collection (Braunschweig and Carballo, 2001).

Exposure to poor housing, hazardous working conditions and social disruption is also common among migrant workers in various parts of Africa (WHO, 2003). In many industrialized countries, asylum seekers who formally lodge application for refugee status are confined in detention centers. These centers are generally overcrowded, increasing the risk of spread of infectious diseases.

Between October 2001 and October 2002, 56 cases of active TB, many with pulmonary involvement, were diagnosed among residents of an overcrowded migrants' shelter in Paris. The outbreak was the result of transmission that had occurred in France, as became evident from the clustering of the cases in time and place, the large number of cases with early-stage disease, and from typing of the isolates (Valin *et al.*, 2005).

Choosing to live in proximity of persons of the same ethnic ancestry can, however, also be one of the coping strategies used by migrants. By living close together, migrants of similar ethnic background can maximize social interaction and maintain group norms and values. Furthermore, a large size and concentration will help ensure the success of ethnic clubs, churches, language newspapers, and specialty stores (Balakrishnan and Maxim, 2005).

Being a migrant can affect the socioeconomic situation in ways different from those experienced by the host population. One example is de-skilling, or 'brain waste,' which relates to the considerable number of highly skilled migrants who work as unskilled labor. University graduates from Africa and Latin America often fail to find jobs in their fields of training after migration to industrialized countries;

doctors or engineers may end up earning a living as cleaners or taxi drivers. Doctors from the former Eastern Block countries face difficulties when seeking recognition of their medical qualifications in western European countries. In Sweden, the unemployment rate for migrants with a tertiary level education is twice as high as that of the native-born population with similar qualifications. De-skilling is assumed to lead to psychosocial and health problems (see following section titled 'Psychosocial problems particular to migrants').

Migration and Gender

Women are marginalized in many societies in respect to education, employment, goods and services, and basic human rights. By migrating to industrialized countries, they may improve their opportunities in personal, educational, and economic terms. However, women with a migration background have a higher probability of working in gender-segregated and unregulated sectors of the economy such as domestic work, entertainment, and sex industries. They are more exposed to forced labor and to sexual abuse by employers or by personnel and inhabitants of refugee camps than men or women of the majority population (UNFPA/IMP, 2004).

Migration can also be stressful and traumatic for women due to the loss of their established social setting and familiar surroundings. Their initial lack of education and occupational experience may limit their social integration in new settings. Moreover, second-generation immigrant girls and women may experience substantial pressure from their parents to conform to traditional values that may not be compatible with the lifestyle of their peers from the majority population. In the case of forced migration (see section 'Irregular Migration and Trafficking in Persons'), women are greatly disadvantaged. In complex emergencies such as war, the social cohesion characteristic of stable societies is disrupted and families are dispersed, increasing people's vulnerability, especially that of women (Carballo *et al.*, 1996; IOM, 2005).

Access to Health Services

In many countries, migrants have limited access to health services in comparison to the majority population. Health-care-seeking behavior is culturally determined, so migrants have to overcome cultural as well as language barriers. People coming from countries or regions of countries where services may have been lacking will have developed coping strategies that make them more fatalistic about disease, more tolerant of pain, and less likely to seek help when ill (Braunschweig and Carballo, 2001; Carballo and Nerukar, 2001). Language problems and lack of information regarding the location and structure of local health services often limit the capacity of

migrants to make optimal use of services. Many migrants cannot communicate with health providers effectively. Few countries routinely use interpreters in health-care facilities or provide multilingual information packs, which also include visual and audiovisual media (Razum and Geiger, 2003).

The different cultural understandings of health and concepts of disease make communication and interaction with migrants more difficult. Culture influences the interpretation and presentation of symptoms, as well as the treatment expected. In many cultures, illness is perceived as coming from 'outside.' Health care in industrialized countries, which is based on a biomedical paradigm, does not adequately respond to the migrants' perception. This can lead to misdiagnoses, inappropriate treatment, and poor compliance on the part of the patients (Braunschweig and Carballo, 2001; Razum and Geiger, 2003).

The legal status of migrants also determines their level of access to health and social services provided in the host country. Legal immigrants, permanent residents, and other long-term migrants often have the same access to health and social services as the local population. The access to health services for asylum seekers varies widely. Most countries provide medical screening to asylum seekers upon arrival, followed by limited access during the processing of their asylum claims. This might take months or years. Although the reasons for these restrictive policies vary, they share one underlying aim: to reduce health and welfare costs (IOM, 2005; Norredam *et al.*, 2005).

Psychosocial Problems Particular to Migrants

Even under the best of conditions, the process of migration often entails uprooting, and separation from family and familiar surroundings, as well as traditional values. Migrants find themselves in new social and cultural situations in which job and legal security may be minimal. Highly educated migrants often consider themselves to be overqualified for the jobs they hold (see the paragraph about de-skilling in the preceding section titled 'Social class'). For many, social integration is difficult. The loss of status and social support can lead to dissatisfaction and depression (Carballo and Nerukar, 2001; Razum and Geiger, 2003).

Persons fleeing war and victims of trafficking may experience posttraumatic stress; this may lead to heightened aggression and health-related problems. Their condition may be aggravated by overcrowding and poor living conditions in migrant detention centers and by the way they are treated. Detention is an additional stressor for asylum seekers that may worsen psychological symptoms. Often, there are no mechanisms to identify victims of torture or sexual abuse in need of specialist care (Braunschweig and Carballo, 2001; Steel and Silove, 2001).

Stigma and discrimination (overt and implicit) can lead to, or aggravate, psychosocial problems. Whereas stigma refers to perceiving certain population groups – for example, because of their ethnic origin – as inferior, discrimination describes the practical consequences of stigmatization in everyday life and in health care. Migrants face stigma and discrimination depending on their country of origin, their religion, and even more so when they are living with stigmatized diseases such as HIV/AIDS.

Working Conditions

Migration for employment is not always safe, and in some cases is not covered by regulations protecting migrant workers. Migrants frequently obtain jobs that are temporary, poorly paid, require low skills, and are therefore unattractive to local labor forces. Carballo and Nerukar (2001) report that the number of industrial accidents and injuries in construction and public works fields is higher among migrant workers than among citizens in many western European countries. Work-related risks are compounded by language barriers, poor communication, a lack of familiarity with the technology used, and by different attitudes to work safety. For example, it is not uncommon that migrant workers are insufficiently protected against exposure to pesticides and other chemical products. Long-term exposure to such products has been linked to depression, neurological disorders, and miscarriages (Carballo and Nerukar, 2001). These problems are compounded where migrant child labor is concerned. Hispanic children of migrant farm workers make up a considerable proportion of farm labor in the United States. These children face even higher risks of injury or death from accidents than their elders (IOM, 2005).

Irregular Migration and Trafficking in Persons

Irregular migration not only poses the highest risk to migrant health; it is also a public health concern in regard to communicable disease control, reproductive health, occupational and environmental health, and sanitation. Undocumented migrants often live in crowded, unsanitary conditions that add to their health risks. When ill, they may not be able to access health services for fear of being reported to immigration authorities and being deported. Providing preventive services for these populations is particularly challenging (Braunschweig and Carballo, 2001; WHO, 2003; Gushulak and MacPherson, 2004; IOM, 2005).

Trafficking, according to the UN General Assembly, is "the recruitment, transportation, transfer, harboring or receipt of persons, either by the threat or use of abduction, force, fraud, deception, coercion, or by the giving of unlawful payments or benefits to achieve the consent of a person having the control over another person for the purpose of exploitation" (UN General Assembly, 1999: 3). Health-related issues are among the most severe consequences of trafficking in persons. Trafficked persons often fall victim to various forms of sexual and physical abuse, which can have devastating and lasting effects on their mental, reproductive, and general physical health and well-being (IOM, 2005). The trafficking of children and adolescents for economical and sexual exploitation demands special attention (Tautz et al., 2006).

Migration and Reproductive Health

Changes in social and economic environment, differential access to health care, changes in sexual behavior and social status affect reproductive health, especially among women. Language or cultural barriers can lead to unfavorable health consequences, for example, during pregnancy. In several EU countries, migrants have a higher proportion of difficult pregnancies, and experience more pregnancy-related illnesses and complications, relative to local women (Razum et al., 1999; Carballo and Nerukar, 2001). In Sweden, for example, Ethiopian and Somali women have an increased perinatal morbidity compared to the general population, while in Denmark ethnic minority and migrant women underuse reproductive checkups (Ackerhans, 2003). In Spain, migrant women from sub-Saharan Africa and Central and South America have particularly high rates of premature births, low birth weight, and complications of delivery (Carballo and Nerukar, 2001).

Perinatal and neonatal mortality rates are frequently higher among immigrants than in the host population. In the UK, perinatal and postnatal mortality rates are higher among immigrants born in Pakistan and the Caribbean than in the general population; a similar gradient is visible among Turkish immigrants in Germany. In Belgium, Turkish immigrants experience perinatal and infant mortality rates that are 3.5 times as high as those of Belgian women (Carballo and Nerukar, 2001; Razum and Geiger, 2003). Conflicting values, as described in the previous section titled 'Migration and gender,' may limit access to contraceptives and to strategies for women to protect themselves against sexually transmitted diseases. A lack of adequate information on contraception, and on where to obtain appropriate advice, is common among immigrant women, in particular among those from the north and sub-Saharan African countries (Carballo and Nerukar, 2001).

Migration and Aging

Due to steady increases in migration and the temporal nature of work migration in many settings, migrant populations are often young in comparison to the host populations. Social and health services are often not prepared for elderly migrants who remain in the host country. Often, the migrants themselves are unprepared, because they had always planned to return to their country of origin. Elderly Turkish work migrants in western European countries, for example, increasingly decide not to return to Turkey where access to health care is more restricted, or where they cannot be close to their children who grew up in the host country and decided to stay there (Razum *et al.*, 2005).

Effects on Health-Care Systems

International migration poses challenges to health-care systems in various ways, both in countries of origin and in host countries of migrants. Developing countries are losing many of their better-educated nationals to richer countries (brain drain). For example, up to 75% of persons emigrating from Africa to the United States, Canada, or to OECD (Organisation of Economic Co-operation and Development) countries are assumed to have completed university-level or equivalent technical training/tertiary education (Saravia and Miranda, 2004). This brain drain includes trained health workers, thus affecting the health-care delivery in countries of origin. Host countries of migrants, however, have to adapt their health-care systems to the needs of heterogeneous minority populations.

Brain Drain in Health Care

Unsatisfactory working conditions, poor remunerations, a high risk of infection, lack of equipment, and lack of further education opportunities are some of the reasons why health-care workers such as physicians, nurses, dentists, and pharmacists leave their countries (Bach, 2003; Diallo, 2004; Saravia and Miranda, 2004; Stilwell *et al.*, 2004). The proportion of trained health workers that has migrated from individual developing countries is not usually known, as the characteristics of emigrants are rarely recorded. Vacancy levels in the health services can serve as a proxy indicator for the brain drain. A 1998 survey of several African countries showed widely varying vacancy levels for medical personnel in the public health sector. For example, a 7.6% vacancy level was reported for doctors in Lesotho compared to 72.9% for specialists in Ghana. Malawi had a vacancy level of 52.9% for nurses. The impact of migration of health-care workers on such countries, which generally have few health workers to start with and whose capacity for reinvestment in education is limited, can be devastating. The loss of health-care professionals almost inevitably leads to inadequate coverage and difficulties in meeting some of the population's health needs. In addition to having to continue working

under poor conditions, the health professionals who stay behind also experience higher workloads and additional stress. This might undermine their motivation to work in their current settings and lead to further migration (WHO, 2003; Stilwell *et al.*, 2004; UNFPA/IMP, 2004). To mitigate effects on the source countries, mechanisms have to be developed so that migration of health workers remains temporary, contributes to their further education, and leads to indirect development support through remittances (Bach, 2003; IOM, 2005).

Brain Gain in Health Care

Doctors and nurses in developed countries also complain of low salaries and poor working conditions in the public sector. More and more of them are joining the private sector or leaving their countries for better-paying jobs. To make up for the loss in manpower, the affected countries are turning to developing countries, mainly in Africa and Asia, for personnel. Examples of this brain gain are as follows: the UK loses about 8000 nurses every year through emigration to Australia, the United States, Canada, Ireland, and New Zealand, and recruits 15 000 from overseas. Without the sustained increase in overseas nurses employed, the United Kingdom would not have been able to reach its 2004 goal of increasing the nursing workforce by 20 000. And, as another example, at least 20% of physicians working in Australia, Canada, and the United States are supposedly from other countries, with a considerable proportion of them from developing countries (Diallo, 2004; Saravia and Miranda, 2004; Stilwell *et al.*, 2004). This phenomenon is not restricted to Europe and the United States: South Africa, which loses almost half of its newly qualified doctors to Canada, the United Kingdom, and Australia, attracts health personnel from poorer countries such as Kenya, Malawi, and Zimbabwe. Eighty percent of the doctors working in South Africa's rural areas come from these three countries (Diallo, 2004).

Challenges for Public Health in Countries of Immigration

Healthy migrants are more likely to be successful in education and employment, and to actively participate in society. Investing in migrant health thus aids their effective integration into communities and makes sense even when seen solely in economic terms (IOM, 2005). Successful integration calls for a comprehensive interpretation of migrant health, comprising not only infectious disease control, but also chronic noncommunicable conditions, mental health concerns, and human rights issues (Grondin, 2004). Providing appropriate services for a minority group such as migrants not only promotes understanding and cohesion in mixed societies; it can also serve as a model for making health systems more responsive to the diverse needs of all clients, irrespective of their nationality or geographic origin (thus employing 'diversity management'). Unfortunately, many politicians see the challenges that migrant health poses to health systems in terms of expenditure rather than investment, and cost rather than benefit.

Health systems, as well as migrant populations, are too diverse, and public health needs too contextual, to offer general advice. There are a number of issues, however, that are pertinent in many different settings. These include:

Health information needs. Reliable data on the health status, behavior, and health resources of migrants need to be collected, analyzed, and reported in a systematic way so that public health policy is based on sufficient information. A relevant practical problem is an appropriate definition of migration status in health statistics. However, information regarding such statistics is often restricted – for example, to nationality or country of birth – thus failing to identify second-generation immigrants.

Language. Health systems in many countries with migrant populations still lack interpreter services and visual aids to lower language barriers in communication. Seemingly 'pragmatic' solutions, such as asking relatives or menial hospital staff of the same origin to act as translators, are unacceptable, both in terms of privacy and of quality of information obtained.

Preventive interventions. Motivating migrants to take up preventive activities is often difficult. A frequent response consists of uncoordinated activities by various well-meaning, and often small, activist groups. Few of the interventions are evidence-based, and sustainability is doubtful after funding runs out. Whereas the importance of such activities should not be denied, networking among the groups is essential. Until interventions and ways of accessing migrant groups have been evaluated, 'best practice' models should be documented and used.

International collaboration. With respect to best practice models, public health scientists and practitioners should also look across national borders to share information and learn from other countries. Research involving countries of origin can help to elucidate reasons for differences in risk between migrants and the majority population, which may be due to such factors as socioeconomic disadvantages, cultural background, or genetic polymorphisms.

Traumatized migrants. The vast majority of health problems experienced by migrants is of the same kind as those of the majority population and can be treated by existing health services. An exception is torture victims, whose condition is often underdiagnosed among refugees and asylum seekers. Most of them require treatment in specialized centers.

In summary, today's decision makers and service providers worldwide are faced with the challenge "to plan and provide effective and accessible health services for communities with diverse languages, cultural backgrounds, migration circumstances and socio-economic status" (Grondin, 2004).

Conclusion

Migration will continue to increase, affecting literally all countries and populations worldwide. Given their minority status and the potential health disadvantages migrants are facing, public health and other sectors should be striving for policies to make migration a healthy and socially productive process. Intervention strategies should be conceptualized and developed within the framework of new public health – that is, they should not just consider migrants as a separate at-risk group, but address them in a systemic approach through which all population groups will benefit. The ultimate goal is the provision of adequate services to *all* persons, irrespective of their nationality or cultural background (diversity management). This requires changes not only in individual attitudes and in health systems, but also in immigration and integration policies. Yet, there is no room for 'unreflected actionism' – interventions should be based on evidence, or at least follow best practice models, and they should be systematically evaluated. Research on migrant health should be based on conceptual models, rather than be driven by the data available.

Citations

Ackerhans M (2003) Health issues of ethnic minority and migrant women: Coping with cultural barriers. *Entre Nous* 55: 9–11 Copenhagen, Denmark: WHO. http://www.euro.who.int/document/ens/en55.pdf (accessed August 2007).

Bach S (2003) *International migration of health workers: Labour and social issues, WP 209.* Geneva, Switzerland: International Labour Office (ILO). http://www.ilo.org/public/english/dialogue/sector/papers/health/wp209.pdf (accessed 2007).

Balakrishnan TR and Maxim P (2005) Residential segregation and socioeconomic integration of visible minorities in Canada. IUSSP Conference. Tours, France, 23 July 23, 2005.

Braunschweig S and Carballo M (2001) *Health and Human Rights of Migrants.* Geneva, Switzerland: International Centre for Migration and Health (ICMH). http://www.dhsantementale.net/cd/biblio/pdf/SM-DH_170.pdf (accessed August 2007).

Carballo M, Grocutt M, and Hadzihasanovic A (1996) Women and migration: A public health issue. *World Health Statistics Quarterly* 49(2): 158–164.

Carballo M and Nerukar A (2001) Migration, refugees, and health risks: Panel summary from the 2000 Emerging Infectious Diseases Conference in Atlanta, Georgia. *Emerging Infectious Diseases* 7(supplement 3): 556–560.

Cookson S, Waldman R, Gushulak B, *et al.* (1998) Immigrant and refugee health. *Emerging Infectious Diseases* 4(3): 427–428.

Diallo K (2004) Data on the migration of health-care workers: Sources, uses, and challenges. *Bulletin of the World Health Organization* 82(8): 601–607.

Grondin D (2004) Editorial: Well-managed migrants' health benefits all. *Bulletin of the World Health Organization* 82(8): 561.

Gushulak BD and MacPherson DW (2004) Globalization of infectious diseases: The impact of migration. *Clinical Infectious Diseases* 38(12): 1742–1748.

IOM (2004) Migration health report 2004. Geneva, Switzerland: International Organization for Migration (IOM). http://www.iom.int/jahia/Jahia/cache/bypass/pid/8?entryId=10142. (accessed August 2007).

IOM (2005) World migration 2005. Costs and benefits of international migration. Geneva, Switzerland: International Organization for Migration (IOM).http://www.iom.int/jahia/Jahia/cache/bypass/pid/8?entryId=932 (accessed August 2007).

Norredam M, Mygind A, and Krasnik A (2005) Access to health care for asylum seekers in the European Union – a comparative study of country policies. *European Journal of Public Health* 16(3): 285–289.

Razum O and Geiger I (2003) Migranten. In: Schwartz FW, Badura B, Busse R, et al. (eds.) *Das Public Health Buch – Gesundheit und Gesundheitswesen*, pp. 686–692. Munich, Germany: Urban and Fischer Verlag.

Razum O, Jahn A, Blettner M, and Reitmaier P (1999) Trends in maternal mortality ratio among women of German and non-German nationality in Germany, 1980 to 1996. *International Journal of Epidemiology* 28(5): 919–925.

Razum O and Twardella D (2002) Time travel with Oliver Twist – towards an explanation for a paradoxically low mortality among recent immigrants. *Tropical Medicine and International Health* 7(1): 4–10.

Razum O, Sahin-Hodoglugil N, and Polit K (2005) Health, wealth, or family ties? Why Turkish work migrants return from Germany. *Journal of Ethnic and Migration Studies* 31(4): 719–739.

Robert Koch-Institut (2005a) Bericht zur epidemiologie der tuberkulose in Deutschland für 2003. Berlin, Germany: Robert Koch-Institut (RKI).

Robert Koch-Institut (2005b) Epidemiologisches bulletin, Sonderausgaben A und B/2005. Berlin, Germany: Robert Koch-Institut (RKI).

Saravia NG and Miranda JF (2004) Plumbing the brain drain. *Bulletin of the World Health Organization* 82(8): 608–615.

Steel Z and Silove DM (2001) The mental health implications of detaining asylum seekers. *Medical Journal of Australia* 175(11–12): 596–599.

Stilwell B, Diallo K, Zurn P, Vujicic M, Adams O, and Dal Poz M (2004) Migration of health-care workers from developing countries: Strategic approaches to its management. *Bulletin of the World Health Organization* 82(8): 595–600.

Tautz S, Bähr A, and Wölte S (2006) Kommerzielle sexuelle Ausbeutung von Kindern und Jugendlichen. In: Razum O, Zeeb H, and Laaser U (eds.) *Globalisierung – Gerechtigkeit – Gesundheit. Einführung in International Public Health*, pp. 245–258. Bern, Switzerland: Huber.

UNFPA/IMP (2004) *Meeting the challenges of migration: Progress since the ICPD*. New York, Geneva, Switzerland: United Nations Fund for Population Activities/The International Migration Policy Programme (UNFPA/IMP). http://www.unfpa.org/upload/lib_pub_file/334_filename_migration.pdf (accessed August 2007).

UN General Assembly (1999) Article 2, revised draft protocol to prevent, suppress and punish trafficking in persons, especially women and children, supplementing the United Nations convention against transnational organised crime. AC/254/4/Add.3/Rev.4. Geneva, Switzerland: UN General Assembly. http://www.unodc.org/unodc/en/trafficking_convention.html (accessed August 2007).

Valin N, Antoun F, Chouaid C, et al. (2005) Outbreak of tuberculosis in a migrants' shelter, Paris, France, 2002. *International Journal of Tuberculosis and Lung Diseases* 9(5): 528–533.

WHO (2003) International migration, health and human rights. *Health and Human Rights Publication Series* vol. 4. Geneva, Switzerland: World Health Organization (WHO). http://www.who.int/hhr/activities/en/intl_migration_hhr.pdf (accessed August 2007).

SECTION 5
BIOSTATISTICS

Biostatistics

P E Leaverton, University of South Florida School of Public Health, Tampa, FL, USA
F V Wilder, The Arthritis Research Institute of America, Clearwater, FL, USA

Introduction

The relatively young discipline of statistics evolved during the last century to become an important aspect of all the sciences. The term statistics now usually includes both descriptive and analytical domains. Those analytical methods that have been found to be particularly useful and prevalent in the design and analysis of medical and public health research studies have been termed biostatistics. The use of these methods will be discussed later in the section titled 'Basic analytical statistics (biostatistics) concepts.' While most readers are unlikely to be practicing biostatisticians, most probably they will be expected to understand and interpret correctly journal articles summarizing research projects relevant to public health practice. Most such articles use statistical techniques in their summaries and analyses (perusal of any recent research journal in medicine or public health verifies this assertion). We review the rationale and interpretation of basic statistical summaries and biostatistical analyses. (Details on many specific statistical methodologies may be found in the several textbooks listed in the section titled 'Further reading.')

Descriptive Statistics

Descriptive Statistics in Public Health

Many nations and all U.S. states mandate that certain data are routinely collected on births, deaths, and other key measures of population health. Under federal law, the U.S. National Center for Health Statistics (NCHS) is required to collect, compile, and disseminate a large number of such health measures. As a result, several important health statistics programs have been developed by NCHS in recent decades to better estimate and understand the status and trends of the health of the American population and several subpopulations. These programs include not only the standard vital statistics (NCHS, 2006) such as births, low birth weights, and deaths, but also national surveys of morbidity and health practices. Naturally the collection of such voluminous amounts of data, by NCHS and other public health organizations, requires suitable methods for summarization, depiction, and interpretation. Collectively labeled descriptive statistics, there are a wide variety of these methods including rates, proportions, and other summary measures.

Several summary descriptive statistics have become the bedrock for assessing population health. As such, they can also provide quantified goals for national and state health programs (U.S. Dept. of Health and Human Services, 2000). For example, the infant mortality rate is widely perceived as the single most important statistic by which to assess the overall health status of large populations. This is the rate at which infants less than one year of age die. In the United States the infant mortality rate for the entire country was 26 per 1000 live births in 1960, which decreased to 6.9 per 1000 live births in 2000, clearly documenting significant progress in maternal and infant health.

Mortality statistics, by age, gender, cause of death, and state are one of the routine, ongoing reports that appear annually in NCHS publications (Heron and Smith, 2006). To account for the aging population, age-adjusted mortality rates are frequently used as the basis for comparing populations, as well as for comparing disease levels and trends. Naturally, the year-to-year changes in such rates usually are not profound. However, one of the most important public health phenomena in the last century was the slow-to-be-recognized turnaround in the age-adjusted mortality rates for coronary heart disease (CHD) that occurred in the late 1960s in the United States. For decades the CHD age-adjusted mortality rate inexorably increased every year. Considered by most as an unavoidable consequence of modernization in all developed countries, CHD had become the leading cause of death with a mortality rate that was gradually worsening every year. But, in the late 1970s, careful examination of this rate by scientists from the NCHS, the National Institutes for Health (NIH), and others, revealed that an unexpected and dramatic change had occurred. It was noted from these data that in the late 1960s, the CHD age-adjusted mortality rate had peaked and had begun a steady decline. This remarkable reversal occurred in both genders, all age groups, and all ethnic categories during a time window of just a few years. Health administrators convened a now famous conference (Havlik and Feinleib, 1979) in 1978 to determine whether this change in the leading cause of death was real or caused by some artifact in the cause of death classification processes.

Once it was determined that the change in the CHD mortality rate was real (i.e., it has continued to decline for decades) several research efforts were launched to determine the cause. While both therapists and those in public health disease prevention were willing to take much of the credit, the lack of accurate CHD morbidity data on a national scale precluded an accurate evaluation of this important finding. Incidence data on first heart attacks were not available and this lack demonstrated the need for accurate morbidity data as well as mortality data on which to prioritize health programs. Public health administrators wanted to know the causes of this important change and, accordingly, promote those practices and programs underlying them. The reasons simply were not clear at that time. Years later, it was generally concluded that both better care after a heart attack as well as increasing CHD prevention activities (which would delay the onset of first attacks) were both instrumental in the decline. Most eventually agreed that prevention activities (e.g., increased public attention to diet, smoking, and blood pressure) were probably responsible for a greater proportion of the decline. This 'data dilemma' in 1978 showed the need for both national morbidity and mortality information to assess health situations. This episode also illustrated how useful routinely collected health data may be in revealing important aspects of a society's changing health patterns by carefully examining the annual collected descriptive statistics on population health.

The NCHS periodically produces a variety of extremely useful public health statistics. They annually summarize infant and general mortality statistics so that public health practitioners may assess absolute and relative changes in population health characteristics. The National Health Interview Survey (HIS) (Pleis and Lethbridge-Çejku, 2006) and the National Health and Nutrition Examination Survey (NHANES) (CDC/NCHS, 2006) have proven extremely useful over the years as a way to evaluate the morbidity and disease prevention risk factor status of the U.S. population. A comprehensive general summary of the nations' health is published every year by NCHS. It is simply called Health United States (NCHS, 2006). In this single volume, one can find detailed information on major diseases as well as risk factors and their trends. The tables, charts, and figures displayed in this annual publication are illustrative of the most efficient and sensible methods of summarizing and conveying large amounts of health information using easily understood descriptive statistics. The World Health Organization (WHO) also produces summary health statistics for the world in which comparable data allow (WHO, 2006). Both the NCHS and WHO websites can be referenced for many more helpful examples of descriptive heath statistics.

Descriptive Statistics – Some Comments on Methods

It is useful to separate data into two major types of measurements, discrete and continuous. Discrete data include counts in which only isolated points on a numerical scale may be observed. Sometimes the counts are converted into percentages. The number of deaths and the percent of

persons dying among those alive at the beginning of a time period are two examples. The percentage of females in a population is another. Prevalence and incidence rates are two categorical data descriptive summaries widely used in epidemiology.

Continuous data are measurements that may theoretically assume any value (limited only by the accuracy of our measuring devices) between two defined points on a numerical scale. Height, weight, blood pressure, and serum cholesterol measurements are common examples. A frequency distribution is usually examined to display the 'picture' of the location and spread of the measurements along a numerical scale. Such distributions come in many shapes. Many but not all data sets display something resembling a bell shape with a grouping of recorded values near or in the center. A statistical model usefully employed to describe such a shape is called the Gaussian or normal distribution model (**Figure 1**).

If this is the case, a simple mean, or arithmetic average, is used to describe this 'central tendency' (or middle grouping) and a standard deviation is calculated to describe the spread of the observations around the mean. Thus only two simply computed statistics can describe a bell-shaped, or relative, frequency distribution very well. The population values for these statistics are usually designated as μ (mean) and σ (standard deviation). We use our sample data to calculate estimates of these population parameters. The mean indicates the central value and the standard deviation efficiently describes the spread of values around this mean. It can be demonstrated that about 68% of the values will lie within one standard deviation from the mean and about 95% will lie within two standard deviations from the mean. If the distribution of measurements is approximated by a normal distribution, then this distribution may be summarized very simply and efficiently in this manner. These two descriptive statistics tell everything about the central tendency and spread of the data.

The symmetry of a normal distribution is important. However, a simple mean may be inappropriate as a measure of central tendency if the data are highly skewed, that

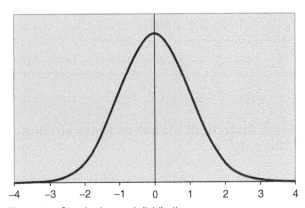

Figure 1 Standard normal distribution.

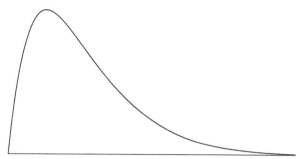

Figure 2 Positive skewed distribution.

is, if the distribution is severely asymmetrical – having a single long tail on either side (**Figure 2**). Blood pressures in untreated populations usually display such a shape.

The median, or middle ranking number, may be the measure of choice in such cases. Another common error is the use of the standard deviation to describe the spread in a set of numbers that clearly are asymmetric. The mean plus or minus two standard deviations will not include 68% of the measurements in these cases. To describe the spread in such distributions, the use of percentiles is usually recommended. Using percentiles in this manner does not require any particular distribution shape for validity.

The reader should consult one of the many basic textbooks on statistics or biostatistics for a review of descriptive statistics methodology (Rosner, 2006). Sometimes these methods are given short shrift compared to analytical methods in courses because of their relative simplicity. However, when summarizing data, it is important to use the most appropriate descriptive statistics, ones that make the points clear for any reader and do not cause a wrongful interpretation of the data. It is easy to convey, intentionally or unintentionally, erroneous messages with poorly chosen descriptive statistics, including poor tables and graphs. One of the best-selling statistics books ever published is entitled *How to Lie With Statistics* (Huff, 1993). This useful work contains many examples that illustrate how even simple descriptive statistics and graphs may mislead. The choice of graph scales is particularly important. Care must be taken in even the seemingly simplest summaries to make certain that the correct informational message is given. It is also recommended that readers examine how reputable public health agencies such as the WHO, the NCHS, and the NIH summarize and display health data. Their publications provide many useful examples of descriptive statistics.

Basic Analytical Statistics (Biostatistics) Concepts

Most of the field of biostatistics and statistics for that matter is devoted to analytical methods for drawing appropriate inferences from research studies, whether they are nonexperimental or experimental. In both types of studies there are five fundamental concepts that are essential to any statistical analysis: population-sample construct, variation, probability, randomness, and causation. An understanding of these ideas is essential to grasp the role of biostatistics in making inferences from our sample data to the population of interest. These concepts and the use of confidence intervals (CIs) and tests of significance are discussed in this section.

Populations and Samples

For a health-related measurement on an individual to have the most meaning, it is desirable to be able to compare it with the distribution on all such measurements in an appropriate reference population. For example, to have the entire measurement distribution for all healthy and the distribution of all sick, untreated persons in the same age and gender group as the individual being measured would be ideal. It would help in making the most informed decision about whether some medical intervention is required. Unfortunately, it is almost never possible to obtain such population distributions for an entire population and we must be satisfied with measurements from a portion of the target population called a sample. Naturally, we want our sample to be representative of the target population and not biased. In this sense, bias may be defined as something that makes a sample different from what it purports to be.

While the population-sample concept is clear when counts or measurements are made in defined human populations, it is useful in other contexts as well. Sometimes such populations are hypothetical. For example, we may consider the population of all total serum cholesterol measurements possible if repeated measurements were made at one time period on one person. Such repeated measurements will differ. The distribution of such measurements in this hypothetical population is due to inherent biological variability (in this case, the within-person variability). If we assume a single value for an individual at one time period, then we may consider the distribution of all such values among a group of persons in a defined population (the between-persons variability). Since we cannot make measurements on the entire population, we use our sample data to make inferences about our target population.

Another important hypothetical distribution comes into play in experimental situations. Here, while we may be able to conduct one experiment, we realize that if we were to conduct the same experiment under the same (as close as possible) conditions we would almost never achieve exactly the same results. Conceptually, the distribution of all such possible experimental results is the target population from which our single observed result is taken. Using this conceptual population-sample idea allows us to use the same statistical inference structure as we would with a very tangible population. We want to make inferences about this hypothetical distribution from our single experiment.

Variation in Health Data

The discipline of statistics developed during the last century in response to a need in all of science to handle variation in measurements. Of course, this is a generic issue, not unique to health data. A brilliant English mathematics professor, Sir Ronald A. Fisher, took the lead in this activity in the 1920s and 30s with much of his work being directed toward improving the design and analysis of experiments in agricultural research, a field that his ideas revolutionized. However, it was soon recognized that many of these concepts and methods had broad utility in the design and analysis of both experimental and nonexperimental studies in any field of science. Fisher and his colleagues showed the world how much of a role randomness played in all studies and suggested methods of analysis using probability methods. As a result, statistical significance tests and confidence intervals (CIs) became a standard for nearly all scientific studies, including public health research. As well, many of the methods were not limited to experimental studies. Statistical methods became recognized as the most appropriate way to handle variation in all research data.

One useful definition of variation is differences between things 'bearing the same label.' Thus, for example, when several similar persons are given the same drug and dosage their measured responses will differ. The degree to which they differ is called response variation. Measurement of a single individual's systolic blood pressure (SBP) will display considerable variation even at one sitting. Variation in SBP readings among different members of a defined population will naturally be even greater. If this measurement is quantitative, such as weight, blood pressure, or cholesterol level, analytical methods involving frequency distributions are used. Often these are based upon the Gaussian or normal distribution models. If the response is categorical, such as improved or unimproved, methods such as a chi-square (χ^2) analysis are usually used in the analysis.

Probability

The definition of probability is still debated among philosophers of science. There is the traditional relative frequency definition and the Bayesian definition, which uses information beyond the scope of this article. Each school of thought has its proponents and each approach has its uses in the analysis of data. However, in most of science, including the health sciences, the most common interpretation is that of relative frequency.

First consider a random process, which is a repetitive process that in a single trial may result in any number of possible outcomes such that the particular outcome is determined by chance and is impossible to predict. The simplest illustrations are often presented using examples from games of chance. We cannot know in advance whether a tossed coin will fall heads or tails, nor can we predict in advance what number will occur when a pair of dice are rolled. That we cannot predict such outcomes is due to the element of chance or randomness. If a random process can result in n equally likely and mutually exclusive outcomes, and if a of these outcomes have attribute A, then the probability of A is said to be the ratio a/n. Thus, symbolically,

$$P(A) = a/n.$$

Two outcomes are said to be mutually exclusive if, when one occurs, the other cannot. Thus, when a coin is tossed, the result is either a head or a tail. The probability of each is one-half. When a single die is rolled, there are six equally likely outcomes, all with a probability of one-sixth. By considering the makeup of coins, dice, or cards, it is easy to determine the long-run probability of such events. We cannot predict the outcome of any specific trial, but we know the relative frequency of the events.

It is easy to comprehend this definition of probability when the mechanisms involved are simple, as in games of chance. When it comes to using this concept in the domain of biological, medical, or public health research, it is not always so clear. The very simple two-group example just cited could easily apply in a simple population question in which everyone could be considered as having been inoculated or not inoculated. The cumulative percent inoculated, seen from repeated sampling from such a defined population, obviously converges toward the true population percentage, the relative frequency. We can call this potentially empirically derived percentage the probability of the event. This relative frequency interpretation of the probability of an event is used throughout the experimental and nonexperimental sciences, including public health research.

Randomness

Although we have previously defined a random process, let us give further consideration to this important notion. Of course, researchers had realized for a long time that variation occurs among persons in similar categories or in response to treatments. Understanding the precise role of randomness in this situation was a major breakthrough in the sciences.

In surveys (e.g., nonexperimental studies) we now know how best to draw a sample from a population so that the sample will be unbiased and will be representative of the parent population. In earlier times samples may have been chosen haphazardly or by methods that seemed free of bias but, in fact, were not. The surest way to ensure unbiasedness is to select a random sample from the population. Sometimes this is easier said than done. Some games of chance seem to have clearly random drawings, whether cards or dice. But when sampling from a large defined human population, stringent attention must be given to the details. A random sample is defined as one selected in such a way that every member of the population has an equal and independent chance of being selected. If this definition is met by our sampling method, then we know our sample is not biased; that, in the long run, our estimate of any population attribute or characteristic will converge toward the true value. (Independence, in this sense, means that the selection of any element in no way influences the selection of any other element.)

Health surveys may be modified, of course, to improve efficiency by taking into account characteristics of the target population. While many national surveys are complex, random selection is at the core of the method. There are two compelling reasons for using random sampling in surveys. First, it assures unbiasedness. Secondly, it allows for the methods of probability to be used in the analyses of the data.

While the design and analysis of experiments is quite different than that of surveys, the role of randomness is no less crucial. Here, it is not random sampling from a defined population; it is random allocation of experimental treatments to subjects (i.e., patients) in clinical trials.

Causation

Like variation, causation is important in the sciences. And, like the concept of variation, the science of statistics plays a major role in 'handling' this frequently controversial topic. The old adage is true – correlation does not imply causation. Just because two variables are associated does not mean that one caused the other. This basic principle is necessary to keep in mind when such observations are made. However, it is frequently ignored. Examples may be seen almost every day in the public arena when two variables, suspected of being causally related, are seen to occur together in a sensible time frame. Do certain medications cause unexpected side effects? Are hormones used in livestock harmful to humans? Are cancers occurring near nuclear or other industrial plants due to being in proximity to such plants? Do certain herbs delay the onset of osteoarthritis? It is so easy, yet often treacherous, to assume two events such as these examples linked in time and/or space are causally related.

Science learned centuries ago (mostly from Galileo's demonstration) that the best way to test, compare, or sort out competing hypotheses is through experimentation. While this is not always possible, due to financial or logistical reasons, it is mandatory when it is possible. It is useful to divide scientific studies into two classes, experimental and nonexperimental. The latter, which include population surveys, are sometimes called observational studies. (This

seems a poor terminology, however, because it implies that observations are not made in experiments.) The difference is that in an experiment, the investigator has control over the major 'independent' or 'predictor' variable(s) under study – that is, drugs, treatments, and so on – and assigns their values to the experimental units. In a nonexperimental study there is no such control and the investigator studies the relationships among variables as they occur in nature.

In nonexperimental studies, researchers look for associations among variables, often in a search for possible cause-and-effect relationships. Because of the complex interactions that may exist among both observed and unobserved variables, however, it is nearly always inappropriate to assume that an association among variables implies that they are causally related. Causal inference is proper only in experiments in which it is possible to rule out other competing hypotheses, at least for most situations encountered in biomedical and public health research.

The basic elements of experimental design may be summarized as follows:

1. Specification of the objectives. This usually requires stating the hypothesis to be tested.
2. Specification of the experimental units (animals, cells, human beings, etc.).
3. Specification of the appropriate experimental design, including the choice of control or comparison group(s).
4. Random allocation of experimental units to study groups.
5. Making every reasonable effort to ensure that study groups are treated as exactly alike as possible throughout the course of the experiment.

Items 4 and 5 above are essential to ensure that any apparent treatment differences in responses are due to (1) true differences in treatment effects, or (2) random processes. When random allocation is properly employed, we ensure that estimates of treatment differences are unbiased and that we may employ analytical statistical methods based on probability in the analysis of the results. Without random allocation such analyses are erroneous.

A clinical trial is an experiment in which the experimental unit is a human being. The same general principles of good experimentation apply, of course, but there are areas of special interest. Ethical and logistical issues are unique to the use of human beings in experiments.

Sampling Variation and Confidence Intervals

When drawing random samples from a defined population, the usual goal is to estimate some specific characteristic, or parameter, of that population. We cannot know that characteristic exactly without observing, or sampling, the whole population. For example, if every member of the population may be classified into one of two mutually exclusive categories, the population may be labeled as binomial. For generality, we may call the two classes, successes (s) and failures (f). The percent of successes in the population may be the characteristic we would like to estimate. We may randomly draw a small sample of size n from a binomial population and count the number of successes. Obviously, the number of successes in our sample divided by the sample size, n, is our (unbiased) estimate. Common sense tells us that if we took another sample of the same size, the new observed sample percentage would not be identical to the first sample. Repeating the same exercise would reveal a distribution of sample percentages. This distribution represents the sampling variation in such an exercise.

One would rightly expect that the mean of this sampling distribution if continued indefinitely would be the same as the underlying target population mean or attribute that we are attempting to estimate. Recognizing the degree of variation in sample results, and quantifying this variation, will allow us to better assess the results from a single sample. It enables us to make a quantified statement about how close our sample estimate is likely to be to the corresponding population value. This knowledge has led to the now common practice of constructing CIs.

Estimates of population values should always be accompanied by a CI. Thus we can understand how to evaluate the point estimate of a population characteristic. Usually, CIs are constructed using a 95% probability statement. Thus, if a sample of size $n = 50$ taken from a binomial population yields 30 successes, the obvious point estimate of the population success percentage is 60%. From statistical tables we find an accompanying 95% CI for this result is 45% to 73%. We state that our best point estimate is 60%. But, unless we are exceptionally lucky, this estimate will not hit the true population value (%) on the nose. The CI is a way of stating how close to the truth we likely are. We can state that we are 95% confident that the true population value (%) is between 45% and 73%. The proper interpretation of this statement is that on repeated samplings of this same size (50), 95% of the time the true value will be included in such intervals. If our sample size is increased to $n = 100$ and we observe the same sample percentage (60%), the corresponding 95% CI shrinks to 50% to 70%. This smaller interval reflects that larger sample sizes increase the chance of obtaining sample estimates that are closer to the true value. The CI method allows researchers to quantify what we all generally knew about sample size. It is now nearly a requirement in all of the sciences that any point estimate from a study be accompanied by a CI.

The above example illustrates how knowledge of sampling variation from a binomial population may be used to construct a useful assessment of quality of a sample percentage through the use of a CI. The same approach may be used to assess sample values from a population of measurements as well. For example, we want to estimate the population mean of a distribution of weights in a defined population of adult males. In this case we know that means calculated from repeated random samples will vary from sample to sample. The sample mean, usually designated as $\bar{x}$, will form a distribution around the true population mean, usually designated μ. The standard deviation of this hypothetical distribution is called the standard error of the mean (SEM), or simply, the standard error (SE). For any such sample from a normal distribution or close to it the sample mean, $\bar{x} \pm 2$ SE will result in an approximate 95% CI for the true mean. That is, about 95% of the time with such sampling, this interval, calculated on the basis of a single random sample, will include the population mean μ. Once again, this allows us to assess the quality of the sample estimate. Shorter intervals obviously imply that the corresponding point estimate is better than one with a wider interval. It is a quantitative method of handling sampling variation.

Confidence intervals are required as part of the display of results from health surveys and experimental results. These intervals must accompany estimates in more complex statistical analyses as well. The basic interpretation remains the same, however. CIs quantify how good our estimates are in the face of inescapable variation.

Tests for Statistical Significance (Testing Hypotheses)

Most medical and public health research involves comparative studies. That is, because of variation in all things biological, control or comparison groups are mandatory. One looks for differences in the means of group measurements, percentages, or some other population characteristic. Usually this comparison takes the form of a hypothesis. A researcher usually suspects a difference between the groups (the reason for the interest) but the hypothesis that a difference exists often includes an infinite number of possibilities. The easiest solution to formulating a probabilistic approach is to state the hypothesis (H) that there is no difference in the population values and then see if the data support that hypothesis. This statement of no difference is called the null hypothesis (H_o). The data from a comparative study are collected and used to examine, or test, this H_o of no difference between the two groups. Thus, we do not directly test the hypothesis of most interest — that of a difference. We test the null hypothesis and make a decision, based on probability, about whether the data are reasonably compatible with that hypothesis. If the observations do not support the null hypotheses, we conclude that there really is a difference between the two groups. In a sense, we set up a straw man that we hope can be knocked down by our study's data. This strategy may seem to be a backward approach but it is the most tenable one, compared to examining the myriad of other possibilities.

Comparing the data from a study with the null hypothesis, H_o, is called a test of that hypothesis. The quantitative issue addressed is that of assessing the compatibility of the observations with H_o. Due to variability we know that there will be a distribution of study results. However, if our procedures were proper (random sampling or random allocation) we know that in most cases the summary results will be close to the null value, if the null hypothesis is true. By bad luck due to variation sometimes the results may be misleading. Quantifying this degree of deviation from H_o, using a probability statement, is called a test of the null hypothesis. If our sample or experimental result is unlikely to have occurred if H_o were true, we do not accept, or we reject, H_o. If our result is likely to have occurred under H_o, we accept H_o. How is 'likely' defined? Convention (starting with Fisher) uses 5% as a demarcation. That is, if our study result is shown to have less than a 5% chance of occurring under H_o, we do not accept H_o. It is usually stated that H_o is rejected. Therefore, we conclude that there is a real difference between the groups. Of course, we may be wrong in rejecting H_o, but we know the probability of this judgment error. This probability assessment of study data has become nearly universal in the sciences. We may use other probabilities, such as 0.01, should we wish. But this chosen value (P-value) should be stated prior to any data collection.

An Example of Hypothesis Testing with Discrete (Binomial) Data

Suppose that we have drawn random samples, each of size 40, from two defined populations. The populations were all men aged 40 to 49 years. We determined one group as current cigarette smokers. The other group is defined as having never been a smoker. Both groups were examined for evidence of coronary heart disease (CHD) and all were found free of CHD. We have the ability to follow each group for several years. After a specified time period, the two groups are reexamined for evidence of CHD during the period of observation. Our null hypothesis in this case is that there is no difference in the CHD rates (incidence) of the two groups. We may classify our sampling results into a 2 × 2 table. (**Table 1**).

The question now is: Could the above sample results have easily occurred by chance alone? Equivalently,

could these results have occurred if the null hypothesis – that is, CHD rates in the two populations were identical – was true? The sample differences ($10/40 = 25\%$ vs. $20/40 = 50\%$) seem large enough that the null hypothesis seems surely false by any assessment of these data. But a statistical analysis is needed to quantify this judgment. (Often such judgments are in error.) A data summary statistic has been found to be a simple and useful way of evaluation of such data. It is the well-known chi-square (χ^2) statistic, which is calculated from such a 2 × 2 table. The distribution of this statistic is known for all 2 × 2 tables under the assumption that the null hypothesis is true. From theoretical and empirical considerations, we know that 95% of chi-square statistics calculated from 2 × 2 tables, when H_o is true, will be less than the value, 3.84. And 5% will exceed this value. In our example, the calculated chi-square is 5.32. The researcher is justified in concluding that these specific results would be unlikely to have occurred if H_o were true. How unlikely? Less than a 5% chance. Usually such a result is expressed at follows; H_o is rejected, or, more precisely, not accepted, at the 5% level. Equivalently, $P < 0.05$. This is also interpreted as having found a statistically significant difference between our two samples at the $P < 0.05$ level. This is a simple example of testing a hypothesis.

Suppose, in our example, that the two sample percentages were closer together, such as 10/40 and 15/40? In this case the calculated chi-square value is 0.93, well below 3.84, so we would accept the H_o. Such a sample result could easily have occurred by chance alone. We would write $P > 0.05$. The observed sample difference is said to be not statistically significant at the 0.05 level.

The above examples are a simple illustration of the difference between a statistically significant difference and one that is not statistically significant. The probability statements are made, assuming that the null hypothesis is true. It should be kept in mind that a statistically significant difference refers only to the reality of a difference. In a statistical test of which the chi-square test is but one of many examples, nothing is said about the magnitude of the difference. Clearly, there are statistically significant differences that are real but too small to be clinically or practically important. That is why a CI should always accompany the results of such a significance test. The accompanying point and interval estimates clarify the likely size of the difference. Actually, if a 95% CI includes the null value, one may use the interval as an equivalent test of H_o. If the null value (zero difference) is included in the 95% CI, we accept H_o. If it is outside the range of the CI we would reject H_o, at the 0.05 level. Because of this fact, some scientists have called for the abandonment of significance testing and the use of P-values in the evaluation of study results. Rather, they argue, the CI gives everything one needs. However, there are more complex

Table 1 Coronary heart disease (CHD) incidence rates: 2 × 2 table

	CHD	Non-CHD	Total
Smokers	20	20	40
Nonsmokers	10	30	40
Total	30	50	80

statistical tests in which a CI is not so easily calculated or interpreted. Tests of significance have become a regular part of data analyses and most scientists seem to prefer the computation of both significance tests and CIs.

There are several ways in which a 2×2 table may arise in research. The above example is one in which two groups of subjects are followed for a period of time to see if illness rates differ in two groups exposed to a suspected causal factor (cigarettes in this case). This is the most elementary example of a cohort epidemiological study. In such an instance an attack rate or incidence rate may be computed for the two groups being compared. From **Table 1**, we can see that the two rates are 50% and 25%. Each of these figures could be construed as the risk of contracting the defined illness in the study's time frame. The two percentages are estimates of the absolute risk. The ratio of the two is labeled the relative risk (RR), a bedrock statistic in epidemiology. In our simple example, the RR is 20/40 divided by 10/40, or 2.0. That is, one is twice as likely to contract CHD when exposed to cigarettes than if there was no such exposure. From our chi-square test, we know that this RR is statistically significant at the 0.05 level. We may wish to construct a CI for our RR estimate as well.

It is important to note the relationship between CIs and tests of hypotheses. If our CI contains the null value, then the null hypothesis is accepted. If our CI excludes the null value, then the null hypothesis is rejected. Thus one may always use the CI as both an indication of how accurate our point estimate is and also to test H_o.

An Example of Hypothesis Testing with Two Sets of Continuous Data

Suppose that we have drawn two random samples not from binomial populations but from two populations of continuous measurements. We have the same two populations as in the previous binomial example, but now (instead of asking a yes/no question) we record a measurement on each member in our two samples. Our single measurement in this case is a simple fasting total cholesterol value. The hypothesis to be tested is that the population mean, μ, is the same in both populations. That is, the two samples essentially come from the same population.

Symbolically, we write the null hypothesis, H_o: $\mu_1 = \mu_2 = \mu$ (the common population mean). Naturally, to investigate this null hypothesis, the first thing to look at is the two sample means. If they are identical, we immediately conclude that the data support H_o. But, of course, this almost never happens. The real question is how far apart must the two sample means be before we reasonably conclude with a precise probability statement that they could not likely have been drawn from the same population? We know that the two samples were actually drawn from two different groups but, if the population means (μ) were identical, then, for our purposes, we are dealing with only one population.

To assess this probability we calculate a summary statistic called the t-statistic. Knowing the distribution of this t-statistic under H_o allows us to test H_o, creating a t-test, as was the case with the chi-square test with binomial data. The t-statistic is a ratio of the difference in the two sample means divided by an estimate of the standard deviation of this difference, called the standard error of the mean difference. If this calculated t-value is close to zero, obviously we are more likely to accept H_o. If the t-value is large (i.e., the sample means are far apart relative to their standard deviation), then we are more likely to reject H_o and conclude that the samples came from two different populations; that is, we would reject H_o. Again, such statements are placed in a probabilistic basis, just as was the case with the chi-square test. The same inferences are drawn with respect to H_o and its likelihood of yielding our observed data – two sets of measurements in this case.

Other Tests of Hypotheses

The previous two examples are among the simplest and most common tests of hypotheses: comparing percentages (discrete data) between two groups and comparing sample means (continuous data) between two groups. Obviously, there are numerous other situations in which a hypothesis may be tested. We may have several groups of means we want to compare. The technique known as the analysis of variance is usually employed in that instance. If we wish to investigate the association between two continuous variables, the methods of regression and correlation are used. The same principles apply; the null hypothesis is stated and a statistic is calculated by which to make a probability statement (test of significance) about the likelihood that our data could have resulted from a situation in which our null hypothesis was true. The same interpretation is used for the resulting significance tests. (For an excellent source of statistical software, including tutorials, for conducting many tests, see under the section titled 'Relevant Websites.')

Sample Size and Statistical Significance

If a properly conducted test for statistical significance reveals a statistically significant result, we trust the probability statement, regardless of the sample size. All tests take into account the size of the samples. As just stated, the researcher must then decide if the difference is large enough to be important. However, if a test result shows that an observed difference is not statistically significant ($P > 0.05$), this result is interpreted as meaning that the observed difference could easily have arisen by chance alone (H_o, true), that is, more than 5% of the time. Is it possible that there is a real difference and that the testing procedure missed it? Are we wrong in accepting H_o in such cases? Whereas our probability statement is correct, the answer is maybe. It is possible to miss real and possibly important differences between the two groups being studied. This can easily happen if our sample size is too small. Although it is beyond the scope of this article, the relationships among the sample size, size of the difference, and the statistical power (probability of rejecting H_o) to detect real differences must be considered in study planning. Sample size calculations should be undertaken as part of the study planning process to ensure that the sample sizes are adequate to detect important differences with a reasonable degree of probability. (See some of the biostatistics references listed for computational details under the section titled 'Further Reading.')

Biostatistics in Public Health

Epidemiology and Clinical Trials

Most epidemiological research is involved in the search for associations, for potential cause-and-effect relationships among variables. Before following up on an observed association, it must first be demonstrated that it could not easily have arisen by chance alone. Obviously, this is where a biostatistical approach is mandated. If you cannot convince your peers that your result is not easily explained by chance, you will not have much success in engendering support for further investigation. Tests of hypotheses and CIs play a basic role in such evaluations.

Once it has been determined that observed differences or associations are unlikely to have been the result of chance alone (i.e., statistically significant), the epidemiologist must evaluate the possibility that the association may be causal. Of course, as we have pointed out, real associations do not imply that two variables are causally related. The surest way to establish causation is by means of an experiment. As we have noted, using human volunteers in an experiment is called a clinical trial. Most clinical trials conducted are in the area of clinical medicine, that is, testing and comparing treatments for persons already diagnosed with an illness. However, in recent years, there have been an increasing number of clinical trials in epidemiology known as prevention trials. The difference between the two approaches is not trivial. Few question the ethics of using volunteers in an experimental search for improved therapies. But if preliminary epidemiological research implicates a possible cause of a disease, it seems unethical to directly test this hypothesis in an experiment. Such a study would mean that some

healthy individuals would be subjected to a variable suspected of causing illness.

Despite the ethical issues involved, there now have been many clinical trials examining the possible cause and effect of variables believed to cause illness. One approach is to find a volunteer population that is already exposed to a suspected cause and randomly remove, or greatly reduce, the exposure to that cause in half of them. Following both groups until some new illnesses occur and comparing the two rates is a logical test of the causal hypothesis. This certainly was the approach in the early cholesterol reduction trials. Such trials showed experimentally that cholesterol reduction was an effective way to reduce the incidence of CHD.

Another aspect of clinical trials among healthy, symptom-free persons is that the time period from initial observation to an adverse health event is usually much longer than would be the case in clinical trials of sick patients. Sample size requirements are correspondingly much higher. And the time of such trials is much longer. One approach to ameliorating this situation is to select volunteers from high-risk subjects, the logic being that such a group would yield more cases of illness in a shorter period of time than from the general population. Thus, when epidemiological research (i.e., an observed association) indicated that beta-carotene supplementation might possibly reduce the risk of lung cancer, trials were begun among smokers who were cancer free. A trial using volunteers from the general population would have been prohibitively expensive and lengthy because the incidence of lung cancer is very low. However, among cigarette smokers, the expected number of cases is much higher. Two well-conducted major trials examining the protective effect of beta-carotene in smokers actually revealed that this supplement was not beneficial and likely increased the risk of lung cancer in smokers. These trials once again demonstrated the need for experimentation to verify a suspected cause-and-effect relationship. It is too easy to assume such a relationship when it has not been proven with sound experimentation.

Some Common Errors in Biostatistics Reasoning

Assuming an observed association implies causality

Epidemiology, the search for variables suspected of being in the causal pathway of disease and disability, is the cornerstone of public health. When such causal variables are found, many public health activities are devoted to reducing their impact. Several successful public health interventions have taken place. These include the reduction of cigarette smoking, serum cholesterol levels, and blood pressure levels. These reductions have had an impact on several diseases seen at the population level, particularly in the area of CHD. In these cases an association was noted between levels of the suspected variables and the onset of disease. However, one cannot be certain that some other perhaps genetic variable may play a role in both the suspected causal variable and a disease. Usually, clinical trials must be employed to rule out other than causal hypotheses.

Of course, there are times when a public health decision must be made in the absence of experimental evidence of causality (i.e., clinical trials). The classic example of such an action is documented in the famous 1964 Surgeon General's Report on cigarette smoking as a cause of lung cancer (U.S. Dept of Health, Education, and Welfare, 1964). It is neither ethical nor logistically feasible to conduct the definitive trial in this situation. However, the sum of the evidence from many nonexperimental studies was consistent enough to result in stating that the association likely was causal and public health action was required. The magnitude of the population effect necessitated this particular action. In most cases, however, experimental evaluation would be required.

Assuming statistical significance equates to practical significance

As we have emphasized, statistical testing relates only to the reality of a group or treatment difference, not to the magnitude of any difference. What does it matter if an analgesic dissolves 5 seconds faster than a competing brand in terms of affecting a headache? That is why many persons prefer to emphasize CIs in biostatistics, rather than statistical tests. A CI allows one to examine the magnitude of an estimated difference along with a significance test. If the interval doesn't include the null value, the null hypothesis may be rejected.

Assuming relative risk is more important than absolute risk

A pharmaceutical advertisement may state simply that the use of their drug will reduce the risk of a heart attack by 25%. By itself, this statement is meaningless. Among what population and over what time period are the first clarifications that come to mind. However, even more important may be the contrast of a reduction in RR versus a reduction in absolute risk. Suppose that the untreated risk of an attack were 4 per 1000 men in a year, and that the treated risk was reduced to 3 per 1000 men in a year. This is a RR reduction of (4-3)/4, or 25%. But the absolute reduction is 1 per 1000 men or 0.1% in a year, which is not as impressive as the RR reduction. Obviously, both risks must be considered and weighed in making a decision about a cost/benefit evaluation regarding embarking on a drug regimen. Oftentimes, the absolute risk is ignored.

See also: Clinical Trials; Health Surveys.

Citations

Centers for Disease Control and Prevention (CDC) and National Center for Health and Statistics (NCHS) (2006) *National Health and Nutrition Examination Survey Data.* Hyattsville, MD: U.S. Department of Health and Human Services, CDC.

Havlik RJ and Feinleib M (eds.) (1979) *Proceedings of the Conference on the Decline in Coronary Heart Disease Mortality,* October 24–25, 1978. NIH Publication No. 79-1610. Washington, DC: National Heart, Lung, and Blood Institute.

Heron MP and Smith BL (2006) *Deaths: Leading Causes for 2003.* National Vital Statistics Reports. Hyattsville, MD: National Center for Health Statistics.

Huff D (1993) *How to Lie with Statistics.* New York: W.W Norton.

National Center for Health Statistics (NCHS) (2006) *Health, United States, 2006: With Chartbook on Trends in the Health of Americans.* Hyattsville, MD: NCHS.

Pleis JR and Lethbridge-Çejku M (2006) Summary health statistics for U.S. adults: National health interview survey, 2005. Vital Health Stat 10(232). Hyattsville, MD: National Center for Health Statistics.

Rosner B (2006) *Fundamentals of Biostatistics,* 6th edn. Belmont, CA: Brooks/Cole.

U.S. Department of Health and Human Services (2000) *Healthy People 2010: Understanding and Improving Health,* 2nd edn. Washington, DC: U.S. Government Printing Office.

U.S. Government (1964) Smoking and Health: *Report of the Advisory Committee to the Surgeon General of the Public Health Service.* Washington, DC: U.S. Department of Health, Education and Welfare.

World Health Organization (2006) *The World Health Report 2006 – Working Together for Health.* Geneva, Switzerland: WHO.

Further Reading

Huff D (1993) *How to Lie with Statistics.* New York: W.W Norton.

National, Center for Health, Statistics (NCHS) (2006) *Health, United States, 2006: With Chartbook on Trends in the Health of Americans.* Hyattsville, MD: NCHS.

Pagano M and Gauvreau K (2000) *Principles of Biostatistics,* 2nd edn. Pacific Grove, CA: Duxbury.

U.S. Department of Health and Human Services (2000) *Healthy People 2010: Understanding and Improving Health,* 2nd edn. Washington, DC: U.S. Government Printing Office.

World Health, Organization (2006) *The World Health Report 2006 – working together for health.* Geneva, Switzerland: WHO.

Relevant Websites

http://www.cdc.gov/nchs – CDC.
http://www.cdc.gov/DataStatistics – CDC, Data and Statistics.
http://www.cdc.gov/epiinfo – CDC Epi Info, What Is Epi Info?
http://www.healthypeople.gov/LHI – Healthy People, Leading Health Indicators.

Meta-Analysis

A Tatsioni and J P A Ioannidis, Tufts University School of Medicine, Boston, MA, USA

General Aspects

Meta-analysis includes a set of methods that can combine quantitatively the evidence from different studies in a mathematically appropriate way. Combining data may improve statistical power, when there are several small studies on a specific question, but each one of them is largely underpowered or has not been designed to address that research question. Meta-analysis may provide a precise and robust summary estimate after a systematic and rigorous integration of the available evidence. In addition, meta-analysis is also useful for listing and possibly exploring sources of bias, quantifying between-study heterogeneity, and proposing some potential explanations for dissecting genuine heterogeneity from bias.

Any type of quantitative data may be combined through meta-analysis. These include, but are not limited to, randomized controlled trials, observational studies, diagnostic test accuracy studies, and prevalence studies. Here we will discuss primarily meta-analyses of randomized controlled trials, and will also touch briefly on issues that pertain to the synthesis of other types of data.

Meta-analysis may be performed retrospectively or prospectively. Most meta-analyses to date have been retrospective. When a prospective meta-analysis is performed, a number of studies are designed and conducted with the anticipation that their data will be combined and analyzed together eventually. The whole procedure is different from a multicenter prospective trial because in prospective meta-analysis, the research protocols of the included studies may be similar but not necessarily identical.

The advent of evidence-based medicine has challenged our understanding about the relative merits of various sources of information. Expert opinion that has had major prestige and influence in clinical and public health decision-making in the past can sometimes be very misleading. Therefore, hierarchies of evidence developed in the 1990s not only displaced expert opinion from its prominent place, but also ranked it at the worst possible tier. Conversely, meta-analysis reached the top tiers of these hierarchies.

The question of whether meta-analyses of many small trials conform with the results of single large trials is important for public health. Theoretically, large trials and meta-analyses should give the same results in the absence of bias. Empirical evidence suggests that for randomized trials, studies with over 1000 subjects tend to have similar results as meta-analyses of smaller studies, but discrepancies that are beyond what can be accounted for by chance may still occur in 10–30% of the cases. In these situations, large trials tend to give more conservative results, but this is not always the case. Differences in the exact estimate of the effect sizes are even more common; in many cases these discrepancies do not reach formal statistical significance probably due to low power. Discrepancies between meta-analyses of small trials and larger trials also tend to be more frequent for secondary than for primary endpoints (Ioannidis *et al.*, 1998).

Background for a Meta-Analysis Protocol

Research Questions

The first important step in conducting a meta-analysis is formulating unambiguous research questions. Well-defined questions help to define the boundaries of the evidence to be reviewed, the literature search strategy, and the inclusion criteria, and may also inform the choice of analytic methods and the interpretation of the results.

The PICO approach (i.e., patient, intervention, comparator, and outcome) to specify parameters to be addressed is a common method to formulate research questions for meta-analysis. For the evaluation of most interventions, the PICO approach assumes that the type of studies to be analyzed is the randomized controlled trial. One might broaden this approach by including experimental as well as observational studies.

Literature Search and Sources of Evidence

Retrospective meta-analysis depends on data that have already been generated, and these data may or may not have been published. Unpublished data may be difficult to retrieve, but even published data may need to be identified and collected from different sources. PubMed is a default source for searching relevant published articles, but depending on the topic other databases may contain articles that are not indexed in PubMed. For clinical trials, the Cochrane Library's Controlled Trials Registry is a valuable source for comprehensive searches.

Bibliographic databases are likely to become more inclusive and even larger in the future. However, electronic search strategies currently fail to identify all pertinent studies. Sensitive strategies will identify a high proportion of relevant literature but at the cost of manually screening through many irrelevant articles. Subject-specific databases, such as BIOSIS, CINAHL, and PsychLit, should be searched when appropriate.

Other methods for identifying information include manually searching through relevant journals, screening reference lists and trial registries, perusal of available trial registries, FDA files in public view or after special request, and personally contacting pharmaceutical and medical device companies, as well as colleagues and researchers who may be aware of other published or unpublished studies. Prospective registration of trials has been adopted since 2004 (DeAngelis et al., 2004) and trial registries may offer an increasingly relevant reference to identify trials that have been completed and others that are ongoing. Registration is increasing and the World Health Organization (WHO) effort brings together the largest current registries that have over 50 000 current and completed studies (Zarin et al., 2007). However, not all trials are being registered as of now, and registration has not been adopted for other types of research where meta-analysis may be applied.

Study Selection

Identified studies and data sets should be evaluated according to a prespecified protocol using parameters defined in the PICO approach discussed earlier. Failure to adhere to a well-defined protocol may produce misleading results, especially if the exclusion of a relevant study or the inclusion of an inappropriate study leads to considerable alteration of the summary estimates. Selection of studies based on availability of reported data for a specific outcome may lead to bias due to selective outcome reporting. Meta-analysts should make efforts to obtain additional information on the relevant outcomes from the primary investigators in these circumstances.

Quality Assessment of the Original Studies

The studies included in a meta-analysis must ideally have sufficient internal validity to produce reliable results. However, large, well-conducted studies with absolutely no biases are not the norm in biomedical research. Issues related to the study quality should be incorporated into the meta-analysis and explored as potential sources of heterogeneity or bias. Sometimes, poor quality may emanate from investigators, sponsors, or other people involved in a study who are aware of these poor choices, but nevertheless they implement them. The typical motive is to inflate treatment effects, and poor quality usually means also a shift in the results in one specific direction. Quality may also be poor due to lack of knowledge and familiarity with research methods. These quality deficits may also be a surrogate of other deficits in the design, conduct, and analysis of a study. In this case, the

effect sizes may be affected in either direction, and actually it may be more common to get deflated rather than inflated effect sizes. Admittedly, separating conflicted knowledge from ignorance is not always easy.

Assessing the quality of a study can sometimes be difficult because it can be inferred only from published information and the relevant information may be poorly reported or unavailable. Many quality scales are circulating in the literature for appraising the reports of primary studies. However, the validity of the use of any quality scales has been questioned (Juni et al., 1999); occasionally, different quality scales can result in different conclusions. Summary scores are popular in the literature but should generally be avoided since they can be misleading. Lack of one quality item is not equivalent to lack of a different one and the composite effects of multiple quality deficits are hard to predict. Whereas early empirical investigations proposed that studies that lack allocation concealment and double-blinding tend to report larger effect sizes, subsequent data suggest that this is not necessarily the case and the effects of quality deficits may vary on a case-by-case basis. Moreover, reported quality is only a surrogate of the true quality of a study, for example, a study may have done something properly but this may not be reported and vice versa. In all, it is prudent to record carefully information on aspects of the design and conduct of studies that are considered as potentially important. Their impact on the results should be examined separately and on a case-by-case basis, without using summary scores. The situation with quality scoring is even more confusing in the observational studies literature and is further compounded by the lack of reporting standards for most observational research until recently.

Statistical Methods: Heterogeneity

There is a widespread misconception that the goal of meta-analyses is to force heterogeneous results from individual studies into a single estimate. Although obtaining a single treatment effect may be appropriate in many circumstances, a more interesting application of meta-analysis is to explore heterogeneity among different trials and to understand possible reasons for these differences. There can be two sources of variability that explain the heterogeneity in a set of studies in a meta-analysis. One of them is the variability due to sampling error, also named within-study variability. The other source of heterogeneity is the between-study variability, which can appear in a meta-analysis when there is true heterogeneity among the population effect sizes estimated by the individual studies. The between-study variability is due to the influence of an indeterminate number of characteristics that vary among the studies, including the characteristics of the samples, variations in the treatment, and variations in the design quality, as well as biases that may affect single studies or the field at large.

The test most commonly used for heterogeneity is the Q statistic, which is based on the chi-square distribution. The Q statistic tends to be insensitive, so significance is claimed at $P < 0.10$, but this does not solve the problem that it still has low power when there are few studies (<20). Conversely, it may have excessive power to detect negligible variability with a high number of studies. Another strategy for quantifying heterogeneity in a meta-analysis consists of estimating the between-study variance. The between-study variance reflects how much the true population effect sizes estimated in the single studies of a meta-analysis differ. The between-study variance depends on the particular effect metric used in a meta-analysis; it is not possible to compare values estimated from meta-analyses that have used different effect-size indices.

The I^2 index of inconsistency is also very popular (Higgins *et al.*, 2002, 2003). The I^2 index can be interpreted as the percentage of the total variability in a set of effect sizes due to true heterogeneity (between-study variability). For example, a meta-analysis with $I^2 = 0$ means that all variability in effect size estimates is due to sampling error within studies. However, a meta-analysis with $I^2 = 50$ means that half of the total variability among effect sizes is caused not by sampling error but by true heterogeneity between studies. With some simplification, percentages of 0–25%, 25–50%, 50–75%, and >75% reflect low, medium, large, and very large inconsistency, respectively (**Table 1**).

An advantage of I^2 is that it is directly comparable across meta-analyses with different numbers of studies and different effect metrics. In this regard, the I^2 index has important advantages with respect to the Q test.

On one hand, it is easily interpretable, because it is a percentage and does not depend on the degrees of freedom. Another advantage is that it provides a way of assessing the magnitude of the heterogeneity in a meta-analysis, whereas the Q test reports about the statistical significance of the homogeneity hypothesis. On the other hand, the confidence interval around I^2 is typically very large when the number of studies is small. With a small number of studies ($k < 20$), both the I^2 index and Q test should be interpreted cautiously (Huedo-Medina *et al.*, 2006).

Statistical Methods: Combining Binary and Dichotomous Data

To summarize the data, each study is given a weight that depends on the precision of its results. The weight is generally estimated as the inverse of the variance of the treatment effect in each study that has two components: the variance of the individual study (the within-study variance) and the variance between different studies (the between-study variance). The simplest approach to thinking about combining different results is to assume that all studies have approximated the same fixed truth and that differences among the observed treatment effects are only the result of chance. In this case, the between-study variance is assumed to be zero, and the calculations are performed with what are called fixed effects models. Fixed effects models are exemplified by the Mantel-Haenszel method and the Peto method in the case of dichotomous data.

In contrast, if the truth itself is not fixed but is believed to vary within a range of values, then each study can be seen as addressing a different true treatment effect, and these treatment effects derive from a distribution of truths

Table 1   Statistical tests for assessing heterogeneity

Statistics	Formula
Q	$$\sum w_i(\Theta_i - \hat{\Theta}_{MH})^2$$
	$$\max\left\{[Q - (k-1)]/\left[\sum w_i - \left(\sum(w_i^2)\right)/\sum w_i\right], 0\right\}$$
$\hat{\tau}^2$	$[Q - (k-1)]/\left[\sum w_i - \left(\sum(w_i^2)\right)/\sum w_i\right]$ for $Q > (k-1)$
	0 for $Q \leq (k-1)$
I^2	$[[Q-(k-1)]/Q] \times 100\%$ for $Q > (k-1)$
	0 for $Q \leq (k-1)$
H^2	$Q/(k-1)$

w_i, weight; Θ: log odds ratio, log relative risk, or risk difference; k, number of studies.

with a variance equal to the between-study variance. In this case, calculations are performed with random effects models, which add the between-study variance to the within-study variance of each study. The most commonly used random effects model is that proposed by DerSimonian and Laird (**Table 2**). More sophisticated, fully Bayesian approaches may also be used to calculate the between-study variance. Fixed and random effects methods have also been developed for continuous outcomes (Hedges and Olkin, 1985).

When the results of the combined studies are significantly heterogeneous or anticipated to be heterogeneous, the fixed effects models are counterintuitive and should be avoided. Conversely, in the absence of between-study heterogeneity, fixed and random effects estimates are identical. Usually, fixed and random effects estimates are similar, but major differences can occur occasionally. In terms of precision, random effects provide larger confidence intervals when heterogeneity is present because between-trial uncertainty is introduced. Compared to the DerSimonian and Laird estimates, fully Bayesian methods may sometimes result in even wider confidence intervals.

Generally, Mantel-Haenszel estimates work well even with small numbers, whereas random effects estimates are unstable. The Peto model may be associated with large bias when the data are unbalanced. Several easy-to-use software programs to combine data have become available. However, the informed researcher should be aware of the preceding caveats and should understand which formulas the software uses.

Bias

Even comprehensive searches of the published literature and all other sources of available data may not produce an unbiased sample of studies when conducting a meta-analysis. Research with statistically significant results is potentially more likely to be submitted, published, or published more rapidly than work with null or nonsignificant results. A meta-analysis of only the identified published studies may lead to an overoptimistic conclusion. This problem is known as publication bias.

Table 2 Statistical methods for fixed- and random-effects model

		Method	Effect size	Weight
Fixed effects model	Binary outcomes	Mantel-Haenszel	$\hat{\Theta}_{MH} = \dfrac{\sum w_i \Theta_i}{\sum w_i}$ Effect size: odds ratio, risk ratio, or risk difference	$w_i = b_i c_i / N_i$ (effect size: odds ratio) $w_i = [c_i/(a_i+b_i)]/N_i$ (effect size: risk ratio) $w_i = n_{1i} n_{2i}/N_i$ (effect size: risk difference)
		Peto's Assumption Free Method	$\hat{OR}_{Peto} = \exp\left\{ \sum w_i \ln(\hat{OR}_i) / \sum w_i \right\}$ Effect size: odds ratio	hypergeometric variance, v_i
	Continuous outcomes	Inverse variance	$\hat{\Theta}_{IV} = \dfrac{\sum w_i \Theta_i}{\sum w_i}$ Effect size: standardized mean difference, or weighted mean difference	$w_i = 1/se(\hat{\Theta}_i)^2$
Random effects model	Binary and continuous outcomes	DerSimonian and Laird	$\hat{\Theta}_{DL} = \left(\sum w_i \Theta_i \right) / \left(\sum w_i \right)$ Effect size: Mantel-Haenszel or the inverse variance estimate	$w_i = 1/se(\hat{\Theta}_i)^2 + \tau^2$

w_i, weight; Θ: log odds ratio, log relative risk, risk difference, standardized mean difference, or weighted mean difference; b_i, intervention subjects without event; c_i, control subjects with event; N_i, total number of study subjects; a_i, intervention subjects with event; n_{1i}, number of subjects in intervention group; n_{2i}, number of subjects in control group; se, standard error; d_i, control subjects without event.

Hypergeometric variance, $v_i = [n_{1i} n_{2i}(a_i + c_i)(b_i + d_i)]/[N_i^2(N_i - 1)]$.

For weighted mean difference, $se = \sqrt{se_{1i}^2/n_{1i} + se_{2i}^2/n_{2i}}$.

Between study variability, $\hat{\tau}^2 = \max\left\{ [Q - (k-1)] / \left[\sum w_i - \left(\sum(w_i^2) \right) / \sum w_i \right], 0 \right\}$.

Funnel plot asymmetry has been proposed as a method to assess the potential for publication bias. Small studies have greater variation in their estimation of the treatment effect and will be found to have more scattering around the mean effect, compared to the larger studies. In a funnel plot, the weight of each study, the sample size, or the inverse of the variance is plotted against the size of its treatment effect in a meta-analysis. This plot should be shaped like an inverted funnel if there is no publication bias; asymmetric funnel plots may suggest publication bias. Nevertheless, there needs to be a range of studies with varying sizes for a funnel plot to be useful. Furthermore, a skewed funnel plot may be caused by factors other than publication bias such as the study quality, the different intensity of intervention, differences in underlying risk, choice of effect measure, and chance. Finally, funnel plot interpretation is subjective and is only an informal method. Funnel plots with plain visual interpretation should be abandoned. Formal statistical tests have also been described regarding funnel plot asymmetry, such as the rank correlation test by Begg and Mazumdar, the linear regression test suggested by Egger, and the more appropriate modified regression method (Peters *et al.*, 2006) as well as the trim and fill method (Duval *et al.*, 2000).

All these methods are based on certain assumptions that hold only in the minority of circumstances (Lau *et al.*, 2006). Empirical evaluations (Ioannidis *et al.*, 2007) suggest that in the vast majority of meta-analyses, these tests should not be applied, as they may yield misleading inferences. A very common misconception is to use these tests and conclude that no publication bias exists simply because the tests don't give a significant signal.

Besides clear-cut publication bias, time-lag bias may cause the delayed publication and dissemination of the least favorable negative results. While trials with formally statistically significant and those with nonsignificant results take the same time to complete – with certain exceptions – the latter trials are delayed publication after their completion (Ioannidis *et al.*, 1998). Another major source of bias is selective reporting of outcomes and analyses (Chan *et al.*, 2004): authors do publish the results of a study, but they selectively present the most favorable analyses and outcomes. This bias is also a major threat for the validity of meta-analysis. Conversely, meta-analysis offers a unique opportunity to examine the consistency of definitions and completeness of reporting of data for specific outcomes.

Language biases have also been described, including a Tower of Babel bias, in which authors selectively publish positive studies in English language journals but negative studies in their native language journals; and a reverse language bias, where studies from certain countries consistently report mostly positive results in their local literatures or even when they publish in the English language. In many medical disciplines, the non-English literature of randomized trials has never been large, is

shrinking even further, or may be of generally dubious quality. Before routinely committing to a specific approach, it would be useful to understand the contribution of different languages to the literature of the potential field.

In the world of nonrandomized evidence, the selective publication forces may be even more prominent. Significance-chasing is probably ubiquitous and may distort the evolving literature over time. A test has been proposed (Ioannidis and Trikalinos, 2007) that tries to evaluate the composite of both publication bias and selective outcome and analysis reporting bias that may result in an excess of statistically significant findings in a specific scientific field. In the absence of study and protocol registration, these biases may be very difficult to address.

Meta-Regression

Meta-regression investigates whether particular covariates (potential effect modifiers) explain any of the heterogeneity of treatment effects between studies. It is not reasonable to assume that all of the heterogeneity is explained, and the possibility of residual heterogeneity must be acknowledged in the statistical analysis. The appropriate analysis is therefore random effects rather than fixed effect meta-regression. Estimating the residual between-study variance is somewhat problematic. The estimate is usually imprecise because it is based on a rather limited number of trials. Different authors have advocated different estimates, for example, empirical Bayes or restricted maximum likelihood estimates. Moreover, conventional random effects methods ignore the imprecision in the between-trial variance estimate. One way to allow for the imprecision is to adopt a Bayesian approach, using, for example, noninformative priors. Whereas this is preferable in principle, especially when the number of trials is small or when the between-trial variance is estimated as zero, the resulting widening of the confidence intervals is rather slight in most practical examples.

Meta-regression analysis uses the individual study as the unit of observation in assessing the relationship between the magnitude of the treatment effect and different predictors. Predictors may be study-specific (e.g., the dose or route of administration of a drug) or ecological variables in which a mean or median value is taken as characteristic of the study group of patients (e.g., mean age or percentage of men or the percentage of participants with an event in the control group [baseline risk]). Ecological meta-regressions may suffer from the ecological fallacy, when the association seen with a group mean does not reflect the association for individual study participants. Given that most meta-analyses in the literature to date have included relatively few studies, it is not unfair to say that most meta-regressions have been misapplied on thin data.

Cumulative Meta-Analysis and Recursive Cumulative Meta-Analysis

The results of a meta-analysis may be seen as a sequential addition of data as more studies appear in a given order, typically chronological. Cumulative meta-analysis addresses the impact of new studies on prior summary estimates, whereas recursive cumulative meta-analysis models the changes in the cumulative treatment effect as a result of new studies, updating of old ones, or retrieval of unpublished ones. Recursive cumulative meta-analysis may be used while a comprehensive meta-analysis is being performed to investigate and present the results as a process of accumulation of missing, updated, and new information.

Effect sizes may fluctuate over time as more evidence appears in the published literature on the same question. Fluctuations of effect size as they may be presented in recursive cumulative meta-analysis may be only an issue of the uncertainty surrounding the summary effect. This uncertainty goes beyond what is conveyed typically by the 95% confidence intervals of a summary estimate by a traditional random effects meta-analysis model. Empirical data suggest that even when we have accumulated data on 2000 randomized subjects, the next trial may change the summary relative risk by about 25% (Trikalinos *et al.*, 2004). Given that most effect sizes are relatively modest, uncertainty for the mere presence of a treatment effect is likely to exist even when several thousand subjects have been randomized. In the majority of clinically important questions, considerable uncertainty is the rule.

In addition, a more problematic type of fluctuation is when effect sizes change in the same direction as more evidence accumulates. In the most common scenario, the addition of more data tends to shrink the treatment effect. Whereas genuine heterogeneity may be operating in some of these cases, the most common explanation is that here we are dealing with biased early estimates of effect that get dissipated as better data gradually accumulate. Many early effects may disappear with more careful scrutiny and additional data. In the epidemiological literature, this phenomenon may be particularly prominent, and in discovery-oriented research with massive hypothesis testing it may be the rule rather than the exception.

Meta-Analysis of Individual Patient Data

Most of the published meta-analyses to date have used summary data from individual studies or subgroups thereof. Meta-analyses using individual patient data from all the pertinent studies are not new, but they represent still a minority. The meta-analysis of individual patient data provides several clear advantages, such as closer involvement of the participating investigators; the ability to verify, clean, standardize, and update the data collected within the included studies; the possibility of more detailed time-to-event analyses; the ability to generate individual-based multivariate models; and the chance to assess the effect of various covariates of interest at the individual patient level avoiding potential ecological fallacies inherent in summary data (Stewart *et al.*, 1995).

The disadvantages of this approach include the potential for retrieval bias when studies whose data are not retrievable are excluded; the potentially lower quality of updated data that have been accumulated after the end of the main follow-up period of a clinical study (e.g., extensive crossovers or incomplete information on many patients); and the time and effort required to obtain data from a multitude of investigators, especially on a retrospective basis. The first two reasons could theoretically make meta-analysis of individual patient data even less reliable than meta-analyses of published group data in some circumstances. Such studies should be encouraged, however, and may eventually become the commonly sought standard, especially with prospective meta-analyses.

Early reports have suggested that the estimates obtained by meta-analysis of individual patient data may occasionally differ from the estimates of conventional meta-analyses of the literature on the same topic. Meta-analyses of individual-level data may then provide more conservative results than conventional meta-analyses. However, the extent and frequency of the discrepancies need to be evaluated in a larger number of examples.

Meta-Analysis of Diagnostic Test Studies

Diagnostic test results are often reported as a numerical quantity on a continuous scale, but are then used as a binary decision tool by defining a threshold above which the test result is positive and below which it is negative. Results may then be summarized in a 2×2 table reflecting the agreement between the test result and the disease state as the number of true positives, false positives, true negatives, and false negatives. Changing this threshold may change the sensitivity and specificity of the test. Test performance is described by the receiver operating characteristic (ROC) curve, which displays the true positive rate (sensitivity) on the vertical axis versus false positive rate (1-specificity) on the horizontal axis for all possible thresholds. This fundamental bivariate structure poses a challenge for constructing a single number summary to describe test performance.

Common single number measures used to describe test performance include accuracy, sensitivity, specificity, positive predictive value, negative predictive value, positive likelihood ratio, negative likelihood ratio, odds ratio, and area under the curve. Only the last four combine information about both sensitivity and specificity. This can be illustrated by the different ROC curves that each measure implies. On one hand, a constant sensitivity implies a horizontal line, a constant specificity implies a vertical line, and a constant likelihood ratio also implies a linear relationship between sensitivity and specificity. The odds ratio, on the other, describes a curve symmetric about the line where sensitivity equals specificity (**Table 3**).

When combining data from several diagnostic tests, the first step should be to plot the sensitivity–specificity pairs in each study on one graph. Because the plot may suggest a curvilinear relationship, the use of summary sensitivity, specificity, or likelihood ratio measures may be inadequate. Combining both sensitivity and specificity independently is approximately appropriate if we believe the test operates at a certain representative combination of sensitivity and specificity. This is usually an oversimplification. Nevertheless, because these summary measures are either proportions or ratios of proportions and so are easily combined using standard meta-analytic techniques, many diagnostic test meta-analyses have reported them. If curvilinearity is detected, it is better instead to summarize with the diagnostic odds ratio using standard methods for combining odds ratios.

The odds ratio is nevertheless still misleading, however, if the ROC curve suggests asymmetry about the line of equal sensitivity and specificity. In this case, the decrease in sensitivity corresponding to increased specificity differs between high and low sensitivity settings. An SROC curve does allow for such asymmetry. It models the linear relationship between the odds ratio and the probability of a positive test and then reexpresses this in terms of the ROC curve. It reduces to the odds ratio if the regression slope is zero so that the odds ratio is invariant to the test positivity threshold. In doing so, however, it treats the observed odds ratios as random effects, but the test positive probabilities as fixed effects. Thus, the resulting summary measure fails to incorporate all the uncertainty in the observed test results. Recently, some analysts have used bivariate random effects models to capture the randomness in both sensitivity and specificity simultaneously (Oei *et al.*, 2003).

In diagnostic studies heterogeneity in sensitivity and specificity can result from a multitude of causes related to definitions of the test and reference standards, operating characteristics of the test, methods of data collection, and patient characteristics. Covariates may be introduced into a regression with any test performance measure as the dependent variable. To date, the most common approach to meta-regression has been to insert covariates into the SROC regression allowing the odds ratio to vary by study characteristics other than test positivity. This implies that performance is described, not by one but by multiple ROC curves.

Meta-Analysis of Observational Studies

Theoretically, randomized controlled trials are susceptible to fewer biases than nonrandomized observational studies in evaluating the efficacy of therapeutic and preventive interventions. However, this does not mean that observational studies are always worse or they lead to necessarily different estimates. For many research questions, data from observational studies may outweigh data from randomized trials, or no data may exist from randomized trials at all. The methods to combine observational data sets follow the same principles as those outlined above for randomized trials. However, more attention is required to the appraisal of biases in single studies and in the field at large – and more conservative interpretation of the summary results is warranted – to avoid falling into the trap of spurious excessive precision offered by the data synthesis. Empirical studies have not agreed on how often the results of randomized trials and observational studies disagree with each other, but one should be aware that

Table 3 Metrics of test performance

Metric	Definition	Advantages	Disadvantages
Accuracy	$(TP + TN)/N$	Intuitive	Depends on prevalence
Sensitivity	TP/N_D	Does not depend on prevalence	Only applies to diseased
Specificity	TN/N_W	Does not depend on prevalence	Only applies to nondiseased
Predictive value positive	TP/N_P	Clinical relevance	Depends on prevalence
Predictive value negative	TN/N_N	Clinical relevance	Depends on prevalence
Likelihood ratio positive	$(TP/N_D)/(FP/N_W)$	Does not depend on prevalence	Only applies to positive tests
Likelihood ratio negative	$(FN/N_D)/(TN/N_W)$	Does not depend on prevalence	Only applies to negative tests
Odds ratio	$TP*TN/FN*FP$	Does not depend on prevalence; combines sensitivity and specificity	Values FP and FN errors equally; not intuitive
Area under curve	area under ROC curve	Does not depend on prevalence; combines sensitivity and specificity	Lack of clinical interpretation

TP, true positive; TN, true negative; FP, false positive; FN, false negative; N, sample size; N_D, TP + FN; N_W, TN + FP; N_P, TP + FP; N_N, TN + FN. Reproduced from Tatsioni A, Zarin DA, Aronson N, Samson DJ, Flamm CR, Schmid C, and Lau J (2005) Challenges in systematic reviews of diagnostic technologies. *Annals of Internal Medicine* 142: 1048–1055.

major disagreements may often be missed due to limited data on one or both types of evidence.

For many important questions in which randomized studies are entirely impossible, for example, the study of harmful exposures and lifestyle factors, or the study of genetic risk factors, meta-analysis of observational studies has been established as a prime method to summarize data from diverse investigators. The same principles and caveats apply to these settings as well.

Quality and Reporting of Meta-Analyses

A large number of meta-analyses are published each year and their overall quality is a concern. Empirical evidence suggests that procedures in meta-analyses are often inadequately reported, and methodological deficiencies that may limit the validity of conclusions are also present (Fishbain *et al.*, 2000; Moher *et al.*, 2007). In an effort to address standards for improving the quality of reporting of meta-analyses of clinical randomized controlled trials, the Quality of Reporting of Meta-Analyses (QUOROM) checklist was published in 1999 based on a conference that was held in October 1996 (Moher *et al.*, 1999). Given the many changes that have happened in the field in the last decade, a new version of QUOROM (called PRISMA) is in the final stages of preparation as this article goes to press. A respective statement for meta-analysis of observational studies (MOOSE, or Meta-Analysis of Observational Studies in Epidemiology) was published in 2000 (Stroup *et al.*, 2000), but may also need updating in the near future. Reporting of meta-analyses of observational studies has also been shown to have common major deficits (Attia *et al.*, 2003).

See also: Measurement and Modeling of Health-Related Quality of Life.

Citations

Attia J, Thakkinstian A, and D'Este C (2003) Meta-analyses of molecular association studies: methodologic lessons for genetic epidemiology. *Journal of Clinical Epidemiology* 56: 297–303.

Chan AW, Hrobjartsson A, Haahr MT, Gotzsche PC, and Altman DG (2004) Empirical evidence for selective reporting of outcomes in randomized trials: Comparison of protocols to published articles. *Journal of the American Medical Association* 291: 2457–2465.

DeAngelis CD, Drazen JM, Frizelle FA, *et al.* (2004) International Committee of Medical Journal Editors. Clinical trial registration: A statement from the International Committee of Medical Journal Editors. *Journal of the American Medical Association* 292: 1363–1364.

Duval S and Tweedie R (2000) Trim and fill: A simple funnel-plot-based method of testing and adjusting for publication bias in meta-analysis. *Biometrics* 56: 455–463.

Fishbain D, Cutler R, Rosomoff HL, and Rosomoff RS (2000) What is the quality of the implemented meta-analytic procedures in chronic pain treatment meta-analysis? *The Clinical Journal of Pain* 16: 73–85.

Hedges LV and Olkin I (1985) *Statistical Methods for Meta-Analysis.* Orlando, FL: Academic Press.

Higgins JP and Thompson SG (2002) Quantifying heterogeneity in a meta-analysis. *Statistics in Medicine* 21: 1539–1558.

Higgins JP, Thompson SG, Deeks JJ, and Altman DG (2003) Measuring inconsistency in meta-analyses. *British Medical Journal* 327: 557–560.

Huedo-Medina TB, Sanchez-Meca J, Marin-Martinez F, and Botella J (2006) Assessing heterogeneity in meta-analysis: Q statistic or I2 index? *Psychological Methods* 11: 193–206.

Ioannidis JPA, Cappelleri JC, and Lau J (1998) Issues in comparisons between meta-analyses and large trials. *Journal of the American Medical Association* 279: 1089–1093.

Ioannidis JP and Trikalinos TA (2007) The appropriateness of asymmetry tests for publication bias in meta-analyses: a large survey. *Canadian Medical Association Journal* 176: 1091–1096.

Ioannidis JP and Trikalinos TA (2007) An exploratory test for an excess of significant findings. *Clinical Trials* 4: 245–253.

Juni P, Witschi A, Bloch R, and Egger M (1999) The hazards of scoring the quality of clinical trials for meta-analysis. *Journal of the American Medical Association* 282: 1054–1060.

Lau J, Ioannidis JP, Terrin N, Schmid CH, and Olkin I (2006) The case of the misleading funnel plot. *British Medical Journal* 333: 597–600.

Moher D, Cook D, Eastwood S, *et al.* (1999) Improving the quality of reports of meta-analysis of randomized controlled trials: The QUOROM statement. *The Lancet* 354: 1896–1900.

Moher D, Tetzlaff J, Tricco AC, Sampson M, and Altman DG (2007) Epidemiology and reports characteristics of systematic reviews. *Public Library of Science Medicine* 4: e78.

Oei EHG, Nikken JJ, Verstignen ACM, Ginai AZ, and Hunink MGM (2003) MR imaging of the minisci and cruciate ligaments: A systematic review. *Radiology* 226: 837–848.

Peters JL, Sutton AJ, Jones DR, Abrams KR, and Rushton L (2006) Comparison of two methods to detect publication bias in meta-analysis. *Journal of the American Medical Association* 295: 676–680.

Stewart LA and Clarke MJ (1995) Practical methodology of meta-analyses (overviews) using updated individual patient data. Cochrane Working Group. *Statistics in Medicine* 14: 2057–2079.

Stroup DF, Berlin JA, Morton SC, *et al.* (2000) Meta-analysis of observational studies in epidemiology: A proposal for reporting. Meta-analysis of Observational Studies in Epidemiology (MOOSE) group. *Journal of the American Medical Association* 283: 2008–2012.

Trikalinos TA, Churchill R, Ferri M, *et al.* (2004) Effect sizes in cumulative meta-analyses of mental health randomized trials evolved over time. EU-PSI project. *Journal of Clinical Epidemiology* 57: 1124–1130.

Zarin DA, Ide NC, Tse T, *et al.* (2007) Issues in the registration of clinical trials. *Journal of the American Medical Association* 297: 2112–2120.

Further Reading

Cook DJ, Mulrow CD, and Haynes RB (1998) *Systematic Reviews.* Philadelphia, PA: American College of Physicians.

Cooper H and Hedges LV (1993) *The Handbook of Research Synthesis.* New York: Russell Sage Foundation.

Egger M, Davey Smith G, and Altman DG (2001) *Systematic Reviews in Health Care. Meta-Analysis in Context,* 2nd edn. London: BMJ Books.

Fleiss JL (1993) The statistical basis of meta-analysis. *Statistical Methods in Medical Research* 2: 121–145.

Ioannidis JP, Ntzani EE, Trikalinos TA, and Contopoulos-Ioannidis DG (2001) Replication validity of genetic association studies. *Nature Genetics* 29: 306–309.

Moses LE, Shapiro D, and Littenberg B (1993) Combining independent studies of a diagnostic test into a summary ROC curve: Data-analytic approaches and some additional considerations. *Statistics in Medicine* 12: 1293–1316.

Petitti DB (1999) *Meta-Analysis, Decision Analysis, and Cost-Effectiveness Analysis: Methods for Quantitative Synthesis in Medicine.* New York: Oxford University Press.

Rothstein H, Sutton AJ, and Borenstein M (2005) *Publication Bias in Meta-Analysis: Prevention, Assessment and Adjustments.* New York: John Wiley.

Rutter CM and Gatsonis CA (2001) A hierarchical regression approach to meta-analysis of diagnostic test accuracy evaluations. *Statistics in Medicine* 20: 2865–2884.

Sutton AJ (2000) *Methods for Meta-Analysis in Medical Research.* New York: John Wiley.

Relevant Websites

http://www.bmj.com/collections/ma.htm — BMJ collections. Meta-analysis: Education and Debate.

http://www.cochrane.org — The Cochrane Collaboration.

http://www.dhe.med.u.org — Department of Hygiene and Edidemiology, University of Ioannia Medical School.

SECTION 6
ETHICAL ISSUES

Ethics of Public Health Research

H A Taylor, R R Faden, and N E Kass, Johns Hopkins University, Baltimore, MD, USA
S Johnson, Albany Medical College, Albany, NY, USA

Introduction

Public health research often involves human subjects. Although some authors have argued that there are significant moral differences between public health research and public health practice (Human Research Protection Office, 1999; National Bioethics Advisory Commission, 2001), few have claimed that public health research presents unique ethical issues from other types of human subjects research. However, a number of examples in the recent history of research ethics, including the Kennedy Krieger Lead Abatement Study (Institute of Medicine, 2005) and the EPA's Children's Environmental Exposure Research Study (CHEERS) (Stokstad, 2004) suggest that, at very least, public health research may bring into sharper focus unresolved issues in the ethics of human research.

Public health research typically has been contrasted with public health practice according to criteria such as performance authority, intent to publish, the funding source, data collection methods, study design or investigator–participant relationship (Bellin and Dubler, 2001; Hodge, 2004). Definitions of public health research have been slow to develop and, it has been suggested, are largely unsatisfying attempts to resolve ethical problems through categorization and redefinition (Fairchild and Bayer, 2004).

In this article, we focus on one type of public health research involving human subjects. Specifically, we consider here the ethics of primary prevention research in which the overall goal is to contribute to our understanding of how to prevent the onset of disease or injury within an otherwise healthy population. In this respect, we focus on population-based research that often involves a specified group or community. The more particular objective of such research may be to characterize the relative health status or health risks of a population (or subgroups within a population), with an eye toward developing a population-based intervention to prevent the onset of disease or injury or to test the effectiveness of a particular population-based intervention.

In some public health research, study populations are referred to as communities. The term community can be defined or circumscribed in many different ways. It is important for public health researchers who conduct community-level research to clearly and carefully define the community within which or about which they will conduct their research. For example, it is meaningful to speak of geographically bounded communities, such as the residents of Soweto, of sociocultural communities, such as Latin American immigrants, and of communities defined by a particular constellation of risk factors, such as injection drug users. Although it is often important for public health researchers to define a population as a community, identifying individuals who can legitimately speak on behalf of the community is a challenge. It may not be possible to find a group of individuals who can speak for a community, much less an entire population under study.

To refine our focus further, the kind of population-based, primary prevention public health research of interest to us needs to be distinguished from standard clinical research. We conceptualize standard clinical research as human subjects research conducted to improve the capacity to treat or cure an active disease or medical condition, or the symptoms of a disease or medical condition (secondary or tertiary prevention of disease). Although the current system of ethical oversight over the conduct of research involving human subjects is in certain respects flawed, its ethical framework is better suited to clinical research than to primary prevention research in public health (National Commission for the Protection of Human Subjects of Biomedical and Behavioral Research, 1979; US Department of Health and Human Services, 2001). The purpose of this article is not to reach definitional clarity about these categories of human research but to highlight the ethical issues related to public health research that traditional human participant regulations and guidelines have not adequately addressed, presumably because the regulations were not written with this type of research in mind. In particular, we argue that the current regulatory framework does not provide adequate moral guidance for investigators conducting primary prevention research in community settings.

Key Ethical Issues

In clinical research, the primary focus of moral attention is the relationship between individual patient-subjects and investigators who are conducting the research. Often these investigators are physicians and nurses who must navigate the complex moral territory of conflicting duties to the medical interests of their patient-subjects and to the scientific objectives of the research (Beauchamp and Childress, 2001). The object of study in clinical research is generally a particular disease state or process. Potential patient-subjects are selected because they have characteristics that are relevant to the disease process under study, not because they are members of a particular community. Thus, the structure of clinical research does not generally create a relational connection between the investigator and any specific community. By contrast, in population-based public health research investigators often have a relationship with a particular community as well as with the individual participants in their research. The object of study is often an entire community at risk of a poor health outcome. When this is the case, arguably, the community itself is a subject of the research. Assuming communities as well as individuals have interests, and perhaps even rights, investigators studying communities should consider these interests and the correlative responsibilities they generate in thinking through the ethics of their research. Specifically, at least three possible kinds of duties to communities need to be considered: The duty to respect the community, the duty not to harm the community, and whether a duty to benefit the community exists.

Duty to Respect the Community

Respect for persons, as one of the three moral principles enshrined in the Belmont Report, is widely accepted as central to the ethics of research involving human subjects (National Commission for the Protection of Human Subjects of Biomedical and Behavioral Research, 1979). However, respect is owed not only to identifiable persons, but also to a wide range of other entities including, where relevant, groups and communities. We can, for example, speak meaningfully of respecting a religious group or a village. The duty to respect the community under study in a public health research project can create a spectrum of obligations for investigators at all phases of research (Popay and Williams, 1996; Chen *et al.*, 2006). For example, some argue that researchers ought to engage the community to inform and consult them about the proposed research and listen to community concerns (Grady, 1995; Wiejer and Emauel, 2000; Israel *et al.*, 2001; Dickert and Sugarman, 2005). Others argue that respectful engagement means that communities ought to be given every opportunity to participate in the development of research, but also requires being respectful of both communities' and individuals' rights not to participate during the course of the study (Wallerstein *et al.*, 2005).

In practice, community engagement can take many forms. Public health researchers can, for example, work with a community to tailor the research agenda to the communities' own health interests and priorities. This approach requires an investment of time and energy and a level of methodological and scientific flexibility that is often beyond most public health investigators. Alternatively, public health researchers can approach a community with an interest in conducting research in a particular area and work with the community to help shape the specifics of the initiative.

For example, a public health researcher interested in developing and testing interventions to prevent childhood injuries could work with the community to specify which childhood injuries are of greatest concern and should be research priorities. Any approach that involves some level of community engagement obviously relies on community cooperation. A community disinterested in being the subjects of public health research or in a particular research proposal can refuse the offer to collaborate which in itself is an opportunity to evidence respect for the community.

In order to engage and inform at the community level, the investigator will have to consider both how best to access the community and how best to deliver information about the planned research. A first step may be to identify and meet with individuals considered leaders, elders, or representatives; stakeholders who can legitimately speak on behalf of some members of the potential study population to seek their support and advice. Admittedly, what is harder is figuring out whether a second step is in order. Do investigators have a responsibility to seek input from members of the community that are not identified as designated stakeholders? In addition to any community-based approach to orient potential subjects to the study, depending on the design of the research, individual consent ought to be obtained as well.

When the entire community rather than individuals within a community is the target of research, there may be little or no role for individual informed consent. For example, a public health investigator may want to assess the effectiveness of a media campaign to increase seat belt use. The study may include randomizing at the community level – two neighborhoods exposed to radio and billboard ads, two other neighborhoods included as control sites. The investigator could measure the impact of the intervention by surveying individuals in the community about their seat belt behavior, in which case the investigator would need to solicit the individual informed consent of each person surveyed regardless of how fully the community endorses the research. Alternatively, the investigator could measure impact by observing seat belt use at random intersections or by accessing injury surveillance records; in these cases she would not have an obligation to obtain individual informed consent.

If the investigator chooses the design in which individual informed consent is not required, this does not mean she is always relieved of a moral obligation to inform the public of her plans and notify them of her presence in the community (e.g., she could utilize media outlets or other methods to reach the study population). As a general rule, investigators conducting research in a defined community ought to, at a minimum, inform the public of their plans and presence. The investigator's obligation to engage the community beyond mere disclosure increases as the potential social harm to the community increases. The absence of community engagement and information sharing in advance of such a study that does result in social harm may compromise the trust the community has in the research enterprise more generally.

In some cases not disclosing the intent of the research in advance may be a necessary component of the chosen research design. While in general deception in research ought to be avoided, it may be morally acceptable to withhold information from the population under certain circumstances, especially when the intent of the research is to improve the public's health and the potential risks to individuals or to the community are small. The seat belt study example above presents no reputational, social, or economic risk to the neighborhoods targeted; therefore the investigator will likely not be required by an IRB to obtain informed consent from each individual in the population to be studied but ought to engage and inform the community of the research to be conducted. In addition, the investigator may not be morally obligated to inform the population of her plan and presence in the community in advance if she can justify the need to withhold information from her subject (the community) in order to obtain a scientifically valid result from her research. In this example, if the community within which seat belt use is to be monitored is told in advance of the intent of the research, the investigators may fail to get an accurate assessment of routine seat belt use. Drivers on alert to observation may be more likely to buckle their belts. In those instances in which it is ethically acceptable to conduct community-based research without providing the community with information about the research, investigators have a special moral obligation to consider whether the research would otherwise be acceptable to the community in which it will be conducted. If, on the other hand, the proposed research may expose the community to reputational, social, or economic risk, the investigator ought to engage and inform the community in advance.

At the conclusion of research, the results from a study ought to be shared with the community, particularly when the knowledge is actionable or interventions are available. This is yet another reason why it is better to err on the side of disclosure to the population. A community unaware of the research underway may be hesitant to embrace the findings of a project conducted without their knowledge.

Duty to Leave Community No Worse Off

Public health research often is justified in terms of potential benefits to a community-at-risk or society at large through findings that contribute to public health practice or policy. When public health investigators intend to conduct research that raises the prospect of harm to the community, they ought to consider such risks in advance and make every reasonable effort to minimize both the likelihood that the risks will materialize and the magnitude of the harm that might result. Public health investigators have a general duty not to set back the interests of others without acceptable offsetting benefits

(Beachamp and Childress, 2001; Kass, 2001; Childress *et al.*, 2002). Moreover, even if the overall balance of potential harms and benefits is favorable, wherever feasible researchers should seek to obtain the agreement of the community stakeholders whose interests are at risk of being harmed. In the ethics of clinical research, the focus of this general duty not to impose harm has been the identifiable research subject. There are certain kinds of public health research where it is not only the interests of research subjects but also the interests of entire communities that may be affected by either the conduct of the research or the research findings.

One example of such community-level harm is social stigma. A study meant to identify predictors of alcoholism among a Native American tribe or a study to measure the prevalence of injection drug use in an inner-city neighborhood may lead to social stigma, which may in turn lead to other community-level harms. A commercial developer, for example, may incorporate the results of either study in deliberations about the advisability of future economic investment. Moreover, when the research community consumes community resources, the very conduct of the research may set the community back as, for example, when a study set in a community hires day care workers to conduct interviews, thus leaving day care centers in the community understaffed.

Public health investigators should consider the possibility of community-based harms in advance of their research, disclose and discuss potential harms with the community wherever possible, and, most importantly, identify and implement strategies to minimize such harms. For example, if an individual enrolled in a randomized placebo-controlled trial of a novel HIV vaccine fails to understand that they may be randomized to a placebo or an intervention with less than 100% effectiveness, he or she may engage in behaviors that increase the likelihood of his or her own exposure to infection, believing that they are protected by their enrollment in the trial ('I have been vaccinated and am therefore protected from infection.'), and increase the exposure risk within their community (Stewart-Brown and Farmer, 1997). Because the behavior of the individual research subject has implications for the health of the community at large, the investigator has an obligation to consider these potential risks in advance of implementation and clearly inform the subject, and the community from which they have been recruited, about the risk of disinhibition as well as about how to minimize risks of infection to themselves and others.

Duty to Leave Community Better Off

That public health researchers have a general obligation to leave communities no worse off as a consequence of their research is likely to be uncontroversial. What is less clear is whether, or to what extent, public health researchers have any positive obligations to leave the communities in which they conduct their work better off after the research is completed. Some have argued that there is a duty to leave such individuals or communities better off, but that this duty is limited and dependent upon a number of factors in the investigator–participant relationship such as participant vulnerability, risk, the intensity and duration of the relationship, and dependence upon the investigator (Richardson and Belsky, 2004). The generally accepted rule in the conduct of clinical trials is that investigators have, at minimum, an obligation at the end of a trial that finds an intervention to be helpful to provide access to the intervention to those to whom it was not provided during the study (i.e., the group that received a placebo is provided with access to the successful intervention). In the context of conducting population-based research, the question becomes how expansive the investigators' obligation becomes. If, for example, the public health researcher finds that a community-based intervention is successful, does the obligation to provide access to the successful intervention extend beyond the control communities within which the study was conducted? The issue seems to arise most often when research is conducted in resource-poor settings (settings that indeed are the target of considerable public health investigation). A related question is whether leaving a population better off extends to interventions beyond the implementation of the successful intervention. In resource-poor contexts, there are likely many unmet public health needs such as access to clean water or condoms or other methods of birth control.

The extent to which the public health investigator has an ethical obligation to secure supplies or funds to provide access to such public health interventions is unclear. Some argue that communities ought to be given the right to negotiate with investigators in what way they would like to be left better off as a result of hosting a clinical trial. Participants in the 2001 Conference on Ethical Aspects of Conducting Research in Developing Countries (2004) argue that populations that host a trial ought to be able to negotiate what benefits are left behind. They argue that host communities ought to be given the power to choose to accept improved access to clean water in addition to or in lieu of broader access to the successful intervention or in exchange for hosting a trial that provides no direct benefit to the individuals enrolled or the community more generally. We argue that, at minimum, public health investigators should make every effort to ensure that a successful public health intervention continues to be available to those communities who participated in the research that established the intervention's effectiveness. In community research in which no intervention is being tested, there also may be circumstances when investigators are obligated to provide goods or services related to the public health problem under study. It remains an open question whether or under what conditions the fair benefits analysis is applicable to community-based public health research. For example, after a study of the impact of an intensive community health education campaign on

HIV transmission rates is completed, if the intervention is determined to be effective, should the investigators' obligations be limited to providing the community with the capacity to sustain the campaign or should the community be able to determine whether it would prefer the distribution of free condoms or the resources to dig a well?

A related debate has to do with the investigators' obligation to provide ancillary care to study participants. The currently accepted definition of ancillary care is "medical care for research participants beyond what is necessary to ensure scientific validity, to prevent study-related harms, or to redress study-related injuries" (Richardson and Belsky, 2004; Dickert et al., 2007). The prevailing view in the field of research ethics holds that researchers working in resource-limited settings have some limited duty to offer ancillary care (Richardson and Belsky, 2004). The current debate in the research ethics literature is about the extent of this limited duty and how best to put it into practice. Limits on this duty could be dictated by the influence the provision of ancillary care may have on the results of the study. That is, the provision of too much ancillary care may mask the efficacy of a particular intervention, resulting in the abandonment of an otherwise beneficial intervention.

The provision of ancillary care is a question often faced by investigators conducting clinical research in resource-poor settings. When investigating the efficacy of a new combination of drugs for HIV for example, investigators are likely to encounter subjects with medical care needs beyond what might be required either scientifically or for patient safety given their subjects' compromised immune status. Public health investigators, because they often enroll thousands of subjects, may be less likely to encounter acute medical needs but are likely to encounter an overwhelming amount of minor health needs. In some settings, public health researchers may be able to exhaust their limited duty to provide ancillary care by arranging for referrals to local health centers where subjects will receive the local standard of care for their condition. In other settings, the public health investigator may not be able to exhaust this limited duty so easily. At least two issues require further thought and deliberation: One, whether it is ethical for public health researchers to conduct research in settings where access to medical care is absent and two, whether sponsors of research in such settings have a limited duty to provide funds to allow for investigators to provide necessary medical care beyond the local standard of care.

Conclusion

The goal of this article was to highlight aspects of public health research that require public health investigators to consider their moral relation to the community, and not only to the individual research participant. While the consideration of community as research subject may not be unique to public health research, the community as potential research subject is at the core of population-based prevention research and therefore at the core of the ethics of public health research.

See also: Codes of Ethics in Public Health.

Citations

Amoroso PJ and Middaugh JP (2003) Research vs. public health practice: When does a study require IRB review? *Preventive Medicine* 36(2): 250–253.

Beauchamp T and Childress JF (2001) *Principles of Biomedical Ethics*, 5th edn. New York: Oxford University Press.

Bellin E and Dubler NN (2001) The quality improvement-research divide and the need for external oversight. *American Journal of Public Health* 91: 1512–1517.

Chen DT, Jone L, and Gelberg L (2006) Ethics of clinical research within a community-academic participatory framework. *Ethnicity and Disease* 16: S118–S135.

Childress JF, Faden RR, Gaare RD, *et al.* (2002) Public health ethics: Mapping the terrain. *Journal of Law, Medicine and Ethics* 30: 170–178.

Dickert N and Sugarman J (2005) Ethical goals of community consultation in research. *American Journal of Public Health* 95: 1123–1127.

Dickert N, DeRiemer K, Duffy PE, *et al.* (2007) Ancillary-care responsibilities in observational research: Two cases, two issues. *Lancet* 369(9564): 874–877.

Fairchild AL and Bayer R (2004) Ethics and the conduct of public health surveillance. *Science* 303: 631–632.

Grady C (1995) *The Search for an AIDS Vaccine: Ethical Issues in the Development and Testing of a Preventive HIV Vaccine.* Bloomington, IN: Indiana University Press.

Hodge JG and Gostin LO with the CTSE Advisory Committee (2004) *Public Health Practice vs. Research: A Report for Public Health Practitioners.* Council of State and Territorial Epidemiologists. http://www.cste.org/pdffiles/newpdffiles/CSTEPHResRptHodgeFinal.5.24.04.pdf.

Human Research Protection Office (1999) *Defining Public Health Research and Public Health Non-Research.* Atlanta, GA: Centers for Disease Control and Prevention.

Institute of Medicine (2005) *Ethical Considerations for Research on Housing-Related Health Hazards Involving Children.* Washington, DC: National Academies Press.

Israel B, Schulz A, Parker E, and Becker AB (2001) Community-based participatory research: Policy recommendations for promoting partnership approach in health research. *Education for Health* 14: 182–197.

Kass NE (2001) An ethics framework for public health. *American Journal of Public Health* 91: 1776–1782.

National Bioethics Advisory Commission (2001) *Ethical and Policy Issues in Research Involving Human Participants.* Washington, DC: National Bioethics Advisory Commission.

National Commission for the Protection of Human Subjects of Biomedical and Behavioral Research (1979) *The Belmont Report: Ethical Principles and Guidelines for the Protection of Human Subjects of Research.* Washington, DC: Department of Health, Education, and Welfare.

Participants in the 2001 Conference on Ethical Aspects of Conducting Research in Developing Countries (2004) Moral standards for research in developing countries: From ''reasonable availability'' to ''fair benefits''. *Hastings Center Report* 34: 17–27.

Popay J and Williams G (1996) Public health research and lay knowledge. *Social Science and Medicine* 42: 759–768.

Richardson H and Belsky L (2004) Medical researchers' ancillary clinical care responsibilities. *British Medical Journal* 328: 1494–1496.

Stewart-Brown S and Farmer A (1997) Screening could seriously damage your health. *British Medical Journal* 314: 533.

Stokstad E (2004) EPA criticized for study of child pesticide exposure. *Science* 306: 961.

US Department of Health and Human Services (2001) *Code of Federal Regulations. 45 (Public Welfare), 46 (Protection of Human Subjects).* Washington DC: US Department of Health and Human Services.

Wallerstein N, Duran B, Minkler M, and Foley K (2005) Developing and maintaining partnerships with communities. In: Israel B, Eng E, Schulz A, and Parker E (eds.) *Methods in Community-Based Participatory Research for Health.* San Francisco, CA: Josey Bass.

Wiejer C and Emanuel EJ (2000) Ethics. Protecting communities in biomedical research. *Science* 289: 1142–1144.

Further Reading

Bayer R, Gostin LO, Jennings B, and Steinbock B (eds.) (2006) *Public Health Ethics: Theory, Policy and Practice.* New York: Oxford University Press.

Beauchamp DE and Steinbock B (eds.) (1999) *New Ethics for the Publics Health.* New York: Oxford University Press.

Soskolne CL, Goodman K, and Coughlin SS (eds.) (1998) *Case Studies in Public Health.* Washington, DC: American Public Health Association.

Relevant Website

http://www.asph.org/UserFiles/EthicsCurriculum.pdf – Association of Schools of Public Health, Ethics and Public Health: Model Curriculum.

Codes of Ethics in Public Health

J C Thomas, University of North Carolina, Chapel Hill, NC, USA
R Gaare Bernheim, University of Virginia, Charlottesville, VA, USA

Introduction

Scholarly and professional interest in public health ethics has increased dramatically in recent years, with new attention on the ethical principles underlying the practice of public health and on a professional code. Public health traditionally has focused more on practice and cases than on developing formal theories of professional ethics.

Nonetheless, particular values, such as social justice and prevention, have animated the day-to-day activities and practice of public health over time. The current interest in naming ethical values demonstrates the field's need for guidance in analyzing, making, and justifying decisions that are becoming increasingly complex and publicly contentious. It also shows the field's commitment to strengthening its professional identity and role, a process that also includes the development of professional competencies, credentialing, and accreditation.

The Need for Codes of Ethics in Professions

Throughout history, many professions such as the medical profession have used codes of ethics, codes of conduct, and oaths to provide a source of guidance and judgment about right and wrong behavior, and good and bad practice. The recent development of a public health code, however, comes at a time when the nature of the professions in society, as well as the usefulness of professional codes, is being challenged – despite a simultaneous proliferation in both the number and variety of codes. A brief consideration of the role of professions and codes provides a helpful context for the discussion of codes of public health ethics.

The term profession generally means a vocation or occupation with the following characteristics: A practice or function grounded in an intellectual tradition that includes specialized knowledge, training, and skill; a commitment to serving clients; and self-regulation. Some describe another feature that involves a public purpose and social function. For example, Mark Frankel (1989) suggests that the professions and society negotiate the terms of their relationship in order to satisfy the profession's desire for autonomy and society's interest in accountability. He states, "Society's granting of power and privilege to the professions is premised on their willingness and ability to contribute to the social well-being and to conduct their affairs in a manner consistent with broader social values" (Frankel, 1989: 110).

Implicit in this traditional social role are ethical challenges for a profession since it owes obligations to a number of parties such as clients, other members of the profession, and the general public. New and even more difficult challenges to the professions today are social, economic, and political pressures that can render professionals mere "technical experts in the service of the political and cultural economy," as stated by Eliot Friedson (2001: 213), writing on professionalism. Friedson explained: "Serving only immediate political, economic, and popular interests cripples both the intellectual development of disciplines and their distinctive moral position that considers the use of their knowledge in light of values that transcend time and place. Should that occur, the character of their responsibility and

their relationship to their societies will have gone through a momentous change" (Friedson, 2001: 213). He believes that professionals should be the moral custodians of their disciplines.

The Functions of Codes of Ethics

A code of ethics is one important way for a profession to create, support, and preserve its moral foundations, its professional integrity, and its relationship of trust with clients and society. Frankel, who believes a code expresses the collective conscience and norms of a profession, identifies three types of codes: An aspirational code that sets ideals to strive for; an educational code that provides commentary and interpretation to help identify and address ethical problems in professional practice; and a regulatory code that sets rules and provides mechanisms for adjudication and enforcement.

Frankel also catalogues eight functions that a code may perform:

1. Enabling document (provides guidance based on collective experience and reflection);
2. Source of public evaluation (provides a basis for public expectation and accountability);
3. Professional socialization (supports group identity and common purpose);
4. Enhance profession's reputation and public trust (persuades the public to trust the profession);
5. Preserve entrenched professional biases (protects dominant values but can censor or restrict important lesser values);
6. Deterrent to unethical behavior (promotes ethical conduct through sanctions);
7. Support system (provides a source of support against improper demands);
8. Adjudication (provides a method for resolving disputes among members).

A profession must decide which type of code and which functions are most appropriate at any point in time, given its relationship with its clients and its relationship with the public. In public health, the professional relationship between the public health professional and client is complex: Public health officials often act both as government officers with public responsibility and police powers, usually authorized through statutes or regulations, on the one hand, and as health professionals, with health as a primary good, on the other. Communities and individuals relate to government officials as both citizens and patients. In a democracy, public health officials may act as physicians with the ethical duty to engage in an informed-consent process, favoring voluntary action over action for which a population has not given its consent (Childress and Bernheim, 2003). In addition, in some circumstances, public health officials act as researchers, yet another relationship that requires public health professionals to follow federal, state, and local laws and ethical principles governing human particpants research.

The Value and Authority of a Code of Ethics

Objections to codes of ethics include their unhelpfulness in guiding conduct or resolving ethical conflict and their potential for misuse as a legalistic document instead of as a reflective tool. This can certainly be true when a profession's organizational structures, culture, education, and leadership do not support the spirit of the code.

Others question the moral authority of a code to guide behavior. Potential sources of authority suggested by Pellegrino (2001) include external sources (e.g, positive public outcomes from the application of a code) and internal sources (e.g., consistency with established beliefs and values of the professionals). Public health activities are generally outcome-oriented. As stated by Childress *et al.* (2003: 170) "the health of the public is the primary end that is sought and the primary outcome for measuring success." In addition, the writing of the U.S. Public Health Code of Ethics began with the identification of values and beliefs inherent to a public health perspective. Thus, the moral authority of the Public Health Code of Ethics derives from both external and internal sources.

Codes of Ethics in Public Health

Codes of ethics in public health are a recent development. While the American Medical Association (AMA) approved its first code of ethics in 1847, the American Public Health Association approved its code in 2002 (Thomas, 2002). The Society of Public Health Educators (SOPHE), representing a constituent discipline of public health, established their code earlier, in 1976. Two other documents relevant to public health are a set of ethics guidelines published in 2000 by the American College of Epidemiology and a code of ethics established by the American College of Healthcare Executives in 2003. Other traditional disciplines within public health either refer to the Public Health Code of Ethics or the codes of related fields. For example, the code of ethics for clinical dieticians applies to aspects of public health nutrition, and codes of ethics pertaining to the environment or to engineering are relevant to environmental health and engineering. Although there is no separate national level code of ethics for environmental health, there are some state level codes.

The late emergence of a code of ethics in public health may reflect that, until recent years, many public health institutions have been commonly led by physicians who would

naturally recognize medical codes of ethics. Moreover, for centuries, physicians have been regarded as the overseers of all health-related matters. Only in the past few decades have nonclinical health professionals begun to assume more authority in health care and prevention. The landmark 1988 Institute of Medicine (IOM) report on public health set the tone for the writing of the U.S. Public Health Code of Ethics. It focused on strengthening federal, state, and local government agencies in their mission of protecting and promoting the health of the public.

Codes of ethics related explicitly to public health in countries other than the U.S. have yet to be written. Instead, one can find lists of values and principles that are often invoked in the context of a particular public health threat. Pandemic influenza planning provides one example. The World Health Organization Project on Addressing Ethical Issues in Pandemic Influenza Planning divided themselves into four working groups:

1. Equitable access to therapeutic and prophylactic measures;
2. Ethics of public health measures in response to pandemic influenza;
3. The role and obligations of health-care workers during an outbreak of pandemic influenza;
4. Issues that arise between governments when developing a multilateral response to a potential outbreak of pandemic influenza (WHO, 2006).

The working group addressing public health measures identified four values: public health necessity (a government should exercise its public health police powers on an individual or group only if the person or group poses a threat to the community such as the likelihood of spreading an infection); reasonable and effective means (the methods by which a threat is addressed should have a reasonable chance of being effective); proportionality (the human burden imposed by a public health regulation should be proportionate to the expected public health benefit); and distributive justice (the risks, benefits, and burdens of public health action should be fairly distributed, thereby precluding the unjustified targeting of an already socially vulnerable population).

Speaking to the tension in public health between the rights of individuals and the good of the community, this group noted *The Siracusa Principles*, which are internationally recognized limitations on human rights established at a meeting in Siracusa, Italy (United Nations Economic and Social Council, 1985). They are as follows:

- The restriction is provided for and carried out in accordance with the law.
- The restriction is in the interest of a legitimate objective of general interest.
- The restriction is strictly necessary in a democratic society to achieve the objective.

- There are no less intrusive and restrictive means available to reach the same objective.
- The restriction is not drafted or imposed arbitrarily, that is, in an unreasonable or otherwise discriminatory manner.

Other lists of values in public health ethics are on websites in the section titled "Relevant websites," below.

Distinctive Characteristics of the U.S. Public Health Code of Ethics

Codes of ethics typically address the situations in which professionals of a particular discipline most commonly encounter ethical challenges. In the case of physicians, it is the patient–physician interaction in a clinical setting. In contrast, the key interaction in public health is between a government agency and the population it serves. For this reason, ethical challenges in public health often have to do with the ways in which a governmental organization, such as a county or state health department, makes decisions and implements policies affecting everyone within a geographical area. In a democratic society, this brings issues of participation and communication to the foreground. Thus, for example, the third of the 12 principles of the Public Health Code of Ethics (**Table 1**) states "Public health policies, programs, and priorities should be developed and evaluated through processes that ensure an opportunity for input from community members." The sixth principle states "Public health institutions should provide communities with the information they have that is needed for decisions on policies or programs and should obtain the community's consent for their implementation" (Thomas *et al.*, 2002)

The U.S. Public Health Code of Ethics is unusual among codes in that it is worded to apply to organizations. Most other codes of ethics, including the code of SOPHE and the ethics guidelines of the American College of Epidemiologists, address the actions of individuals within the profession. Of the 12 principles of the Public Health Code of Ethics, five state obligations of public health institutions, four state responsibilities of public health, and three state ethical principles of public health policies and programs. For example, the eleventh principle in the Code states "Public health institutions should ensure the professional competence of their employees."

In a population, one person's action or condition affects others. This is perhaps clearest in the case of an infectious disease where an infected person can transmit the infection to others. Thus, the role of patient autonomy, so prominent in medical ethics, takes a back seat to the role of interdependence in public health. Interdependence dictates that in some instances an individual's autonomy or freedom must be restricted to protect the health of others. Perhaps

Table 1   The US Public Health Code of Ethics

1. Public health should address principally the fundamental causes of disease and requirements for health, aiming to prevent adverse health outcomes
2. Public health should achieve community health in a way that respects the rights of individuals in the community
3. Public health policies, programs, and priorities should be developed and evaluated through processes that ensure an opportunity for input from community members
4. Public health should advocate and work for the empowerment of disenfranchised community members, aiming to ensure that the basic resources and conditions necessary for health are accessible to all
5. Public health should seek the information needed to implement effective policies and programs that protect and promote health
6. Public health institutions should provide communities with the information they have that is needed for decisions on policies or programs and should obtain the community's consent for their implementation
7. Public health institutions should act in a timely manner on the information they have within the resources and the mandate given to them by the public
8. Public health programs and policies should incorporate a variety of approaches that anticipate and respect diverse values, beliefs, and cultures in the community
9. Public health programs and policies should be implemented in a manner that most enhances the physical and social environment
10. Public health institutions should protect the confidentiality of information that can bring harm to an individual or community if made public. Exceptions must be justified on the basis of the high likelihood of significant harm to the individual or others
11. Public health institutions should ensure the professional competence of their employees
12. Public health institutions and their employees should engage in collaborations and affiliations in ways that build the public's trust and the institution's effectiveness

Available on the website of the Public Health Leadership Society, http://www.phls.org (accessed September 2007).

the key ethical challenge of public health in a democratic society, then, is the tension between individual rights and the health of the community. The Public Health Code of Ethics acknowledges but does not resolve this tension by stating in its second principle: "Public health should achieve community health in a way that respects the rights of individuals in the community." Notes on the individual principles that accompany the Code underscore that in the tension between the individual and the community, the starting place for public health is the community.

Relations Between Various Codes Within Public Health

The codes of the constituent disciplines of public health narrow in on particular concerns within the profession.

In doing so, they enumerate more principles than does the code for public health. The Code of Ethics of the American College of Healthcare Executives consists of 39 principles grouped into six responsibilities: to the profession, to patients, to the organization (i.e., an employer), to employees, to the community, and to report violations of the Code. The SOPHE Code of Ethics consists of 38 sections or principles categorized into six articles or responsibilities. The responsibilities are to the public, the profession, employers, the delivery of health education, research and evaluation, and professional preparation. As an example of the level of detail, the first section of the third article (pertaining to responsibilities to employers) states "Health Educators accurately represent their qualifications and the qualifications of others whom they recommend."

None of the principles in the three codes for constituent organizations (ACE, ACHE, SOPHE) disagrees with the Public Health Code of Ethics. Each affirms accountability, equity, confidentiality, professional competence, and more. One potential area for disagreement between the codes for epidemiologists and public health relate to advocacy. Some epidemiologists assert that advocating for certain groups or needs compromises scientific objectivity. Yet, the Public Health Code states that "Public health should advocate and work for the empowerment of disenfranchised community members." The ACE avoided this controversy by stating both sides of the issue: "In confronting public health problems, epidemiologists sometimes act as advocates on behalf of members of affected communities. Advocacy should not impair scientific objectivity."

A few principles in the Public Health Code of Ethics are not addressed in the other codes. The Public Health Code, for example, emphasizes the importance of prevention and addressing the fundamental causes of disease. It also speaks clearly of the need to allow communities to have input into policies affecting them, and for collaboration among institutions and organizations. The absence of these principles from the other codes does not represent a disagreement. Rather it highlights the value of a code that transcends the perspectives of the constituent disciplines within public health, one that maintains a broader, interdisciplinary perspective. The agreement and complementarity of the codes demonstrate that one code does not supersede another. A professional needs both the global perspective of the Public Health Code and the particularity of the code of his or her narrower profession.

Research Ethics

Principles and rules for research ethics have developed along a path separate from codes of ethics. They have evolved out of recommendations resulting from high-profile research abuses such as Nazi war crimes and the Tuskegee study of untreated syphilis. The principal concerns in research ethics are informed consent and the protection of vulnerable individuals such as prisoners and minors. To ensure compliance with prescribed procedures in federally funded research, there exists an institutional infrastructure reaching from the federal government to individual institutions such as universities. Institutions found not to comply with the prescribed procedures can lose their license to conduct federally funded research until they are found to be compliant once again.

Codes of ethics for the practice of public health do not have the enforcement structures seen in research ethics. Rather, the codes are aspirational, articulating the values and expectations of the profession. They are a means of being transparent and enabling the public they serve to hold them accountable for their actions. In addition, they serve as a tool for identifying and addressing ethical issues. For example, ethical issues in the application of genomics to public health were identified by considering genomics in light of each principle of the Public Health Code of Ethics in turn (Thomas, 2005).

Conclusion

Codes of ethics are important to the degree they lead to trust in public health institutions. The effectiveness of public health institutions depends heavily on the trust of the populations they serve. Distrust results in passive resistance and in some cases active resistance to policies and programs. A code of ethics reminds an institution of what it must do to maintain that trust.

See also: Ethics of Health Promotion; Ethics of Public Health Research; Ethics of Screening.

Citations

Childress JF, Faden RR, and Gaare RD (2002) Public health ethics: Mapping the terrain. *Journal of Law Medicine & Ethics* 30: 170–178.

Childress JF and Gaare Bernheim R (2003) Beyond the liberal and communitarian impasse: A framework and vision for public health. *Florida Law Review* 55: 1191–1215.

Frankel MS (1989) Professional codes: Why, how, and with what impact? *Journal of Business Ethics* 8: 109–115.

Friedson E (2001) *Professionalism: The Third Logic*. Chicago, IL: University of Chicago Press.

Institute of Medicine (1988) *The Future of the Public Health*. Washington DC: National Academy Press.

Pellegrino ED (2001) Professional Codes. In: Sugarman J and Sulmasy DP (eds.) *Methods in Medical Ethics*. Washington DC: Georgetown University Press.

Thomas JC, Sage M, Dillenberg J, and Guillory VJ (2002) A code of ethics for public health. *American Journal of Public Health* 92: 1057–1059.

Thomas JC, Zuiker E, Millikan R, and Rockhill B (2005) Genomics and public health ethics. *American Journal of Public Health* 95: 2139–2143.

United Nations Economic and Social Council (1985) Siracusa principles on the limitation and derogation provisions in the International Covenant on Civil and Political Rights. http://www.who.int/csr/resources/publications/WHO_CDS_EPR_GIP_2007_2c.pdf (accessed April 2008).

World Health Organization (2006) World Health Organization Project on addressing ethical issues in pandemic influenza planning, draft paper for working group two: Ethics of public health measures in response to pandemic influenza. http://www.who.int/entity/eth/ethics/PI_Ethics_draft_paper_WG2_6_Oct_06.pdf (accessed October 2006).

Further Reading

Bernheim RG (2003) Public health ethics: The voices of practitioners. *Journal of Law Medicine & Ethics* 31: S104–S107.

Higgs-Kleyn N and Kapelianis D (1999) The role of professional codes in regulating ethical conduct. *Journal of Business Ethics* 19: 363–374.

Kass N (2001) An ethics framework for public health. *American Journal of Public Health* 91: 1776–1782.

Morrison EE (2006) *Ethics in Health Administration: A Practical Approach for Decision Makers*. London: Jones and Bartlett Publishers.

Thomas JC (2005) Skills in the ethical practice of public health. *Journal of Public Health Management and Practice* 11: 260–261.

Weed DL and McKeown RE (2003) Science and social responsibility in public health. *Environmental Health Perspectives* 111: 1804–1808.

Relevant Websites

http://acepidemiology2.org/policystmts/EthicsGuide.asp – American College of Epidemiology Ethics Guidelines.

http://www.ache.org/ABT_ACHE/code.cfm – American College of Healthcare Executives Code of Ethics.

http://www.cdc.gov/od/science/phec/ – Centers for Disease Control, public health ethics.

http://ethics.iit.edu/codes/ – Center for the Study of Ethics in the Professions, Illinois Institute of Technology, Codes of Ethics Online.

http://www.ecdc.eu.int/Health_topics/Pandemic_Influenza/Pandemic_Planning.html – European Centre for Disease Prevention and Control, National Pandemic Influenza Plans.

http://www.neac.health.govt.nz/moh.nsf/indexcm/neac-resources-publications-getting through together/ – National Ethics Advisory Committee of New Zealand. Ethical Values for Planning for and Responding to a Pandemic in New Zealand-A Statement for Discussion.

http://www.phls.org – Public Health Code of Ethics and accompanying documents, Public Health Leadership Society.

http://www.sophe.org/about/ethics.html. – Society for Public Health Education Code of Ethics.

http://www.utoronto.ca/jcb/home/documents/pandemic.pdf – University of Toronto Joint Centre for Bioethics. Stand on Guard for Thee: Ethical Considerations in Preparedness Planning for Pandemic Influenza.

Ethics of Screening

S S Coughlin, Centers for Disease Control and Prevention, Atlanta, GA, USA

Published by Elsevier Inc.

Introduction

Over the past few decades, there has been substantial interest among bioethicists and public health practitioners in identifying, analyzing, and addressing ethical issues in screening (Mant and Fowler, 1990; Burke *et al.*, 2001; Hodge, 2004). Screening is the presumptive identification of an unrecognized disease or condition by the use of tests, examinations, or other procedures that can help identify apparently well individuals who have a disease or disease precursor. Persons with positive or suspicious findings then undergo further evaluation or treatment. The ultimate objective of screening is to reduce the morbidity and mortality from a disease among the persons screened. When screening tests are applied to large, unselected populations, the process is referred to as mass screening (Fletcher, 1988). Several frameworks for analyzing and addressing ethical and policy issues in public health screening programs have been proposed over the years.

General Principles for Mass Screening Programs

In 1968, Wilson and Jungner proposed ten principles for mass screening programs (**Table 1**) (Wilson and Jungner, 1968). These principles, which were partly derived from reports about screening programs for breast cancer and other chronic conditions in the 1950s and 1960s, are often cited in the planning and evaluation of population screening programs. These principles relate to the adequacy of the scientific evidence, the balance of risks and benefits, the availability of an effective treatment, the acceptability of the screening test to the population, and the costs and resources required (Burke *et al.*, 2001). Refinements have been proposed over the years with further specification of the principles of screening (Cole and Morrison, 1980; Cadman, *et al.*, 1984; Miller, 1985; Sox, 1994; Harris *et al.*, 2001). For example, guidelines for assessing the effectiveness of community screening programs were proposed by Cadman *et al.* in 1984. These guidelines consider whether

Table 1   Principles for mass screening programs

1. The condition sought should be an important health problem
2. There should be an accepted treatment for patients with recognized disease
3. Facilities for diagnosis and treatment should be available
4. There should be a recognizable latent or early symptomatic stage
5. There should be a suitable test or examination
6. The test should be acceptable to the population
7. The natural history of the condition, including development from latent to declared disease, should be adequately understood
8. There should be an agreed policy on whom to treat as patients
9. The cost of case-finding (including diagnosis and treatment of patients diagnosed) should be economically balanced in relation to possible expenditure on medical care as a whole
10. Case-finding should be a continuing process and not a once and for all project

Adapted from Wilson JMG and Jungner F (1968) *Principles and Practice of Screening for Disease. Public Health Papers No. 34.* Geneva: World Health Organization.

the program's effectiveness has been demonstrated in a randomized trial, whether efficacious treatments are available, whether the burden of suffering from the condition warrants screening, whether there is a good screening test, whether the health system can cope with the screening program, and other issues. Criteria for the effectiveness of clinical preventive services have been developed by the Canadian Task Force on the Periodic Health Examination (1994) and by the U.S. Preventive Services Task Force (1996; Harris *et al.*, 2001).

Ethical Considerations in Screening

Screening raises a number of important ethical issues, including provisions for obtaining informed consent, protecting privacy and confidentiality, and balancing risks and potential benefits, and issues pertaining to targeted screening of higher-risk persons. Other ethical considerations relate to costs and how best to allocate finite public resources for screening.

Informed Consent and Informed Decision Making

The principle of respect for the autonomy of persons supports the right of individuals to informed consent prior to screening (Hodge, 2004). Provisions for informed consent ensure that persons undergoing screening make free choices and encourage providers to act responsibly in their interactions with patients. The focus should be placed not only on the obligation of providers to disclose information, but also on the quality

of the understanding and consent of the person undergoing screening. Individuals should be given information about the procedure, the meaning of a positive or negative test result, and any appreciable risks or potential harms and benefits before undergoing screening (Hodge, 2004). In order for persons to give informed consent for screening, they need to understand the risk of a false-positive (or false-negative) test result and the procedures that may follow it (Lee, 1993).

Principles of informed consent for screening have some features in common with emerging models of informed decision making and shared decision making for screening and other health-care services (Whitney *et al.*, 2003). An emphasis is placed on ensuring that persons are provided with balanced and relevant information to allow them to make informed decisions about their choices concerning screening options (Briss *et al.*, 2004; Sheridan *et al.*, 2004; Hewitson and Austoker, 2005). As discussed by Briss *et al.* (2004), informed decision making occurs

> when an individual understands the nature of the disease or condition being addressed; understands the clinical service and its likely consequences, including risks, limitations, benefits, alternatives, and uncertainties; has considered his or her preferences as appropriate; has participated in decision making at a personally desirable level; and either makes a decision consistent with his or her preferences and values or elects to defer a decision to a later time.

Shared decision making occurs when a patient and his or her health-care provider, in a clinical setting, both express preferences and participate in making treatment decisions (Briss *et al.*, 2004; Sheridan *et al.*, 2004). Characteristics of an informed and joint decision identified by Sheridan *et al.* (2004) are shown in **Table 2**.

Voluntary Versus Mandatory Screening

Public health screening is generally voluntary. For example, public health programs for HIV testing and counseling

Table 2   Characteristics of an informed and joint decision

The patient must:
1. Understand the risk or seriousness of the disease or condition
2. Understand the preventive service, including the risks, benefits, alternatives, and uncertainties
3. Have weighed his or her values regarding the potential harms and benefits associated with the service
4. Have engaged in decision making at a level he or she desires and feels comfortable with the decision

Adapted from Sheridan SL, Harris RP, Wooll SH, *et al.* (2004) Shared decision making about screening and chemoprevention. A suggested approach from the U.S. Preventive Services Task Force. *American Journal of Preventive Medicine* 26: 56–66.

are voluntary because mandatory HIV testing would not adequately respect individual autonomy. In addition, mandatory testing in clinical settings would likely deter people from seeking health care and hinder the public health goal of increasing the number of persons who learn their HIV status. The latter goal is vital for reaching high-risk sero-negative people to help them to stay uninfected, and for detecting HIV infection when the potential for transmission is greatest and the need for prevention and treatment are greatest (NCHS, Healthy People 2010).

Some examples of mandatory screening can be cited. For example, most states require the screening of infants for certain genetic disorders such as phenylketonuria (PKU). Persons must participate in the screening program unless the parents of the child opt out for religious or philosophical reasons (Hodge, 2004). Public health officials may justify mandatory newborn screening programs, even without parental consent, under utilitarian principles authorizing state governments to protect children (Hodge, 2004). A 1975 National Research Council report concluded that mandatory screening was justified only if there was evidence that it would prevent death or other serious harm to the affected individual (NRC, 1975; Grosse et al., 2006).

Benefits and Risks of Screening

General principles of biomedical ethics such as beneficence (protect the welfare of patients and promote the general welfare) and nonmaleficence (do no harm) can be further specified to identify specific ethical principles and rules relevant to screening. The potential benefits of screening include the early detection of disease and the prevention of serious illness or disability and improved survival. The societal benefits of screening were highlighted in the Second Edition of the *Guide to Clinical Preventive Services* (1996):

> Preventive services for the early detection of disease have also been associated with substantial reductions in morbidity and mortality. Age-adjusted mortality from stroke has decreased by more than 50% since 1972, a trend attributed in part to earlier detection and treatment of hypertension. Dramatic reductions in the incidence of invasive cervical cancer and in cervical cancer mortality have occurred following the implementation of screening programs using Papanicolaou testing to detect cervical dysplasia. Children with metabolic disorders such as phenylketonuria and congenital hypothyroidism, who once suffered severe irreversible mental retardation, now usually retain normal cognitive function as a result of routine newborn screening and treatment.

The U.S. Preventive Services Task Force considers benefits from both population and individual perspectives (Harris et al., 2001). For the benefit from a screening test or other clinical intervention to be considered substantial, the service must have at least a small relative impact on a frequent condition with a substantial population burden, or a large impact on an infrequent condition that poses a significant burden at the individual level (Harris et al., 2001).

Screening is undertaken for conditions that are important public health problems in terms of morbidity and mortality, and for conditions for which early detection and treatment has been shown to be effective in reducing mortality or serious disability. If early treatment is not effective, then early detection alone merely extends the length of time the disease is known to exist, without providing benefits to individuals in terms of increased survival (Fletcher, 1988). Screening leads to some diagnostic procedures that otherwise would never be done (Cole and Morrison, 1980). Screening may also lead to earlier or more debilitating treatment of persons with incurable disease (Cole and Morrison, 1980). Public health policy makers rely on information from randomized controlled trials and other scientific evidence to evaluate the effectiveness, potential benefits, and risks or potential harms of screening. Scientific evidence is also used to evaluate the costs of screening programs and to decide how best to allocate limited resources.

The potential harms and risk associated with screening also have to be taken into account, especially since screening programs are aimed at large numbers of apparently healthy individuals. Minor complications or infrequent adverse effects that would be acceptable in the treatment of a severe illness take on greater importance in the screening of asymptomatic persons and require careful evaluation to determine whether the potential benefits exceed risks (USPSTF, 1996). There may be risks associated with the test itself such as the potential for bowel perforation with colonoscopy. There may be risks associated with false-positive or false-negative test results. The potential harms of screening may also include labeling effects and the psychological impact of test results or a diagnosis on individuals. If prognosis is not improved by presymptomatic detection, screening for a disease can cause anxiety without providing any benefit (Sox, 1994). Overdiagnosis can sometimes occur with screening; overdiagnosis is the identification of disease that would not have produced signs or symptoms before death (Black, 2000).

Medical information collected as part of screening should be rigorously protected in order to protect patient privacy and confidentiality and to minimize risks or potential harms such as stigmatization or discrimination. Only a few specific exceptions exist such as mandatory partner notification laws for HIV infection that physicians are legally required to follow in some states (Khalsa, 2006).

The U.S. Preventive Services Task Force considers all types of potential harms of a service such as screening, both direct harms of the service itself and indirect harms that may be a consequence of the initial intervention (Harris *et al.*, 2001). Benefits and harms are then weighed by the Task Force, a process which includes value judgments (Harris *et al.*, 2001).

The balance of risks and benefits from screening may be different for older adults than for younger adults (American Geriatrics Society Ethics Committee, 2003). For persons who have a short life expectancy, clinical care should focus on conditions for which treatment is likely to be of immediate benefit rather than on screening for asymptomatic disease.

Ethics of Targeted Screening

Targeted screening efforts assist public health officials in identifying a disease or condition that affects subgroups of persons differentially (Hodge, 2004). Through targeted screening, it may be possible to lower costs while retaining most or all of the benefits of a screening program by screening a population with increased prevalence of the disease or condition (Cole and Morrison, 1980). Targeted screening programs aimed at high-risk individuals may increase the specificity of the screening test and minimize the number of false-positive results (Cole and Morrison, 1980). There are also potential drawbacks to targeted screening such as a possible increased potential for stigmatization of persons targeted for screening. As with all screening programs, facilities for diagnosis and treatment should be accessible and affordable.

Distributive Justice

The equitable distribution of health-care resources such as screening services is grounded in ethical principles of justice (Beauchamp, 1996). Utilitarian theories of justice emphasize a mixture of criteria so that public utility is maximized. From this perspective, a just distribution of screening benefits is determined by the utility to all affected by it. An egalitarian theory of justice holds that each person should share equally in the distribution of the potential benefits of health-care resources such as screening services. Other theories of justice hold that society has an obligation to correct inequalities in the distribution of resources, and that those who are least well off should benefit by having access to affordable screening services and other resources. Such theories of justice provide considerable support for maximizing benefits to medically underserved persons, especially if providing services to socially disadvantaged persons ultimately benefits society as a whole (Beauchamp, 1996).

Ethical Issues in Genetic Testing and Screening

A number of important ethical issues arise in genetic testing for disease susceptibility among adults. Genetic information, unlike other health information, is both personal and private and familial. The information obtained through genetic testing and screening may have implications for health professionals and patients as both may need to consider whether they have an obligation to inform at-risk relatives (Burke and Press, 2006; Loud *et al.*, 2006).

Examples of genetic testing for susceptibility to adult-onset conditions include *BRCA1* and *BRCA2* gene testing for susceptibility to breast and ovarian cancer and genetic testing for susceptibility to hereditary colorectal cancer syndromes (Coughlin and Miller, 1999; Coughlin *et al.*, 1999; USPSTF, 2005). Genetic testing for disease susceptibility raises ethical and social concerns related to the adequacy of informed consent, the availability of pre- and posttest counseling, and the avoidance of genetic discrimination (Hodge, 2004). Other ethical and social issues relate to the cost of and access to genetic testing, especially among those who are socioeconomically disadvantaged or uninsured. The disclosure of genetic test results can have psychological and economic ramifications for the person screened and his or her relatives (Lerman and Croyle, 1994). Some persons screened may experience anxiety or other adverse psychological effects or disrupted personal relationships. Reproductive choices may also be affected. The provision of genetic information without proper counseling and follow-up can lead to psychological distress (Geller *et al.*, 1997). To make an informed decision about whether to request genetic testing, persons must understand the potential benefits as well as the limitations of current options for disease prevention and early detection (Geller *et al.*, 1995, 1997). An important role of genetic counseling is to ensure that persons considering undergoing genetic testing understand the limited nature of information about genetic risk.

In European countries, the United States, and other countries, legal and regulatory safeguards to prevent genetic discrimination have been strengthened in recent years. However, existing laws and regulations are still inadequate to prevent problems associated with genetic discrimination, such as loss of employment or insurance (Hodge, 2004). The potential for discrimination by health insurers is an important risk associated with genetic testing.

Newborn Screening and Prenatal Diagnosis

There has been ongoing discussion of newborn screening programs in the United Kingdom, the United States, Canada, Australia, New Zealand, and other countries

(Webster *et al.*, 2003; Eggertson, 2005; Patch, 2006; Southern *et al.*, 2007). Newborn screening programs in the United States are run by state public health departments (Botkin, 2006). Newborn screening commonly refers not only to laboratory testing but also to a comprehensive system that includes parent and provider education, dried-blood-spot specimen collection, and follow-up, diagnosis, and treatment (Godard *et al.*, 2003; Grosse *et al.*, 2006). Newborn screening for PKU, which began in the United States in the 1960s, allows for the prevention of severe disability since the initiation of a low-phenylalanine diet immediately after birth can prevent severe neurologic damage and mental retardation (Grosse *et al.*, 2006). The number of conditions currently tested for in newborn screening programs varies considerably by place of residence. In the United States, most states require that infants be screened for treatable genetic disorders such as phenylkentonuria (PKU), although parents may sometimes refuse on religious or philosophical grounds. In addition to PKU, almost all states screen newborns for hemoglobinopathies such as sickle cell disease and for galactosemia (Botkin, 2006).

Prenatal diagnosis raises somewhat different ethical issues than those posed by newborn screening (Clayton, 1999). Prenatal diagnosis requires that informed consent be obtained and that potential benefits and risks be explained. As noted by Hodge (2004):

> Principles of autonomy strongly support an individual's right to informed consent prior to genetic testing or screening... Prior to the administration of a test, patients are entitled to explanations of the nature and scope of the information to be gathered, the meaning of positive test results, the underlying disease or condition, and any appreciable risks involved in the testing or activities following a positive result.

Examples of genetic screening or testing in the delivery of clinical care include prenatal carrier screening for Tay-Sachs or cystic fibrosis, and prenatal testing to detect Down syndrome in higher-risk pregnancies (Hodge, 2004).

Summary

In summary, frameworks for addressing ethical and policy issues in public health screening programs consider the adequacy of the scientific evidence, the balance of risks and benefits, the availability and affordability of an effective treatment, the acceptability of the screening test to the population, patient preferences, and the costs and resources required as well as additional ethical considerations. The latter include provisions for obtaining informed consent, protecting privacy and confidentiality, and avoiding discrimination and stigmatization. The benefits of screening include the prevention of serious illness or disability and improved survival. Public health policy makers rely on information from randomized controlled trials and other scientific evidence to evaluate the effectiveness, potential benefits, and risks or potential harms of screening. On a societal scale, there is a potential for the production of a population of worried well individuals through mass screening. In addition, genetic screening programs may create the illusion that all diseases ultimately are genetic, to the detriment of other public health approaches for decreasing morbidity and mortality. Other ethical and social issues relate to the cost of screening and access to screening, especially among socioeconomically disadvantaged or uninsured persons.

Citations

American Geriatrics Society Ethics Committee (2006) Health screening decisions for older adults: AGS position paper. *Journal of the American Geriatrics Society* 51: 270–271.

Beauchamp TL (1996) Moral foundations. In: Coughlin SS and Beauchamp TL (eds.) *Ethics and Epidemiology*, pp. 24–52. New York: Oxford University Press.

Black WC (2000) Overdiagnosis: an underrecognized cause of confusion and harm in cancer screening. *Journal of the National Cancer Institute* 92: 1280–1282.

Briss P, Rimer B, Reilley B, *et al.* (2004) Promoting informed decisions about cancer screening in communities and healthcare systems. *American Journal of Preventive Medicine* 26: 67–80.

Burke W and Press N (2006) Ethical obligations and counseling challenges in cancer genetics. *Journal of the National Comprehensive Cancer Network* 4: 185–191.

Burke W, Coughlin SS, Lee NC, *et al.* (2001) Application of population screening principles to genetic screening for adult-onset conditions. *Genetic Testing* 5: 201–211.

Cadman D, Chambers L, Feldman W, and Sackett D (1984) Assessing the effectiveness of community screening programs. *Journal of the American Medical Association* 251: 1580–1585.

Canadian Task Force on the Periodic Health Examination (1994) *Canadian Guide to Clinical Preventive Health Care*. Ottawa, Canada: Canada Communication Group.

Clayton EW (1999) What should be the role of public health in newborn screening and prenatal diagnosis? *American Journal of Preventive Medicine* 16: 111–115.

Cole P and Morrison AS (1980) Basic issues in population screening for cancer. *Journal of the National Cancer Institute* 64: 1263–1272.

Coughlin SS and Miller DS (1999) Public health perspectives on testing for colorectal cancer susceptibility genes. *American Journal of Preventive Medicine* 16: 99–104.

Coughlin SS, Khoury MJ, and Steinberg KK (1997) BRCA1 and BRCA2 gene mutations and risk of breast cancer. Public health perspectives. *American Journal of Preventive Medicine* 16: 91–98.

Eggertson L (2005) Canada lags on newborn screening. *Canadian Medical Association Journal* 173: 23.

Fletcher RH, Fletcher SW, and Wagner EH (1988) *Clinical Epidemiology: The Essentials*, 2nd edn. Baltimore, MD: Williams & Wilkins.

Geller G, Bernhardt BA, Helzlsouer K, *et al.* (1995) Informed consent for BRCA1 testing. *Nature Genetics* 11: 364.

Geller G, Botkin JR, Green MJ, *et al.* (1997) Genetic testing for susceptibility to adult-onset cancer. The process and content of informed consent. *Journal of the American Medical Association* 277: 1467–1474.

Godard B, Kate L, Evers-Kiebooms G, *et al.* (2003) Population genetic screening programmes: Principles, techniques, practices, and policies. *European Journal of Human Genetics* 11(supplement 2): S49–S87.

Grosse SD, Boyle CA, Kenneson A, *et al.* (2006) From public health emergency to public health service: The implications of evolving criteria for newborn screening panels. *Pediatrics* 117: 923–929.

Harris RP, Helfand M, Woolf SH, *et al.* (2001) Current methods of the U.S. Preventive Services Task Force: a review of the process.

American Journal of Preventive Medicine 20(supplement 3): 21–35.

Hewitson P and Austoker J (2005) Patient information, informed decision-making and the psycho-social impact of prostate-specific antigen testing. *British Journal of Urology International* 95(supplement 3): 16–32.

Hodge JG (2004) Ethical issues concerning genetic testing and screening in public health. *American Journal of Medical Genetics* 125C: 66–70.

Kerruish NJ and Robertson SP (2006) Newborn screening: New developments, new dilemmas. *Journal of Medical Ethics* 31: 393–398.

Khalsa AM (2006) Preventive counseling, screening, and therapy for the patient with newly diagnosed HIV infection. *American Family Physician* 15: 271–280.

Lee JM (1993) Screening and informed consent. *New England Journal of Medicine* 328: 438–440.

Lerman C and Croyle R (1994) Psychological issues in genetic testing for breast cancer susceptibility. *Archives of Internal Medicine* 154: 609–616.

Loud JT, Weissman NE, Peters JA, *et al.* (2006) Deliberate deceit of family members: A challenge to providers of clinical genetics services. *Journal of Clinical Oncology* 24: 1643–1646.

Mant D and Fowler G (1990) Mass screening: Theory and ethics. *British Medical Journal* 300: 916–918.

Miller AB (1985) Principles of screening and of the evaluation of screening programs. In: Miller AB (ed.) *Screening for Cancer*, pp. 3–24. San Diego, CA: Acadamic Press.

National Center for Health Statistics (2007). *Healthy People 2010*. Chapter 13: HIV. Centers for Disease Control and Prevention. http://healthypeople.gov/Document/HTML/Volume1/13HIV.htm (accessed September 2007).

National Research Council (1975) *Committee for the Study of Inborn Errors of Metabolism. Genetic Screening: Programs, Principles, and Research*. Washington, DC: National Academy of Sciences.

Patch C (2006) Newborn screening policy in the United Kingdom and the United States: Two different communities of practice. *MCN American Journal of Maternal Child Nursing* 31: 164–168.

Sheridan SL, Harris RP, Woolf SH, *et al.* (2004) Shared decision making about screening and chemoprevention. A suggested approach from the U.S. Preventive Services Task Force. *American Journal of Preventive Medicine* 26: 56–66.

Southern KW, Munck A, Pollitt R, *et al.* (2007) A survey of newborn screening for cystic fibrosis in Europe. *Journal of Cystic Fibrosis* 6: 57–65.

Sox HC (1994) Preventive health services in adults. *New England Journal of Medicine* 330: 1589–1595.

U.S. Preventive Services Task Force (1996) *Guide to Clinical Preventive Services*. Baltimore, MD: Williams & Wilkins.

U.S. Preventive Services Task Force (2005) *Genetic Risk Assessment and BRCA Mutation Testing for Breast and Ovarian Cancer Susceptibility*. September 2005. http://www.ahrq.gov/clinic/uspstf/uspsbrgen.htm (accessed September 2007).

Webster D (2003) Newborn screening in Australia and New Zealand. *Southeast Asian Journal of Tropical Medicine and Public Health* 34 (supplement 3): 69–70.

Whitney SN, McGuire AL, and McCullogh LB (2003) A typology of shared decision making, informed consent, and simple consent. *Annals of Internal Medicine* 140: 54–59.

Wilson JMG and Jungner F (1968) *Principles and Practice of Screening for Disease. Public Health Papers No. 34*. Geneva, Switzerland: World Health Organization.

Ethics of Health Promotion

N Guttman, Tel Aviv University, Tel Aviv, Israel

Introduction

Health promotion activities are inevitably fraught with moral and ethical issues (Seedhouse, 2002). The issues they address typically relate to sensitive topics, deeply held beliefs, and moral judgments (Doxiadis, 1987). Even the most benevolent or seemingly benign activities constitute an attempt to influence people's lives, whether at the individual, community, or national level. Key ethical concerns in health promotion range from issues related to paternalism or interference with people's autonomy and privacy for the sake of promoting the health of individuals or society as a whole, to concerns regarding equity and distributive justice, where health promotion interventions may inadvertently widen health gaps. Ethical issues invariably arise in issues related to personal responsibility and the role and obligation of government in influencing people's health-related practices through engineering methods, incentives and educational programs, or persuasive media campaigns (Beauchamp, 1988). Because of limited resources, ethical issues also emerge as they relate to decisions about which population will be the target of the intervention, and which will not.

Addressing ethical issues in health promotion is important not only because any benevolent attempt to contribute to the well-being of people should be ethical but also because of pragmatic implications: Interventions that are sensitive to ethical concerns are more likely to gain people's trust and respect. With the proliferation of sophisticated and intrusive activities that aim to influence intimate practices and fundamental social values (e.g., sexuality, parent–child relations), identifying ethical issues in health promotion has become an imperative. In multicultural settings, members of diverse populations may hold beliefs or engage in practices considered by health promoters as 'unhealthy' but that have important cultural significance. Because health promoters increasingly embrace commercial marketing tactics and new communication technologies, issues arise concerning the ethics of persuasion strategies and respect for people's autonomy (Andreasen, 2001).

In some cases, the ethical issues that emerge in health promotion activities are explicit and elicit a debate, while in other cases, pertinent ethical issues may be more difficult to recognize in the wide range of health promotion activities. Therefore, it is important to identify and elucidate them. The range of ethical issues in health promotion is as broad as the types of issues addressed. Ethical issues can be found in each component of the intervention, from conception of goals and the challenge of informed consent to assessment of outcomes. Ethical issues can be identified as they relate to how problems and responsibilities are defined, which type of influence approaches and strategies are employed, and what the direct and indirect impacts of the intervention are.

Ethical Issues Embedded in Defining Problems and Responsibilities

Implicit in health promotion activities are ideological and moral approaches, in particular regarding the definition of the health problem and the responsibility of the individual. A health problem can be identified as a result of economic deprivation or inequity or, in contrast, as a result of lack of personal motivation. Each type of problem definition and the type of health promotion intervention that is chosen raises ethical issues (Guttman, 2000).

Personal Responsibility and Health Promotion

Personal responsibility is believed to be a powerful factor in health promotion but is an issue that elicits contrasting views and ethical concerns (Minkler, 1999). One important assumption is that individuals are free to make certain choices about many health-related practices, and therefore should be encouraged to be responsible for those choices. People are urged to make prudent and responsible choices in their food consumption, leisure activities, sexual relations, and lifestyle in general. Emphasis on personal responsibility is often viewed as an effective means to promote desired behaviors and to enhance people's sense of efficacy and autonomy. Whereas the notion of personal responsibility might serve to empower individuals and populations and promote a sense of agency or care for others, it may also inadvertently become 'victim blaming' when messages attribute blame or shame to those who do not adopt them. In particular, this can occur when people's choice to engage in or to refrain from certain practices depends to a large extent on factors outside their control or on limited economic opportunities (Marantz, 1990). Also, even when health messages do not explicitly blame individuals for taking full responsibility for their health, these messages may frame the notion of responsibility for disease or injury prevention as if it were primarily under the control of individuals. This can de-emphasize the role of structural

and institutional factors such as the work environment, housing conditions, or pollution in the etiology of many health-related problems (Wikler, 2004). An emphasis on personal responsibility in health promotion messages might reinforce unfair distinctions between what society accepts as justified risks to one's health and unjustified or immoral ones. Further, the notion of personal responsibility also relates to conceptions of social roles and obligations that may differ across groups and populations. For example, people may be called upon to promote or protect the health of significant others (e.g., children, spouses). Thus, appealing to people's sense of obligation can help reinforce moral commitments such as caring, solidarity, and compassion, but it might also place a burden on people who have limited control over others' behaviors.

Harm Reduction Approaches and Health Promotion

Numerous health promotion programs draw on what has been called a 'harm reduction' approach, described by some of its advocates as 'compassionate pragmatism.' According to this approach, there is an ethical imperative to help people to reduce their vulnerability to risk from engaging in particular practices that are not morally condoned by certain groups or society as a whole. They are not asked to discontinue these practices, but mainly to reduce the risk of harm. Proponents often justify this approach on the basis of the obligation of health promoters to help people with special needs to avoid serious harm, as well as on the basis of its utility. This approach has been applied in the prevention of substance abuse and sexually transmitted infections among young adults and in syringe-exchange programs for injection drug users to prevent HIV infection. It is also found in programs that promote the use of a 'designated driver' when people intend to consume large amounts of alcoholic beverages. In fact, many health promotion programs that aim to minimize the harm of indoor and outdoor pollution, sedentary work places, long work hours, and various environmental hazards can be seen as adopting a modified variation of the harm-reduction approach: to reduce – but not eliminate – the risk of people exposed to various hazards, whether voluntarily or not. An implicit ethical consideration is the obligation of health promoters to help people to reduce their risk from harm, regardless of whether or not they engage in socially sanctioned practices (Sachs, 1996). There is also an implicit social judgment regarding which risks or which environmental hazards are socially acceptable and which are not. This further raises ethical issues regarding the obligation of health promoters either to change social and physical environments characterized as 'unhealthy' or mainly to help people adapt to them.

The Challenge of Informed Consent in Health Promotion Activities

In a medical care context, before certain medical procedures are done on patients who may experience adverse consequences, it is an ethical and often a legal requirement to obtain their informed consent. Because health promotion activities are often viewed as relatively unobtrusive and are mainly implemented in the context of populations, the question of whether informed consent is required is contested. Yet health promotion activities, by definition, aim to influence people's practices, and it is argued that certain standards or procedures are needed to ensure that an informed consent is obtained on behalf of diverse populations. On a national scale, health promotion may reflect policies formulated as a result of a political democratic process, but on the local or organizational level, the question arises as to who represents the community residents. The issue is of particular importance when programs serve as 'social experiments' to prove the efficacy of one type of method over another. Some interventions engage advisory boards, but it may be uncertain to what extent these members represent the varied community perspectives. Another ethical concern arises when programs aim to address sensitive issues with populations that may be reluctant to discuss them. Disclosing from the outset the purpose of the program – before gaining the trust of the population – may jeopardize the program.

Ethical Issues in Strategic Approaches

There are a wide array of strategic approaches and tactics used in health promotion for the purpose of promoting the health of individuals and populations, among them the use of engineering approaches and incentives, harm reduction approaches, targeting particular population segments, the use of social marketing methods and collaborations with various organizations, some with commercial interests, and the use of various communication tactics and cultural themes. Other issues relate to the reliability of the knowledge and information transmitted and obtaining informed consent of individuals and communities toward whom the activities are aimed.

Ethical Issues in Engineering Approaches

An underlying assumption in public health is that people's behaviors can be influenced by shaping their physical environment in a way that facilitates or prescribes a particular course of action. Sometimes this may occur without them even being aware that they have engaged in health promotion activities, for example, the fluoridation of drinking water, pedestrian bridges on cross roads, and automatic seat belts. The central ethical issue that emerges is respect for the autonomy of the individual and the moral argument that people should be entitled to make their own decisions regarding their actions, and not be compelled to adopt certain practices. Proponents of engineering approaches cite various arguments in favor of using engineering strategies. One is that engineering approaches are more egalitarian because they help those with limited economic means to adopt the recommended practices. Another is that they can be more efficient and serve the wider public good by ensuring that most people will adhere to them. Proponents suggest that engineering methods are democratic when the public expresses their support for these measures.

Ethical Issues in Targeting and Segmentation

To effectively utilize resources by choosing to focus on particular segments of the population is accepted as an essential strategic approach in health promotion. It is considered an ethical approach because it requires the provision of equivalent but culturally appropriate messages to populations with different sociocultural backgrounds and levels of literacy. Yet, the mere decision to 'segment' a population according to certain parameters and allocate limited resources to 'tailor' promotion activities to certain populations raises ethical issues regarding equity as well as utility: It may be decided to target those who are most likely to adopt recommendations or who seem to possess a higher degree of readiness to do so (following a utilitarian approach). Or it may be decided to focus the efforts on those with the greatest need, who are considered 'hard to reach' and less likely to adopt the recommendations, thus raising concerns associated with utility and of the inefficient use of limited resources that are available for health promotion.

Ethical Issues in the Adoption of Social Marketing Approaches for Health Promotion

Commercial marketing strategies have been shown to be hugely successful in influencing people to purchase various products and services and to adopt particular lifestyle trends. This has prompted many health promotion programs to adopt methods and tactics used in commercial marketing as a means to enhance the reach of their programs and to influence intended populations to adopt certain practices. The application of commercial marketing strategies, including using manipulative tactics and advancing commercialism (for example, by using prizes and incentives), raises a host of ethical concerns (Andreasen, 2001).

Ethical Issues in Communication Tactics and Persuasive Appeals

In order to get people to voluntarily change their behaviors for the purpose of promoting their health, they may need to be convinced that it is worthwhile for them as individuals or for society as a whole. By implication, health promotion activities need to be persuasive. Yet highly persuasive appeals can be emotionally manipulative, and may rely on exaggeration, omission, or misrepresentation of risks or of potential benefits (Hastings *et al.*, 2004). Proponents argue that it is justified to use such tactics because they are effective in getting people to adopt recommended health-related practices. The dilemma of whether to use highly persuasive tactics is particularly vexing when members from the intervention's population suggest using them, and it thus could be argued that they have consented to the use of a manipulative strategy. Alternative approaches are to present pertinent information and to use a dialogical approach. But these may be viewed as more complex and less appealing to particular populations. Furthermore, people from different cultures may differ in their values regarding what a moral method to influence people is. Some may prefer emphasizing personal responsibility, whereas others may want to stress social solidarity, respect for elders, or harmony with nature.

The Reliability of Current Knowledge on How to Promote Health

Various ethical issues arise when considering the validity and reliability of current knowledge of how to promote health, considering the constant flow of contradictory information and contrasting approaches. There are growing concerns among health promoters about the reliability of information regarding new findings or recommendations that are based on tentative evidence or may prove later on to be inaccurate. A common dilemma is how to present such recommendations, because people may be wary of accepting them if they are not communicated with a strong sense of certainty.

Cultural Sensitivity and Moral Relativism

An important tenet is respect for cultural heritage and sensitivity to cultural beliefs and customs. Health promotion programs often incorporate cultural values, symbols, and themes in health messages, and this can reflect cultural sensitivity and serve as a way to encourage the adoption of the health recommendations. Interventions may aim to promote behaviors or attitudes that contradict certain cultural values or may be viewed by members of a certain group as offensive. Health promoters may consider overriding the consideration of cultural sensitivity because they believe that the health promotion activity is essential. In certain cases, they may view certain cultural practices to be immoral and feel that they should be abolished; thus, in these situations, they do not accept a cultural relativism ethical approach.

Ethical Issues Associated with Direct and Indirect Detrimental Impact

Although health promotion aims to be beneficial to its intended population or to society as a whole, inadvertent detrimental impact can take place, which raises ethical concerns. This can be on the social level, associated with concerns with equity and causing inadvertent harm, or on the cultural level, by turning health into an overriding value.

Increasing Social Gaps

Health promotion activities are typically committed to the moral obligation to promote equity in terms of health promotion opportunities across social groups. Yet health promotion activities that achieve significant improvements in the adoption of healthier practices among large populations may inadvertently reinforce, rather than reduce, existing social disparities. It has been found that large-scale programs that aim to influence lifestyle behaviors including smoking cessation and physical activities are more likely to have an impact on individuals with greater economic resources. This has raised concern regarding equity in health promotion; and in order to benefit lower-income populations, health promotion programs increasingly focus on activities that are tailored to specific communities and aim to enhance their resources rather than focus on providing information for individual behavior change.

Labeling and Stigmatization

A prominent concern in health promotion is that its activities may inadvertently label individuals or groups in a way that can negatively affect their identity, cause them to feel shame, or even stigmatize them. Thus, the challenge of health promotion programs is to avoid labeling, stigmatizing, or making negative attributions about the people or populations who have detrimental medical conditions that the health promotion programs are trying to prevent.

Denial of Gratifications

Health promotion activities often call upon people to relinquish practices they enjoy, which may serve as stress-coping practices or which have become part of their identity or daily routine. These practices may have cultural significance or emotional importance, even when they may be viewed as risky or even immoral. Such practices might offer members of vulnerable groups not only pleasure but also an important coping mechanism that is not easily substituted. Those less economically or socially privileged may have fewer options for healthier substitutions. An ethical issue is whether health promoters are morally obligated to help find alternative practices when they aim to eliminate practices that serve social or emotional functions, particularly among members of diverse cultural or economically disadvantaged groups.

Turning Health into an Overriding Value

Even ardent proponents of health promotion have noted with concern the moral impact of health promotion messages on culture and society as people and governments conceptualize health as an overriding value. Critics maintain that industrialized societies have become obsessed with the promotion and protection of health and that the pursuit of health has turned into a crusade with moral overtones. When health becomes an overriding value, it can turn into something people pursue relentlessly at the expense of other things in their lives or, in turn, people may feel inadequate when they do not do so (Callahan, 2000). An emphasis on good health as a value can turn those who have no serious health problems into the 'worried well' and may contribute to people's escalating expectations from medicine and the health-care system. This may raise concerns regarding equity, because the more powerful groups will be able to demand that the health-care system meet their needs (Becker, 1993). Another concern is that a cultural preoccupation with personal health practices may distract people from other social issues and causes of ill health. It is feared that an emphasis on personal health as a value may serve to promote self-interest at the expense of concern for others and equity (Buchanan, 2000).

Conclusion

A central ethical dilemma in health promotion is the contradiction between the obligation to respect people's autonomy, privacy, and cultural beliefs and the employment of restrictions and persuasive activities for health promotion, which may infringe on people's autonomy or conflict with their cultural beliefs (McLeroy *et al.*, 1987). On one hand, according to the ethical principle of respect for autonomy, people should be free to make their own decisions regarding health-related practices. On the other hand, because individual choices and behaviors often take place within social or physical environments that can be detrimental to people's health, health promoters believe they are obligated to find the most effective strategies to influence them (Cribb and Duncan, 2002). These strategies, especially those considered the most effective, raise ethical dilemmas that require a systematic ethical analysis to elucidate value considerations and require scrutiny of health promotion messages for ethical issues as a routine part of health promotion activities.

See also: Codes of Ethics in Public Health.

Citations

Andreasen AR (ed.) (2001) *Ethics in Social Marketing.* Washington, DC: Georgetown University Press.

Beauchamp DE (1988) *The Health of the Republic: Epidemics, Medicine, and Moralism as Challenges to Democracy.* Philadelphia, PA: Temple University Press.

Becker MH (1993) A medical sociologist looks at health promotion. *Journal of Health and Social Behavior* 34: 1–6.

Buchanan DR (2000) *An Ethic for Health Promotion: Rethinking the Sources of Human Well-Being.* Oxford, UK: Oxford University Press.

Callahan D (ed.) (2000) *Promoting Healthy Behavior: How Much Freedom? Whose Responsibility?* Washington, DC: Georgetown University Press.

Cribb A and Duncan P (2002) *Health Promotion and Professional Ethics.* Oxford, UK: Blackwell Publishing.

Doxiadis S (ed.) (1987) *Ethical Dilemmas in Health Promotion.* New York: Wiley & Sons.

Guttman N (2000) *Public Health Communication Interventions: Values and Ethical Dilemmas.* Thousand Oaks, CA: Sage.

Hastings G, Stead M, and Webb J (2004) Fear appeals in social marketing: Strategic and ethical reasons for concern. *Psychology and Marketing* 21(11): 961–986.

Marantz PR (1990) Blaming the victim: The negative consequence of preventive medicine. *American Journal of Public Health* 80: 1186–1187.

McLeroy KR, Gottlieb NH, and Burdine JN (1987) The business of health promotion: Ethical issues and professional responsibilities. *Health Education Quarterly* 14: 91–109.

Minkler M (1999) Personal responsibility for health? A review of the arguments and the evidence at century's end. *Health Education and Behavior* 26: 121–140.

Sachs L (1996) Causality, responsibility and blame-core issues in the cultural construction and subtext of prevention. *Sociology of Health and Illness* 18(5): 632–652.

Seedhouse D (2001) Health promotion's ethical challenge. *Health Promotion Journal of Australia* 12: 135–138.

Wikler D (2004) Personal and social responsibility for health. In: Anand S, Peter F and Sen A (eds.) *Public Health, Ethics, and Equity,* pp. 109–134. Oxford, UK: Oxford University Press.

Further Reading

Verweij M (1999) Medicalization as a moral problem for preventive medicine. *Bioethics* 13: 89–105.

Subject Index

Notes

The index is arranged in set-out style with a maximum of three levels of heading. Major discussion of a subject is indicated by bold page numbers. Page numbers suffixed by T and F refer to Tables and Figures respectively. vs. indicates a comparison.

Printed and bound by CPI Group (UK) Ltd, Croydon, CR0 4YY

03/10/2024

01040314-0019